NEUROLOGIC COMPLICATIONS OF CRITICAL ILLNESS

SECOND EDITION

Series Editor
Sid Gilman, M.D., F.R.C.P.
William J. Herdman Professor of Neurology
Chair, Department of Neurology
University of Michigan Medical Center

Contemporary Neurology Series

NEUROLOGIC COMPLICATIONS OF CRITICAL ILLNESS

SECOND EDITION

EELCO F. M. WIJDICKS, M.D., Ph.D., F.A.C.P.

Professor of Neurology, Mayo Medical School,
Consultant, Department of Neurology, and
Medical Director, Neurological/Neurosurgical Intensive Care Unit,
Saint Marys Hospital and Mayo Medical Center
Rochester, Minnesota

OXFORD

UNIVERSITY PRESS

2002

OXFORD
UNIVERSITY PRESS

Oxford   New York
Athens   Auckland   Bangkok   Bogotá   Buenos Aires   Cape Town
Chennai   Dar es Salaam   Delhi   Florence   Hong Kong   Istanbul   Karachi
Kolkata   Kuala Lumpur   Madrid   Melbourne   Mexico City   Mumbai   Nairobi
Paris   São Paulo   Shanghai   Singapore   Taipei   Tokyo   Toronto   Warsaw

and associated companies in
Berlin   Ibadan

Copyright © 2002 by Mayo Foundation for Medical Education and Research

Published by Oxford University Press, Inc.
198 Madison Avenue, New York, New York 10016
http://www.oup-usa.org

Oxford is a registered trademark of Oxford University Press.

Library of Congress Cataloging-in-Publication Data
Wijdicks, Eelco F. M., 1954–
Neurologic complications of critical illness / Eelco F. M. Wijdicks.—2nd ed.
p. ; cm. — (Contemporary neurology series; 64)
Previous ed. entitled Neurology of critical illness.
Includes bibliographical references and index.
ISBN 0-19-514079-6
1. Neurological intensive care.   2. Neurologic manifestations of general diseases.
I. Wijdicks, Eelco F.M., 1954–   .
Neurology of critical illness. II. Title.   III. Series.
[DNLM: 1. Critical Illness.   2. Neurologic Manifestations.   3. Intensive Care.
WL 340   W662n 2002]   RC350.N49 W55 2002   616.8'0428—dc21   2001036168

Nothing in this publication implies that Mayo Foundation endorses any of the products mentioned in this book. Care has been taken to confirm the accuracy of the information presented and to describe generally accepted practices. However, the authors, editors, and publisher are not responsible for errors or omissions or for any consequences from application of the information in this book and make no warranty, express or implied, with respect to the contents of the publication. The authors, editors, and publisher have exerted every effort to ensure that drug selection and dosage set forth in this text are in accordance with current recommendations and practice at the time of publication. However, in view of ongoing research, changes in government regulations, and the constant flow of information relating to drug therapy and drug reactions, the reader is urged to check the package insert for each drug for any change in indications and dosage and for added warnings and precautions. This is particularly important when the recommended agent is a new or infrequently employed drug. Some drugs and medical devices presented in this publication have Food and Drug Administration (FDA) clearance for limited use in restricted research settings. It is the responsibility of health care providers to ascertain the FDA status of each drug or device planned for use in their clinical practice.

1 2 3 4 5 6 7 8 9

Printed in the United States of America
on acid-free paper

To my wife, Barbara-Jane,
and my children,
Coen and Marilou—my everything

FOREWORD TO THE FIRST EDITION

Neurologic intensive care has indeed come far as a distinctive specialty in its 15 or so years of existence. When critical care was in its adolescence, few internists felt the need to have neurologic assistance for their patients with hepatic or renal encephalopathies or seizures. Even the practice of asking neurologists to see comatose patients after cardiac arrest is relatively new and arises from the perception that these clinical states are too complex to understand confidently and that alternative and secondary neurologic problems potentially complicate the management picture. The current situation is quite different. As the neurologic aspects of medicine have been omitted from many medical training programs and the tools of neurology, particularly imaging and electrophysiology, have been refined, the neurologic state has become even more mysterious to the non-neurologist. Moreover, a panoply of new neurologic problems has been produced by organ transplantation. The system has stayed balanced, however, as neurologists have assumed the task of educating themselves about aspects of acute medical illness that affect neurologic care and, recently, about neurologic features of acute but primarily systemic diseases. Neurologists like Dr. Wijdicks are to be found heading large neurologically and neurosurgically oriented intensive care units and playing a large role in the clinical advice and procedures in other critical care units throughout the hospital. They have become the arbiters of such diverse problems as brain death, postoperative neurologic complications, and respiratory and medical decisions in patients with Guillain-Barré syndrome and myasthenia gravis.

By building on the impressive advances of the original field of neurointensive care, involving intracranial pressure and acute stroke management, from what was essentially a subsidiary part of neurosurgical practice, Dr. Wijdicks has greatly expanded the purview of the neurologist with this book and provided for the first time a comprehensive guide to neurologic problems in general intensive care. A recent survey by Dr. Thomas Bleck and colleagues (Crit Care Med 21:98–103, 1993) emphasizes the importance of this subject by pointing out that 12% of 1758 consecutive patients in a general intensive care unit had major neurologic complications of their illness, many unrecognized.

The chapters herein are comprehensive and very practical and provide the reader with ample citations to pursue finer points of management. The style of giving sensible advice when any of several courses of action is possible is commendable, particularly because so much of the material is original work that addresses crucial problems in the field. This book will be devoured not only by clinically oriented neurologists but also, it is hoped, by intensive care specialists of every sort, so that the field will be viewed as more unified than before the book was written and a new basis for neurologic practice in medical and surgical intensive care will be established.

Allan H. Ropper, M.D.
Chief of Neurology
St. Elizabeth's Hospital
Boston, Massachusetts

PREFACE TO THE SECOND EDITION

Since the first edition of *Neurologic Complications of Critical Illness* (previously titled *Neurology of Critical Illness*) appeared in 1995, much has changed in this field of acute neurology. Abundant new information has become available on neurologic complications in organ transplant recipients, on muscle and nerve injury in critical illness, and on prognostication. More definitional clarity and precision have ensued thanks to the use of magnetic resonance imaging and electrophysiologic tests. I have used the material of the first edition but have updated, corrected, expanded, and refined the text. I have added new chapters on the evaluation of coma focusing on structural causes, neurologic complications in the critically ill pregnant patient, and a long overdue discussion of withdrawal of life support from a neurologist's perspective. Much of the new material is original, including figures. Mayo Clinic is one of the most creative places at which to work; thus, the material came to me naturally.

My aim has been to produce a comprehensive text about a newly developed field in acute neurology. The arduous task of covering all complexities of critical illness that are associated with neurologic conditions could be accomplished only by ruthless selection and rejection of material to make the chapters readable and useful for clinicians. I have added brief discussions of pathophysiology (set off from the rest of the text) that should not distract the reader from the main content.

Many people have contributed to the composition, assembly, and editing of this book. It is no exaggeration to say that I could not have achieved the writing of this book without the hard work of the Mayo Clinic Section of Scientific Publications (Roberta Schwartz, John Prickman, Sharon Wadleigh, and Reneé VanVleet), the Section of Media Support Services, and the medical illustrator, David Factor. I specifically thank the staff of Oxford University Press (Fiona Stevens) and Sid Gilman for reviewing the entire text with much enthusiasm.

I hope this book will stimulate research and better understanding of neurologic complications in critically ill patients. The hurdles of research in this high-wrought environment should be taken as challenges. Doing so would make owning this book more meaningful. To paraphrase Sir Henry Wade, "The wards [intensive care units] are the greatest of all research laboratories" (Sir Henry Wade, 1871–1955).

E. F. M. Wijdicks, M.D.

PREFACE TO THE FIRST EDITION

Neurologic critical care has emerged from the practical management issues of acute stroke care, increased intracranial pressure, and neuromuscular weakness. At Saint Marys Hospital, one of the hospitals affiliated with the Mayo Clinic, the neurology critical care service provides primary care for all neurology patients in the neurology–neurosurgery intensive care unit. Operating under the aegis of the Department of Neurology and the Division of Pulmonary and Critical Care Medicine, the service also manages neurologic complications in critically ill patients in medical and surgical intensive care units. Many anesthesiologists and pulmonologists in critical care play a major part in the daily care of these very sick patients. It is unfortunate that even today, many excellent textbooks and monographs on critical care tend to be superficial (and certainly not focused) in their discussion of neurologic complications.

This monograph introduces the neurology of critical illness within the field of neurologic critical care and reflects the continuing shift in the orientation of the field. The orientation of this book is clinical, and the management protocols in each clinical chapter should emphasize this orientation. The book is divided into four parts. The first part focuses on general clinical neurologic problems in patients in intensive care units. It deals with the most frequent consultations in critically ill patients. Parts II and III, the core of the book, provide full accounts of major clinical syndromes organized by specialized intensive care units. Every experienced neurologist knows that a neurologic complication in a critically ill patient occurs in a complex clinical situation that requires a broad basic knowledge of many of the subspecialties. Every chapter provides a representative selection of the state of the art in the intensive care unit, necessary for an understanding of critical care medicine. The chapters attempt to be comprehensive but concentrate on the most important issues in critical care medicine. The diagnostic approach is the theme of each chapter, but emergency management and salvation of the patient with a neurologic catastrophe are also considered.

A common misunderstanding is that a serious neurologic complication will put an end to the aggressive care of the very sick patient. In many instances, neurologists do not share this pessimism. It is true that at times no recovery can be anticipated, but the outcome need not always be grim. Thus, Part IV of the book covers the prognostication of neurologic complications and provides guidelines in common clinical neurologic problems facing the intensive care specialist and consulting neurologist in everyday decisions.

A good deal of what follows is new. I hope this book is useful to neurologists, medical and surgical intensive care specialists, critical care nurses, and many other specialized physicians who manage the pressing problems in intensive care units.

E. F. M. Wijdicks, M.D.

CONTENTS

Part I

General Clinical Neurologic Problems in the Intensive Care Unit

Part I

General Clinical Neurologic Problems in the Intensive Care Unit

COMA AND OTHER STATES OF ALTERED AWARENESS

Critically ill patients are hardly ever sharp, and their attention tends to fade away. These very sick patients must deal with the contin- uing deterioration in organ functions and struggle to beat fatigue. This precarious wakefulness becomes even more fragile in patients blanketed by sedative drugs or an- tipsychotic agents.

The central nervous system can be part of a critical illness, and when it is involved three themes dominate: failure of patients to fully awaken after recuperation from a major sur- gical procedure, acute loss of consciousness or agitation, and, occasionally, coma in a de- veloping but as yet undiagnosed illness. If we were to select one area of neurology for which consulting neurologists show a singu- lar aptitude, it would be altered awareness or coma. But in dealing with critically ill pa- tients who have become comatose, one comes to realize that different judgments are required because unique problems may sur- face.

This chapter discusses causes of coma in evolving critical illness. It also juxtaposes coma with other types of disturbances of alertness and cognition. Here the main anatomical and neuropharmacologic con- tributors of consciousness are characterized, different states of altered consciousness are defined, and major causes of coma in the in- tensive care unit (ICU) are listed.

DEFINITIONS OF ALTERED STATES OF CONSCIOUSNESS

Normal consciousness implies a condition of being awake and aware of self and envi- ronment. It requires an arousal stimulus (reticular formation) and intact content, coherence of thought, and mental activity (cerebral hemispheres). Arousal disturbances lead to diminished alertness. Content disturbances lead to diminished awareness and inattention, disorientation, and lack of integration of perception and processing memory. In a sense, altered arousal involves altered state of awareness, and these two components are interrelated but sometimes dissociated. One can be awake and aware, awake but not aware, and not awake and not aware. Some clinicians are still ill at ease with the classification of different disorders of consciousness. These disorders are listed here to facilitate conversations in day-to-day practice.

Locked-in Syndrome

In *locked-in syndrome* ("imprisoned mind"), patients have normal consciousness but complete body paralysis except voluntary vertical eye movements. They thus cannot move their limbs, grimace, or swallow. Structural lesions in the base of the pons spare the pathways to the oculomotor nuclei in the mesencephalon, so that patients continue to communicate through vertical eye movements and blinking. The medulla oblongata is spared. Central chemoreceptors in the ventral surface of the medulla are intact, and thus there is normal respiratory drive. Hearing is intact, but vocalizing is not possible through a capped tracheostomy cannula. Consciousness may be reduced when the tegmentum is involved. Variants of this classic syndrome are common. It should be differentiated from paralysis of all muscle movement by neuromuscular junction blocking agents.

Hypersomnia

Hypersomnia is an increase in sleeping time with normal sleep patterns, a situation often caused by sleep deprivation, metabolites of sedative drugs, or acute hepatic or renal failure. Acute brain stem lesions involving the tegmentum or bilateral lesions of the paramedian dorsal thalamus may also dampen arousal.

Acute Confusional State

Impairment of attention, memory, and logical thinking; lack of recall of parts of the day and location; no coherent conversation; and prominent distractability are the features of confusion. When systemic manifestations, hallucinations, and confusion are combined, the term *delirium* is used. Signs of autonomic hyperactivity, including tachycardia, hypertension, and sweating, may occur.

Coma

Coma is a state of unresponsiveness (sleeplike) in which the undisturbed patient lies with eyes closed and cannot be aroused to stimuli. Self-awareness and sleep–wake cycles are absent.[1] Movement toward objects and verbal response (if the patient is not intubated) do not exist, and the patient experiences no suffering. Pathologic motor responses or no response at all is commonly observed.

Persistent Vegetative State

Persistent vegetative state may evolve from coma due to extensive injury to the brain. This condition of complete unawareness becomes associated with sleep–wake cycles and opening of the eyes but without any expression or recognition of external stimuli. Visual tracking to shown objects is absent. Brain stem function (including respiratory drive) is largely preserved.

Brain Death

Brain death is the vernacular expression for irreversible loss of all brain and brain stem function. Being a matter of certitude after excluding confounders, this implies documentation of permanently lost consciousness, no motor response to pain stimuli, absent brain stem reflexes, and absent respiratory drive when the respiratory centers are maximally stimulated at an arbitrarily set target of P_{CO_2} of 60 mm Hg.[2]

NEUROANATOMY AND NEUROPHARMACOLOGY OF CONSCIOUSNESS

The processes that govern normal consciousness are only minimally understood, but the critical anatomical parts have been defined under the term *ascending reticular activating system*. This system, located in the rostral brain stem, targets the thalamus, which in turn disperses connections to the cortex and vice versa, creating a thalamic–cortical circuitry.[3] One column of the system projects to the medial thalamic nuclei, interlaminar nuclei, and ventromedial nuclei; another column remains ventral and courses through the lateral hypothalamus to reach the basal forebrain neurons, which in turn modulate cortical activity as well.[4]

The function discharged by the ascending reticular activating system is arousal. Another major system, the limbic system, contributes not to arousal but to mood, affect, motivation, and memory. Amnestic syndromes are mostly a consequence of involvement of the hippocampus, an important component that projects to the mamillary body and anterior thalamic nucleus.

Arousal is determined not only by intact connections but also by neurotransmitters (Fig. 1–1). Exciting glutaminergic neurons of the reticular formation project to the nonspecific thalamocortical systems. The retinal nucleus of the thalamus may be a key component in gating interchange and in regulating sleep–wake cycles and depth of sleep.[5] The retinal nucleus also contains a large set of inhibitory γ-aminobutyric acid (GABA) that can be recruited to further modulate neuronal traffic and control excitability. Noradrenergic neurons also modulate arousal. These cells are located in the locus ceruleus, a small group of pigmented cells localized in the lateral part of the upper pons. The role of this structure is currently thought to be enhancement of vigilance, particularly with unexpected stimuli. If damaged, it prevents the development of rapid eye movement sleep and reduces total sleep time. Other monoamines, such as serotonin and histamine, originating from raphe nuclei in the median brain stem and from

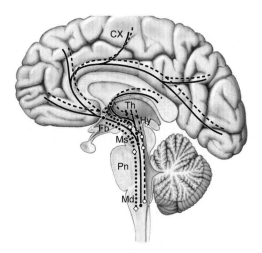

Figure 1–1. Sagittal drawing of the brain showing the regions most critically involved in generating and maintaining cortical activation and the waking state. These areas, maximally active during waking, include the *ascending reticular activating system* of the dorsal brain stem, the midline-medial and intralaminar *thalamocortical projection system*, and the *basal forebrain*. Within these regions are glutamatergic neurons of the reticular formation (diamonds), which project to the nonspecific thalamocortical projection system, noradrenergic neurons of the locus ceruleus as well as other catecholaminergic neurons (open circles), which project in a diffuse manner to subcortical relays and directly to the cerebral cortex, and cholinergic neurons (filled circles), which project from the pontomesencephalic tegmentum to subcortical relays and from the basal forebrain to the cerebral cortex in a widespread manner. CX, cortex; Fb, forebrain; Hy, hypothalamus; Md, medulla; Ms, mesencephalon; Pn, pons; Th, thalamus. (Modified from Jones BE. Basic mechanisms of sleep–wake states. In: Kryger MH, Roth T, Desment WE [eds]. Principles and Practice of Sleep Medicine, 2nd ed. WB Saunders, Philadelphia, 1994, pp 145–162. By permission of the publisher.)

the hypothalamus, enhance wakefulness through ascending projections to the thalamus, basal forebrain, and cortex.

The cholinergic system projects from the dorsal pontomesencephalic tegmentum to subcortical relays and from the basal forebrain to the cerebral cortex. Its function is not only to enhance attention but also to retain recent memories and to create rapid eye movement sleep.

PATHOPHYSIOLOGIC MECHANISMS

This model (in Figure 1–1), albeit oversimplified, may be used to explain disorders of consciousness discussed in other chapters of this book. For example, benzodiazepines, barbiturates, and propofol specifically enhance GABA activity and lower excitation, inducing drowsiness, sleep, and coma. Benzodiazepines act on endogenous receptors in the cortex and midbrain and on opioid target receptors throughout the brain. In hepatic encephalopathy, GABA-mediated inhibition has been suggested as a mechanism, as well as down-regulation of glutamate N-methyl-D-aspartate receptors, both of which disrupt a sensible balance of excitation and inhibition.

Structural lesions interrupt the cortical stimulation by the reticular formation and generate an altered state of consciousness as long as the bilateral thalamocortical circuits are affected. Coma can be predicted when structural destructive or compressive lesions interrupt these synapsing fibers, which extend from the trigeminal nerve entry in midpons to the thalamus, or involve both cerebral hemispheres. Common lesions are occlusion of the basilar artery, causing ischemia of the brain stem central core; pontine hemorrhage involving the tegmentum; and compression from acute, mostly hemorrhagic, cerebellar lesions.

Bilateral lesions in the thalamus are commonly from infarcts due to basilar artery occlusion, from extending midbrain-pontine hemorrhage or cerebral vein occlusion, or from occlusion of the thalamic perforators due to fulminant meningitis. Cerebral hemisphere lesions reduce alertness only if bilateral. The cause may be either mass effect from tissue shift or associated hydrocephalus (for example, cerebral parenchymal hematoma extending into the ventricular system).

NEUROLOGIC EXAMINATION OF THE ACUTELY CONFUSED PATIENT

Assessment of acute confusion, albeit a psychiatric disorder, is a frequent incentive for intensive care specialists to consult a neurologist.

Acute confusional state and delirium are conceptually related but differ in severity. Both conditions commonly affect elderly patients, who may be notably susceptible because of an underlying (and not earlier recognized) dementia.[6,7] In these instances, family members confirm a gradual decline in performance, productivity, and creativity, with earlier episodes of disconcerted behavior in demanding circumstances.

Patients with a critical illness are at high risk for delirium. The term "ICU psychosis" has waned in popularity and may not be useful if it suggests that ICU deprivation is the major cause. Risk factors for delirium have been identified and are consistent throughout studies. These include dementia, Parkinson's disease, surgery, fever, infections (particularly in the urinary tract), visual impairment, polypharmacy, and use of psychoactive drugs.[8–14]

Confusion or delirium in any acutely hospitalized patient could be due to withdrawal of alcohol or drugs. Drugs that can produce delirium are listed in Table 1–1.[11–13] Postoperative delirium may occur in 25% to 50% of elderly patients, most commonly in orthopedic surgery or with use of anticholinergics and barbiturates as anesthetic drugs.[11,14] Postoperative pain emerged as a major factor in one prospective observational study, and such pain may increase the risk of delirium by early disturbance of the sleep–wake cycle.[15] There is no conclusive evidence of a significant association of hypoxemia or hypocapnia with delirium.

Delirium after transplantation is most commonly related to cyclosporine or tacrolimus neurotoxicity and occurs in 20% to 30% of transplant recipients.[16] Delirium is more common in patients who undergo liver transplantation for alcoholic disease. Alcohol withdrawal seems not a good explanation for this, because serum alcohol levels measured before transplantation have been normal in these patients when they have been in a rehabilitation program. The pathogenesis of delirium needs further study because agitation may jeopardize safety through dislodgment of lines.

Delirium is more commonly associated with intra-aortic balloon pump procedures and may occur in one-third of these patients.[17] However, incidence studies in delirium after cardiac surgery are complicated, and results are probably not reliable because

Table 1–1. **Categories of Drugs Associated with Delirium Commonly Used in the Intensive Care Unit**

Adrenocorticosteroids*	Opioid agonists*
α-adrenergic agonists	Penicillins
α-adrenergic blockers	Phenothiazines
Aluminum-containing antacids*	Quinolone antibiotics
Aminoglycoside antibiotics	Sulfonamides
β-adrenergic blockers*	Tacrolimus*
Butyrophenones	Tetracyclines
Calcium channel blockers	Thiazide diuretics
Cephalosporins	Tricyclic and tetracyclic antidepressants
Cyclosporine*	
Digitalis	
Histamine receptor antagonists*	

*If delirium is present, administration of these drugs should be discontinued first.
Modified from Brust JCM. Neurotoxic Side Effects of Prescription Drugs. Boston, Butterworth-Heinemann, 1996, pp 313–316. By permission of the publisher.

of small sample size, changing classification over time, and heterogeneous patient diagnosis.[18,19]

Acute confusional state is characterized by impairment of all mental faculties and a condition of being out of touch with surroundings. Thus attention and memory, logical thinking, orientation, and mathematical skill are abnormal, and a chaotic perception of medical illness is evident. The capacity to recall parts of the day, procedures, discussions with physicians, and visits by family is lost, and patients often look bewildered at their restraints. Patients may yell and swear, are generally noisy, and will try to get out of bed. Coherent conversation is not possible, and directions are not followed. Although sleep hygiene in ICUs is generally fragmented, sleep and wake patterns for these patients are notably disturbed and more random. Snoring during the day becomes excessive from taking sedative drugs the night before and being interrupted by nocturnal agitation.

In the *Diagnostic and Statistical Manual of Mental Disorders, Fourth Edition*, delirium is defined as "disturbance of consciousness with reduced ability to focus, sustain, or shift attention. Dementia must be excluded as a reason to explain change in cognition or perceptual disturbance. The disorder develops over time, and there must be evidence that delirium is caused by medical disorder."

Delirium is characterized by profound perceptual disturbances and hallucinations. Persecutory delusions are common. The level of awareness fluctuates and systemic manifestations emerge. Hallucinations are vivid and frightening. Warning signs of delirium tremens have been identified (Table 1–2).

Delirium tremens poses complex management issues that are beyond the scope of these guidelines and requires psychiatric consultation. It typically begins on the third or fourth day after a patient stops drinking.[20] Delirium tremens is characterized by involuntary tugging at sheets, picking at imaginary objects, intensified tremor and severe confusion, often accompanied by agitation and hallucinations (typically, visual or tactile tachycardia, sweating, and hypertensive episodes). It is relatively rare (with estimates ranging from 0.1% to 1% of persons, 5% of patients withdrawing from alcohol) but life-threatening, especially in critically ill patients. This syndrome typically lasts for approximately 5 days once it begins, and duration probably is not affected by treatment.

Neurologic examination of cognition in patients in the ICU is frustrating and often fragmentary. Only patients with mild manifestations can give reliable responses to the testing questions. Acute confusional states, however, can be graded by testing recall (naming of three unrelated objects: "car," "Mr. Johnson," "tunnel"), attention (repeat-

Table 1–2. **Warning Signs in Developing Delirium Tremens**

Pulse ≥120/min

Systolic blood pressure >160 mmHg

Respirations >30/min or <10/min

Temperature >38.5°C

Seizures

Difficult to arouse

Cumulative dose during first 24 hr of 400 mg of chlordiazepoxide orally, 8 mg of lorazepam intravenously, or 16 mg of lorazepam orally

ing a series of digits, telephone number), or calculation (counting down from 100 by subtracting 7). Writing and reading a complete sentence, copying a cube, and following complex commands (for example, take this paper, fold it in half, and put it to the left of your body) test agraphia, apraxia, and alexia as more specific neurobehavioral disorders.

In any newly confused or delirious patient, other clues may be detected that suggest a structural lesion rather than more common physiologic brain dysfunction. These may include neglect of the left side, hemiparesis, and denial of blindness.

NEUROLOGIC EXAMINATION OF COMATOSE PATIENTS

It is often difficult to determine the state of awareness in critically ill patients. They may look about, be distracted and detached, fidget constantly, and not focus on anything until at last they catch sight of the doctor or nurse entering the room.

The impact of sedation on the state of awareness of the critically ill patient varies substantially. In some patients, a dream-like state exists, with temporary awakening occurring during procedures that cause pain. Many pharmacologic sedating agents (Chapter 2) not only produce a calming effect but also distort sounds with an echoing effect. Some physicians' and nurses' remarks may be irrelevant in content for the patient but nonetheless become amplified, suggesting danger to the patient. Patients may feel "closed in" when high doses of sedative agents are used, or they may lack any urge to signal discomfort or fear. Invasive proce-

dures are perceived by some patients as painless manipulations, prodding, or sticking, and this effect may explain the patient's easy compliance with the attending staff; in other patients, because of the perception of impending pain, any close contact causes agitation.

Although neurologic examination of the critically ill patient with altered consciousness may necessarily be truncated in the ICU, it should include the most essential components (Table 1–3). The following clinical neurologic findings should be documented for any comatose patient: meningismus, subhyaloid hemorrhages or papilledema, pupillary reactions and size, oculocephalic responses, corneal responses, facial asymmetry to pain, motor tone, any abnormal movements (tonic–clonic seizures, myoclonus, asterixis), and neuro-ophthalmologic findings. These components need to be documented in a disciplined manner and be followed by classification of coma (Table 1–4). The main purpose of the neurologic examination is to recognize telltale signs that determine not only the location of the lesion but also the direction of further diagnostic laboratory evaluation.

Generally, the Glasgow coma scale is the most useful means of conducting such an examination, although motor response may be the only reliable test in ventilated patients. In a certain number of these patients, the eyes may be swollen shut from excessive fluid replacement or direct trauma and speech muted from endotracheal intubation. Although neurologic examination of a small number of critically ill patients requiring multiple devices and infusions, among other things, may seem pared down to almost less than the essentials, the examination of spontaneous eye movements, position of the eyes with eyelid opening, and eye movements after head turning or cold water irrigation in the ear can be quite localizing.

Our understanding of eye movements is as follows: Brief, rapid voluntary conjugate horizontal movements are fired from the frontal lobe. Bundles from this eye field in the frontal lobe descend to the midbrain and cross at the location of the trochlear nerve to synapse with the paramedian pontine reticular formation and sixth nerve nucleus. Rapid voluntary vertical movements are fired from bilateral frontal and occipital

Table 1–3. **Neurologic Examination in Critically Ill Patients with Impaired Consciousness**

Clinical Features	Attributes to Check
Eye responses (GCS)	No eyelid opening to pain Eyelids open to pain Eyelids open to voice Eyes open spontaneously (and fixating on objects)
Motor responses (GCS)	No motor response to pain Localizing to pain stimuli Withdrawal to pain stimuli Pathologic flexion to pain stimuli Pathologic extension to pain stimuli Following two-step commands (e.g., hand signs)
Verbal responses (GCS)	No speech or endotracheal intubation Incomprehensible speech or sounds only Inappropriate speech Confused conversation Oriented speech
Neck movement	Rigidity Meningeal irritation
Ophthalmoscopy	Subhyloid hemorrhage Papilledema
Pupillary size	Unilateral or bilateral mydriasis Unilateral or bilateral miosis Midposition
Pupillary light response	Absent Sluggish
Eye movement and gaze	Oculocephalic or caloric response to cold water Nystagmus Gaze preference Absent caloric responses or disconjugate gaze
Corneal reflexes	Absent unilaterally or bilaterally
Eyelid position and facial muscles	Ptosis Asymmetrical grimacing to pain supraorbitally
Oropharyngeal responses	Gag reflex absent Cough reflex absent
Speech	Muted Aphasia Dysarthria
Motor tone	Rigidity Paratonic Flaccid
Tendon reflexes	Absent Increased Clonus
Sensation	Absent pin prick responses in limbs Sharp level at trunk Neglect

(continued)

Table 1–3. **Neurologic Examination in Critically Ill Patients with Impaired Consciousness (*cont.*)**

Clinical Features	Attributes to Check
Twitches	Eyelid twitching
	Trismus
	Myoclonus
	Generalized tonic–clonic seizures
	Clonic limb shaking
	Tremors
	Dystonia
	Dyskinesia

GCS, Glasgow coma scale.

eye fields synapsing at the junction of midbrain and thalamus, predominantly in the tegmentum, and connecting to oculomotor nuclei. The resting eye positions, illustrated in Figure 1–2, indicate lesions in the supranuclear pathways of conjugate eye movements.

Horizontal conjugate deviation indicates a hemispheric lesion. The gaze is directed toward the lesion. With a lesion of the frontal lobe, the eyes tonically turn toward the abnormality because one eye field is unopposed. The oculomotor nuclei are localized between mesencephalon and pons; thus lesions in the pons below this level of crossing fibers may produce tonic deviation away from the lesion. Persistent horizontal gaze preference indicates a substantial hemispheric lesion. Intermittent horizontal gaze preference may indicate seizures, often with eyelid myoclonus and nystagmoid movements during resolution. When the thalamus is directly damaged or involved because of compression from a central type of brain herniation, the eyes are directed the opposite way ("wrong-way eyes").

Midbrain lesions at the tegmentum interrupt vertical eye movements and may cause tonic downward movement. Downward eye deviation localizes either in the thalamus or in the dorsal midbrain, often from a massive thalamic hemorrhage extending into the mesencephalon. Upward deviation, on the other hand, is less precisely localized anatomically but indicates bilateral hemispheric damage, such as that seen with extensive hypoxic–ischemic insult after cardiac resuscitation or asphyxia. Brief upward gaze spasm (oculogyric crisis) may be caused by neuroleptic drugs or cyclosporine toxicity.

Skew deviation in the resting position is indicative of a primary brain stem lesion, possibly in the region of the interstitial nucleus of Cajal. The higher eye is often at a site similar to that of the midbrain or pons lesion. Brain stem lesions may interrupt the medial longitudinal fasciculus. Caloric stimulation with ice water stimulates horizontal canals with the head elevated 30° and produces a tonic deviation toward the ear, but it may bring out an adduction paralysis (internuclear ophthalmoplegia). Poor responses may occur in patients treated with vestibulotoxic drugs, such as aminoglycosides and vancomycin.

Spontaneous eye movements rarely have localizing value and are most commonly seen with hypoxic–ischemic insults producing coma. Certain abnormalities do indicate brain stem involvement. They are summarized in Figure 1–3.

Table 1–4. **Major Categories of Coma**

Hemispheric lesion with brain shift

Diffuse bihemispheric structural lesion

Diencephalon lesion involving both thalami

Cerebellar lesion with brain stem compression or ischemia

Primary brain stem (mesencephalon–pons) lesion

Diffuse physiologic brain dysfunction from acute metabolic derangement, drugs, or intoxication

Psychogenic unresponsiveness

Nystagmus may indicate an acute lesion in the brain stem or cerebellum. However, nonstructural and reversible causes, particularly drug intoxication, should be considered. Vertical nystagmus may be due to morphine administered in any dose epidurally or by patient control or to magnesium deficiency, antiepileptic agents, ketamine, or Wernicke-Korsakoff syndrome.[25–27]

Change in pupil diameter is often the only indication of neurologic deterioration in critically ill patients receiving muscle relaxants. Pupil size may vary considerably in mechanically ventilated patients.[28] Any anisocoria should be taken seriously and not be attributed to physiologic fluctuations or, worse, to interobserver variability among critical care nursing staff. One study of experienced nursing personnel found that interobserver agreement with simple pupil measurements at bedside was excellent, and only agreement on pupillary reaction to light was poor.[29] Anisocoria, defined as difference in pupil size of >1 mm, should be further evaluated. A simplified chart for bedside testing is given in Figure 1–4.

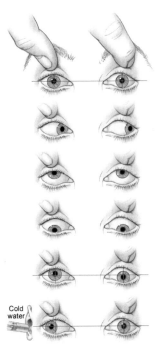

Figure 1–2. Common abnormal eye positions. From top to bottom: normal, lateral horizontal gaze, upward gaze, downward gaze, skew deviation, internuclear ophthalmoplegia (see text for its significance).

Bilateral miosis with preserved light reflex is frequently encountered in critically ill patients. A large proportion of patients in the ICU have miosis from treatment with narcotic agents by any route of administration.[30,31] This action can be proven after antagonization with naloxone. Small pupils have been reported in a patient with nonketotic hyperglycemia.[32] Pinpoint pupils in a structural lesion are traditionally seen in patients with large pontine hemorrhages, but the additional presence of coma, skew deviation, or intranuclear ophthalmoplegia is more helpful in establishing the diagnosis.

Unilateral miosis almost always represents Horner's syndrome from sympathetic denervation of the pupil. This anisocoria may be less apparent in brightly illuminated ICU rooms, and thus should be exaggerated by examination in the dark, which causes the normal pupil to widen. Horner's syndrome may have causes at any level of the sympathetic pathway, but in medical and surgical ICUs, internal jugular vein catheterization, acute brachial plexopathies, and extensive thoracic surgery are the most frequently associated conditions (see Chapter 5).

Sudden unilateral fixed, dilated pupil is evidence of third nerve dysfunction through direct compression or from brain stem distortion caused by a rapidly expanding intracranial mass. However, accidental unilateral pupillary dilatation has been reported in several cases in association with aerosolized anticholinergics in which the mist condenses on the eyelids.[33]

Bilateral mydriasis with normal light responses in patients receiving neuromuscular blockade may signal anxiety, or they may have a florid delirium. When associated with tachycardia, mydriasis may be a sign of inadequate sedation. Pharmacologic agents are frequent causes of bilateral mydriasis but obviously do not result in unresponsiveness to bright light. Truly fixed dilated pupils are uncommonly due to intoxication but are present in some instances of massive overdose of carbamazepine, tricyclic antidepressants, or amphetamines.[34] However, extreme cases of fixed, dilated pupils have been reported in patients with antibiotic-induced paralysis. Systemically administered atropine in standard doses (0.03 mg/kg) may cause some pupillary dilatation, but the effect is of-

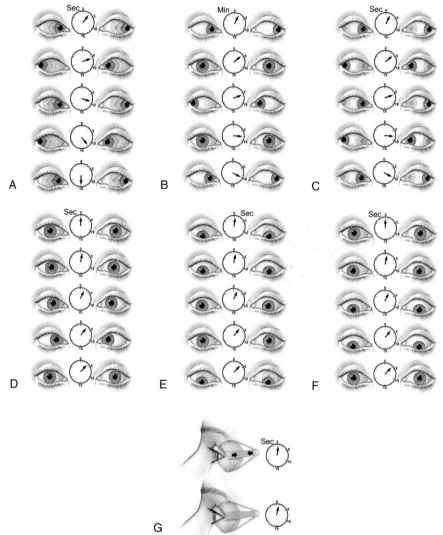

Figure 1–3. Common eye movement abnormalities. (A) *Roving:* Conjugate or dysconjugate slow eye movements in drowsy state without particular significance; they disappear with brain stem lesions. (B) *Periodic alternating gaze:* Horizontal conjugate deviations of the eyes alternating every few minutes. Hepatic encephalopathy but also bihemispheric midbrain or vermis lesions can be responsible.[22-24] (C) *Ping-pong:* Horizontal conjugate deviation of the eyes alternating every few seconds (nonlocalizing bihemispheric damage or vermis lesion).[21] (D) *Convergence nystagmus:* Ocular divergence in slow motion followed by a rapid convergence jerk signifies a lesion in the mesencephalon. (E) *Bobbing:* Rapid downward conjugate movement with slower return to baseline position is found mostly in pontine lesions (primary or due to compression from lesions in the cerebellum). (F) *Dipping:* Slow downward conjugate movement with rapid return to baseline position corresponds to bihemispheric damage, often hypoxic–ischemic. (G) *Retractory nystagmus:* Jerking of the eye back into the orbit due to simultaneous contraction of all ocular muscles signifies a lesion in mesencephalon.

ten too small to be appreciated clinically.[35,36] After cardiac resuscitation, bilateral mydriasis may have its origin in large doses of atropine or dopamine and in the adrenergic stress response. Excessive doses of dopamine in four patients were reported to dilate and fix the pupils, but more often, pupillary reactions remain normal in patients treated with dopamine regardless of the dosage. The pupillary signs encountered in the ICU are shown in Figure 1–5. Bilateral fixed pupils often maintain a middle position and may indicate extensive brain destruction and the final stage of herniation, sometimes even brain death.

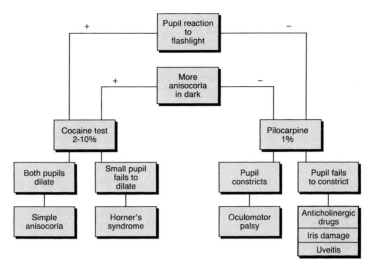

Figure 1–4. Bedside test for anisocoria in the intensive care unit. Further localization of Horner's syndrome can be done with the use of 1% hydroxyamphetamine. Adie's (tonic) pupil, common in the general population, should be considered if no cause is found; it can be investigated by slit-lamp examination (sector palsy of sphincter), or its supersensitivity can be examined with diluted pilocarpine 0.1%. (Modified from Thompson HS, Pilley SFJ. Unequal pupils: a flow chart for sorting out the anisocorias. Surv Ophthalmol 21:45–48, 1976. By permission of Elsevier Science Publishing.)

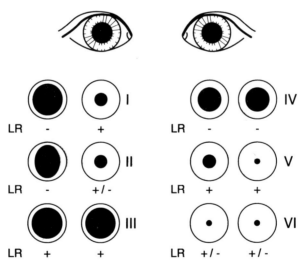

Figure 1–5. Pupillary signs in the intensive care unit. Top pupils represent normal reference. LR, light response. I: Unilateral dilated pupil: third nerve palsy from acute intracranial mass, brain stem contusion, or, rarely, postoperative pituitary apoplexy; acute glaucoma; sympathomimetics (cocaine, amphetamines), antihistamines, tricyclic antidepressants (if pupil does not constrict with pilocarpine, consider local trauma or topical anticholinergic agent). II: Oval pupil (often transitory appearance of pupils signaling increased intracranial pressure). III: Mydriasis (anxiety, delirium, pain, seizures, botulism, atropine, aerosolized albuterol, amyl nitrite, magnesium excess, norepinephrine, dopamine, aminoglycoside, and tetracycline overdose). IV: Pupils fixed in midposition (typical in end-stage brain herniation syndromes and brain death). V: Horner's syndrome (traumatic carotid dissection, brachial plexopathy, trauma from internal jugular vein catheter placement, major thoracic surgery). VI: Miosis (opioids, cholinergic toxicity, organophosphate toxicity, clonidine, phenothiazines, pilocarpine, acute pontine lesion); light response should be present but may be very difficult to appreciate, even with the use of a magnifying glass.

Visual fields can be tested by moving one's hand suddenly toward the patient's eye, causing blinking, and asymmetries indicate hemianopia. Facial grimacing should be examined after forceful compression of the supraorbital nerve or temporomandibular joint. It is important to distinguish between a central facial and a peripheral facial palsy. Central facial palsy involves weakness of the lower face with asymmetry of the mouth angle. Asymmetrical grimacing may involve the orbicularis oculi in central facial paralysis but not the frontal muscles. Frontal muscle asymmetry points to peripheral facial nerve damage and, in the appropriate situation, often indicates basal skull fracture or mastoiditis.

The snout, jaw, and glabellar reflexes may be increased and are elicited by tapping the upper lip, chin, and root of the nose, respectively. A positive reaction merely indicates a bilateral supranuclear lesion and is not further localizing. It is common in bihemispheric damage from trauma or anoxia. Chvostek's sign, elicited by tapping over the facial nerve anterior to the ear, is seen in tetany, and in a comatose patient may indicate a postictal state from severe hypocalcemia.

Twitching of the face and mouth may indicate subtle subclinical seizures but more often is a forme fruste of myoclonus status epilepticus. Biting of the endotracheal tube in this situation is common, but clenching of the jaw (almost pathognomonic for tetanus) is rare.

Repetitive blinking may also indicate a forme fruste of generalized myoclonus status epilepticus. With every blink, an upward gaze is noted, but blinking may be isolated. We noted this phenomenon in a comatose patient with bithalamic damage after cardiac resuscitation. The pathways and pathophysiology of blinking in coma remain unknown.

Finally, the uvula reflex may be difficult to assess in intubated patients, and it is more important to obtain a cough reflex with tracheal suctioning. Absence of a cough reflex may be due to potent anesthetics (for example, propofol) or brain death.

Motor responses in critically ill patients clearly indicate the severity of bihemispheric or brain stem damage and may change with deepening of coma. These motor responses indicate structural lesions in both cerebral hemispheres or in the brain stem and typically evolve during brain herniation, and it is crucial to differentiate motor reflex responses from abnormal movements induced by medication, seizures, or acute metabolic derangements (Fig. 1–6). One should be aware that flaccidity and failure to withdraw to pain are common in critically ill patients. Major causes of this condition are prolonged use of neuromuscular blocking agents (Chapter 2), critical illness polyneuropathy from sepsis, and lack of pain perception due to accumulation of anesthetic agents. Hemiplegia is detected by asymmetrical withdrawal to pinching, but there are other corroborating signs, such as a pseudothickened leg from hypotonia, hyperflexia, and Babinski's sign.

Decreased level of consciousness is often associated with an occasional jerk in an extremity, barely displacing it, and may involve only the fingers. It disappears when the patient is aroused. Myoclonus, asterixis, and seizures (partial or generalized) may be

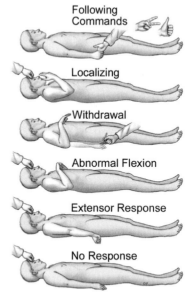

Figure 1–6. Motor responses documented in the Glasgow coma scale (see also Table 1–3): following commands and hand positions (victory sign, thumbs up), localizing pain stimulus after compression of the supraorbital nerve, withdrawal to pain, abnormal flexion (coordinated slow flexion and adduction in arms and wrists), abnormal extensor responses (adduction of arms, extended and hyperpronation), and no response to pain (flaccidity).

observed during progression of symptoms. Myoclonus can be generalized or multifocal and typically occurs after an extensive anoxic–ischemic insult but may be associated with certain drugs (see Chapter 2; Fig. 2–5). The asynchronic twitching of multiple muscle groups may include face and trunk. If segmental myoclonus occurs, it may indicate an additional spinal cord lesion (for example, after thoracoabdominal aorta repairs). Action myoclonus is evident with movement to a certain target and disappears at rest (Chapter 19).

General appearance of the comatose patient may point toward a certain cause. One should specifically examine the patient for denotative signs such as tongue bite (seizure), bruising over the mastoid (basal skull fracture), and petechiae on the face (asphyxia). Conversely, certain physical signs (Table 1–5) unexplained by critical illness may indicate a heretofore unrecognized neurologic disorder.

BRAIN HERNIATION SYNDROMES

An acute supratentorial mass is often recognized by signs of brain herniation. Two ma-

Table 1–5. **Physical Signs in Patients with Impaired Consciousness**

Eyelid Edema
Myxedema
Trauma
Cavernous sinus thrombophlebitis

Fever
Meningoencephalitis
Epidural abscess
Sympathetic storms ("diencephalic seizures")

Hypertension
Subarachnoid hemorrhage
Intracerebral hematoma (with intraventricular extension)
Eclampsia

Hypotension
Brain death
Spinal cord injury

---

jor types of brain herniation occur: uncal herniation and central herniation.[22,37]

The volume of tissue and fluids inside the skull is constant (Monro-Kellie doctrine). Introduction of additional volume (for example, mass, increased cerebrospinal fluid from hydrocephalus, diffuse brain swelling) leads to compensatory measures (displacement of cerebrospinal fluid to spinal compartment, collapse of venous compartment) but then goes on to displacement of abnormal and normal brain tissue.

Uncal herniation refers to displacement of the uncal gyrus, which is part of the temporal lobe, into the tentorial opening. The midbrain displaces horizontally and may rotate if the compression is off center. The surrounding (ambient) cistern opens and allows further filling with brain tissue. Progression of the process can occur only in a more vertical direction or the brain stem buckles. Downward herniation of the brain stem has been considered a final common pathway and leads to irreversible destruction of vital parts of the brain stem. Damage to the vertically displacing brain stem occurs because fixation of the posterior circulation to the circle of Willis leads to stretching or even severing of the penetrating pontine vessels.

The clinical manifestations parallel the damage to the brain stem and exiting third cranial nerve.[22,37] The proximity of the third nerve to the swollen uncus leads to sudden dilatation of the pupil with loss of the light reflex. Another mechanism of damage may be compression against the clivus from brain stem displacement.[38] Midbrain involvement leads to a decrease in pupil size and emergence of light-fixed, midposition pupils 3 to 5 mm in diameter, sustained tachypnea, and motor responses evolving to pathologic withdrawal. Oculocephalic reflexes may fail when the pons becomes involved, and apnea occurs when the medulla fails.

Central herniation refers to a centrally located supratentorial mass that causes compression of the diencephalon and downward displacement of the midbrain through the tentorial opening. Therefore, the mesencephalon is involved early in the course. Decrease in level of consciousness with midposition pupils is not so dramatic in presentation as sudden pupillary enlargement, and the gradual progression, often over days, may be less noticed. The early diencephalon stage to the midbrain–pons stage commonly produces progressively more drowsiness, Cheyne-Stokes breathing, or tachypnea with pathologic flexion responses. Breathing may remain adequate without respiratory support because the damage may halt at a pontine level.[22,37]

Destructive lesions in the posterior fossa produce brain stem signs at presentation and fairly symmetrical motor responses, rapidly evolving into bilateral extensor responses. The pretectal compression leads to downward deviation or failure of upgaze of the eyes. Clinical features include pinpoint pupils due to pontine involvement, reduced horizontal oculocephalic responses, and corneal reflexes. When this pressure cone compresses the medulla, it may produce apnea.

NEUROLOGIC EXAMINATION IN BRAIN DEATH

Brain death may evolve from traumatic brain injury, a severe ischemic–anoxic injury (prolonged cardiac resuscitation, smoke inhalation), catastrophic parenchymal hematoma or massive hemispheric infarct, rapidly progressive bacterial meningitis, or fulminant hepatic failure. Progression to brain death in medical ICUs may be signaled by a marked reduction in blood pressure or sudden appearance of poikilothermy in a patient with acute onset of coma.

Brain death is equivalent to irreversible loss of all brain stem functions. This definition implies (*1*) documentation of loss of consciousness, (*2*) no motor response to pain stimuli, (*3*) no brain stem reflex, and (*4*) apnea.[2,39] A structural central nervous system abnormality compatible with brain death should be demonstrated by computed tomography (CT) scan. The diagnosis of brain death must be in doubt if results of CT scan or cerebrospinal fluid studies are normal unless an obvious pathophysiologic mechanism for brain death is present. However, in patients critically ill from a medical or surgical condition, the proportion of patients with initially normal CT findings may be higher because cardiac arrest or asphyxia is common.

Pitfalls of diagnosing brain death should be recognized. First, hypothermia may blunt brain stem responses when core temperatures are below 32°C and may mimic brain death below 27°C (Chapter 16). Second, drugs that confound the clinical assessment should be excluded, and some may even produce isoelectric electroencephalograms (barbiturates, tricyclic antidepressants, neuromuscular blocking agents, methaqualone, opiates, benzodiazepines, mecloqualone, meprobamate, and bretylium).[40,41]

The clinical diagnosis of brain death may be very difficult immediately after surgery. Volatile anesthetic agents usually wash out in several minutes, but when clearance is in doubt, they can be measured in end-tidal volume. Prolonged activity of neuromuscular junction blocking agents can be determined with a peripheral nerve stimulator. Large doses of narcotics are typically used in complicated operations (for example, cardiovascular repairs). Naloxone reverses the manifestations of opioids. The effects of benzodiazepines can be reversed with flumazenil.

To overcome the possible pitfalls of making the diagnosis of brain death, the directions outlined in Figure 1–7 are proposed. Testing for apnea can proceed only after certain precautions have been taken.[42] Clinical examination of the brain stem includes testing of brain stem reflexes, evaluation of motor response to pain, and evaluation of the patient's inability to trigger breathing (apnea test).

Brain Stem Reflexes

The pupillary response to bright light should be absent in both eyes. Round, oval, or irregularly shaped pupils are all compatible with brain death. Most pupils are in mid position (4 to 6 mm), but dilated pupils (6 to 8 mm) are compatible with brain death. Many drugs can influence the size of the pupil, but the response to light often remains intact. Topical instillation of drugs and trauma to the cornea or bulbus oculi

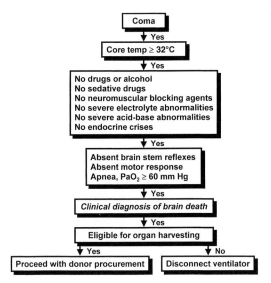

Figure 1–7. Proposed guidelines for the clinical diagnosis of brain death.

may cause reactive mydriasis, but more often reactive miosis is present in the acute stage of direct trauma. Obviously, preexisting anatomical abnormalities of the iris should be excluded. Neuromuscular blocking drugs do not noticeably influence pupil size, because nicotine receptors are absent in the iris.

Ocular movements should be absent after caloric testing with ice water. Caloric testing should ideally be done with the head elevated to 30°. In this position, the horizontal canal becomes vertical. A cold stimulus causes sedimentation of the endolymph, stimulating the hair cells. The tympanum is irrigated with 50 mL of ice water on each side. The procedure is best accomplished by connecting a 50 mL syringe filled with ice water to a small suction catheter that is then inserted into the external auditory canal. To facilitate assessment of subtle eye movements, a pen mark should be placed on the lower eyelid at the level of the center of the pupil before cold water irrigation. No tonic deviation of the eyes toward the cold caloric stimulus should be demonstrated after 1 min of observation, and at least 5 min should be allowed between sides.

Many drugs may diminish but rarely completely abolish the caloric response (aminoglycosides, tricyclic antidepressants,

anticholinergics, antiepileptic drugs, and chemotherapeutic agents).[43] In closed head injury, eyelid edema and chemosis of the conjunctiva may restrict movement of the globes. Clotted blood or cerumen may diminish the caloric response; perforation of the tympanum enhances the response.

Corneal reflexes, which should be absent, are tested with a throat swab. Grimacing to pain can be tested by application of pressure on the supraorbital ridge or deep pressure on both condyles at the level of the temporomandibular joint.

Lack of cough response to bronchial suctioning should be demonstrated. To and fro movement of the endotracheal tube is not a sufficient stimulus.

Motor Examination

Motor responses of the arms to pain stimuli should be absent after forceful supraorbital nerve, nail bed, or temporomandibular pressure. Motor response other than decorticate or decerebrate response can be present in arms and legs and may indicate a spinal reflex. It usually consists of some flexion movement.

Some clinical observations can cause delayed assessment of donors, mainly because the insignificance of the findings is not appreciated by non-neurologists. Deep tendon reflexes and plantar reflexes (including clonus and Babinski's sign) are compatible with the diagnosis of brain death. Spontaneous movements of the limbs, more frequent in young adults, include rapid flexion in the arms and raising the arms off the bed, and respiratory-like movements consist of shoulder elevation and adduction, back arching, and intercostal retraction characteristic of an agonal breathing pattern.[44–47]

Apnea Test

The apnea test procedure is based on the disconnection of the ventilator and apneic oxygenation.[48] The apnea test precautions and procedure are summarized in Figure 1–8. The procedure is facilitated when the apnea test is begun with a baseline Pa_{CO_2} of 35 to 45 mm Hg and, after preoxygenation,

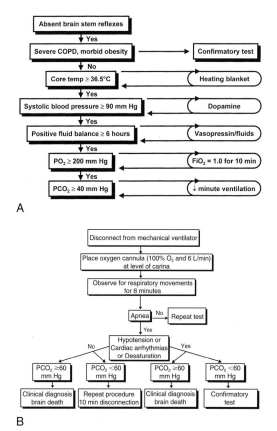

Figure 1–8. Apnea testing in brain death. *A:* Precautions. *B:* Procedure. COPD, chronic obstructive pulmonary disease.

Pa_{O_2} is increased more than 200 mm Hg. With a median increase of 3 mm Hg/hr, the target level Pa_{CO_2} of 60 mm Hg, or an increase of 20 mm Hg above normal baseline P_{CO_2}, is usually reached 8 min after disconnection.[2,49,50] Oxygenation with 100% O_2 through a catheter at the level of the carina (6 L/min) secures adequate oxygenation during the test.[51] Oxygenation prevents hypoxia in the test period, but because preexisting severe pulmonary disease, bilateral pneumonia, acute respiratory distress syndrome, or neurogenic edema creates a large dead space, oxygenation may be inadequate in patients with these conditions.

Respiratory acidosis, an expected result during the apnea test, is usually tolerated without hypoxia but may potentially cause arrhythmias in susceptible patients. The most common manifestations are ventricular premature contractions, ventricular tachycardia, and mild hypotension, but they invariably oc-

cur in patients without preoxygenation.[42] However, with adequate precautions, complications are minimal.

NEUROIMAGING IN COMA

Computed tomography (CT) scanning is a mandatory diagnostic test and has a current acquisition time of less than 10 min. It can document generalized edema, cerebral hemorrhage, and ischemic stroke with swelling, but its diagnostic yield is low in ischemic–anoxic injury, environmental injuries, and the period early after trauma. Structural damage should be excluded in any patient with a decreased level of consciousness. If damage is present, it should be correlated to the depth of coma and stage of herniation. Typically, significant shift of the midline structures (septum pellucidum), calcified pineal gland, hydrocephalus, or intraventricular hemorrhage should be found.

Magnetic resonance imaging (MRI) has come to the forefront as a diagnostic tool, and when anesthesia support is available, it may identify or exclude structural damage. Its prognostic value has not yet been established.

The abnormalities on neuroimaging studies of coma are summarized in Table 1–6, and examples are shown in Figure 1–9. When results of CT scanning are initially normal, MRI may be helpful, but often the conditions listed in Table 1–7 should be considered.

SPECIAL CLINICAL SITUATIONS AND PROBLEMS

It may be practical to broaden the spectrum of disorders of consciousness beyond the traditional categories and discuss them as they appear at clinical rounds.

Failure to Awaken after Discontinuation of Sedation

Failure of patients to fully awaken after discontinuation of sedatives, narcotic agents, or combinations is common. These patients are frequently jaundiced (with documented

Table 1–6. **Abnormalities on Neuroimaging Studies of Coma**

	Findings	Suggested Disorders
Computed tomography scanning	Mass lesion (brain shift, herniation)	Hematoma, infarct, abscess, metastasis, glioma, lymphoma
	Hemorrhage in basal cisterns	Aneurysmal subarachnoid hemorrhage
	Intraventricular hemorrhage	Coagulopathy, trauma, AVM
	Multiple hemorrhagic infarcts	Cerebral venous thrombosis from DIC
	Multiple cerebral infarcts	Endocarditis, cholesterol embolization, postcardiac surgery emboli
	Diffuse cerebral edema	Cardiac arrest, relapse of CNS leukemia, fulminant meningitis, acute hepatic necrosis
	Acute hydrocephalus	Acute bacterial meningitis
	Pontine or cerebellum hemorrhage	Hypertension, coagulopathy
Magnetic resonance imaging	Hyperintense lesions in white matter and basal ganglia	Acute chemotherapy-induced toxic leukoencephalopathy (e.g., methotrexate), PML
	Pontine trident-shaped lesion	Central pontine myelinolysis
	Thalamus, occipital, pontine lesion	Acute basilar artery occlusion
	Temporal, frontal lobe hyperintensities	Herpes simplex encephalitis
	Parietal–occipital lesions	Cyclosporine, tacrolimus neurotoxicity, hypertensive encephalopathy
	Multiple rounded lesions	*Toxoplasma*, cryptococcoma, *Aspergillus* abscesses

AVM, arteriovenous malformation; CNS, central nervous system; DIC, diffuse intravascular coagulation; PML, progressive multifocal leukoencephalopathy.

liver function abnormalities) and recently have been given a benzodiazepine (midazolam) or a narcotic drug (fentanyl). Both drugs are cleared through the liver and therefore accumulate. Typically, prolonged sedation occurs from many days of accumulation of metabolites, and further observation over time is required. In other patients, the reason for unresponsiveness or failure to awaken is obvious by localizing neurologic findings and confirmatory neuroimaging. However, the cause of bilateral hemispheric dysfunction remains puzzling and vexing, particularly when results of the initial CT scan are normal. Further diagnostic considerations are listed in Table 1–7.

Failure to Awaken after Surgery

Failure of a patient to awaken after a major cardiovascular repair is an ominous sign. A devastating ischemic stroke involving multiple arterial territories is a frequent cause of failure to awaken. Its mechanism may be hypotension or multiple emboli. Patients with postoperative ischemic strokes may have had pronounced hypotension during unclamping of the aorta, but it can be implicated only if it persists for a certain period. In addition to perioperative hypotension and cardiac resuscitation during surgery, multiple embolic events are possible reasons for multiple cerebral infarction. The risk of embolization is significant in patients with severe atherosclerotic disease of the ascending aorta and it almost certainly occurs at the time of clamping.

Air embolism may occur during orthopedic operations. Air entrapment in open veins or bone can occur when patients are in Trendelenburg's position (for example, pelvic operations) or when the patient's hip is elevated above the level of the heart during hip

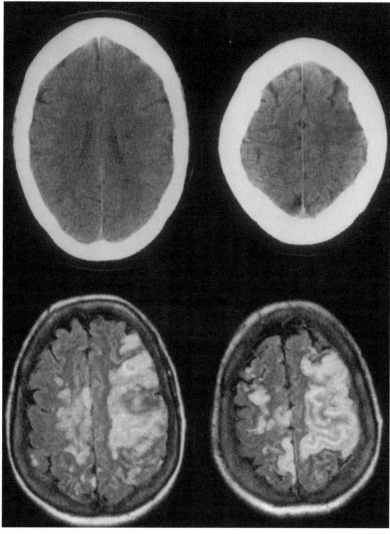

Figure 1–9. Examples of destructive lesions causing coma by interruption of the anatomical structures of the reticular formation and projection. Computed tomography scans are barely abnormal, but magnetic resonance images show multiple hemispheric infarcts after cardioversion (*A*). (*Continued*)

operations. Cardiac collapse, acute broncho-spasm, and pulmonary edema usually occur in association with air embolism but may all be bypassed in a patient with a patent foramen ovale.

If failure to awaken occurs after trauma and the patient has been admitted directly to the operating room from the emergency department, intracranial contusion or extraparenchymal hematoma should be considered. Patients taken directly to the oper-

ating room with life-threatening blunt abdominal trauma may have additional head injury, subdural hematoma, or epidural hematoma that was not apparent on initial examination.[52] A unilateral fixed pupil may suddenly occur during surgical repair of a vascular injury or abdominal exploration for trauma (pupillary light reflexes are the only brain stem reflexes that can be monitored during general anesthesia).

Acute electrolyte imbalance is a relatively

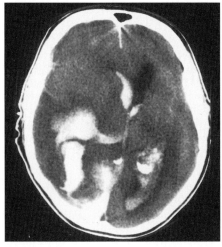

B

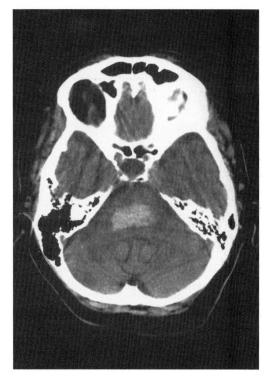

C

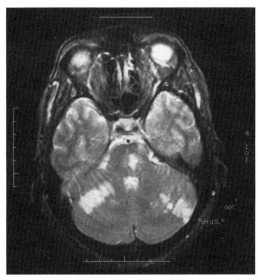

D

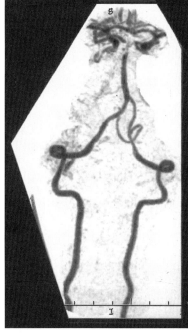

Figure 1–9. (*Continued*) Examples of destructive lesions causing coma by interruption of the anatomical structures of the reticular formation and projection. Lobar hematoma producing acute hemoventricle and hydrocephalus from ruptured mycotic aneurysm (*B*); and pontine tegmental hemorrhage from use of tissue plasminogen activator (*C*). Signal abnormality in pons (magnetic resonance image, *D*) and occlusion of distal basilar artery (magnetic resonance angiogram, *E*) following cardiac surgery (cerebellar lesions are also shown).

E

Table 1-7. Causes of Coma in Critically Ill Patients with Normal Initial Computed Tomography Findings

Anoxic–ischemic encephalopathy

Drug overdose

Neurotoxicity from immunosuppressive agents, chemotherapeutic agents

Diffuse axonal brain injury

Acute central nervous system infection

Fat embolization

Acute basilar artery occlusion

Cholesterol embolization

Central pontine myelinolysis

Diffuse intravascular coagulation

Thrombotic thrombocytopenic purpura

Central nervous system vasculitis (with connective tissue disease)

Prolonged hypoglycemia

Acute severe hyponatremia

Acute severe hypercalcemia

Acute nonketotic hyperglycemia

Metabolic acidosis

Acute hypercapnia with hypoxemia

Adrenal crises

Myxomatous coma

Thyrotoxic coma

Acute uremia

Acute increase in arterial ammonia

Hyperthermia

frequent cause of postoperative confusion, progressive drowsiness, or coma. Increased levels of antidiuretic hormone associated with decreased serum osmolality and hyperosmolar urine are typical during the first postoperative days. When free water is used, renal handling of free water is impaired, because renal function is decreased after the use of inhalational anesthetics, barbiturates, and opioids. Hyponatremia can occur rapidly and is a life-threatening condition that may result in seizures, apnea, and cardiac arrhythmias, often at levels below 110 mEq/L.[53,54]

Other common causes of acute postoperative hyponatremia are administration of large doses of hypotonic fluid to patients with impaired ability to excrete water after transurethral prostatectomy[55] and administration of oxytocin to patients during obstetric procedures.[53]

Failure to awaken after heart transplantation is less commonly due to a structural lesion in the central nervous system. Without localizing neurologic findings, the most common cause of unresponsiveness is drug-induced coma. Narcotic agents are often used liberally in cardiac transplant recipients to decrease pain and to overcome postoperative hypertension.[56] These agents (usually morphine and fentanyl) may cause significant postoperative sedation. Typically, high doses of narcotic agents are given intraoperatively, and many anesthesiologists use fentanyl (with diazepam) or sufentanil (with lorazepam). Naloxone reverses the effects of narcotic agents.

However, failure of patients to awaken may originate with the marked hypotension that occurs intraoperatively, with episodes of significant hypoxemia, or, more often, with cardiac resuscitation for asystole or ventricular fibrillation. Cardiac arrest can occur in the immediate postoperative phase and be devastating. In these patients, the most common clinical problems associated with perioperative cardiac arrest are hypovolemia, tamponade, and overdose of potent vasodilators.

Neurologic complications in the early postoperative phase have decreased in recent years. Much of this decrease has been due to meticulous care in removing all residual atrial tissue or thrombus. Also, the use of a more precise everting anastomosis may have decreased intracardiac thrombus formation on the suture interface and the resultant massive embolic showers and cerebral infarcts.

Neurologic evaluation in the first days after lung transplantation is extremely difficult, because most patients are sedated, paralyzed, and mechanically ventilated. Some programs dictate continuing mechanical ventilation to decrease stress on the critical tracheal anastomosis, but most patients are rapidly weaned within 36 hr.[57] Pulmonary hemorrhage and infection may dominate the early postoperative course.[57] Impaired consciousness, therefore, may reflect the hypoxemia associated with pulmonary edema from reperfusion injury to the graft.

Impaired consciousness and acute confusional state occur in a large proportion of patients with liver transplantation. Many metabolic abnormalities are present, but none significantly contributes to the diminished alertness of the patients. With a new functioning liver, the level of alertness should improve rapidly.

An important subset of patients who almost invariably are drowsy after liver transplantation are patients with fulminant hepatic failure. Patients with fulminant hepatic failure are prone to increased intracranial pressure because of brain edema (Chapter 10). Return of consciousness to baseline level takes days, and these patients typically have a more prolonged awakening in the postoperative phase. In addition, the use of barbiturates perioperatively to control increased intracranial pressure may contribute substantially to a postoperative altered consciousness.

Central pontine myelinolysis should be considered in patients who do not awaken after liver transplantation. Impaired consciousness can be explained by damage to the thalamus as an extrapontine manifestation of osmotic demyelination or extension of demyelination to the pontine tegmentum.[58]

A rare cause of postoperative stupor is pituitary apoplexy.[59–61] We have treated two such patients in 2 years after prostate and cardiac operations. Clinical clues leading logically to the pituitary gland are visual loss from lifting of the chiasm, unilateral ptosis and fixed dilated pupil from compression of the third nerve in the adjacent cavernous sinus, and loss of pituitary function. Dexamethasone and usually urgent neurosurgical treatment are indicated. Blood loss, hemodynamic fluctuations from cardiopulmonary bypass, or anticoagulation may predispose to hemorrhage in the tumor.

Acute Loss of Consciousness in Evolving Critical Illness

Patients who become acutely comatose while critically ill commonly have a catastrophic neurologic illness. In our experience, a large

proportion of patients have a devastating intracerebral hematoma or subarachnoid hemorrhage.[62] These disorders (which may be the inaugural presentation) typically occur in patients with systemic fungemia, coagulopathies, and a ruptured mycotic aneurysm from endocarditis. Acute basilar artery occlusion due to an embolus can complicate dissection of the thoracic aorta, valve repair, and cardiac transplantation.

Rapidly deepening stupor in patients with multiple traumatic injuries should point to fat embolization,[63] evolving epidural or subdural hematoma, or enlarging hemorrhagic contusions with mass effect and edema. Multiple cerebral infarcts are a common cause of coma in the medical ICU.[62]

Acute lapse into coma can occur after correction of hyponatremia, cardiac resuscitation, and carbon monoxide intoxication, all of which are manifestations of a dramatic extensive demyelination of both hemispheres. These patients seem to do very well but suddenly unexpectedly deteriorate to a deep coma and succumb.

APPROACH TO THE ACUTELY CONFUSED AND DELIRIOUS PATIENT

The drug of choice in the delirious patient is lorazepam, 0.04 mg/kg intravenously every 2 to 4 hr as needed.[64] One may use midazolam at 0.03 mg/kg to initiate therapy if a rapid effect is desired. Optimal benzodiazepine therapy results in amelioration of the signs and symptoms of autonomic hyperactivity. The usual maintenance dosage is 1 to 10 mg of lorazepam per hour. Once the patient is stable, benzodiazepine therapy should be tapered gradually.

If the patient has received optimal benzodiazepine therapy and is confused or suffering from delirium tremens, one can add haloperidol to manage agitation.[65] Haloperidol is administered intravenously at an initial dose of 0.5 to 2.0 mg for mildly agitated patients and 5 to 10 mg for those who are severely agitated. If control is not achieved in 30 min, the initial dose is repeated. If the patient's condition remains unstable, the initial dose is doubled every 30 min until control is established. Once control of agitation is achieved with the loading dose, 50% of the total loading dose is given as a maintenance dose divided into intervals of 6 to 8 hr. Titration is to the lowest dose that controls symptoms. Administration is tapered gradually according to the clinical status of the patient. Dosages may be reduced in the elderly and those with hepatic failure. Patient response may vary widely, and doses of up to 50 or 60 mg of haloperidol have been needed to control agitation. A psychiatry consultation may be obtained to assist in management.

APPROACH TO THE COMATOSE PATIENT

Localization should be attempted and requires practical knowledge. In the ICU, bihemispheric dysfunction is common, but brain stem or cerebellar lesions can be mapped out using key clinical pointers, as described before.

With a plethora of potential causes of coma, there are major challenges in elucidating the cause of coma; a disciplined approach is shown in Table 1–8. A systemic approach to prolonged sedation includes reconstruction of the pharmacodynamics and pharmacokinetics (Chapter 2). Often alkalosis, drug interactions, and large doses of sedative drugs change elimination to zero-order kinetics, directly contributing to prolonged sedation. Drug levels should be measured if possible. For any drug, one should obtain the metabolic half-life and calculate the time remaining to clearance, assuming full elimination.

Recent laboratory values should be obtained, and the medical records should be scrutinized for trends. Spinal fluid examination is needed when meningitis is suspected. It should be considered in patients with previous spinal anesthesia, trauma, and evidence of paranasal sinusitis in an attempt to document bacterial meningitis. Because of common triggers such as hypotension and coagulopathies, neurologists should place their interpretive emphasis on structural causes. Computed tomography scanning or

Table 1–8. Diagnostic Approach to Coma in Critical Illness

- Chart sedative drugs and doses
- Assess function of the liver and kidneys, body temperature, serum albumin concentration, and acid–base balance
- Reconstruct plausible drug interactions
- Consider antagonists for benzodiazepines (flumazenil, 1 mg), narcotics (naloxone, 0.1 to 0.4 mg), and nondepolarizing muscle relaxants (neostigmine, 0.035 to 0.070 mg/kg, with atropine, 1 mg)
- Localize examination findings to one main category (Table 1–4)
- Obtain computed tomography scan of the brain
- Consider magnetic resonance imaging (T2-weighted, fluid attenuation, inversion recovery)
- Obtain electroencephalogram and somatosensory potentials (optional)
- Obtain spinal fluid for cell count, glucose, Gram's stain, and cultures (optional)

MRI may be done but may not be rewarding without localizing neurologic findings. The role of electroencephalography, including its place in the detection of nonconvulsive status epilepticus, is discussed in separate sections of this monograph, but it has generally lost its practical value here to neuroimaging, particularly diffusion-weighted MRI. Possible abnormalities on electroencephalography are shown in Table 1–9.

If a cause of coma remains unknown, the following disorders should be considered: cholesterol embolization (Chapter 3), thrombotic thrombocytopenic purpura (Chapter 11), central nervous system vasculitis due to vasculitic syndrome (Chapter 12), or isolated angiitis. Management of specific disorders is discussed in other chapters.

APPROACH TO BRAIN DEATH

It is advised to repeat clinical diagnosis after an (arbitrary) interval of at least 6 hr. A confirmatory test is not mandatory in the

Table 1–9. **Classification of the Electroencephalogram in Coma**

Category	Subcategory	Possible Interpretation
I. Delta or theta >50% of record (not theta coma)	A. Reactivity B. No reactivity	Sedation, meningitis, encephalitis, ADEM
II. Triphasic waves		Acute hepatic or renal failure, penicillin intoxication, MOF
III. Burst-suppression	A. With epileptiform activity B. Without epileptiform activity	Bartiturates, anoxic damage, any drug-induced coma
IV. Alpha, theta, or spindle coma (unreactive)		Anoxic or septic encephalopathy, sedation
V. Epileptiform activity (not in burst-suppression pattern)	A. Generalized B. Focal or multifocal	Nonconvulsive status epilepticus, cyclosporine toxicity, encephalitis

Guidelines

1. Burst-suppression pattern should have generalized flattening at standard sensitivity for ≥1 sec at least every 20 sec.
2. Suppression: voltage criteria should be met for the entire record; there should be no reactivity.
3. When >1 category applies, select the most critical:
   - Suppression is the most serious category.
   - Burst-suppression is more important than triphasic waves, which are more significant than dysrhythmia or delta.

ADEM, acute disseminated encephalomyelitis; MOF, multiorgan failure.

Modified from Young GB, McLachlan RS, Kreeft JH, Demelo JD. An electroencephalographic classification for coma. Can J Neurol Sci 24:320–325, 1997. By permission of the journal.

United States except in patients who are not amenable to reliable evaluation of specific components of clinical testing. Throughout the world, major differences exist in the number of physicians, expertise, specialty requirement, and recommendations in confirmatory tests.

In many reports on confirmatory tests, blind assessment and interobserver variation are not consistently addressed. Clinical experience with confirmatory tests other than cerebral angiography, nuclear scanning, electroencephalography, and transcranial Doppler ultrasonography is limited.[66–70]

Organ procurement can proceed if the family accepts donation and the vital organs and tissue are viable. The ventilator and any supportive therapy are discontinued if organ or tissue donation is not allowed.

CONCLUSIONS

The evaluation of coma in a critically ill patient is complex, and the differential diagnosis is broad. The clinical spectrum of the neurologic aspects of critical illness has become better defined. The cause of coma is never obvious, and particular attention should be paid to acute changes in laboratory values, recent invasive procedures, documented hypoxemic periods, cardiac arrhythmias, any recent change in medication, drug interactions of sedative agents, and drug intoxication, particularly from immunosuppressive agents such as cyclosporine and tacrolimus. All laboratory test results need to be carefully reviewed. The "one trigger, one cause of coma" model may not apply to every case, but an overriding cause is often found.

REFERENCES

1. Plum F. Coma and related global disturbances of the human conscious state. In: Peters A, Jones EG (eds). Normal and altered states of function, Vol. 9, Cerebral Cortex series. Plenum Press, New York, 1991, pp 359–425.
2. Wijdicks EFM. The diagnosis of brain death. N Engl J Med 344:1215–1221, 2001.
3. Zeman A. Consciousness. Brain 124:1263–1289, 2001.
4. Kolmac CI, Mitrofanis J. Patterns of brainstem projection to the thalamic reticular nucleus. J Comp Neurol 396:531–543, 1998.
5. Guillery RW, Feig SL, Lozsadi DA. Paying attention to the thalamic reticular nucleus. Trends Neurosci 21:28–32, 1998.
6. O'Keeffe ST, Ni Chonchubhair A. Postoperative delirium in the elderly. Br J Anaesth 73:673–687, 1994.
7. Parikh SS, Chung F. Postoperative delirium in the elderly. Anesth Analg 80:1223–1232, 1995.
8. Lipowski ZJ. Delirium: Acute Confusional States. Oxford University Press, New York, 1990.
9. Brown TM. Drug-induced delirium. Semin Clin Neuropsychiatry 5:113–124, 2000.
10. McGuire BE, Basten CJ, Ryan CJ, Gallagher J. Intensive care unit syndrome: a dangerous misnomer. Arch Intern Med 160:906–909, 2000.
11. Dyer CB, Ashton CM, Teasdale TA. Postoperative delirium. A review of 80 primary data-collection studies. Arch Intern Med 155:461–465, 1995.
12. Freiberger JJ, Marsicano TH. Alprazolam withdrawal presenting as delirium after cardiac surgery. J Cardiothorac Vasc Anesth 5:150–152, 1991.
13. Picotte-Prillmayer D, DiMaggio JR, Baile WF. H₂ blocker delirium. Psychosomatics 36:74–77, 1995.
14. Golden WE, Lavender RC, Metzer WS. Acute postoperative confusion and hallucinations in Parkinson disease. Ann Intern Med 111:218–222, 1989.
15. Lynch EP, Lazor MA, Gellis JE, Orav J, Goldman L, Marcantonio ER. The impact of postoperative pain on the development of postoperative delirium. Anesth Analg 86:781–785, 1998.
16. de Groen PC, Aksamit AJ, Rakela J, Forbes GS, Krom RA. Central nervous system toxicity after liver transplantation. The role of cyclosporine and cholesterol. N Engl J Med 317:861–866, 1987.
17. Sanders KM, Stern TA. Management of delirium associated with use of the intra-aortic balloon pump. Am J Crit Care 2:371–377, 1993.
18. Kuhn WF, Myers B, Brennan AF, et al. Psychopathology in heart transplant candidates. J Heart Transplant 7:223–226, 1988.
19. van der Mast RC, Roest FH. Delirium after cardiac surgery: a critical review. J Psychosom Res 41:13–30, 1996.
20. Mayo-Smith MF. Pharmacological management of alcohol withdrawal. A meta-analysis and evidence-based practice guideline. JAMA 278:144–151, 1997.
21. Senelick RC. "Ping-pong" gaze. Periodic alternating gaze deviation. Neurology 26:532–535, 1976.
22. Plum F, Posner JB. The Diagnosis of Stupor and Coma, 3rd ed. FA Davis, Philadelphia, 1980.
23. Lapresle J, Said G. Forced downward and convergent deviation of the eyes and periodic ocular movements in aneurysmal hemorrhage of the mesencephalic tegmentum [in French]. Rev Neurol (Paris) 133:497–503, 1977.
24. Stewart JD, Kirkham TH, Mathieson G. Periodic alternating gaze. Neurology 29:222–224, 1979.
25. Saul RF, Selhorst JB. Downbeat nystagmus with magnesium depletion. Arch Neurol 38:650–652, 1981.
26. Henderson RD, Wijdicks EFM. Downbeat nystagmus associated with intravenous patient-controlled administration of morphine. Anesth Analg 91:691–692, 2000.
27. Stevens RA, Sharrock NE. Nystagmus following epidural morphine (letter). Anesthesiology 74:390–391, 1991.
28. Ohtsuka K, Asakura K, Kawasaki H, Sawa M. Respiratory fluctuations of the human pupil. Exp Brain Res 71:215–217, 1988.
29. Wilson SF, Amling JK, Floyd SD, McNair ND. Determining interrater reliability of nurses' assessments of pupillary size and reaction. J Neurosci Nurs 20:189–192, 1988.
30. Bromage PR, Camporesi EM, Durant PA, Nielsen CH. Nonrespiratory side effects of epidural morphine. Anesth Analg 61:490–495, 1982.
31. Murray RB, Adler MW, Korczyn AD. The pupillary effects of opioids. Life Sci 33:495–509, 1983.
32. Boutros G, Insler MS. Reversible pupillary miosis during a hyperglycaemic episode: case report. Diabetologia 27:50–51, 1984.
33. Helprin GA, Clarke GM. Unilateral fixed dilated pupil associated with nebulised ipratropium [letter]. Lancet 2:1469, 1986.
34. Cordova S, Lee R. Fixed, dilated pupils in the ICU: another recoverable cause. Anaesth Intensive Care 28:91–93, 2000.
35. Goetting MG, Contreras E. Systemic atropine administration during cardiac arrest does not cause fixed and dilated pupils. Ann Emerg Med 20:55–57, 1991.
36. Greenan J, Prasad J. Comparison of the ocular effects of atropine or glycopyrrolate with two I.V. induction agents. Br J Anaesth 57:180–183, 1985.
37. Wijdicks EFM. Neurologic Catastrophes in the Emergency Department. Butterworth-Heinemann, Boston, 2000.
38. Ropper AH, Cole D, Louis DN. Clinicopathologic correlation in a case of pupillary dilation from cerebral hemorrhage. Arch Neurol 48:1166–1169, 1991.
39. Wijdicks EFM. Determining brain death in adults. Neurology 45:1003–1011, 1995.
40. Thompson AE, Sussmane JB. Bretylium intoxication resembling clinical brain death. Crit Care Med 17:194–195, 1989.
41. Yang KL, Dantzker DR. Reversible brain death. A manifestation of amitriptyline overdose. Chest 99:1037–1038, 1991.
42. Goudreau JL, Wijdicks EFM, Emery SF. Complications during apnea testing in the determination of brain death: predisposing factors. Neurology 55:1045–1048, 2000.
43. Snavely SR, Hodges GR. The neurotoxicity of antibacterial agents. Ann Intern Med 101:92–104, 1984.
44. Jordan JE, Dyess E, Cliett J. Unusual spontaneous movements in brain-dead patients [letter]. Neurology 35:1082, 1985.
45. Jørgensen EO. Spinal man after brain death. The

unilateral extension–pronation reflex of the upper limb as an indication of brain death. Acta Neurochir 28:259–273, 1973.

46. Mandel S, Arenas A, Scasta D. Spinal automatism in cerebral death [letter]. N Engl J Med 307:501, 1982.

47. Ropper AH. Unusual spontaneous movements in brain-dead patients. Neurology 34:1089–1092, 1984.

48. Ropper AH, Kennedy SK, Russell L. Apnea testing in the diagnosis of brain death. Clinical and physiological observations. J Neurosurg 55:942–946, 1981.

49. Belsh JM, Blatt R, Schiffman PL. Apnea testing in brain death. Arch Intern Med 146:2385–2388, 1986.

50. Benzel EC, Gross CD, Hadden TA, Kesterson L, Landreneau MD. The apnea test for the determination of brain death. J Neurosurg 71:191–194, 1989.

51. Marks SJ, Zisfein J. Apneic oxygenation in apnea tests for brain death. A controlled trial. Arch Neurol 47:1066–1068, 1990.

52. Bucci MN, Phillips TW, McGillicuddy JE. Delayed epidural hemorrhage in hypotensive multiple trauma patients. Neurosurgery 19:65–68, 1986.

53. Arieff AI, Llach F, Massry SG. Neurological manifestations and morbidity of hyponatremia: correlation with brain water and electrolytes. Medicine (Baltimore) 55:121–129, 1976.

54. Arieff AI. Hyponatremia, convulsions, respiratory arrest, and permanent brain damage after elective surgery in healthy women. N Engl J Med 314: 1529–1535, 1986.

55. Jensen V. The TURP syndrome. Can J Anaesth 38: 90–96, 1991.

56. Bolman R III, Saffitz J. Early postoperative care of the cardiac transplantation patient: routine considerations and immunosuppressive therapy. Prog Cardiovasc Dis 33:137–148, 1990.

57. Meyers BF, Patterson GA. Current status of lung transplantation. Adv Surg 34:301–318, 2000.

58. Wijdicks EF, Blue PR, Steers JL, Wiesner RH. Central pontine myelinolysis with stupor alone after orthotopic liver transplantation. Liver Transpl Surg 2:14–16, 1996.

59. Slavin ML, Budabin M. Pituitary apoplexy associated with cardiac surgery. Am J Ophthalmol 98: 291–296, 1984.

60. Savage EB, Gugino L, Starr PA, Black PM, Cohn LH, Aranki SF. Pituitary apoplexy following cardiopulmonary bypass: considerations for a staged cardiac and neurosurgical procedure. Eur J Cardiothorac Surg 8:333–336, 1994.

61. Absalom M, Rogers KH, Moulton RJ, Mazer CD. Pituitary apoplexy after coronary artery surgery. Anesth Analg 76:648–649, 1993.

62. Wijdicks EF, Scott JP. Stroke in the medical intensive-care unit. Mayo Clin Proc 73:642–646, 1998.

63. Levy D. The fat embolism syndrome. A review. Clin Orthop 261:281–286, 1990.

64. Fish DN. Treatment of delirium in the critically ill patient. Clin Pharm 10:456–466, 1991.

65. Seneff MG, Mathews RA. Use of haloperidol infusions to control delirium in critically ill adults. Ann Pharmacother 29:690–693, 1995.

66. Kurtek RW, Lai KK, Tauxe WN, Eidelman BH, Fung JJ. Tc-99m hexamethylpropylene amine oxime scintigraphy in the diagnosis of brain death and its implications for the harvesting of organs used for transplantation. Clin Nucl Med 25:7–10, 2000.

67. Hadani M, Bruk B, Ram Z, Knoller N, Spiegelmann R, Segal E. Application of transcranial Doppler ultrasonography for the diagnosis of brain death. Intensive Care Med 25:822–828, 1999.

68. Bennett DR. The EEG in determination of brain death. Ann N Y Acad Sci 315:110–120, 1978.

69. Petty GW, Mohr JP, Pedley TA, et al. The role of transcranial Doppler in confirming brain death: sensitivity, specificity, and suggestions for performance and interpretation. Neurology 40:300–303, 1990.

70. Ropper AH, Kehne SM, Wechsler L. Transcranial Doppler in brain death. Neurology 37:1733–1735, 1987.

Chapter 2

NEUROLOGIC MANIFESTATIONS OF PHARMACOLOGIC AGENTS COMMONLY USED IN THE INTENSIVE CARE UNIT

less accurate, but with knowledge of the pharmacokinetics and pharmacodynamics of each agent, some reasonable estimate of its effect is possible. In the ideal situation, sedation is simply briefly discontinued or pharmacologically reversed, but the severity of illness can dictate prolonged use, and suggesting termination of sedation may be inappropriate. As a plain matter of fact, multipharmacy in a certain patient may invoke a feeling of reluctance by neurologists to assess prognosis in these patients. Sedation aside, many drugs are used in the intensive care unit (ICU). These drugs have direct neurotoxic effects, and this chapter summarizes those that are commonly used to manage critical illness but that in addition affect neurologic function. Also addressed is the interaction of drugs that causes prolonged sedation.

Critically ill patients are sedated to facilitate mechanical ventilation, overcome anxiety, protect against myocardial stress and ischemia, and support sleep. The desired depth may vary from "conscious sedation," which creates a comfort level to allow nursing procedures without pain, to levels approaching general anesthesia. Many agents (for example, midazolam and propofol) are administered by continuous infusion. Neurologic assessment in sedated patients is unmistakably

PRINCIPLES OF PHARMACODYNAMICS AND PHARMACOKINETICS IN CRITICAL ILLNESS

Pharmacodynamics is the comprehension of the relationship between the drug concentration and pharmacologic efficacy (what drugs do to the body). The study of pharmacodynamics has qualitative aspects (for example, specific chemical receptors, active sites of enzymes, and selective target tissue sites) and quantitative aspects (for example, dose responsiveness, potency, therapeutic efficacy, and tolerance).

Generally used anesthetic agents act unselectively or by binding to receptors. Drug receptor effects are complex, have been partially elucidated, and may involve control of membrane ion channels in the proximity of the receptor. Important receptors in the pharmacodynamics of anesthetic drugs are γ-aminobutyric acid (GABA), N-methyl-D-aspartate (NMDA), and opioids (μ, δ, and κ). Barbiturates, benzodiazepines, and propofol bind to the GABA receptors and activate them because they resemble the natural transmitter, but they also have a greater capacity to resist degradation and act longer than the endogenous substances.[1] The number of receptors changes from exposure and may decrease with continuous exposure (down-regulation), resulting in a loss of efficacy (tachyphylaxis). This so-called acquired tolerance is especially known with opioids at their receptor sites. They may also have an increased effect from prolonged contact with antagonists (up-regulation). The application of these pharmacodynamic principles is relevant in the ICU. For example, when a benzodiazepine is administered, tolerance may occur with excessive doses and extended duration. Most typically, patients who are tolerant of the effects of alcohol have a similar physiologic response to benzodiazepines and barbiturates, so that a higher dose is required to achieve sedation.

The quantitative aspects of pharmacodynamics include potency and efficacy. *Potency* is the amount of drug in relation to its effect, and *therapeutic efficacy* is the capacity of a drug to produce an often maximum effect. An important concept is the *therapeutic index*, which is the maximum tolerated dose divided by the minimum desired therapeutic effect. Drugs with a small therapeutic window cause adverse effects well below the amount that produces the maximum effect.

Pharmacokinetics studies the relationships of dose administration, concentration of the drug over time, and rate at which the drug enters, diffuses within, and leaves the body (what the body does to the drug). Most drugs are subject to *first-order* processes of ab-

sorption, distribution within the central compartment (predominantly the blood volume and any highly vascularized organ), metabolism, and excretion. The rate at which these occur is directly proportional to the concentration of the drug. In first-order (exponential) processes, it can be predicted that, for example, a 50% increase in dose will lead to an increase in steady-state plasma concentration by the same percentage.

Zero-order processes (saturation) are much slower than first-order processes, and elimination occurs independent of concentration. This process requires enzymatic elimination and thus is limited in speed. Many drugs exhibit saturation, or zero-order, kinetics when a high enough dose is administered, and this effect explains delay in recovery from drug overdose. Phenytoin is a typical example. At low doses, elimination can match an increase in dose, but gradually with higher doses, the enzymatic process reaches saturation and the plasma concentration rises disproportionately into toxic territory.

Many drugs are administered intravenously. In about five times the half-life, the mean plasma concentration is constant and at a plateau; the plasma concentration decreases to zero in five times the half-life when infusion is stopped.

The pharmacokinetics of drugs used in critically ill patients, however, undergoes significant changes. These alterations, which can be substantial, are summarized in Figure 2–1.

Clearance of benzodiazepines occurs primarily through liver metabolism, which involves both microsomal oxidation and glucuronide conjugation. Hepatic metabolism depends on hepatic blood flow, enzyme activity, and protein binding. Hepatic blood flow can be reduced in late-stage sepsis and hemorrhagic shock. In fact, hepatic blood flow is reduced threefold in sepsis during the hypodynamic phase; in one study, reduction was up to 71% in hemorrhagic shock.[2] However, the pharmacokinetics of benzodiazepines becomes normal after adequate and rapid fluid resuscitation.[3,4] Hepatic drug metabolism can be reduced by positive end-expiratory pressure (as little as 10 mm Hg),[5,6] reducing hepatic blood flow 20% to 50%; by α-adrenergic receptor agents, such

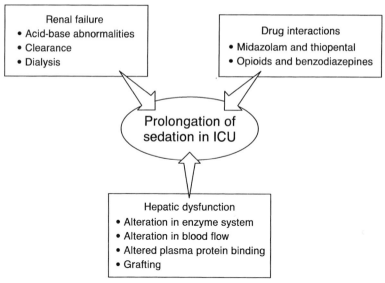

Figure 2–1. Factors leading to prolonged effect of drugs used in the intensive care unit (ICU).

as norepinephrine and epinephrine; and by high doses of dopamine, resulting in vasoconstriction of hepatic venous and arterial systems.

Alterations in the activity of cytochrome P-450 have been documented not only after burns[7,8] but also after any other type of critical illness. With traumatic injury, such as leg fractures[9] and limb ischemia, alteration is probably a result of acute-phase response interleukins on P-450 function.[10,11] Depressed P-450 enzyme systems were also noted in a preliminary study on head injury.[12]

Altered protein binding remains a crucial component in hepatic drug metabolism associated with critical illness and may last up to 4 weeks after the critical illness has been controlled. With hypoalbuminemia, a greater proportion of benzodiazepines is unbound and thus active. Finally, after liver transplantation, liver function (monitored by bile output and liver function tests) can be marginal, and accumulation of benzodiazepines can be very rapid. Thus, hepatic dysfunction in critically ill patients is a major contributor to prolonged sedation and may be underappreciated.

Renal failure is very common in critical illness, predominantly affecting the clearance of morphine and midazolam metabolites.[13]

Commonly, the proposed mechanism is reduced perfusion of the kidney, but metabolic acidosis and respiratory alkalosis in this condition may also change the pH difference between tissue and plasma compartments, leading to a change in tissue distribution.

Important drug interactions are summarized in Table 2–1. Anesthetic drugs and sedative agents administered simultaneously may amplify the sedative effect (synergism). Examples are propofol, midazolam, and alfentanil and the combination of midazolam and thiopental, opioids, and benzodiazepines. The mechanism proposed for the midazolam-thiopental synergism is an allosteric alteration caused by the barbiturate in the GABA receptor that enhances benzodiazepine binding to the GABA molecule. The use of adjunctive neuroactive agents, such as tricyclic antidepressants, phenothiazines, opiates, and sedatives, additively increases sedation but does not necessarily increase half-life or prolong effect.

Endocrine changes may reduce metabolism, particularly conditions such as hypothyroidism and hypothermia. Other factors that may influence clearance of the drug are old age,[14] major surgery, and underlying chronic disease, such as cirrhosis.

Table 2–1. **Drugs Prolonging Clearance of Sedatives and Analgesic Agents Commonly Used in the Intensive Care Unit**

Drug	Causative Agent
Midazolam	Cimetidine
	Clarithromycin
	Delavirdine
	Diltiazem
	Erythromycin
	Fluconazole
	Grepafloxacin
	Indinavir
	Itraconazole
	Ketoconazole
	Nefazodone
	Nelfinavir
	Omeprazole
	Probenecid
	Ranitidine
	Ritonavir
	Roxithromycin
	Saquinavir
	Troleandomycin
	Verapamil
Lorazepam	Clozapine
	Loxapine
	Probenecid
	Quetiapine
	Valproic acid?
Propofol	Bupivacaine
	Diazepam?
	Lidocaine (IM)
Morphine	Cimetidine
	Metoclopramide
	Monoamine oxidase inhibitors
Fentanyl	Clonidine
	Methohexital
	Ritonavir
Diazepam	Cimetidine
	Cisapride
	Clarithromycin
	Disulfiram
	Erythromycin
	Fluoxetine
	Itraconazole
	Ketoconazole
	Omeprazole
	Oral contraceptives
	Paroxetine
	Propoxyphene
	Ritonavir
	Sertraline
	Troleandomycin

IM, intramuscularly.

EFFECT OF DRUGS ON NEUROMUSCULAR FUNCTION

The need for neuromuscular blocking (NMB) agents is controversial.[15,16] Use in medical and surgical ICUs is limited by the serious potential for disuse muscle atrophy and the complexity of nursing care. Neuromuscular blocking agents may also pose a significant danger to the patient if the ventilator inadvertently becomes disconnected. Neurologic examination is limited to examination of pupils that remain normal in size, because nicotinic receptors are absent and the pupillary light reflex therefore remains intact.[17] In many patients, however, miosis is seen from additional use of narcotic agents and not as a consequence of NMB agents. In ICU practice, muscle relaxation with NMB agents is considered in patients with severe pulmonary disease who have high airway pressures and decreased pulmonary compliance during mechanical ventilation, patients with tetanus, and patients with tenuous surgical repairs. In patients with severe hypothermia, the NMB agents eliminate intense shivering that increases oxygen consumption and myocardial work.

When the drug is withdrawn, recovery from paralysis is seen within 1 hr, but prolonged paralysis may occur when drugs that may potentiate neuromuscular blockade are administered. Clindamycin, metronidazole, tetracycline, furosemide, corticosteroids,[18] anticholinesterase drugs, local anesthetics, and most antiarrhythmic agents are well known to produce interactions with nondepolarizing NMB agents[19] (see Chapter 4, Fig. 4–1). Respiratory acidosis, metabolic alkalosis, and electrolyte disorders may increase the blocking effect of nondepolarizing drugs on the neuromuscular junction as well, but the clinical significance in all these circumstances is less clear. Aminoglycosides, but not penicillin or cephalosporins, prolong neuromuscular blockade, probably by inhibition of presynaptic acetylcholine release.[20] Under these conditions, weaning from neuromuscular blockade may take additional hours. In contrast, previous long-term use of antiepileptic drugs, phenytoin, carbamazepine,[21] and aminophylline may diminish the effects of muscle relaxants, probably because of long-term induction of the cytochrome P-450 system.

Table 2–2. **Nondepolarizing Muscle Relaxants**

Agent	Initial Dose (mg/kg)	Initial Drip Rate (mg/kg/hr)	Duration (min)
Metocurine	0.3	0.1	60–90
Pancuronium	0.1	0.025	60–90
Atracurium	0.4	0.7	30–60
Vecuronium	0.08	0.07	30–60

From Coyle JP, Cullen DJ. Anesthetic pharmacology and critical care. In: Chernow B (ed). The Pharmacologic Approach to the Critically Ill Patient, 2nd ed. Williams & Wilkins, Baltimore, 1988, pp 241–253. By permission of Lippincott, Williams & Wilkins.

Most reports of prolonged muscle weakness are linked to pancuronium and vecuronium.[22,23] Table 2–2 shows commonly used doses and duration of clinical effect for four nondepolarizing muscle relaxants. Duration of action after a single bolus is usually 90 min. Therefore, 25% of the initial dose is usually repeated every 45 to 90 min.

Atracurium has a propensity to release histamine, apparently dose related, but with the introduction of an isomer, *cis*-atracurium, this effect most likely has been eliminated. Fewer problems can be expected with use of atracurium. Atracurium is very expensive, however, and a propensity to increasing doses during use results in formidable total costs. Rocuronium, a derivative of vecuronium, is less potent than vecuronium[24,25] but has been developed for its rapid onset of action.

Mivacurium has distinct pharmacologic characteristics because its recovery is due to metabolism by plasma cholinesterase. It does not accumulate and is not in any way influenced by age or organ failure.[26]

Nondepolarizing drugs should be monitored in the ICU with the use of peripheral nerve stimulators[27-30] (Fig. 2–2). Like many procedures and monitoring devices, the peripheral nerve stimulator was introduced in ICUs after being used successfully for years in the operating room. This technique of estimating the neuromuscular transmission is easily applied at the bedside and is now standard care. The response of the twitching thumb is manually assessed after the ulnar nerve is stimulated supramaximally at the wrist through cutaneous electrodes. Abduction of the thumb creating some preload also facilitates the tactile evaluation by the rater. Depth of neuromuscular blockade can be assessed by objective criteria, such as post-tetanic potentiation, but the train-of-four method (four twitches every 0.5 sec with supramaximal stimuli) is more practical. Frequent use of the peripheral nerve stimulator should guide the infusion rate of neuromuscular blocking agents and the need for an additional bolus. Standard practice is to titrate to one or two twitches, and the absence of twitches suggests a muscle relaxant overdose.[31]

PATHOPHYSIOLOGIC MECHANISMS

The muscle relaxants act on the alpha unit of the postjunctional nicotinic cholinergic receptor. The cholinergic receptor spans the membrane of the muscle cell and consists of two alpha protein subunits and one of beta, delta, and epsilon.[32] Only when both alpha sites are occupied does a conformational change occur that opens the central canal. This allows a flux of cations, which depolarizes the cell membrane and leads to muscle contraction. *Depolarizing neuromuscular blockade* refers to depolarizing of the motor end plate, mimicking the action of acetylcholine (for example, succinylcholine, decamethonium) and preventing repolarization and normal action of acetylcholine. Depolarization is not maintained with prolonged or repeated use, and succinylcholine develops a so-called phase II block characterized by fading response and potential for reversal of its effect by anticholinesterases. This phenome-

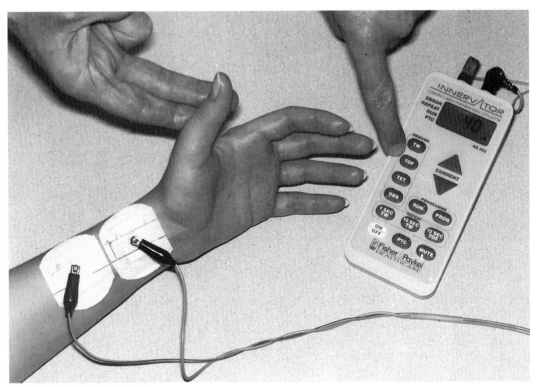

Figure 2–2. Peripheral nerve stimulator. Two fingers abduct the thumb and sense the twitches. TOF, train of four; 40 mA is a sufficient current.

non may represent desensitization but may reflect ion channel block.

Nondepolarizing blockade (e.g., pancuronium, vecuronium, atracurium) refers to a competition of the agent with acetylcholine for its receptor site, but the motor end plate is not depolarized, leaving opportunity for terminating the effect with an anticholinesterase, such as neostigmine or edrophonium.[33] The result is reaccumulation of acetylcholine and competition with the nondepolarizing agent. The effects of NMB agents can be tested by peripheral stimulation. Four supramaximal stimuli produce a "fade" response in which the responses after the first one decrease.[34] Depolarizing agents cause all four to decrease simultaneously.

Recovery of muscle weakness after vecuronium or pancuronium use has a stereotypical pattern. The diaphragm is relatively more resistant to muscle relaxants.[35] Therefore, resumption of diaphragmatic work, ev-ident by triggering of the ventilator, usually comes first and is soon followed by improved head lift and recovery of oropharyngeal, proximal, and distal muscles. Without the ability to routinely measure plasma levels of NMB agents, it may be difficult to know whether active metabolites have blocked the neuromuscular junction. Segredo and colleagues[36] found that metabolites of vecuronium may accumulate in patients with renal failure, metabolic acidosis, and hypermagnesemia. This finding may superficially indicate that metabolites of NMB agents would prolong its effect, but electrophysiologic data in this study were not available; therefore, a cause-and-effect relationship was not clearly established. However, it is very likely that before control of neuromuscular blockade with bedside peripheral nerve stimulators was available, overdose may have significantly prolonged paralysis in many patients. For example, in one patient who had no administration of pancuronium 6 days before death, large doses of the drug were found in muscles at biopsy.[37]

Therefore, persistent muscle paralysis after discontinuation of muscle relaxants usually implies overdose or enhancement from other drugs. Approximately 0.04% of patients have a gene defect that reduces the effect of plasma cholinesterase through an increase in the inhibiting dibucaine substance. As a result, these patients are unable to metabolize succinylcholine and have a prolonged action instead of the typical brief duration from rapid metabolism. Other gene defects have been characterized—the fluoride-resistant gene and silent gene—with even lower prevalence.[38,39] In most patients, this condition is immediately evident by persistence of train-of-four abnormalities after withdrawal of the paralytic agent.

It is appropriate here to point out that pancuronium and vecuronium have been associated with muscle weakness lasting for weeks to months after discontinuation.[36,40–44] Prolonged muscle paralysis has also been linked to atracurium.[45] Therefore, it has been argued that the steroid nucleus of vecuronium and pancuronium is not essential in prolonged weakness. Systemic electrophysiologic studies are not available in these patients with prolonged muscle weakness without prior sepsis and corticosteroids. Finally, prolonged use of neuromuscular agents without measures that protect peripheral nerves from compression may also cause multiple entrapment neuropathies. Bilateral peroneal and ulnar palsies from prolonged immoblization and insufficient protection at compression points may occur, but no study of prevalence in the ICU is available. A comprehensive discussion of causes of generalized weakness can be found in Chapter 4.

EFFECT OF DRUGS ON LEVEL OF CONSCIOUSNESS

Many patients need sedation to achieve a desired level of relaxation, but the metabolism of drugs in critically ill patients is uncertain and patient response may vary. Pharmacodynamics and pharmacokinetics are sparsely studied in critically ill patients. Even if results were available, it would be difficult to extrapolate them to another critically ill population, often so clearly characterized by het-

Table 2–3. **Ramsay Scale**

1. Anxious and agitated or restless, or both
2. Cooperative, oriented, and tranquil
3. Responding to commands only
4. Brisk response to light glabellar tap or loud auditory stimulus
5. Sluggish response to light glabellar tap or loud auditory stimulus
6. No response to glabellar tap or auditory stimulus

Data from Ramsay et al.[47]

erogeneity and an unpredictable clinical course.

Scales may be useful to avoid oversedation, and the modified Ramsay scale allows assessment of level of consciousness. The interrater proportion of agreement was 0.93 for this scale[46] (Table 2–3). Clearly, a better (more practical and reliable) scale is needed for neurologists. For the moment, both the Ramsay and the Glasgow coma scales (Chapter 1) may reflect depth of sedation.

Narcotic Agents

Narcotic agents may effectively relieve pain (Table 2–4). Epidural administration of narcotics has recently been introduced as a pain-relieving measure in patients with major thoracic surgery. Narcotic analgesia is very helpful in surgical ICUs and additionally may mute stress-related cardiac ischemia. To overcome prolonged awaking times with benzodiazepines, short-acting opioids have also been used to induce sedation, but

Table 2–4. **Opioid Agents Commonly Used in the Intensive Care Unit**

Agent	Elimination Half-life (hr)
Morphine	1.5–4
Fentanyl	2–5
Sufentanil	2–3
Alfentanil	1.5–3.5
Phenoperidine	1.5–4
Pethidine	3–6.5
Nalbuphine	3.5–4

depression of the level of consciousness is not particularly pronounced with standard doses.

Most patients in the ICU are treated with intermittent doses of morphine. Alternative narcotic drugs, such as alfentanil and sufentanil, are generally used to induce anesthesia.[48,49] Intravenous morphine drips of 1 to 3 mg/hr produce minimal side effects. The most pronounced are miosis[50–52] and vertical nystagmus[53] (see Chapter 1). Seizures or seizure-like movements have been observed after induction with opioids. Anesthesiologists more often than neurologists are aware of these movements induced by opioids. Many patients experience sudden onset of rigidity of abdominal and chest wall muscles,[54] flexion in the neck, and myoclonic jerks[55] in the upper and lower limbs, which may be associated with flexion at the elbows and fingers and extension at the hips and knees, mimicking pathologic flexion or decorticate posturing.[55–58]

The time course of these "convulsions" may also strongly resemble that of generalized tonic–clonic seizures, but electroencephalographic recordings during these manifestations have not revealed specific epileptiform activity.[59,60] Generally, the risk of tonic–clonic seizures after opioid administration is low in patients with no history of epilepsy. Conversely, as noted in Chapter 3, narcotic agents may be associated with new-onset seizures after sudden withdrawal.

Midazolam

Patients requiring mechanical ventilation need adequate sedation to overcome the distress of being in an ICU environment.[61] Benzodiazepines are widely used in ICUs, but pharmacokinetics are changed in critical illness.[62,63] Claims of short-elimination half-life for some of the recently introduced benzodiazepines may not always apply in this category of patients. In addition, metabolites of midazolam (conjugated α-hydroxymidazolam) may penetrate the cerebrospinal fluid, causing prolonged sedation, particularly in patients with renal failure. In one study, even when the concentration of midazolam was below the detectable range, a good response to an antagonist was seen.[13] A recent study

suggested that midazolam (or fentanyl) may cause worsening of a previous neurologic deficit, but this may be a more general property of centrally acting drugs.[64]

Midazolam, a water-soluble imidazole benzodiazepine, is twice as potent as diazepam. After a single dose of midazolam, an elimination half-life of 1 to 4 hr can be expected. Mechanically ventilated patients with multiorgan failure, however, have reduced clearance,[65] causing midazolam to accumulate. Shelly and colleagues[66,67] found that the elimination half-life was greater than 12 hr in half of their patients despite the claim of rapid clearance from the circulation. A randomized study that compared midazolam with propofol found more realistic data.[68] Patients receiving mechanical ventilation had a return of spontaneous ventilation and adequate response to command an average of 6.5 hr after administration of midazolam was discontinued. Isolated reports of extremely prolonged recovery time (up to 3 days) may be related to associated liver disease. Pentobarbital and thiopental enhance the effects of midazolam. Small doses of opioids and cimetidine, frequently used in the ICU, may increase the plasma concentration of midazolam. If the drug is given by continuous infusion for prolonged periods without intermittent assessment of the level of consciousness, accumulation in tissues may occur,[67] but others have presented contradictory data.[69]

Several studies compared midazolam with lorazepam. These studies showed some conflicting data on efficacy, but lorazepam compared favorably with midazolam when costs were considered (four to six times less expensive than midazolam).[70,71]

The effects of midazolam can be transiently reversed by the benzodiazepine antagonist flumazenil. Flumazenil is a competitive antagonist at the benzodiazepine receptor.[72] After administration, onset of reversal is very rapid, within 1 to 2 min, and usually a dose of 0.4 to 1.0 mg produces complete antagonism. The duration is dose dependent and ranges from 15 min to 2.5 hr. Flumazenil may be given in doses of up to 1 mg at 20–min intervals, but in patients with suspected benzodiazepine overdose, a continuous infusion of 1 mg/hr may be used. Seizures have been reported and tend to occur in patients who have been receiving benzodiazepines for long-term sedation and probably also in patients with other propensities for seizures (for example, prior seizure disorder). Use of flumazenil in reversal of hepatic encephalopathy is controversial (see Chapter 10).

Lorazepam

Lorazepam is a short-acting benzodiazepine, although its half-life may be nearly 10 to 20 hr. Clearance is largely through the kidney; therefore, it is a good alternative to midazolam in patients with liver failure. Withdrawal of lorazepam may induce seizures or, as it would with any other benzodiazepine, nonconvulsive status epilepticus. Lorazepam is most often used for long-term sedation for any medical reason, be it delirium, anxiety, or long-term mechanical ventilation. Its low comparative cost makes it the preferred drug for long-term sedation.

Propofol

Propofol, an agent frequently used for induction of anesthesia, has become commonplace in ICUs.[73–75] The pharmacokinetics of propofol elimination is weight-dependent.[76] This agent may become a preferred drug for sedation but is already acceptable as a suitable agent for short procedures, such as endotracheal intubation. Neurologic examination in patients who have received propofol is unreliable, and most brain stem reflexes may disappear except for pupillary light response. High doses of propofol (5 to 7 mg/kg/hr) may produce burst suppression on the electroencephalogram.[77]

A randomized study of propofol (1 to 3 mg/kg/hr) and midazolam (0.1 to 0.2 mg/kg/hr) showed that propofol had important advantages over midazolam in many respects.[68] The half-life of propofol, even in mechanically ventilated patients,[78] is short (1.5 to 12.4 hr), and many patients awaken almost immediately after discontinuation of the intravenous infusion. In general, patients awaken within 30 min, but time to extubation may range from 11 to 205 min.[79] In addition, the terminal half-life after a 10-day infusion of propofol is even more prolonged and may approach 1 to 3 days. Clinical experience in the ICU population is extensive. Side effects are green discoloration of urine and adrenocortical suppression, although only at extremely high doses. Acid–base abnormalities (particularly metabolic acidosis) without a good correlation with dose or duration of infusion have been noted in children. In the reported cases, however, sepsis was a possible confounder.[80] Other side effects are choreoathetoid movements, myoclonus, opisthotonus (with high doses), increased triglyceride levels from the lipid emulsion formula, decrease in plasma cortisol, and possible inhibition of the immune system.

The use of propofol in traumatic head injury has increased substantially in the past decade. A recent multicenter trial resolved many of the questions about safety and efficacy.[81] Propofol in mechanically ventilated patients with head injury was compared with morphine. Intracranial pressure was similar between these groups, although after 3 days, on average, mean daily intracranial pressure was lower in the propofol group. Other methods to lower intracranial pressure were significantly less often used in the propofol group (for example, pentobarbital, cerebrospinal fluid drainage). Outcome could not be assessed, partly because of major differences in Glasgow coma scale scores between the groups on admission.[81] Therefore, propofol may be a useful sedative agent in traumatic brain injury, although its role in control of intracranial pressure remains undetermined. Initial experience with propofol in brain edema associated with fulminant hepatic failure is encouraging (Chapter 10).

COMMONLY USED DRUGS WITH DIRECT NEUROTOXIC EFFECTS

The neurologic manifestations of drugs frequently used in the ICU are listed in Table 2–5. Drug intoxication more commonly occurs in patients with multiorgan failure or multiple drug regimens, and neurologic manifestations then are obviously more

Table 2–5. **Neurologic Manifestations of Drugs Frequently Used in the Intensive Care Unit**

Agent	Neurologic Manifestations
Amiodarone[82–84]	Optic neuropathy, tremor, gait ataxia, peripheral neuropathy (4 or more months of treatment)
Amphotericin B[85]	Headache, tremor, confusion, akinetic mutism
Aminophylline	Seizures, headache, insomnia
Cimetidine[86]	Myokymias, seizures, dysarthria, drowsiness, hallucinations
Hydralazine	Distal axonopathy
Hydrocortisone	Acute myopathy
Ketamine	Myoclonus
Lidocaine	Myokymias, myoclonus, paresthesias
Local anesthetics[87,88]	Seizures
Metoclopramide[89]	Oculogyric crises, torticollis, trismus, parkinsonism
Metronidazole[90]	Distal axonopathy, cerebellar lesions, visual hallucinations
Neuroleptic agents	Malignant neuroleptic syndrome
Penicillin derivatives	Multiple myoclonus, asterixis, coma
Sodium nitroprusside	Muscle spasm, convulsions
Succinylcholine	Malignant hyperthermia

prevalent. The most common neurologic manifestations are seizures, decreased level of response, and prolonged blockade of the neuromuscular junction or myopathy.

Acute Steroid Myopathy

A well-recognized complication of intravenously administered corticosteroids is acute myopathy.[91–94] Acute quadriplegic myopathy must be seriously entertained in a patient with status asthmaticus treated intravenously with pancuronium and large doses of corticosteroids (usually up to 1 g/day) who has markedly increased creatine kinase levels.[92,95–101] Possibly, disuse atrophy contributes because an increase in the number of cytoplasmic corticosteroid receptors in this condition increases the corticosteroid exposure.[102] Complete ophthalmoplegia and severe proximal limb weakness have been described as part of a corticosteroid and pancuronium myopathy,[103] but acute steroid myopathy does not involve respiratory muscles. Muscle biopsy may show necrotic changes and vacuolar changes in all fiber types, which also reflect the increased creatine kinase values and occasional myoglobinuria in these patients. Characteristic findings, however, are selective loss of the thick filaments (myosin) and absence of myosin mRNA.[104]

Acute myopathy during intravenous treatment with high doses of corticosteroids and neuromuscular blocking agents typically documents type II fiber atrophy with characteristic selective loss of myosin. Myosin is targeted, but the reason for this preferential destruction is speculative.[104,105] One study documented enhanced expression of calpains.[106] This proteolytic system is calcium-activated protease, which rarely is expressed by corticosteroids. This finding suggests that corticosteroids may not be important in its genesis, and, indeed, several cases without corticosteroid use but with well-documented muscle biopsy study[107] have been reported, suggesting other pathways generated through critical illness, such as sepsis. Up-regulation of glucocorticoid receptors or endogenous steroid production has been suggested. Further insight was obtained with an animal study[108] in which the sciatic nerve was removed from a steroid-treated and denervated rat. This study documented reduction in skeletal muscle type I sodium channels and thus reduced excitability. Reduced excitability appeared in this study from depolarization of the resting membrane potential that was later followed by increased inactivation of sodium channels.

Malignant Hyperthermia

Malignant hyperthermia is not an exclusively anesthesiologic disorder. The incidence is 1:50,000 in adults receiving general anesthesia.[109] The consulting neurologist can assess subtle changes in the neurologic condition and, more important, is familiar with associated myopathies.[110] Malignant hyperthermia frequently occurs in the operating room, and the anesthesiologist determines whether further action (particularly dantrolene infusion) should be undertaken.

Clinical presentation of malignant hyperthermia (Table 2–6) is a consequence of elevated myoplasmic calcium, hypermetabolism, and rhabdomyolysis.[109,111,112] The most common muscle manifestation is masseter muscle rigidity or trismus.[112,113] Very often, flaccidity, caused by succinylcholine, occurs, but generalized muscle rigidity may soon follow.[112,113] Masseter spasm is dramatic in presentation and may be associated with cyanosis, labile blood pressure, and marked tachycardia. Fasciculations are frequently

Table 2–6. Clinical Features of Malignant Hyperthermia

Fever (≥41°C)
Masseter trismus and skeletal muscle rigidity
Metabolic and respiratory acidosis
Cardiac arrhythmias
Marked hyperkalemia
Marked increase in serum creatine kinase concentration (>20,000 IU/L)
Myoglobinuria
Hypercalcemia (fulminant type)
Intravascular coagulopathy (fulminant type)

Data from Rosenberg.[113]

seen, and masseter trismus seriously hampers intubation. Masseter muscle rigidity subsides within minutes after discontinuation of the triggering anesthetic.

Interpretation of masseter muscle rigidity may be difficult, especially because many patients, if not all, given halothane and succinylcholine have a slight increase in jaw muscle tone.[114] Masseter spasm, more common in children, occurs in 1 in 12,000 anesthetic procedures in which suxamethonium is administered. Whether anesthesia should be continued in patients with rigid masseter muscles is a persistent dilemma, especially in emergency surgery. Progression to fulminant malignant hyperthermia rarely occurs with discontinuation, and treatment with dantrolene may prevent further exacerbation. Masseter spasm is often associated with an increased serum creatine kinase value and myoglobinuria, but the increased concentration of creatine kinase may also be related to an underlying myopathy.

Fulminant malignant hyperthermia is clinically characterized by rapid development of metabolic acidosis and hyperthermia. Myoglobinuria from rhabdomyolysis is an almost obligatory finding. An early sign in a significant number of patients is tachycardia, often accompanied by labile blood pressure. As a consequence of increased carbon dioxide production, tachypnea occurs but may be considerably hampered by rigidity of chest wall muscles. Laboratory findings include respiratory and metabolic acidosis; increased serum concentrations of creatine kinase, potassium, calcium, and magnesium; and hyperglycemia.[115] A massive potassium flux from the sarcoplasm may cause heart block and ultimately cardiac arrest.

Malignant hyperthermia has been associated with congenital myopathies, most often Duchenne's muscular dystrophy, central core disease, myotonia congenita, and myotonic dystrophy.[110]

Several skeletal muscle relaxants (for example, succinylcholine chloride, decamethonium, gallamine) and inhalation anesthetics (for example, halothane, enflurane, isoflurane) are capable of inducing hyperthermic reactions. New anesthetics have not been adequately tested; propofol probably is harmless. Desflurane, a potential inhalation anesthetic, appeared to trigger malignant hyperthermia in susceptible swine.[116]

PATHOPHYSIOLOGIC MECHANISMS

The pathophysiologic mechanism in malignant hyperthermia is complex.[111] In brief, the most impressive biochemical disturbance is an abrupt increase in the intracellular ionized calcium concentration in muscles followed by extreme depletion of adenosine triphosphate reserves that results in rigor and dysfunction of cell membranes. The current view is that malignant hyperthermia is a myopathy in which an impaired calcium regulation mechanism exists.[111] Increased intracellular calcium results in uncoupling of oxidative phosphorylation and enhanced glycolysis. The net effect is an increase in oxygen consumption, a marked decrease in high-energy phosphate metabolites, and production of large amounts of lactate and heat. The underlying defect is a mutation in the ryanodine receptor *RYR1* gene, a calcium release channel localized in the membrane of the sarcoplasmic reticulum.[117,118]

Treatment is summarized in Table 2–7. Hyperventilation with 100% oxygen and discontinuation of inhalational anesthesia are immediately followed by dantrolene infusion.[119] Dantrolene may have been responsible for aborting crises and reducing mortality in 60% of patients.[109] Administration of sodium bicarbonate should be guided by arterial blood gas analysis. Cooling the pa-

Table 2–7. **Drug Treatment of Malignant Hyperthermia**

Dantrolene, 2 mg/kg every 5 min to total dose of 10 mg/kg

Bicarbonate, 2 to 4 mEq/kg

Glucose and insulin IV (if hyperkalemia)

Heparin IV (if disseminated intravascular coagulation)

Data from Harrison.[119]

tient is an essential part of treatment, and vaporization with fans is very effective.

Neuroleptic Malignant Syndrome

Neuroleptic malignant syndrome is associated with use of neuroleptic agents and closely parallels clinically malignant hyperthermia and lethal catatonia.[120] Many patients have schizophrenia or affective disorder. The exact neurochemical changes in neuroleptic malignant syndrome are unclear, but multiple neurotransmitter systems are involved. Hyperthermia and autonomic instability herald the abrupt onset of rapidly progressive deterioration.[121–125] Autonomic dysfunction is characterized by tachycardia, wide swings in blood pressure, tachypnea, and diaphoresis. The typical increasing rigidity may take some days. Mutism is characteristic. Rigidity is reflected by increased creatine kinase levels, but these levels can be extremely variable and normal at the time of fever[126] (Table 2–8).

Management consists of discontinuing administration of any neuroleptic agent, reinstitution of a dopa agonist if recently withdrawn (particularly in parkinsonian patients), cooling, and liberal amounts of fluid to minimize kidney damage.[127] Bromocriptine and amantadine have been used in addition to dantrolene. Clear benefit has also been noted with high doses of benzodiazepines (lorazepam or clonazepam). A large retrospective review of 734 previously reported cases found that amantadine, bromocriptine, and dantrolene, alone or in combination, resulted in improvement and decreased rates of relapse and that use of bromocriptine or dantrolene, or both, led to a significant decrease in mortality.[127]

Lethal (Malignant) Catatonia

Lethal, or malignant, catatonia most likely is an identical disorder without the association with neuroleptic agents and more severe dysautonomia. This disorder may follow any neurologic catastrophe (for example, postresuscitation encephalopathy or meningitis), and signs could be falsely attributed

Table 2–8. Research Criteria for Neuroleptic Malignant Syndrome

A. The development of severe muscle rigidity and elevated temperature associated with the use of neuroleptic medication
B. Two (or more) of the following:
Diaphoresis
Dysphagia
Tremor
Incontinence
Changes in level of consciousness, ranging from confusion to coma
Mutism
Elevated or labile blood pressure
Leukocytosis
Laboratory evidence of muscle injury (e.g., elevated creatine kinase levels)
C. The symptoms in criteria A and B are not caused by another substance (e.g., phencyclidine) or a neurologic or other general medical condition (e.g., viral encephalitis)
D. The symptoms in criteria A and B are not better accounted for by a mental disorder (e.g., mood disorder with catatonic features)

From American Psychiatric Association: Diagnostic and Statistical Manual of Mental Disorders, 4th ed., Text Revision. American Psychiatric Association, Washington, DC, 2000, p 798. By permission.

to the primary disorder (Fig. 2–3). The medical complications can be substantial, including aspiration, myocardial stunning, disseminated intravascular coagulation, upper gastrointestinal tract bleeding, and pulmonary emboli. In severe cases, electroconvulsive therapy is lifesaving in malignant catatonia, for which it should be first-line treatment.[128] Daily bilateral electroconvulsive therapy up to 12 treatments may be needed for symptoms to resolve. Recovery may be protracted, taking months.

Serotonin Syndrome

With the introduction of selective serotonin reuptake inhibitors (for example, sertraline, fluoxetine, paroxetine) comes a new syndrome labeled "serotonin syndrome" (attributed to excessive 5-hydroxytryptamine

stimulation). Its presentation is virtually the same as that of neuroleptic malignant syndrome, with marked dysautonomic features. In addition to agitation, delirium, hallucinations, and manic behavior, the syndrome includes hyperthermia, diaphoresis, diarrhea, lacrimation, shivering, and profound myoclonus. Rigidity is much less pronounced in this syndrome.[129,130] Poisoning with anticholinergic agents, amphetamines, cocaine, and lithium should be excluded by drug screens. The entity resolves spontaneously within 3 days, but certain symptoms may need immediate intervention. Success has been claimed with cyproheptadine, 4 mg/hr, for myoclonus; esmolol, 50 to 200 μg/kg/min, for tachycardia; and methysergide, 2 mg twice a day, for all manifestations.[131,132] Supportive measures such as benzodiazepine therapy, cooling, airway protection, and hydration may be effective. Because some studies suggest that dantrolene enhances central serotonin metabolism, it should be avoided.[133,134] This finding reemphasizes the importance of clinically distinguishing between serotonin syndrome and neuroleptic malignant syndrome.

CONCLUSIONS

It is common to find that patients in the ICU have numerous drugs listed on their daily medication chart. Familiarity with currently used medication in the ICU is crucial for further evaluation of patients who fail to fully recover their level of consciousness. Fortunately, newer pharmacologic agents are short-acting, and awakening can be expected in a matter of minutes. Nonetheless, the most common cause of alteration of consciousness in critically ill patients is related to previous administration of sedative drugs that accumulate over days because of diminished clearance or pharmacologic interactions. Sometimes its washout is the cause of mysterious awakening.

Neurologic manifestations of commonly used drugs in the ICU have been repeatedly documented. Elimination of the drug is typically associated with full resolution of signs and symptoms.

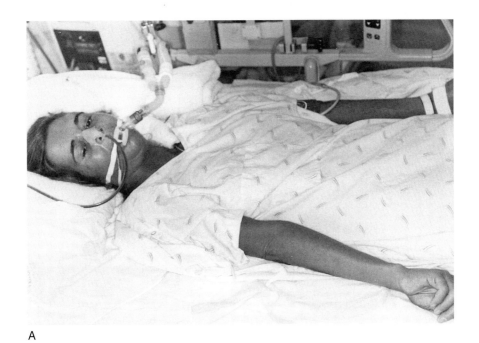

A

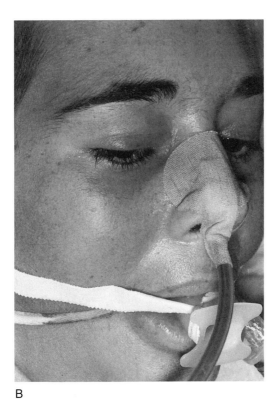

B

Figure 2–3. Malignant catatonia with brief periods (minutes) of mydriasis, tachycardia, tachypnea, and stupor. Note posturing (*A*). In addition, wetting of the skin (*B*) is evident from the glistening reflection of flash photography. Note pearls of sweat and collection in nasolabial fold. The tone became flaccid after this spell, but consciousness remained markedly decreased. Electroconvulsive therapy was successful.

REFERENCES

1. Chernow B (ed). The Pharmacologic Approach to the Critically Ill Patient, 3rd ed. Williams & Wilkins, Baltimore, 1994.
2. McKindley DS, Hanes S, Boucher BA. Hepatic drug metabolism in critical illness. Pharmacotherapy 18:759–778, 1998.
3. Adams P, Gelman S, Reves JG, Greenblatt DJ, Alvis JM, Bradley E. Midazolam pharmacodynamics and pharmacokinetics during acute hypovolemia. Anesthesiology 63:140–146, 1985.
4. Macnab MS, Macrae DJ, Guy E, Grant IS, Feely J. Profound reduction in morphine clearance and liver blood flow in shock. Intensive Care Med 12:366–369, 1986.
5. Bersten AD, Gnidec AA, Rutledge FS, Sibbald WJ. Hyperdynamic sepsis modifies a PEEP-mediated redistribution in organ blood flows. Am Rev Respir Dis 141:1198–1208, 1990.
6. Richard C, Berdeaux A, Delion F, et al. Effect of mechanical ventilation on hepatic drug pharmacokinetics. Chest 90:837–841, 1986.
7. Ciaccio EI, Fruncillo RJ. Decreased aryl hydrocarbon hydroxylase after a 15% burn injury. Biochem Pharmacol 28:3151–3152, 1979.
8. Fruncillo RJ, Di Gregorio GJ. Pharmacokinetics of pentobarbital, quinidine, lidocaine, and theophylline in the thermally injured rat. J Pharm Sci 73:1117–1121, 1984.
9. Griffeth LK, Rosen GM, Tschanz C, Rauckman EJ. Effects of model traumatic injury on hepatic drug metabolism in the rat. I. In vivo antipyrine metabolism. Drug Metab Dispos 11:517–525, 1983.
10. Ferrari L, Kremers P, Batt AM, Gielen JE, Siest G. Differential effects of human recombinant interleukin-1 beta on cytochrome P-450-dependent activities in cultured fetal rat hepatocytes. Drug Metab Dispos 20:407–412, 1992.
11. McKindley DS, Boucher BA, Hess MM, Rodman JH, Feler C, Fabian TC. Effect of acute phase response on phenytoin metabolism in neurotrauma patients. J Clin Pharmacol 37:129–139, 1997.
12. Toler SM, Young AB, McClain CJ, Shedlofsky SI, Bandyopadhyay AM, Blouin RA. Head injury and cytochrome P-450 enzymes. Differential effect on mRNA and protein expression in the Fischer-344 rat. Drug Metab Dispos 21:1064–1069, 1993.
13. Bauer TM, Ritz R, Haberthur C, et al. Prolonged sedation due to accumulation of conjugated metabolites of midazolam. Lancet 346:145–147, 1995.
14. Harper KW, Collier PS, Dundee JW, Elliott P, Halliday NJ, Lowry KG. Age and nature of operation influence the pharmacokinetics of midazolam. Br J Anaesth 57:866–871, 1985.
15. Durbin CG Jr. Neuromuscular blocking agents and sedative drugs. Clinical uses and toxic effects in the critical care unit. Crit Care Clin 7:489–506, 1991.
16. Fiamengo SA, Savarese JJ. Use of muscle relaxants in intensive care units [editorial]. Crit Care Med 19:1457–1459, 1991.
17. Gray AT, Krejci ST, Larson MD. Neuromuscular blocking drugs do not alter the pupillary light reflex of anesthetized humans. Arch Neurol 54:579–584, 1997.
18. Kindler CH, Verotta D, Gray AT, Gropper MA, Yost CS. Additive inhibition of nicotinic acetylcholine receptors by corticosteroids and the neuromuscular blocking drug vecuronium. Anesthesiology 92:821–832, 2000.
19. Wright EA, McQuillen MP. Antibiotic-induced neuromuscular blockade. Ann N Y Acad Sci 183:358–368, 1971.
20. Sokoll MD, Gergis SD. Antibiotics and neuromuscular function. Anesthesiology 55:148–159, 1981.
21. Spacek A, Neiger FX, Krenn CG, Hoerauf K, Kress HG. Rocuronium-induced neuromuscular block is affected by chronic carbamazepine therapy. Anesthesiology 90:109–112, 1999.
22. Darrah WC, Johnston JR, Mirakhur RK. Vecuronium infusions for prolonged muscle relaxation in the intensive care unit. Crit Care Med 17:1297–1300, 1989.
23. Hansen-Flaschen J, Cowen J, Raps EC. Neuromuscular blockade in the intensive care unit. More than we bargained for. Am Rev Respir Dis 147:234–236, 1993.
24. Sparr HJ, Beaufort TM, Fuchs-Buder T. Newer neuromuscular blocking agents: how do they compare with established agents? Drugs 61:919–942, 2001.
25. Mayer M, Doenicke A, Hofmann A, Peter K. Onset and recovery of rocuronium (Org 9426) and vecuronium under enflurane anaesthesia. Br J Anaesth 69:511–512, 1992.
26. Savarese JJ, Ali HH, Basta SJ, et al. The clinical neuromuscular pharmacology of mivacurium chloride (BW B1090U). A short-acting nondepolarizing ester neuromuscular blocking drug. Anesthesiology 68:723–732, 1988.
27. Ali HH, Savarese JJ. Monitoring of neuromuscular function. Anesthesiology 45:216–249, 1976.
28. Isenstein DA, Venner DS, Duggan J. Neuromuscular blockade in the intensive care unit. Chest 102:1258–1266, 1992.
29. Pedersen T, Viby-Mogensen J, Bang U, Olsen NV, Jensen E, Engboek J. Does perioperative tactile evaluation of the train-of-four response influence the frequency of postoperative residual neuromuscular blockade? Anesthesiology 73:835–839, 1990.
30. Rudis MI, Sikora CA, Angus E, et al. A prospective, randomized, controlled evaluation of peripheral nerve stimulation versus standard clinical dosing of neuromuscular blocking agents in critically ill patients. Crit Care Med 25:575–583, 1997.
31. Shapiro BA, Warren J, Egol AB, et al. Practice parameters for sustained neuromuscular blockade in the adult critically ill patient: an executive summary. Society of Critical Care Medicine. Crit Care Med 23:1601–1605, 1995.
32. Hubbard JI. Mechanism of transmitter release. Prog Biophys Mol Biol 21:33–124, 1970.
33. Bevan DR, Donati F, Kopman AF. Reversal of neuromuscular blockade. Anesthesiology 77:785–805, 1992.
34. Ali HH, Utting JE, Gray TC. Quantitative assessment of residual antidepolarizing block (parts 1 and 2). Br J Anaesth 43:473–485, 1971.

35. Chauvin M, Lebrault C, Duvaldestin P. The neuromuscular blocking effect of vecuronium on the human diaphragm. Anesth Analg 66:117–122, 1987.
36. Segredo V, Matthay MA, Sharma ML, Gruenke LD, Caldwell JE, Miller RD. Prolonged neuromuscular blockade after long-term administration of vecuronium in two critically ill patients. Anesthesiology 72:566–570, 1990.
37. Vandenbrom RH, Wierda JM. Pancuronium bromide in the intensive care unit: a case of overdose. Anesthesiology 69:996–997, 1988.
38. Kalow W, Genest K. A method for the detection of atypical forms of human serum cholinesterase: determination of debucaine numbers. Can J Biochem Physiol 35:339–346, 1957.
39. Whittaker M. Plasma cholinesterase variants and the anaesthetist. Anaesthesia 35:174–197, 1980.
40. Haas JL, Shaefer MS, Miwa LJ, Wood RP, Shaw BW Jr. Prolonged paralysis associated with long-term pancuronium use. Pharmacotherapy 9:154–157, 1989.
41. Kupfer Y, Namba T, Kaldawi E, Tessler S. Prolonged weakness after long-term infusion of vecuronium bromide. Ann Intern Med 117:484–486, 1992.
42. Partridge BL, Abrams JH, Bazemore C, Rubin R. Prolonged neuromuscular blockade after long-term infusion of vecuronium bromide in the intensive care unit. Crit Care Med 18:1177–1179, 1990.
43. Rossiter A, Souney PF, McGowan S, Carvajal P. Pancuronium-induced prolonged neuromuscular blockade. Crit Care Med 19:1583–1587, 1991.
44. Vanderheyden BA, Reynolds HN, Gerold KB, Emanuele T. Prolonged paralysis after long-term vecuronium infusion. Crit Care Med 20:304–307, 1992.
45. Davis NA, Rodgers JE, Gonzalez ER, Fowler AA III. Prolonged weakness after cisatracurium infusion: a case report. Crit Care Med 26:1290–1292, 1998.
46. Riker RR, Picard JT, Fraser GL. Prospective evaluation of the Sedation–Agitation Scale for adult critically ill patients. Crit Care Med 27:1325–1329, 1999.
47. Ramsay MA, Savage TM, Simpson BR, Goodwin R. Controlled sedation with alphadone-alphadolone. Br Med J 2:656–659, 1974.
48. Sear JW, Fisher A, Summerfield RJ. Is alfentanil by infusion useful for sedation on the ITU? Eur J Anaesthesiol Suppl 1:55–61, 1987.
49. Yate PM, Thomas D, Sebel PS. Alfentanil infusion for sedation and analgesia in intensive care [letter]. Lancet 2:396–397, 1984.
50. Asbury AJ. Pupil response to alfentanil and fentanyl. A study in patients anaesthetised with halothane. Anaesthesia 41:717–720, 1986.
51. Murray RB, Adler MW, and Korczyn AD. The pupillary effects of opioids. Life Sci 33:495–509, 1983.
52. Rabinowitz R, Korczyn AD. The specificity of the pupillary actions of morphine and naloxone. J Ocul Pharmacol 3:17–21, 1987.
53. Henderson RD, Wijdicks EFM: Downbeat nystagmus associated with intravenous patient-controlled administration of morphine. Anesth Analg 91:691–692, 2000.
54. Benthuysen JL, Smith NT, Sanford TJ, Head N, Dec-Silver H. Physiology of alfentanil-induced rigidity. Anesthesiology 64:440–446, 1986.
55. Parkinson SK, Bailey SL, Little WL, Mueller JB. Myoclonic seizure activity with chronic high-dose spinal opioid administration. Anesthesiology 72:743–745, 1990.
56. Bowdle TA. Myoclonus following sufentanil without EEG seizure activity. Anesthesiology 67:593–595, 1987.
57. Bromage PR, Camporesi EM, Durant PA, Nielsen CH. Nonrespiratory side effects of epidural morphine. Anesth Analg 61:490–495, 1982.
58. Viscomi CM, Bailey PL. Opioid-induced rigidity after intravenous fentanyl. Obstet Gynecol 89:822–824, 1997.
59. Scott JC, Sarnquist FH. Seizure-like movements during a fentanyl infusion with absence of seizure activity in a simultaneous EEG recording. Anesthesiology 62:812–814, 1985.
60. Smith NT, Benthuysen JL, Bickford RG, et al. Seizures during opioid anesthetic induction—are they opioid-induced rigidity? Anesthesiology 71:852–862, 1989.
61. Veselis RA. Sedation and pain management for the critically ill. Crit Care Clin 4:167–181, 1988.
62. Park GR, Miller E. What changes drug metabolism in critically ill patients—III? Effect of pre-existing disease on the metabolism of midazolam. Anaesthesia 51:431–434, 1996.
63. Park GR, Miller E, Navapurkar V. What changes drug metabolism in critically ill patients?—II Serum inhibits the metabolism of midazolam in human microsomes. Anaesthesia 51:11–15, 1996.
64. Thal GD, Szabo MD, Lopez-Bresnahan M, Crosby G. Exacerbation or unmasking of focal neurologic deficits by sedatives. Anesthesiology 85:21–25, 1996.
65. Shafer A, Doze VA, White PF. Pharmacokinetic variability of midazolam infusions in critically ill patients. Crit Care Med 18:1039–1041, 1990.
66. Shelly MP, Mendel L, Park GR. Failure of critically ill patients to metabolise midazolam. Anaesthesia 42:619–626, 1987.
67. Shelly MP, Sultan MA, Bodenham A, Park GR. Midazolam infusions in critically ill patients. Eur J Anaesthesiol 8:21–27, 1991.
68. Aitkenhead AR, Pepperman ML, Willatts SM, et al. Comparison of propofol and midazolam for sedation in critically ill patients. Lancet 2:704–709, 1989.
69. Michalk S, Moncorge C, Fichelle A, et al. Midazolam infusion for basal sedation in intensive care: absence of accumulation. Intensive Care Med 15:37–41, 1988.
70. Cernaianu AC, DelRossi AJ, Flum DR, et al. Lorazepam and midazolam in the intensive care unit: a randomized, prospective, multicenter study of hemodynamics, oxygen transport, efficacy, and cost. Crit Care Med 24: 222–228, 1996.
71. McCollam JS, O'Neil MG, Norcross ED, Byrne TK, Reeves ST. Continuous infusions of lorazepam, midazolam, and propofol for sedation of the critically ill surgery trauma patient: a prospective, randomized comparison. Crit Care Med 27:2454–2458, 1999.

72. Pepperman ML. Double-blind study of the reversal of midazolam-induced sedation in the intensive care unit with flumazenil (Ro 15-1788): effect on weaning from ventilation. Anaesth Intensive Care 18:38–44, 1990.

73. Carrasco G, Molina R, Costa J, Soler JM, Cabre L. Propofol vs midazolam in short-, medium-, and long-term sedation of critically ill patients. A cost–benefit analysis. Chest 103:557–564, 1993.

74. Hall RI, Sandham D, Cardinal P, Tweeddale M, Moher D, Wang X, Anis AH. Propofol vs midazolam for ICU sedation: A Canadian multicenter randomized trial. Chest 119:1151–1159, 2001.

75. Harris CE, Grounds RM, Murray AM, Lumley J, Royston D, Morgan M. Propofol for long-term sedation in the intensive care unit. A comparison with papaveretum and midazolam. Anaesthesia 45:366–372, 1990.

76. Schuttler J, Ihmsen H. Population pharmacokinetics of propofol: a multicenter study. Anesthesiology 92:727–738, 2000.

77. Illievich UM, Petricek W, Schramm W, Weindlmayr-Goettel M, Czech T, Spiss CK. Electroencephalographic burst suppression by propofol infusion in humans: hemodyanamic consequences. Anesth Analg 77:155–160, 1993.

78. Beller JP, Pottecher T, Lugnier A, Mangin P, Otteni JC. Prolonged sedation with propofol in ICU patients: recovery and blood concentration changes during periodic interruptions in infusion. Br J Anaesth 61:583–588, 1988.

79. Fulton B, Sorkin EM. Propofol: an overview of its pharmacology and a review of its clinical efficacy in intensive care sedation. Drugs 50:636–657, 1995.

80. Susla GM. Propofol toxicity in critically ill pediatric patients: show us the proof. Crit Care Med 26:1959–1960, 1998.

81. Kelly DF, Goodale DB, Williams J, et al. Propofol in the treatment of moderate and severe head injury: a randomized, prospective double-blined pilot trial. J Neurosurg 90:1042–1052, 1999.

82. Charness ME, Morady F, Scheinman MM. Frequent neurologic toxicity associated with amiodarone therapy. Neurology 34:669–671, 1984.

83. Coxon A, Pallis CA. Metronidazole neuropathy. J Neurol Neurosurg Psychiatry 39:403–405, 1976.

84. Mansour AM, Puklin JE, O'Grady R. Optic nerve ultrastructure following amiodarone therapy. J Clin Neuroophthalmol 8:231–237, 1988.

85. Walker RW, Rosenblum MK. Amphotericin B–associated leukoencephalopathy. Neurology 42:2005–2010, 1992.

86. McGuigan JE. A consideration of the adverse effects of cimetidine. Gastroenterology 80:181–192, 1981.

87. Davison R, Parker M, Atkinson AJ Jr. Excessive serum lidocaine levels during maintenance infusions: mechanisms and prevention. Am Heart J 104:203–208, 1982.

88. Modica PA, Tempelhoff R, White PF. Pro- and anticonvulsant effects of anesthetics (part I). Anesth Analg 70:303–315, 1990.

89. Dingwall AE. Oculogyric crisis after day case anaesthesia [letter]. Anaesthesia 42:565, 1987.

90. Bradley WG, Karlsson IJ, Rassol CG. Metronidazole neuropathy. Br Med J 2:610–611, 1977.

91. Bachmann P, Gaussorgues P, Piperno D, Fussy A, Jaboulay JM, Robert D. Acute myopathy after status asthmaticus [letter]. Presse Med 16:1486, 1987.

92. Brun-Buisson C, Gherardi R. Hydrocortisone and pancuronium bromide: acute myopathy during status asthmaticus [letter]. Crit Care Med 16:731–733, 1988.

93. Van Marle W, Woods KL. Acute hydrocortisone myopathy. Br Med J 281:271–272, 1980.

94. Williams TJ, O'Hehir RE, Czarny D, Horne M, Bowes G. Acute myopathy in severe acute asthma treated with intravenously administered corticosteroids. Am Rev Respir Dis 137:460–463, 1988.

95. Knox AJ, Mascie-Taylor BH, Muers MF. Acute hydrocortisone myopathy in acute severe asthma. Thorax 41:411–412, 1986.

96. Kupfer Y, Okrent DG, Twersky RA, Tessler S. Disuse atrophy in a ventilated patient with status asthmaticus receiving neuromuscular blockade. Crit Care Med 15:795–796, 1987.

97. MacFarlane IA, Rosenthal FD. Severe myopathy after status asthmaticus [letter]. Lancet 2:615, 1977.

98. Subramony SH, Carpenter DE, Raju S, Pride M, Evans OB. Myopathy and prolonged neuromuscular blockade after lung transplant. Crit Care Med 19:1580–1582, 1991.

99. Leatherman JW, Fluegel WL, David WS, Davies SF, Iber C. Muscle weakness in mechanically ventilated patients with severe asthma. Am J Respir Crit Care Med 153:1686–1690, 1996.

100. Hanson P, Dive A, Brucher J-M, Bisteau M, Dangoisse M, Deltombe T. Acute corticosteriod myopathy in intensive care patients. Muscle Nerve 20:1371–1380, 1997.

101. Faragher MW, Day BJ, Dennett X. Critical care myopathy: an electrophysiological and histological study. Muscle Nerve 19:516–518, 1996.

102. DuBois DC, Almon RR. Disuse atrophy of skeletal muscle is associated with an increase in number of glucocorticoid receptors. Endocrinology 107:1649–1651, 1980.

103. Sitwell LD, Weinshenker BG, Monpetit V, Reid D. Complete ophthalmoplegia as a complication of acute corticosteroid- and pancuronium-associated myopathy. Neurology 41:921–922, 1991.

104. Larsson L, Li X, Edstrom L, et al. Acute quadriplegia and loss of muscle myosin in patients treated with nondepolarizing neuromuscular blocking agents and corticosteroids: mechanisms at the cellular and molecular levels. Crit Care Med 28:34–45, 2000.

105. Gutmann L, Blumenthal D, Schochet SS. Acute type II myofiber atrophy in critical illness. Neurology 46:819–821, 1996.

106. Yeh JY, Ou BR, Forsberg NE. Effects of dexamethasone on muscle protein homeostasis and on calpain and calpastatin activities and gene expression in rabbits. J Endocrinol 141:209–217, 1994.

107. Helliwell TR, Wilkinson A, Griffiths RD, McClelland P, Palmer TE, Bone JM. Muscle fibre atrophy in critically ill patients is associated with the loss of myosin filaments and the presence of lysosomal enzymes and ubiquitin. Neuropathol Appl Neurobiol 24:507–517, 1998.

108. Rich MM, Pinter MJ, Kraner SD, Barchi RL. Loss

of electrical excitability in an animal model of acute quadriplegic myopathy. Ann Neurol 43:171–179, 1998.

109. Jurkat-Rott K, McCarthy T, Lehmann-Horn F. Genetics and pathogenesis of malignant hyperthermia. Muscle Nerve 23:4–17, 2000.

110. Brownell AK. Malignant hyperthermia: relationship to other diseases. Br J Anaesth 60:303–308, 1988.

111. Gronert GA, Mott J, Lee J. Aetiology of malignant hyperthermia. Br J Anaesth 60:253–267, 1988.

112. Larach MG, Rosenberg H, Larach DR, Broennle AM. Prediction of malignant hyperthermia susceptibility by clinical signs. Anesthesiology 66:547–550, 1987.

113. Rosenberg H. Clinical presentation of malignant hyperthermia. Br J Anaesth 60:268–273, 1988.

114. Schwartz L, Rockoff MA, Koka BV. Masseter spasm with anesthesia: incidence and implications. Anesthesiology 61:772–775, 1984.

115. Heffron JJ. Malignant hyperthermia: biochemical aspects of the acute episode. Br J Anaesth 60:274–278, 1988.

116. Wedel DJ, Iaizzo PA, Milde JH. Desflurane is a trigger of malignant hyperthermia in susceptible swine. Anesthesiology 74:508–512, 1991.

117. Brandt A, Schleithoff L, Jurkat-Rott K, Klingler W, Baur C, Lehmann-Horn F. Screening of the ryanodine receptor gene in 105 malignant hyperthermia families: novel mutations and concordance with the in vitro contracture test. Hum Mol Genet 8:2055–2062, 1999.

118. Gencik M, Bencik A, Mortier W, Epplen JT. Novel mutation in the *RYR1* gene (R2454C) in a patient with malignant hyperthermia. Hum Mutat 15:122, 2000.

119. Harrison GG. Malignant hyperthermia. Dantrolene—dynamics and kinetics. Br J Anaesth 60:279–286, 1988.

120. Fink M. Neuroleptic malignant syndrome and catatonia: one entity or two? [editorial]. Biol Psychiatry 39:1–4, 1996.

121. Anderson WH. Lethal catatonia and the neuroleptic malignant syndrome [editorial]. Crit Care Med 19:1333–1334, 1991.

122. Granner MA, Wooten GF. Neuroleptic malignant syndrome or parkinsonism hyperpyrexia syndrome. Semin Neurol 11:228–235, 1991.

123. Kellam AM. The neuroleptic malignant syndrome, so-called. A survey of the world literature. Br J Psychiatry 150:752–759, 1987.

124. Keyser DL, Rodnitzky RL. Neuroleptic malignant syndrome in Parkinson's disease after withdrawal or alteration of dopaminergic therapy. Arch Intern Med 151:794–796, 1991.

125. Nierenberg D, Disch M, Manheimer E, et al. Facilitating prompt diagnosis and treatment of the neuroleptic malignant syndrome. Clin Pharmacol Ther 50:580–586, 1991.

126. Velamoor VR. Neuroleptic malignant syndrome. Recognition, prevention and management. Drug Safety 19:73–82, 1998.

127. Sakkas P, Davis JM, Hua J, Wang Z. Pharmacotherapy of neuroleptic malignant syndrome. Psychiatr Ann 21:157–164, 1991.

128. Philbrick KL, Rummans TA. Malignant catatonia. J Neuropsychiatry Clin Neurosci 6:1–13, 1994.

129. Sternbach H. The serotonin syndrome. Am J Psychiatry 148:705–713, 1991.

130. Bodner RA, Lynch T, Lewis L, Kahn D. Serotonin syndrome. Neurology 45:219–223, 1995.

131. Sandyk R. L-dopa induced "serotonin syndrome" in a parkinsonian patient on bromocriptine [letter]. J Clin Psychopharmacol 6:194–195, 1986.

132. Lappin RI, Auchincloss EL. Treatment of the serotonin syndrome with cyproheptadine [letter]. N Engl J Med 331:1021–1022, 1994.

133. Nisijima K, Ishiguro T. Does dantrolene influence central dopamine and serotonin metabolism in the neuroleptic malignant syndrome? A retrospective study. Biol Psychiatry 33:45–48, 1993.

134. Mason PJ, Morris VA, Balcezak TJ. Serotonin syndrome. Presentation of 2 cases and review of the literature. Medicine (Baltimore) 79:201–209, 2000.

SEIZURES IN THE INTENSIVE CARE UNIT

The circumstances that surround critical illness make patients more vulnerable to seizures. Aside from acute metabolic alterations, drug toxicity and drug withdrawal are common precipitating factors.[1] However, seizures in critically ill patients may indicate a new catastrophic neurologic event, such as intracerebral hematoma, or herald an emerging central nervous system infection, particularly in the immunocompromised transplant population.

Seizures in the intensive care unit (ICU) are observed by staff who may be less experienced in recognizing different types of seizures. There may also be a tendency to mistake movements such as extensor posturing, dystonia, shivering, or single myoclonic jerks for epileptic fits.

The broad categories of causes of seizure in the ICU are discussed in this chapter. Further details can be found in the chapters on cardiac arrest (Chapter 7), electrolyte disorders (Chapter 8), hypertensive encephalopathy (Chapter 9), eclampsia (Chapter 13), polytrauma (Chapter 17), and transplantation (Chapter 18).

GENERALIZED TONIC–CLONIC SEIZURES

Most seizures in critical illness can be classified as generalized tonic–clonic seizures or partial (focal) seizures. Focal seizures involving the face and one limb, alone or together, producing continuous clonic movement with retained consciousness point to a structural lesion. Generalized tonic–clonic seizures do not escape attention unless muted by sedation or neuromuscular blocking agents.

Usually, sudden stiffening (tonic phase) is followed by rapid breathing or bucking of the ventilator and then by rhythmic jerking of extremities (clonic phase), jaw clenching, and tongue biting. Eventually, postictal confusion or prolonged sleep occurs. More subtle presentations may involve transient gaze preference, nystagmoid jerking, eyelid twitching with simultaneous jerks of the globe, brief recurrent twitching in one limb, or nose-rubbing after resolution of the seizure.[2] These clinical manifestations are fragments of a generalized tonic–clonic seizure but may occur with corresponding generalized spike and wave pattern on a simultaneously registered electroencephalogram.

PATHOPHYSIOLOGIC MECHANISMS

None of the conventional explanations seems to explain convincingly why structural or metabolic changes result in epilepsy. Epileptogenesis in structural lesions, such as traumatic brain injury, involvement of the cerebral cortex due to hemorrhage with iron deposition, or ischemia, remains speculative. Possible mechanisms in the acute phase of head injury are loss of inhibitory interneurons due to shearing, progressive depolarization due to changes in a damaged cell membrane, and ferric cations, one component of hemoglobin, resulting in formation of free radicals. Late seizures may be a consequence of dendritic deformation or synaptic remodeling increasing excitation.[3,4]

The proconvulsant effect of antibiotics is linked to antagonism of γ-aminobutyric acid (GABA) activity.[5] Imipenem, cephalosporins, and, probably, penicillin directly prevent GABA from binding to the receptor that produces central nervous system excitation through inhibition of inward chloride currents. Penicillin binds within the GABA chloride channel to prevent chloride influx.[6,7] Alcohol-related seizures may be common in any ICU, and a specific N-methyl-D-aspartate (NMDA) action has been suggested, with inhibition of the glutamate receptors of the NMDA type during drinking, resulting in up-regulation and supersensitivity during withdrawal.[8]

The pathophysiologic consequences of status epilepticus are selective death of distinct neuronal populations, predominantly the CA_1 and CA_3 hippocampal neurons. One particularly prevailing concept is the $GluR_2$ hypothesis. Within 24 hr of status epilepticus, the expression of glutamate receptor 2 ($GluR_2$) is down-regulated and its role of preventing influx of calcium and possibly zinc diminishes, permitting delayed neurodegeneration.[9,10] Nevander and colleagues[11] found abnormalities in central parts of the globus pallidus, amygdala, and thalamic nuclei after 45 min of seizures.

DRUG-INDUCED AND DRUG-WITHDRAWAL SEIZURES

Many drugs commonly prescribed in the ICU decrease the threshold for seizures[12,13] (Table 3–1). Antibiotic agents, hypoglycemic agents, methylxanthines, antipsychotic drugs, and, in particular, lidocaine are the most commonly involved drugs in seizures. A direct epileptogenic effect from the drug is assumed, but in some instances an electrolyte disorder is produced that in turn causes the seizure.

In most instances, renal failure or recent sudden increase in dosage could be identified as the precipitating event. In a study at San Francisco General Hospital,[17] drug-associated seizures, such as those linked to isoniazid, bronchodilators, insulin, psychotropic drugs, and lidocaine, accounted for most of the seizures. Seizures, however, occurred in a fraction of patients admitted to various wards, including ICUs.[17,18]

Even though drug toxicity is an established cause of seizures, in a published se-

Table 3–1. **Drug-Associated Seizures in the Intensive Care Unit***

Antiarrhythmic agents	Lidocaine
	Flecainide
	Esmolol
Antibiotics	Imipenem
	Norfloxacin
	Ciprofloxacin
	Cefepime
	Penicillin derivatives
Antidepressants	Amitriptyline
	Doxepin
	Nortriptyline
Antipsychotics	Chlorpromazine
	Haloperidol
	Thioridazine
	Perphenazine
	Trifluoperazine
Bronchodilators	Theophylline
	Aminophylline
	Terbutaline
Immunosuppressive and chemotherapeutic agents	Cyclosporine, tacrolimus
	Busulfan
	Cyclophosphamide

*Seen mostly with documented drug toxicity.[13–16]

ries of new-onset seizures in the ICU, only 8 of 55 patients (15%) could be identified[19] (Table 3–2). Five patients had documented toxicity to antibiotics and three to antiarrhythmic drugs. All five patients with toxic levels of antibiotics had renal failure. Sudden withdrawal of drugs, particularly narcotic agents and benzodiazepines, was more prevalent as a cause of new-onset seizures in the ICU.[19] Repeated intramuscular injections for at least 7 days, with daily doses that range from 12 to 30 mg in patients given morphine, could trigger seizures when suddenly withheld. Benzodiazepines are frequently used for maintenance of sedation in ventilated patients, and sudden withdrawal after prolonged infusion may sporadically produce single epileptic seizures or precipitate nonconvulsive status epilepticus.

Withdrawal in drug addicts or alcoholics may be a cause of tonic–clonic seizures. In most patients, dependence on these substances is known, but seizures soon after hospital admission may be the first indication of physical dependence.

Alcohol-related seizures occur only in patients with a history of heavy drinking and inevitable sobriety due to ICU admission.[20–23] Delirium tremens may follow but

Table 3–2. **Causes of New-Onset Seizures in Critical Illness**

Causes	Patients (n)
Drug withdrawal	18
Morphine	11
Propoxyphene	5
Midazolam	1
Meperidine	1
Metabolic abnormalities	18
Hyponatremia	10
Hypocalcemia	4
Acute uremia	2
Hyperglycemia	1
Hypoglycemia	1
Drug toxicity	8
Antibiotics	5
Antiarrhythmics	3
Stroke	5
Unknown	6
Total	55

From Wijdicks and Sharbrough.[19] By permission of the American Academy of Neurology.

can be absent in patients after alcohol withdrawal seizures. A single generalized tonic–clonic seizure or, in about one-fourth of the patients, a flurry of seizures may strike within 6 hr after admission to the hospital. In 97% of patients, seizures occur within 3 days of the last drink.[23] The seizures are self-limited, but status epilepticus is not unusual. In the San Francisco General Hospital experience of 249 adults with status epilepticus, 27 patients (11%) had alcohol-related seizures, and 12 of these (44%) presented with status epilepticus.[24]

There is evidence that lorazepam (2 mg intravenously) substantially reduces (to 3%) the risk of recurrent seizures connected to alcoholism,[25] and its use is superior to that of other antiepileptic drugs.[26] Physicians, however, should remain properly dubious about linking alcohol use to seizures. A clinically significant intracranial lesion was reported in 6.2% of 259 patients with a first alcohol withdrawal seizure, and in half of these patients, a potential neurosurgical lesion (for example, subdural hematoma) was found.[27] At Mayo Clinic hospitals, from 1982 to 1999, 21 patients with new-onset seizures in ICUs had a history of heavy alcohol use. However, in 15 of these 21 patients, other possible triggers (antibiotic or aminophylline toxicity or hyponatremia) were identified (E.F.M. Wijdicks, unpublished observations).

Seizures in patients undergoing transplantation are often related to cyclosporine.[28,29] Although seizures can occur in patients with therapeutic cyclosporine levels without any other precipitating factor, the risk of seizures after transplantation is increased in cyclosporine-treated patients with any of the following features: high-dose methylprednisolone therapy, aluminum overload, hypertension, hypomagnesemia, low serum cholesterol levels, and structural central nervous system lesions (Chapter 18).[28,29]

Seizures in organ transplant recipients are most common in heart and liver transplantation, probably a reflection of the more complicated postoperative course. The predominant factor contributing to new-onset seizures in the modern era remains immunosuppression neurotoxicity of cyclosporine, tacrolimus, and, less commonly, a recently introduced microemulsion of cyclosporine (Neoral).[30,31] Seizures due to immunosuppression neurotoxicity are commonly associated with other manifestations, such as visual hallucinations, cortical blindness, and profound tremors (Chapter 18).

SEIZURES AND ACUTE METABOLIC DERANGEMENTS

Seizures occur typically in overt acute metabolic derangements.[5] The threshold serum levels in acute metabolic derangement are never absolute, and the case for a causative link remains difficult to prove. Generally, the rapidity of the change in serum values makes the association more compelling.

Hypocalcemia may be caused by radical neck dissection with sacrifice of the parathyroid glands or may result from suppression of parathyroid function by extensive burns, sepsis, pancreatitis, aminoglycosides, or cimetidine. Seizures are not a typical manifestation of hypocalcemia. More commonly, hypocalcemic patients complain of muscle cramps and irregular twitching, which should not be interpreted as focal seizures. Nonetheless, seizures occur in patients who have clinical manifestations of severe hypocalcemia, such as Chvostek's and Trousseau's signs (Chapter 8).

Hypophosphatemia is primarily caused by gram-negative sepsis and less often associated with malnutrition in patients receiving parenteral nutrition. A considerable decrease in the serum level of phosphate is necessary to trigger seizures (Chapter 8).

Hypoglycemia usually results from insulin overdose in parenterally fed patients. Tonic–clonic seizures associated with hypoglycemia may be focal but often become generalized. Prompt treatment in patients with suspected hypoglycemia may raise blood levels rapidly. Therefore, the finding of low normal glucose values in patients with seizures who are treated by intravenous administration of glucose on the assumption they have hypoglycemia may nevertheless indicate that hypoglycemia was the main trigger of seizures. In addition, finger stick-reflectance meter determinations are less accurate in the lower end of the reading scale.

Dilutional hyponatremia, a very common electrolyte disturbance in surgical ICUs, is seen in the first postoperative days. Seizures occur in patients who have a sudden acute decrease in serum sodium concentration, often to less than 120 mEq/L. Virtually all patients have a decrease in the level of consciousness, possibly due to development of cerebral edema, but it can be explained by prolonged postictal state, particularly if hyponatremia is not immediately corrected. Postoperative antidiuretic hormone stimulation and thus water retention in typical cases of severe hyponatremia and excess intravenous fluid infusion have contributed. Hyponatremia has also been recognized as a potential precipitating factor of seizures after severe burns (Chapter 16) and liver transplantation[32] (Chapter 18); in both conditions hyponatremia was generated by massive fluid shifts. In our study in patients with new-onset seizures, hyponatremia was the most frequent metabolic abnormality.[19] Ten of the 18 patients had severe hyponatremia (ranging from 114 to 125 mmol/L).

SEIZURES AND STRUCTURAL CENTRAL NERVOUS SYSTEM ABNORMALITIES

Structural central nervous system abnormalities, some of which may have been previously unrecognized, may be a cause of seizures in the ICU. At both Mayo Clinic hospitals in Rochester, Minnesota, new-onset seizures from structural causes in critically ill patients were most often linked to polytrauma with brain injury.[19] Other structural central nervous system lesions that may cause seizures in critical illness are fungal or parasitic infection in patients who are immunosuppressed (Chapter 18) or have acquired immunodeficiency syndrome (AIDS), air embolism (Chapter 5), bacterial meningitis (Chapter 6), and intracerebral hematoma with severe coagulopathy (Chapter 11).

CONVULSIVE STATUS EPILEPTICUS

Recurrence of a tonic–clonic seizure in an ICU is frequently encountered despite therapy, and approximately one-third of patients with new-onset seizures have a second or third seizure.[19] Tonic–clonic status epilepticus is commonly defined as repetitive seizures without full recovery between the episodes, usually with seizure intervals of 5 to 10 min.[33] Convulsive status epilepticus consists of repeated symmetrical contractions of the face and limbs and may have focal onset. Status epilepticus may begin with adversive movements of the head and eyes, flexion of the ipsilateral arm, extension of the ipsilateral leg, and repeated vocalizations. Over time, both tonic and clonic phases decrease in duration in patients with continuing seizures, and they may even fade into solitary multifocal twitches in all limbs.

It is uncommon for tonic–clonic status epilepticus to appear in patients without a history of epilepsy.[34] In a critical care unit, status epilepticus can develop when a well-known precipitating factor (for example, acute severe hyponatremia or drug-induced neurotoxicity) is not recognized or the seriousness of the trigger is not appreciated, but a massive brain injury could perpetuate seizures, too.

Possible triggers for tonic–clonic status epilepticus are iatrogenic drug overdose and, more predictably, severe acute metabolic derangements and impaired absorption of antiepileptic drugs in patients with a seizure disorder after major abdominal surgical procedures. Quite tentative factors that could potentially contribute are sleep deprivation during long stays in an ICU and fever from any type of infection or sepsis.

Status epilepticus is a neurologic emergency and poses an immediate problem.[34–36] The first priority in treatment is to act quickly to prevent neuronal dropout from prolonged seizure activity.

Laboratory Evaluation and Therapeutic Consequences

Blood tests to search for hyperglycemia, hypoglycemia, hyponatremia, hypocalcemia, and hypomagnesemia should be done immediately. Blood samples should be obtained to screen for toxic drug levels. Acid–base abnormalities seen after a cluster of seizures normalize spontaneously, and all categories of acid–base disorders have been reported.[37–39] Metabolic (lactic) acidosis oc-

curs because of excessive muscular contraction, which results in glycogen depletion and anaerobic glycolysis, promoting lactic acid formation from pyruvic acid. Metabolic acidosis, at least with pH values of about 7.20, was not significantly associated with potential life-threatening cardiac arrhythmias in one study.[39] Respiratory acidosis alone or in combination with metabolic acidosis is equally common.[39] The mechanism by which P_{CO_2} may increase after status epilepticus is shown in Figure 3–1. Causes for hypoventilation are central depression of respiratory control from benzodiazepines, reduced respiratory drive as a consequence of preceding seizure activity on the central respiratory neurons, and diaphragmatic contraction during seizures followed by peripheral respiratory muscle fatigue.

Severe lactic acidosis should be treated only if blood gas values have not improved within 1 hr, if the pH is consistently lower than 7.20, and if it is associated with hypotension. Sodium bicarbonate (100 mEq, intravenously) usually suffices to correct the acidosis. The concerns regarding lactic acidosis in this situation are probably inflated, and indiscriminate use of sodium bicarbonate may result in alkalemia that decreases the seizure threshold.

The electroencephalogram may have diagnostic value in patients with a random seizure, but the chance of capturing spike–wave discharges is not great. Nonetheless, documentation of potential epileptiform discharges probably can be expected in 50% of cases. The predictive value of these electroencephalographic findings for a second seizure in this population is not known. Ic-

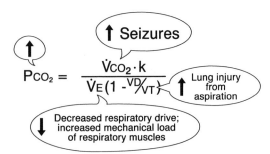

Figure 3–1. Mechanism of respiratory acidosis in status epilepticus. P_{CO_2}, arterial carbon dioxide tension; k, constant; $\dot{V}_{CO_2}$, carbon dioxide production; $\dot{V}E$, expired minute ventilation; VD/VT, anatomical dead space.

tal patterns may include a series of arrhythmic waves, mixture of spikes and waves, or diffuse, generalized polyspikes.[40] Periodic lateralized epileptiform discharges may support a structural lesion, but their significance, ictal or interictal (and thus therapeutic intervention or observation), remains uncertain, particularly when no clinical accompaniment exists.[40] One may argue that an electroencephalogram should be obtained in patients with prolonged (>30 min) postictal unresponsiveness to differentiate postictal coma or confusion from continuing seizure activity.

The value of continuous electroencephalographic monitoring is currently being investigated. A recent prospective study of continuous electroencephalographic monitoring in head injury documented seizures in 22% of 94 patients, with six episodes of status epilepticus, within the first week of admission despite therapeutic levels of phenytoin for prophylaxis.[41] The incidence in this study was twice as high as that in studies with only clinically witnessed seizures, raising the important question of whether continuous electroencephalographic monitoring should be considered in severe brain injury during the first week.

The cerebrospinal fluid may show changes due to seizures. The interpretation of the cerebrospinal fluid formula becomes important when a lumbar puncture is done to exclude meningitis.[42] A mild increase in erythrocytes and leukocytes with a variable percentage of polymorphonuclear cells may occur after seizures.[42] In a study by Edwards and colleagues,[43] 2 of 98 patients had a transient pleocytosis (up to 65 leukocyte counts) that normalized within 3 days. However, although the duration of seizures may be important in the generation of pleocytosis in cerebrospinal fluid, patients with intractable status epilepticus may have repeatedly normal findings in the fluid. Therefore, an increased cell count in the cerebrospinal fluid should prompt further search for an infectious cause of seizures.

In new-onset status epilepticus, structural brain lesions should be actively sought.[19] Computed tomography (CT) scanning and cerebrospinal fluid examination do not sufficiently exclude an acute new insult to the central nervous system. Often, CT scanning in status epilepticus in the ICU yields normal findings. Contrast CT is discouraged because rhabdomyolysis associated with repetitive muscle contractions may transiently impair renal function and additional contrast agent exposure may adversely affect renal function.

Magnetic resonance imaging (MRI) may have a much higher yield in unexplained seizures and may document posterior leukoencephalopathy indicating immunosuppression neurotoxicity, hypertensive encephalopathy, cortical laminar necrosis from anoxic–ischemic damage, multiple small abscesses, or contusional lesions not imaged on CT. Finally, it should be pointed out that seizures alone may cause magnetic resonance abnormalities.[44] Conventional MRI techniques have shown transient T2-weighted hyperintensities. Increased cortical perfusion corresponding to the discharging focus has been reported on diffusion-weighted and perfusion MRI in convulsive, nonconvulsive, and focal status epilepticus.[45–48] All changes were reportedly reversible and possibly due to a hypermetabolic, hyperexcitable state requiring hyperperfusion.

Medical Complications

Hypertension and cardiac arrhythmias are common sequelae of recurrent seizures or status epilepticus. At the onset of status epilepticus, a striking increase in systolic blood pressure, generally accompanied by marked sinus tachycardia, is found. Both responses are the result of increased sympathetic activity. Increase in venous return associated with motor activity during the tonic phase does not contribute, because cardiovascular responses have been demonstrated to be identical in paralyzed animals.[49] After control of the seizures, blood pressure rapidly returns to normal.

Cardiac stunning may be an important manifestation after status epilepticus. A decrease in left ventricular contractility has been documented in an experimental study with neonatal pigs in status epilepticus.[50] Increased catecholamine output with subsequent subendocardial or myocardial damage has been suggested, but severe lactic acidosis may also cause a reduction in myocardial contractional forces.

Cardiac arrhythmias are very common during seizures.[50–52] Any type of tachyarrhythmia may occur, but sinus tachycardia or paroxysmal supraventricular tachycardia is more usual. In addition, single cases have been reported of prolonged sinus arrest alternating with episodes of bradycardia at the time of a complex partial seizure,[51,53] but these cardiac arrhythmias are seldom life threatening. Cardiac arrhythmias may become difficult to manage at the time status epilepticus is terminated with intravenous administration of phenytoin. The introduction of fosphenytoin has not reduced the incidence of cardiac arrhythmias.

A well-recognized complication after status epilepticus is neurogenic pulmonary edema,[54,55] but most cases of pulmonary edema after seizures are caused by aspiration. In an earlier study, Terrence and colleagues[55] postulated that neurogenic pulmonary edema may be a cause of unexpected death in young epileptic patients. In an autopsy study of eight patients, they noted gross hemorrhagic pulmonary edema without any pathologic findings in the heart.

The patient may rapidly become severely hypoxemic and in need of mechanical ventilation using increasing doses of positive end-expiratory pressure. Chest radiographs may be normal in the very early phase, but diffuse areas of opacities ("whiteout") develop in time.

The onset of pulmonary edema usually coincides with resolution of the seizure and postictal drowsiness. The hallmark of neurogenic pulmonary edema is proteinaceous bloody, foamy sputum with an increased ratio of alveolar edema to plasma protein concentration. These findings suggest increased pulmonary vascular permeability. Pulmonary wedge pressures are normal. Therapy is directed toward optimal oxygenation, and the use of positive end-expiratory pressure, usually within the range of 10 to 15 cm H_2O, is of major importance. On the basis of a few anecdotal cases, outcome is good with prompt institution of therapy.

Disseminated intravascular coagulation is exceedingly uncommon but has been reported in status epilepticus associated with sustained muscle injury.[56] The pathophysiologic pathway is unclear. Patients may display signs and symptoms that reflect the consequences of both diffuse microvascular thrombosis and hemorrhagic diathesis. These signs include acute renal failure, adult respiratory distress syndrome, skin ecchymosis, venipuncture oozing, and gastrointestinal hemorrhage, but in most patients, only laboratory abnormalities exist. Thrombocytopenia, afibrinogenemia, schistocytes on peripheral blood smear, increased fibrin degradation products, and abnormal coagulation test results should be present to confirm the diagnosis. Usually, all routine reaction times (activated partial thromboplastin, prothrombin, and thrombin) are prolonged. Acute disseminated coagulation should be treated initially with a bolus of 10,000 U of heparin and then by intermittent intravenous administration of heparin. Transfusion of platelets and fresh frozen plasma to replenish clotting factors should be started immediately.

Tonic–clonic seizures may damage muscle.[57–60] A slight increase in serum creatine kinase concentration is invariably found after a single seizure, but creatine kinase levels may reach enormous proportions within a day. Some laboratory values may point to rhabdomyolysis. These are metabolic acidosis not entirely explained by lactate accumulation, hyperkalemia, increased serum aldolase, hypocalcemia, and certainly myoglobinuria. Most cases associated with status epilepticus reported in the literature are mild and temporary.

Fractures of the long bones and vertebral bodies may occur after status epilepticus, and elderly patients, because of osteoporosis, may be more susceptible.[61–64] A virtually pathognomonic fracture after seizures is bilateral posterior fracture-dislocation of the humeral head. An example of a typical dislocation commonly resulting in failure to move the arm freely and causing pain is shown in Figure 3–2A. It remains an unusual occurrence, also seen in electrocution.[61] Excluding patients with associated trauma, Finelli and Cardi[62] found that 7 of 3000 hospital admissions were for seizures and fractures. In a study by Vernay and colleagues,[63] 2.5% of 227 consecutive hospitalized patients had compression fractures that could be attributed to seizures alone. The salient point was made that a compression fracture of the first four lumbar bodies without evidence of compression fractures at other lo-

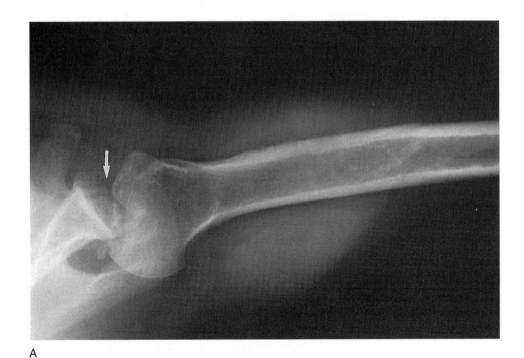

A

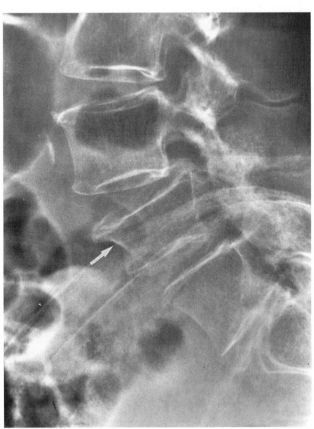

B

Figure 3–2. *A*: Radiograph of shoulder documenting posterior dislocation in a patient who failed to move an arm after a seizure. The anterior portion of the humerus head is off center and impacted against the glenoid (arrow). *B*: Compression fracture of lumbar vertebral body (arrow) in a patient who recovered from status epilepticus before first noticing back pain.

53

cations is very unusual in osteoporosis. In a series of patients with status epilepticus seen at the Mayo Clinic, one patient had lumbar spine compression fracture[39] (Fig. 3–2B).

NONCONVULSIVE STATUS EPILEPTICUS

Confusion, diminished awareness, perseverated speech, and fluctuating responsiveness may signal nonconvulsive status epilepticus.[65–67] Its incidence in the ICU is not known exactly, but it remains a frequent reason for consultation in patients who do not awaken. It is premature to suggest that it may be underdiagnosed, and in our experience, documentation of nonconvulsive status epilepticus in patients with critical illness is rare. Nonconvulsive status epilepticus commonly follows a clearly defined generalized tonic–clonic seizure or occurs in elderly patients with a major irreversible brain injury,[68] after sudden withdrawal of antiepileptic therapy,[69] or in patients with sudden withdrawal of benzodiazepines, such as midazolam and propofol.[70] Many other triggers have been reported, as listed in Table 3–3.

Patients in nonconvulsive status epilepticus invariably have a waxing and waning conscious state rather than total unresponsiveness. This cyclic clouding of consciousness is the most apparent clinical expression of nonconvulsive status epilepticus. Trance-like staring has been noted. In some patients, this expression may be accompanied by a catatonic-like posture, which may come on abruptly.[75] Automatism may appear preferentially in complex partial status epilepticus. These automatisms may include pinching on blankets, face or nose rubbing, stereotypical speech phrases, and verbal perseveration. Many patients, however, are simply in a twilight state. Eyelid flutter and myoclonic jerks in jaw muscles are at times the first telltale signs of nonconvulsive status epilepticus.

Diagnosis of nonconvulsive status epilepticus can be confirmed with an electroencephalographic recording that demonstrates diffuse spike or polyspike and wave complexes at frequencies of 1 to 3 Hz. Frontocentral polyspike waves, however, may occur in bursts of rapid generalized spikes mixed with slow activity[71] (Fig. 3–3).

Nonconvulsive status epilepticus in the ICU occurred in a surprisingly high percentage (8%) of comatose patients who did not have overt clinical signs of seizure activity, but the depth of coma was insufficiently documented. Mortality reached 50%, and the effect of antiepileptic drugs was not known in all instances. In this series of patients with a high occurrence of anoxic–ischemic injury, the electroencephalographic manifestations of rhythmic sharp waves, slow spike–wave complexes, or generalized periodic discharges may have reflected structural damage rather than a potentially treatable ictal phenomenon.[76] Response to intravenously administered benzodiazepines should be assessed in patients with dubious electroencephalographic findings. If the diagnosis is correct, intravenous administration of diazepam in a dose of 2 mg/min up to 20 mg/min aborts the ictus in most patients.

MANAGEMENT OF SEIZURES AND STATUS EPILEPTICUS

Antiepileptic treatment must be considered after a single tonic–clonic seizure. It is very reasonable to administer a loading dose of phenytoin and continue treatment for 1 month in critically ill patients with a flurry of new-onset seizures, in patients with increased intracranial pressure, and in patients in a barely compensated cardiovascular state. It should be clearly appreciated that another generalized tonic–clonic seizure may further imperil the critically ill patient. Unrestrained

Table 3–3. **Potential Triggers for Nonconvulsive Status Epilepticus in the Intensive Care Unit**[69–74]

Generalized tonic–clonic seizure

Antiepileptic drug withdrawal

Benzodiazepine withdrawal

Psychotropic drugs (lithium carbonate, neuroleptics, tricyclic antidepressants)

Metabolic abnormalities (hyponatremia, hypocalcemia)

Miscellaneous (e.g., cerebral angiogram, electroconvulsive therapy)

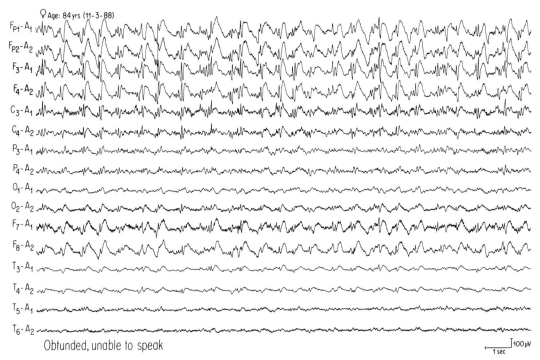

Figure 3–3. Electroencephalographic example of polyspikes and wave complexes consistent with nonconvulsive status epilepticus. (Courtesy of Dr. B. F. Westmoreland.)

movements may result in injury to the patient, dislodgment of catheters providing essential drugs (such as vasopressors), or pulmonary aspiration. Hypermetabolism associated with seizures may produce hemodynamic compromise by exceeding the body's ability to deliver oxygen to vital organs. In all these conditions, it is prudent to allow a brief period of treatment with antiepileptic drugs, such as phenytoin.

In patients with a seizure associated with an acute metabolic derangement that can be quickly corrected, it is prudent to withhold antiepileptic drugs while correcting the metabolic derangement. However, when recurrent seizures take place, intravenous administration of phenytoin, 20 mg/kg, is warranted to bridge the period during which the metabolic derangement is corrected.

Treatment with antiepileptic drugs calls for meticulous attention to changes in the underlying condition of the critically ill patient. Changes in pharmacokinetics occur mainly through drug interactions and may result in subtherapeutic or toxic levels. The most common drug interactions with phenytoin are summarized in Table 3–4. Phenytoin

must be administered intravenously because the absorption of phenytoin remains poor with tube feeding.[77] In some patients, there is no absorption at all.

Equally important, monitoring of total serum phenytoin can be misleading in patients with hypoalbuminemia. In addition, the high propensity of phenytoin binding to albumin may be altered by drugs. In patients with multiorgan failure, hepatic failure may contribute to a decrease in clearance of the unbound drug. Unfamiliarity with these pharmacologic changes may prompt an increase in the dose of phenytoin in a patient with a normal total serum phenytoin level who in fact has an increased free phenytoin level. Severe phenytoin intoxication in four patients as a result of hypoalbuminemia[78] is shown in Figure 3–4. Increased free phenytoin concentration indicates toxicity better than total concentration. In these patients, phenytoin toxicity was manifested by a combination of cerebellar signs, nystagmus, and diplopia, but a gradual decrease in level of consciousness or, paradoxically, an increase in the number of seizures may occur.[79]

Many successful protocols have been de-

Table 3–4. **Drug Interactions with Phenytoin**

Increase phenytoin serum level
Amiodarone
Chloramphenicol
Chlorpromazine
Cimetidine
Isoniazid
Propoxyphene
Sulfonamide

Decrease phenytoin serum level
Carbamazepine
Clonazepam, diazepam
Cyclosporine
Digitoxin
Doxycycline
Glucocorticoids
Oral anticoagulants
Phenobarbital
Theophylline
Valproic acid

signed for the initial treatment of status epilepticus,[80–88] but the different approaches for refractory status epilepticus have not been compared in a controlled study. Fosphenytoin has been of recent interest.[86]

Benzodiazepines are the first-line drugs, but the choice of one over another is a matter of debate. Clonazepam, lorazepam, and diazepam are equally effective and have similar side effects.[87] Many experts consider lorazepam to be one of the first options in the treatment of repeated seizures, and comparative trials have shown lorazepam to be superior to phenytoin.[89]

Initial treatment of status epilepticus is probably most effectively accomplished with intravenously administered lorazepam or diazepam. The initial doses of lorazepam, 0.1 mg/kg, and diazapam, 0.15 mg/kg, are equally effective, and 60% to 70% of seizures may cease. Treatment with intravenously administered phenytoin should begin as rapidly as possible, usually within 5 to 10 min after the first intravenous dose of lorazepam or diazepam. Typically, a loading dose of phenytoin of 18 to 20 mg/kg at a rate of 50 mg/min is instituted (Table 3–5). Lower in-

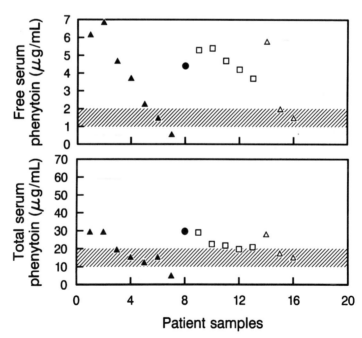

Figure 3–4. Matched pairs of free and total serum phenytoin levels in four critically ill patients with hypoalbuminemia. Each kind of symbol represents one patient. The normal range is shaded. (From Lindow and Wijdicks.[78] By permission of the American College of Chest Physicians.)

Table 3–5. **Intravenously Administered Drugs Used in the Treatment of Status Epilepticus**[87,88,90–105]

Drug	Loading Dose	Rate of Administration	Therapeutic Level
Diazepam	10–20 mg	Push	0.5–0.8 μg/mL
Lorazepam	4–8 mg	Push	Not available
Phenytoin	18–20 mg/kg	50 mg/min	10–20 μg/mL
Phenobarbital	10–60 mg/kg	100 mg/min	10–40 μg/mL
Thiopental	2–4 mg/kg	3–5 mg/kg/hr	NS on EEG
Pentobarbital	10 mg/kg	1–3 mg/kg/hr	NS on EEG
Lidocaine	2–3 mg/kg	3–10 mg/kg/hr	Not available
Propofol	1–3 mg/kg	6–10 mg/kg/hr	Not available
Midazolam	10 mg	0.4 mg/kg/hr	Not available

EEG, electroencephalogram; NS, no seizure activity.

fusion rates should be tried when hypotension or prolongation of the QRS interval occurs. If seizures have not halted at the end of the infusion, an additional one-third of the initial loading dose of phenytoin can be administered.

Fosphenytoin, a water-soluble prodrug of phenytoin, most likely will replace phenytoin, but its cost remains prohibitive in many institutions (the average dose of generic intravenous phenytoin [1500 mg] costs approximately $7, whereas the equivalent dose of fosphenytoin is $162). Fosphenytoin can be given at 100 to 150 mg of phenytoin-equivalent (PE) units per minute, two to three times faster than phenytoin.

Phenobarbital remains a very attractive option for first-line treatment in critically ill patients with a history of cardiac arrhythmias and may be equally effective in control of status epilepticus.[84] Phenobarbital (initial dose, 10 mg/kg; rate, 100 mg/min) should be considered the drug of choice in patients in the ICU who continue to have seizures after loading doses of benzodiazepine and phenytoin. Aggressive treatment with high doses of phenobarbital (60 mg/kg) may obviate pentobarbital coma, but results of studies in adult patients are not available.

Currently, midazolam and propofol are used as second-line therapy, although effectiveness is unproven and a controlled comparative trial with barbiturates has not been performed.[102–105] The major attractiveness of midazolam or propofol is its short-acting

pharmacologic characteristic. Weaning from these drugs should be accomplished quickly, giving them an advantage over barbiturates with longer elimination times. Prolonged infusion (3 or more days), however, may lead to marked prolongation of half-life in midazolam (from 2 to 6 hr to 53 hr in one example).[106]

A difficult situation arises if seizures are not controlled by this management protocol. Pentobarbital can be administered in a bolus of 10 mg/kg followed by an infusion of 1 to 3 mg/kg/hr[107] or, alternatively, thiopental, 3 to 5 mg/kg/hr infusion rate (Table 3–5). If an electroencephalogram is without spike–wave activity, increasing the dosage of barbiturate until a burst suppression pattern is reached is not needed and will lead to a substantial cardiodepressant effect. Therapy is continued for at least 24 hr. Phenytoin therapy should be continued, but an increase in dosage may be required (Table 3–4). Long-term administration of barbiturates (5 days or more) is strongly discouraged, because pulmonary edema, skin edema, and ileus may occur. More important, the risk of *Pseudomonas* and *Staphylococcus* pneumonia is increased from a direct effect of barbiturates on ciliary function. Fortunately, in many patients, seizures are fully controlled with midazolam, propafol, or barbiturates, and third-line treatments are not necessary.

The efficacy of third-line therapies in intractable status epilepticus is derived from a few case reports and small series. Side effects are major, and usually these drugs eventually fail to control the seizures.

Lidocaine has been reported to be effective in refractory convulsive status epilepticus,[97] although it may paradoxically produce seizures and, more important, cardiac arrhythmias. Good control was reported with a single intravenous dose of lidocaine of 2 mg/kg followed by a maintenance dose of 3 to 4 mg/kg/hr.

Use of anesthetic agents in the ICU may cause problems because efficient scavenging of volatile agents in the ICU is difficult. Isoflurane (3%) may be tried as a last resort, but the outcome in treated patients is not impressively better. A reasonable approach to status epilepticus is shown in Figure 3–5.

Weaning from these drugs can probably be initiated after 24 hours, preferably under electroencephalographic monitoring. Patients who relapse with seizures after propofol, midazolam, or barbiturates have been discontinued are best served by a second, longer course. In these patients, it is likely that secondary brain damage perpetuates status epilepticus, and recovery cannot be expected.

OUTCOME

Mortality from a cluster of seizures or status epilepticus varied from 1% to 6% in a large series[108,109] but was much higher (34%) in patients admitted to medical or surgical ICUs. Prognosis for good recovery was

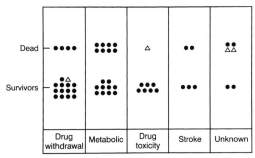

Figure 3–6. Outcome according to etiologic categories in critically ill patients with new-onset seizures. Triangles represent patients with status epilepticus. (From Wijdicks and Sharbrough.[19] By permission of the American Academy of Neurology.)

guarded in patients with seizures associated with acute metabolic changes, but largely because of the underlying illness (Fig. 3–6). Seizures in association with immunosuppression did not recur after administration of antiepileptic drugs was discontinued.[31]

Prognostic factors for poor outcome in patients with status epilepticus treated with barbiturates have been identified.[33] Among these factors are multiorgan failure, age less than 40 years, and hypotension requiring pressors after barbiturate treatment. In a 1990 prospective study of 143 patients with epilepsy, status epilepticus rarely had an adverse effect on neuropsychologic function,[110] and if it was present, only subtle abnormalities were found. Careful review of the literature shows that long-term morbidity is very uncommon in nonconvulsive status epilepticus, and other medical illnesses may have played a role in studies claiming abnormal results of neuropsychologic tests.[111,112] Presence of periodic epileptiform discharges on postictal electroencephalograms in status epilepticus may predict poor outcome.[113]

CONCLUSIONS

Many patients in the ICU may become transiently jittery, but few truly have seizures. Brief myoclonic jerks are probably more common than seizures simply because myokymias and myoclonus are well-known side effects of drugs frequently used in the ICU (for example, ketamine, lidocaine, penicillin derivatives).

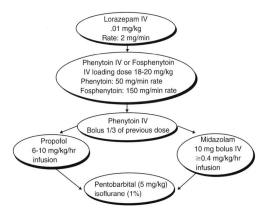

Figure 3–5. Algorithm to treat a flurry of seizures or status epilepticus.

Although it has intuitively been said that in critical illness several interdependent factors are active, new-onset seizures can be classified in major categories of causes. In addition, the diagnostic evaluation of new-onset seizures in critically ill patients depends on the population in which they occur. For example, in transplantation units, immunosuppressive agents such as cyclosporine and tacrolimus and antibiotics given prophylactically should be excluded first as major causes. In surgical trauma units, however, a new-onset seizure may signify associated head injury or alcohol or drug withdrawal that led to the injury. In medical or surgical ICUs, new-onset seizures can be due to drug toxicity, drug withdrawal, and acute metabolic derangements (most often hyponatremia). Withdrawal of narcotic agents has been found in one-third of the patients.

Although short-term administration of antiepileptic drugs (for example, phenytoin) can be considered, the clinical situation is far more complex. Hypoalbuminemia may increase free levels of phenytoin up to toxic levels, and phenytoin may cause changes in other drug levels in both directions. It is prudent to defer antiepileptic drugs in a correctable situation (for example, acute metabolic derangement) but to use anticonvulsants when seizures are posing an additional risk to the patient.

Every intensive care specialist and consulting neurologist should have a prefixed idea of the choice of antiepileptic drugs in status epilepticus. The sequence is generally lorazepam, phenytoin, and possibly midazolam, propofol, or barbiturates. An ineffective approach may possibly increase the risk of long-term sequelae.

REFERENCES

1. Vasko MR, Brater DC. Drug interactions. In: Chernow B (ed). Essentials of Critical Care Pharmacology (abridged from The Pharmacologic Approach to the Critically Ill, 2nd ed). Williams & Wilkins, Baltimore, 1989, pp 1–26.
2. Geyer JD, Payne TA, Faught E, Drury I. Postictal nose-rubbing in the diagnosis, lateralization, and localization of seizures. Neurology 52:743–745, 1999.
3. Willmore LJ. Post-traumatic epilepsy: cellular mechanisms and implications for treatment. Epilepsia 31 (Suppl 3):S67–S73, 1990.
4. Willmore LJ, Sypert GW, Munson JB. Recurrent seizures induced by cortical iron injection: a model of posttraumatic epilepsy. Ann Neurol 4:329–336, 1978.
5. Delanty N, Vaughan CJ, French JA. Medical causes of seizures. Lancet 352:383–390, 1998.
6. Tsuda A, Ito M, Kishi K, Shiraishi H, Tsuda H, Mori C. Effect of penicillin on GABA-gated chloride ion influx. Neurochem Res 19:1–4, 1994.
7. Wallace KL. Antibiotic-induced convulsions. Crit Care Clin 13:741–762, 1997.
8. Liljequist S. The competitive NMDA receptor antagonist, CGP 39551, inhibits ethanol withdrawal seizures. Eur J Pharmacol 192:197–198, 1991.
9. Pellegrini-Giampietro DE, Gorter JA, Bennett MVL, Zukin RS. The GluR2 (GluR-B) hypothesis: Ca^{2+}-permeable AMPA receptors in neurological disorders. Trends Neurosci 20:464–470, 1997.
10. Grooms SY, Opitz T, Bennett MV, Zukin RS. Status epilepticus decreases glutamate receptor 2 mRNA and protein expression in hippocampal pyramidal cells before neuronal death. Proc Natl Acad Sci USA 97:3631–3636, 2000.
11. Nevander G, Ingvar M, Auer R, Siesjo BK. Status epilepticus in well-oxygenated rats causes neuronal necrosis. Ann Neurol 18:281–290, 1985.
12. Bader MB. Role of ciprofloxacin in fatal seizures [letter]. Chest 101:883–884, 1992.
13. Chernow B (ed). Essentials of Critical Care Pharmacology (abridged from The Pharmacologic Approach to the Critically Ill, 2nd ed). Williams & Wilkins, Baltimore, 1989.
14. Anastasio GD, Menscer D, Little JM Jr. Norfloxacin and seizures [letter]. Ann Intern Med 109:169–170, 1988.
15. Modica PA, Tempelhoff R, White PF. Pro- and anticonvulsant effects of anesthetics (part I). Anesth Analg 70:303–315, 1990.
16. Dixit S, Kurle P, Buyan-Dent L, Sheth RD. Status epilepticus associated with cefepime. Neurology 54:2153–2155, 2000.
17. Messing RO, Closson RG, Simon RP. Drug-induced seizures: a 10-year experience. Neurology 34:1582–1586, 1984.
18. Report from Boston Collaborative Drug Surveillance Program. Drug-induced convulsions. Lancet 2:677–679, 1972.
19. Wijdicks EFM, Sharbrough FW. New-onset seizures in critically ill patients. Neurology 43:1042–1044, 1993.
20. Morris JC, Victor M. Alcohol withdrawal seizures. Emerg Med Clin North Am 5:827–839, 1987.
21. Ng SK, Hauser WA, Brust JC, Susser M. Alcohol consumption and withdrawal in new-onset seizures. N Engl J Med 319:666–673, 1988.
22. Simon RP. Alcohol and seizures [editorial]. N Engl J Med 319:715–716, 1988.
23. Victor M, Brausch C. The role of abstinence in the genesis of alcoholic epilepsy. Epilepsia 8:1–20, 1967.
24. Alldredge BK, Lowenstein DH. Status epilepticus related to alcohol abuse. Epilepsia 34:1033–1037, 1993.
25. D'Onofrio G, Rathlev NK, Ulrich AS, Fish SS, Freedland ES. Lorazepam for the prevention of recurrent seizures related to alcohol. N Engl J Med 340:915–919, 1999.
26. Mayo-Smith MF. Pharmacological management of

alcohol withdrawal. A meta-analysis and evidence-based practice guideline. American Society of Addiction Medicine Working Group on Pharmacological Management of Alcohol Withdrawal. JAMA 278:144–151, 1997.

27. Earnest MP, Feldman H, Marx JA, Harris JA, Biletch M, Sullivan LP. Intracranial lesions shown by CT scans in 259 cases of first alcohol-related seizures. Neurology 38:1561–1565, 1988.

28. Gilmore RL. Seizures and antiepileptic drug use in transplant patients. Neurol Clin 6:279–296, 1988.

29. Wszolek ZK, Aksamit AJ, Ellingson RJ, et al. Epileptiform electroencephalographic abnormalities in liver transplant recipients. Ann Neurol 30:37–41, 1991.

30. Wijdicks EFM, Dahlke LJ, Wiesner RH. Oral cyclosporine decreases severity of neurotoxicity in liver transplant recipients. Neurology 52:1708–1710, 1999.

31. Wijdicks EFM, Plevak DJ, Wiesner RH, Steers JL. Causes and outcome of seizures in liver transplant recipients. Neurology 47:1523–1525, 1996.

32. Estol CJ, Lopez O, Brenner RP, Martinez AJ. Seizures after liver transplantation: a clinicopathologic study. Neurology 39:1297–1301, 1989.

33. Yaffe K, Lowenstein DH. Prognostic factors of pentobarbital therapy for refractory generalized status epilepticus. Neurology 43:895–900, 1993.

34. Aminoff MJ, Simon RP. Status epilepticus. Causes, clinical features and consequences in 98 patients. Am J Med 69:657–666, 1980.

35. Brodie MJ. Status epilepticus in adults. Lancet 336:551–552, 1990.

36. Delgado-Escueta AV, Swartz B. Status epilepticus. In: Dam M, Gram L (eds). Comprehensive Epileptology. Raven Press, New York, 1991, pp 251–270.

37. Orringer CE, Eustace JC, Wunsch CD, Gardner LB. Natural history of lactic acidosis after grandmal seizures. A model for the study of an anion-gap acidosis not associated with hyperkalemia. N Engl J Med 297:796–799, 1977.

38. Uthman BM, Wilder BJ. Emergency management of seizures: an overview. Epilepsia 30 (Suppl 2): S33–S37, 1989.

39. Wijdicks EFM, Hubmayr RD. Acute acid-base disorders associated with status epilepticus. Mayo Clin Proc 69:1044–1046, 1994.

40. Sundaram M, Sadler RM, Young GB, Pillay N. EEG in epilepsy: current perspectives. Can J Neurol Sci 26:255–262, 1999.

41. Vespa PM, Nuwer MR, Nenov V, et al. Increased incidence and impact of nonconvulsive and convulsive seizures after traumatic brain injury as detected by continuous electroencephalographic monitoring. J Neurosurg 91:750–760, 1999.

42. Schmidley JW, Simon RP. Postictal pleocytosis. Ann Neurol 9:81–84, 1981.

43. Edwards R, Schmidley JW, Simon RP. How often does a CSF pleocytosis follow generalized convulsions? Ann Neurol 13:460–462, 1983.

44. De Carolis P, Crisci M, Laudadio S, Baldrati A, Sacquegna T. Transient abnormalities on magnetic resonance imaging after partial status epilepticus. Ital J Neurol Sci 13:267–269, 1992.

45. Wieshmann UC, Symms MR, Shorvon SD. Diffusion changes in status epilepticus [letter]. Lancet 350:493–494, 1997.

46. Hisano T, Ohno M, Egawa T, Takano T, Shimada M. Changes in diffusion-weighted MRI after status epilepticus. Pediatr Neurol 22:327–329, 2000.

47. Flacke S, Wullner U, Keller E, Hamzei F, Urbach H. Reversible changes in echo planar perfusion- and diffusion-weighted MRI in status epilepticus. Neuroradiology 42:92–95, 2000.

48. Lansberg MG, O'Brien MW, Norbash AM, Moseley ME, Morrell M, Albers GW. MRI abnormalities associated with partial status epilepticus. Neurology 52:1021–1027, 1999.

49. Meldrum BS, Vigouroux RA, Brierley JB. Systemic factors and epileptic brain damage. Prolonged seizures in paralyzed, artifically ventilated baboons. Arch Neurol 29:82–87, 1973.

50. Young RS, Fripp RR, Yagel SK, Werner JC, McGrath G, Schuler HG. Cardiac dysfunction during status epilepticus in the neonatal pig. Ann Neurol 18:291–297, 1985.

51. Kiok MC, Terrence CF, Fromm GH, Lavine S. Sinus arrest in epilepsy. Neurology 36:115–116, 1986.

52. Meldrum BS, Horton RW. Physiology of status epilepticus in primates. Arch Neurol 28:1–9, 1973.

53. Smith-Demps C, Jagoda A. A case of seizure-related bradycardia and asystole. Am J Emerg Med 16:582–584, 1998.

54. Darnell JC, Jay SJ. Recurrent postictal pulmonary edema: a case report and review of the literature. Epilepsia 23:71–83, 1982.

55. Terrence CF, Rao GR, Perper JA. Neurogenic pulmonary edema in unexpected, unexplained death of epileptic patients. Ann Neurol 9:458–464, 1981.

56. Felcher A, Commichau C, Cao Q, Brown MJ, Torres A, Francis CW. Disseminated intravascular coagulation and status epilepticus. Neurology 51: 629–631, 1998.

57. Engel JN, Mellul VG, Goodman DB. Phenytoin hypersensitivity: a case of severe acute rhabdomyolysis. Am J Med 81:928–930, 1986.

58. Os I, Lyngdal PT. General convulsions and rhabdomyolysis. Case reports. Acta Neurol Scand 79: 246–248, 1989.

59. Singhal PC, Chugh KS, Gulati DR. Myoglobinuria and renal failure after status epilepticus. Neurology 28:200–201, 1978.

60. Spengler RF, Arrowsmith JB, Kilarski DJ, Buchanan C, Von Behren L, Graham DR. Severe soft-tissue injury following intravenous infusion of phenytoin. Patient and drug administration risk factors. Arch Intern Med 148:1329–1333, 1988.

61. Brackstone M, Patterson SD, Kertesz A. Triple "E" syndrome: bilateral locked posterior fracture dislocation of the shoulders. Neurology 56:1403–1404, 2001.

62. Finelli PF, Cardi JK. Seizure as a cause of fracture. Neurology 39:858–860, 1989.

63. Vernay D, Dubost JJ, Dordain G, Sauvezie B. Seizures and compression fracture [letter]. Neurology 40:725–726, 1990.

64. Spitz MC. Injuries and death as a consequence of seizures in people with epilepsy. Epilepsia 39:904–907, 1998.

65. Hersch EL, Billings RF. Acute confusional state with status petit mal as a withdrawal syndrome—and five year follow-up. Can J Psychiatry 33:157–159, 1988.

66. Lee SI. Nonconvulsive status epilepticus. Ictal confusion in later life. Arch Neurol 42:778–781, 1985.

67. Somerville ER, Bruni J. Tonic status epilepticus presenting as confusional state. Ann Neurol 13:549–551, 1983.

68. Litt B, Wityk RJ, Hertz SH, et al. Nonconvulsive status epilepticus in the critically ill elderly. Epilepsia 39:1194–1202, 1998.

69. Dunne JW, Summers QA, Stewart-Wynne EG. Nonconvulsive status epilepticus: a prospective study in an adult general hospital. Q J Med 62:117–126, 1987.

70. Thomas P, Beaumanoir A, Genton P, Dolisi C, Chatel M. 'Denovo' absence status of late onset: report of 11 cases. Neurology 42:104–110, 1992.

71. Guberman A, Cantu-Reyna G, Stuss D, Broughton R. Nonconvulsive generalized status epilepticus: clinical features, neuropsychological testing, and long-term follow-up. Neurology 36:1284–1291, 1986.

72. Jagoda A, Riggio S. Nonconvulsive status epilepticus in adults. Am J Emerg Med 6:250–254, 1988.

73. Varma NK, Lee SI. Nonconvulsive status epilepticus following electroconvulsive therapy. Neurology 42:263–264, 1992.

74. Vickrey BG, Bahls FH. Nonconvulsive status epilepticus following cerebral angiography. Ann Neurol 25:199–201, 1989.

75. Hauser P, Devinsky O, De Bellis M, Theodore WH, Post RM. Benzodiazepine withdrawal delirium with catatonic features. Occurrence in patients with partial seizure disorders. Arch Neurol 46:696–699, 1989.

76. Towne AR, Waterhouse EJ, Boggs JG, et al. Prevalence of nonconvulsive status epilepticus in comatose patients. Neurology 54:340–345, 2000.

77. Au Yeung SC, Ensom MH. Phenytoin and enteral feedings: does evidence support an interaction? Ann Pharmacother 34:896–905, 2000.

78. Lindow J, Wijdicks EFM. Phenytoin toxicity associated with hypoalbuminemia in critically ill patients. Chest 105:602–604, 1994.

79. Osorio I, Burnstine TH, Remler B, Manon-Espaillat R, Reed RC. Phenytoin-induced seizures: a paradoxical effect at toxic concentrations in epileptic patients. Epilepsia 30:230–234, 1989.

80. Chapman MG, Smith M, Hirsch NP. Status epilepticus. Anaesthesia 56:648–659, 2001.

81. Lowenstein DH, Alldredge BK. Status epilepticus. N Engl J Med 338:970–976, 1998.

82. Lowenstein DH, Aminoff MJ, Simon RP. Barbiturate anesthesia in the treatment of status epilepticus: clinical experience with 14 patients. Neurology 38:395–400, 1988.

83. Porter RJ. Epilepsy: 100 elementary principles. Major Probl Neurol 20:1–186, 1989.

84. Shaner DM, McCurdy SA, Herring MO, Gabor AJ. Treatment of status epilepticus: a prospective comparison of diazepam and phenytoin versus phenobarbital and optional phenytoin. Neurology 38:202–207, 1988.

85. Treiman DM. Pharmacokinetics and clinical use of benzodiazepines in the management of status epilepticus. Epilepsia 30 (Suppl 2):S4–S10, 1989.

86. Heafield MTE. Managing status epilepticus: new drug offers real advantages [editorial]. BMJ 320:953–954, 2000.

87. Leppik IE, Derivan AT, Homan RW, Walker J, Ramsay RE, Patrick B. Double-blind study of lorazepam and diazepam in status epilepticus. JAMA 249:1452–1454, 1983.

88. Shorvon S. The management of status epilepticus. J Neurowl Neurosurg Psychiatry 70 Suppl 2:II22–II27, 2001.

89. Treiman DM, Meyers PD, Walton NY, et al. A comparison of four treatments for generalized convulsive status epilepticus. Veterans Affairs Status Epilepticus Cooperative Study Group. N Engl J Med 339:792–798, 1998.

90. Chilvers CR, Laurie PS. Successful use of propofol in status epilepticus [letter]. Anaesthesia 45:995–996, 1990.

91. Cranford RE, Leppik IE, Patrick B, Anderson CB, Kostick B. Intravenous phenytoin in acute treatment of seizures. Neurology 29:1474–1479, 1979.

92. Kofke WA, Snider MT, Young RS, Ramer JC. Prolonged low flow isoflurane anesthesia for status epilepticus. Anesthesiology 62:653–656, 1985.

93. Kofke WA, Young RS, Davis P, et al. Isoflurane for refractory status epilepticus: a clinical series. Anesthesiology 71:653–659, 1989.

94. Lockman LA. Other antiepileptic drugs: paraldehyde. In: Levy RH, Dreifuss FE, Mattson RH, et al. (eds). Antiepileptic Drugs, 3rd ed. Raven Press, New York, 1989, pp 881–886.

95. Mackenzie SJ, Kapadia F, Grant IS. Propofol infusion for control of status epilepticus. Anaesthesia 45:1043–1045, 1990.

96. Orlowski JP, Erenberg G, Lueders H, Cruse RP. Hypothermia and barbiturate coma for refractory status epilepticus. Crit Care Med 12:367–372, 1984.

97. Pascual J, Ciudad J, Berciano J. Role of lidocaine (lignocaine) in managing status epilepticus. J Neurol Neurosurg Psychiatry 55:49–51, 1992.

98. Rashkin MC, Youngs C, Penovich P. Pentobarbital treatment of refractory status epilepticus. Neurology 37:500–503, 1987.

99. Van Ness PC. Pentobarbital and EEG burst suppression in treatment of status epilepticus refractory to benzodiazepines and phenytoin. Epilepsia 31:61–67, 1990.

100. Walker JE, Homan RW, Vasko MR, Crawford IL, Bell RD, Tasker WG. Lorazepam in status epilepticus. Ann Neurol 6:207–213, 1979.

101. Wood PR, Browne GP, Pugh S. Propofol infusion for the treatment of status epilepticus [letter]. Lancet 1:480–481, 1988.

102. Kumar A, Bleck TP. Intravenous midazolam for the treatment of refractory status epilepticus. Crit Care Med 20:483–488, 1992.

103. Brown LA, Levin GM. Role of propofol in refractory status epilepticus. Ann Pharmacother 32:1053–1059, 1998.

104. Stecker MM, Kramer TH, Raps EC, O'Meeghan R, Dulaney E, Skaar DJ. Treatment of refractory status epilepticus with propofol: clinical and pharmacokinetic findings. Epilepsia 39:18–26, 1998.

105. Holtkamp M, Tong X, Walker MC. Propofol in

subanesthetic doses terminates status epilepticus in a rodent model. Ann Neurol 49:260–263,2001.

106. Naritoku DK, Sinha S. Prolongation of midazolam half-life after sustained infusion for status epilepticus. Neurology 54:1366–1368, 2000.

107. Osorio I, Reed RC. Treatment of refractory generalized tonic–clonic status epilepticus with pentobarbital anesthesia after high-dose phenytoin. Epilepsia 30:464–471, 1989.

108. Hauser WA. Status epilepticus: epidemiologic considerations. Neurology 40 (Suppl 2):9–13, 1990.

109. Sung CY, Chu NS. Status epilepticus in the elderly: etiology, seizure type and outcome. Acta Neurol Scand 80:51–56, 1989.

110. Dodrill CB, Wilensky AJ. Intellectual impairment as an outcome of status epilepticus. Neurology 40 (Suppl 2):23–27, 1990.

111. Drislane FW. Evidence against permanent neurologic damage from nonconvulsive status epilepticus. J Clin Neurophysiol 16:323–331, 1999.

112. Kaplan PW. No, some types of nonconvulsive status epilepticus cause little permanent neurologic sequelae (or: "the cure may be worse than the disease"). Neurophysiol Clin 30:377–382, 2000.

113. Nei M, Lee JM, Shanker VL, Sperling MR. The EEG and prognosis in status epilepticus. Epilepsia 40:157–163, 1999.

Chapter 4

GENERALIZED WEAKNESS IN THE INTENSIVE CARE UNIT

GENERAL CONSIDERATIONS
DISORDERS OF THE SPINAL CORD
DISORDERS OF PERIPHERAL NERVES
DISORDERS OF THE NEUROMUSCULAR
  JUNCTION
DISORDERS OF SKELETAL MUSCLE
ELECTRODIAGNOSTIC STUDIES
CONCLUSIONS

Generalized weakness, an inherently ambiguous designation, has long been seen as an obstacle to recovery in patients whose critical illness has begun to subside. Disuse atrophy develops quickly, even more so if the patient is in a catabolic state. In one study of normal persons, muscle strength decreased 5% a day and 7% to 26% after 5 weeks of bedrest.[1] Whether a debilitated patient in fact has a neuromuscular disorder can be difficult to assess. Many patients are too ill to undergo adequate assessment of their neuromuscular condition. Results of muscle testing can be misleading in fatigued patients with severe sleep deprivation from the fragmented sleep patterns that are very common in intensive care units (ICUs).[2] In patients with severe cardiac and respiratory failure, muscle testing may result in immediate oxygen desaturation whenever a movement of limbs is initiated. It becomes of great concern to critical care physicians when patients have marked wasting of muscle, are unable to signal with their arms, and are not weaned from the ventilator despite several attempts.

There are large gaps in our knowledge of causes of "generalized weakness" in ICUs. Prospective studies of neuromuscular weakness in the ICU are not available, and cohort studies have largely focused on so-called critical illness polyneuropathy.[3,4] A recent important study that reviewed the spectrum of neuromuscular weakness was selective toward patients who were referred for electrophysiologic studies.[5] This study found a myopathy in 46% of 92 patients, peripheral neuropathy in 28%, motor neuron disease in 7%, and myasthenic syndromes in 3%.

As evidence accrues, one can expect in all likelihood that most patients with generalized weakness in medical or surgical ICUs have so-called critical illness neuropathy or myopathy, persistent weakness after administration of neuromuscular blocking agents, or a previously undiagnosed neuromuscular disorder that first became apparent with acute respiratory failure. Certainly, a number of neuromuscular disorders may rapidly progress into involvement of respiratory or bulbar muscles and lead to aspiration pneumonia or mechanical respiratory failure. In one study, five of seven patients with motor neuron disease had the diagnosis made at presentation in an ICU.[5]

This chapter provides an overview of causes of generalized weakness associated with a myelopathy, neuropathy, neuromuscular junction disorder, or myopathy in the ICU to facilitate diagnostic thinking. More comprehensive data can be found in subsequent chapters.

GENERAL CONSIDERATIONS

It can take some time before a neuromuscular disorder is appreciated in a critically ill patient and triggers a neurologic consultation. The ICU nurses may have already noted that the patient fails to move limbs spontaneously or against minimal resistance during daily hygiene routines. Other patients cannot tolerate weaning from the mechanical ventilator, and this failure suggests a previously undiagnosed neurologic disorder. Commonly, rapidly developing hypercapnia points to a diaphragmatic weakness. In these patients, one should recognize clinical telltale signs of two comparatively frequent disorders: myotonic dystrophy (frontal baldness, temporal muscle wasting, bilateral facial palsy causing a "depressed" expression [Jammergestalt], and myotonia with grasping) and amyotrophic lateral sclerosis (signs of upper and lower motor neuron involvement, such as widespread fasciculations, tongue fibrillations and atrophy, prominent atrophy of the interossei, and brisk reflexes).

Neurologic examination of the weak patient should include inspection of spontaneous movements (fasciculations, myokymia) and skin (erythema, purpura, ulcerations). Muscle weakness can be graded, but strength often is an approximation because of little cooperation from the sick patient. Bilateral flaccid paralysis of the arms and legs or of the arms more than the legs may indicate a spinal origin, certainly if the anal reflex is lost, body temperature is low, the skin is warm, and priapism and dysautonomia are present. Distal weakness is common in neuropathies, and proximal weakness is common in inflammatory polyneuropathies. Sensory loss may be suggested by failure of the patient to grimace or retract, but careful evaluation of sensory level is not always reliable. The patient needs to display adequate attention for the physician to search for a possible thoracic level of pinprick analgesia. Neurologic examination also requires evaluation of areflexia, atrophy causing prominence of the hand tendons and tibia (for example, in polyneuropathy, amyotrophic lateral sclerosis), fatigability of upward gaze producing worsening ptosis, and weakness of the masseter muscle (myasthenia gravis).

DISORDERS OF THE SPINAL CORD

Quadriplegia may have its origin in the spinal cord. Hypotonia, failure to control bladder and bowel sphincters, areflexia, and a distinct sensory level to pin prick are found initially (Chapter 17). The odds favor spinal cord damage as a potential cause of acute generalized limb weakness in critically ill patients if the patient has traumatic spinal cord injury (closed or penetrating) or spinal cord infarction associated with thoracoabdominal aneurysm repairs. Infectious causes of spinal cord injury occasionally occur, particularly in patients who have been admitted with acute lung injury necessitating mechanical ventilation. Causes of acute lung infection associated with myelitis may include groups A and B coxsackievirus, cytomegalovirus, *Mycoplasma*, and *Legionella*.[6]

In immunosuppressed patients, cytomegalovirus, herpes zoster, and *Aspergillus* infection can involve the spinal cord. *Listeria* may occasionally cause a spinal cord abscess.[7] Vacuolar myelopathy should be considered in patients infected with human immunodeficiency virus (HIV), although *Toxoplasma*, cytomegalovirus, syphilis, myelitis, and spinal cord lymphoma are alternative causes in patients with acquired immunodeficiency syndrome (AIDS). Presentation in most of these cases is rarely acute and is more likely to be gradual progression to a clinical syndrome with spastic paraparesis with loss of joint position sense due to myelin loss in the lateral and posterior columns. The clinical findings are virtually the same as those in subacute combined degeneration. Magnetic resonance imaging (MRI) does not show intrinsic signal abnormality but more commonly reveals atrophy in the thoracic segments.[8,9]

Bacterial infection of the spinal cord (epidural abscess) occurs most often after wound infection (Chapter 6) and may be a major diagnostic challenge because initial signs before weakness may simulate sepsis. Spinal cord compression from epidural hematoma, predominantly in patients with overt coagulopathies, has been repeatedly reported (Chapter 11).

A rare disorder discovered after acute asthma in children has been reported in over 20 patients (Hopkins' syndrome).[10,11] Flaccid paralysis of a single extremity without involvement of sensation but with fever, increased cerebrospinal fluid protein, and, less commonly, pleocytosis has characterized the disorder. Motor deficit, probably secondary to anterior horn cell involvement, never completely disappeared.

Generally, MRI of the spine is the most useful imaging technique in spinal cord involvement, and if the suspicion of spinal cord involvement is high, the neurologist should press for timely transport to the radiology suite.

DISORDERS OF PERIPHERAL NERVES

Causes of acute hospital-acquired polyneuropathy are few. Systemic illness (for example, vasculitis, acute porphyria) may concomitantly afflict peripheral nerves, and in very occasional circumstances, recently instituted drugs may induce a toxic polyneuropathy. As expected, patients with drug-induced polyneuropathy have a gradual mode of onset, but several months of treatment may be sufficient to produce objective findings of sensory and motor nerve involvement. It is important to distinguish between axonal and demyelinating polyneuropathies, which can be done with bedside electrophysiologic studies.

Axonal polyneuropathies in critically ill patients are either drug induced (neuromuscular blocking agents or corticosteroids, or both) or, much more commonly, due to sepsis[3,4] (Chapter 6). In addition, because critical illness is prevalent in patients with cancer, toxic neuropathies in the ICU can be associated with prior use of chemotherapy (platinum, taxanes, vinca alkaloids, and suramin).[12]

Sensorimotor neuropathies after relatively short intervals of treatment (3 months) have been noted with amiodarone and metronidazole, all with nerve biopsy confirmation. Metronidazole has been implicated as a frequent cause of neuropathy, but its role in causing axonal neuropathy in ICUs is probably overestimated.[13] All other drugs used in ICUs produce only transient paresthesias, fleeting numbness, and no diffuse weakness.

Abrupt onset of paresthesias and progressive quadriparesis with notable areflexia may indicate the emergence of an acute inflammatory demyelinating polyneuropathy (Guillain-Barré syndrome). Guillain-Barré syndrome may occur after any type of surgery, epidural anesthesia, administration of fibrinolytic agents, and, paradoxically, high doses of methylprednisolone for asthma. Guillain-Barré syndrome very rarely complicates a critical illness. Several cases associated with hematopoietic stem cell transplantation and graft-versus-host disease have been reported (see Chapter 18). The clinical features of Guillain-Barré syndrome are distinct from those of critical illness polyneuropathy (Chapter 6). Cranial nerve deficits are conspicuously absent in critical illness polyneuropathy, even in patients with complete quadriplegia. Electrodiagnostic tests in Guillain-Barré syndrome invariably show evidence of demyelination with reduced compound muscle action potential, increased F-wave latency, conduction block, and increased distal latency.

In critically ill patients with AIDS, a progressive disabling polyradiculopathy related to cytomegalovirus has been described. In these patients, polymorphonuclear pleocytosis is found in the cerebrospinal fluid and cytomegalovirus cultures are positive.[14] The incidence of cytomegalovirus radiculopathy may increase because the prevalence of cytomegalovirus-related infections has increased in patients who have had *Pneumocystis carinii* pneumonia prophylaxis. In a series of 15 patients with acute lumbosacral polyradiculopathy due to cytomegalovirus, progression was halted in most patients treated with ganciclovir, although many became paraplegic and lost bladder and bowel control during the first 2 weeks of therapy.[15] However, a progressive polyneuropathy due to HIV with electromyographic characteristics of a demyelinating neuropathy has also been described and became plausible when electron micrography demonstrated viral capsids inside the nerve.[16]

DISORDERS OF THE NEUROMUSCULAR JUNCTION

Neuromuscular blocking agents, when used for at least 2 days, may produce prolonged (hours to weeks) muscular weakness when discontinued. The mechanism of profound weakness other than continued blockade of the neuromuscular junction by active metabolic products is not known (details are discussed in Chapter 2). In addition, drugs that inhibit neuromuscular function are seldom solely responsible for profound generalized weakness, and an underlying neuromuscular junction disorder should be suspected. However, some drugs may increase the sensitivity to neuromuscular blocking agents or unveil a myasthenic disorder[17] (Table 4–1). Electromyographic evidence of a neuromuscular junction defect on electrodiagnostic testing must be present before weakness can be attributed to neuromuscular blockade from drugs. For example, antibiotic-induced paralysis from aminoglycosides and polymyxin antibiotics has been described.[18] Anticholinesterase administration has very often been unsuccessful, and antibiotic-induced paralysis therefore remains an unclear entity.

The most common disorders seen in the ICU are myasthenia gravis and Lambert-Eaton syndrome.

Myasthenia gravis is an autoimmune disorder due to antibodies directed against acetylcholine receptor on the postsynaptic end-plate membrane.[19] Fluctuation in muscle weakness and fatigability when provoked, diplopia, and ptosis are hallmarks. Respiratory muscle weakness typically is seen in a myasthenic crisis and may be the presenting feature. Tests to confirm myasthenia gravis include increased serum acetylcholine receptor–binding antibodies (normal, ≤ 0.02 mmol/L) and striational antibodies (normal, $<1:60$) and gradually decreasing response on 2 Hz stimulation or increased jitter on single-fiber electromyography. Therapy is a

series of intravenous immunoglobulin infusions or plasma exchange.[20]

Lambert-Eaton myasthenic syndrome, an autoimmune channelopathy, is diagnosed in patients with proximal muscle weakness, commonly in the legs, dry mouth, constipation, and decreased reflexes. Antibody-induced reduction of the presynaptic voltage-gated calcium channels is the main pathophysiologic defect. Electromyography shows reduced amplitude of the compound muscle action potential with a gradual decrease at 2 Hz but a severalfold increase after tetanic stimulation.[21] A clinical correlate is the improvement of strength after maximal muscle activation. Lambert-Eaton syndrome may point to a small cell lung carcinoma, thymoma, or lymphoproliferative disease. The drug 3,4-diaminopyridine is effective.[22]

Rapidly ascending flaccid paralysis from tick paralysis (finding a tick in the hair and removing it with a tweezers leads to dramatic improvement) and rapidly descending paralysis from botulism (early onset of gastrointestinal discomfort, profound blurred vision from dilated pupils, oropharyngeal weakness but intact sensation;[23] see Chapter 6) are rare causes of generalized weakness but commonly associated with respiratory failure.

Severe electrolyte disorders (for example, hypermagnesemia) probably can produce severe weakness, most likely from a block at the neuromuscular junction, but in hypophosphatemia and hypokalemia, the pathophysiologic mechanism is less clear (see Chapter 8).

DISORDERS OF SKELETAL MUSCLE

Loss of muscle mass is expected in immobilized critically ill patients. Prolonged immobilization may lead to muscle wasting due to depressed insulin-induced glucose transport.[24] Disuse of skeletal muscle rapidly produces atrophy. Muscle biopsy shows intact architecture, little change in type I muscle fibers, and mostly degeneration of type II fibers.[25,26] In a landmark 1998 study involving several muscle biopsy specimens in critically ill patients, muscle atrophy was noted

Table 4–1. Drugs Enhancing the Effect of Neuromuscular Blocking Agents

Antiarrhythmic agents (procainamide, quinine, quinidine, lidocaine)

Antibiotics (aminoglycosides, polymyxin B, clindamycin, imipenem-cilastatin)

Phenytoin or fosphenytoin

Beta-blockers (propranolol, timolol)

Calcium channel blockers

Anesthetic drugs (ketamine, midazolam)

Psychotropic agents (lithium, chlorpromazine, promazine)

Immunosuppressing agents (corticosteroids, cyclosporine)

Table 4–2. **Causes of Rhabdomyolysis in the Intensive Care Unit**

Ischemia (occlusion of brachial or femoral artery)

Infection (septic shock, influenza A, *Mycoplasma*, coxsackievirus)

Environmental or crush injury (heat stroke, mechanical)

Status epilepticus

Malignant neuroleptic syndrome

Drugs (amphotericin B, ϵ-aminocaproic acid, theophylline*)

*May cause seizures, which are the more likely mechanism.

within 10 days after ICU admissions and in almost 70% of the second specimens.[27] Prolonged immobilization of limbs in patients with neuromuscular blockade may produce pressure necrosis in dorsally located muscles but probably never as striking as that in compartment syndromes.

Rhabdomyolysis may be a cause of weakness in critically ill patients (Table 4–2). The prevalence of rhabdomyolysis is not known, but it may be much higher than appreciated because its triggers are so common in critical illness. The most common causes are probably trauma and ischemia of large fleshy muscles from arterial occlusion, but the condition may also be due to infections such as *Mycoplasma* pneumonia.[28] Myoglobinuria can be found when rhabdomyolysis is massive. Most patients have considerable muscle weakness and pain when tested. Biceps, quadriceps, and gastrocnemius muscles are tender on palpation and may appear swollen. Rapid resolution of weakness and decrease in creatine kinase level, often from initial serum levels of around 10,000 IU, are expected within 2 to 3 days.[29] Thus the initial increase in creatine kinase may go unnoticed, and only muscle biopsy may be able to document the diagnosis.

Nutritional deficiency may also contribute to loss of muscle bulk when a catabolic state is not balanced by high caloric intake. This state can be expected in any patient with sepsis, trauma, burns, or previous malnourishment from alcohol or drug abuse. Specific vitamin deficiencies have not consistently been shown to produce myopathic changes

on biopsy examinations except for vitamin E in malabsorption syndromes.

Muscle weakness may be due to an acute quadriplegic myopathy.[30] Many synonyms have been introduced, including "critical illness myopathy."[30] Acute myopathy does exist, but its circumstances have not been clearly delineated and corticosteroids have a major part in its genesis[31,32] (see Chapter 2 for steroid-induced necrotic myopathy). Acute myopathy in liver transplantation is more common than critical illness polyneuropathy.[33,34]

The major diagnostic features for critical illness myopathy proposed by Lacomis and co-workers[35] are (1) sensory nerve action potential amplitudes >80% of the lower limit of normal in two or more nerves, (2) needle electromyographic findings of short-duration, low-amplitude motor unit potentials with early or normal full recruitment, with or without fibrillation potentials, (3) absence of a decremental response on repetitive nerve stimulation, and (4) muscle histopathologic findings of myopathy with loss of myosin. Their proposed supportive features are (1) compound muscle action potential amplitudes <80% of the lower limit of normal in two or more nerves without conduction block, (2) increased serum creatine kinase concentration (best assessed in the first week of illness), and (3) demonstration of muscle inexcitability. By definition, patients are or were critically ill, and weakness should have begun after the onset of critical illness.

The category of drug-induced myopathies is poorly defined in the ICU. These drugs are listed in Table 4–3 for consideration, but specific well-documented cases are very scarce.[36] Another group of diseases to be considered in patients with generalized weakness consists of primary myopathies associated with respiratory failure.[37] There are many incidental reports of respiratory failure as the initial manifestations of dermatomyositis, polymyositis, mitochondrial myopathy, and myotonic dystrophy.[37–39]

Endocrine causes of myopathies are discussed in Chapter 8. Progressive muscle weakness can be expected in thyrotoxic myopathy, myxedema myopathy, osteomalacia myopathy, and myopathies associated with adrenal and pancreatic diseases. All these

Table 4–3. Drugs That Can Induce Myopathy in the Intensive Care Unit

Corticosteroids
Penicillamine
Procainamide
Amiodarone
Streptokinase
Colchicine
Clofibrate
Zidovudine

Data from Pascuzzi.[36]

disorders, however, affect a minority of patients with muscle weakness in the ICU.

Along with an expected increase in critically ill patients with AIDS comes a higher incidence of AIDS-associated muscle wasting. Most admissions of AIDS patients to the ICU are related to mechanical ventilation for *Pneumocystis carinii* pneumonia. After recovery from respiratory failure, many patients are weak and wasted from undernutrition, AIDS-wasting syndrome, or zidovudine treatment. Zidovudine myopathy is considered when serum creatine kinase levels are elevated severalfold, and examination of muscle biopsy specimens may reveal mitochondrial changes suggested by ragged red fibers and endomysial inflammation.[40] Recovery can be expected after administration of zidovudine is discontinued or replaced by dideoxycytidine or treatment is begun with corticosteroids.[41]

ELECTRODIAGNOSTIC STUDIES

Clinical differentiation of a myopathy, a polyneuropathy, and a neuromuscular disorder from one another is very difficult when all four limbs are flaccid and other signs are lacking (Fig. 4–1). Electrodiagnostic evaluation can be diagnostic, but interpretation requires expertise. Muscle biopsy may bring a more definitive classification.

Table 4–4. Electrophysiologic Features of Major Neuromuscular Disorders Associated with Any Critical Illness

Disorder	NCV and EMG	Special Considerations
Critical illness myopathy	Reduced CMAP amplitude, short duration, early recruitment	Lack of direct stimulation of muscle may be diagnostic
Critical illness polyneuropathy	Reduced CMAP SNAP amplitude, decreased recruitment, fibrillation potentials, positive sharp waves	Reduced sensory potentials may be due to ankle edema or underlying systemic illness, such as diabetes Phrenic nerve stimulation abnormalities are diagnostic
MG or prolonged NMBA effect	Reduced CMAP amplitude, decremental response with 2 or 3 Hz repetitive stimulation	Higher yield with proximal muscles than with distal muscles High yield with axillary, musculocutaneous, and facial stimulation
Acute polyradiculopathy (GBS or CIDP)	Prolonged distal latency, reduced motor velocities, conduction block	Absence of blink responses and prolonged F-wave latency may be diagnostic
Motor neuron disease	Polyphasic waveforms with late components, poor recruitment, widespread fibrillation potentials, normal SNAP	Typical asymmetrical distributions, early abnormal phrenic nerve CMAP and diaphragm denervation

CIDP, chronic inflammatory demyelinating polyneuropathy; CMAP, compound muscle action potential; EMG, electromyogram; GBS, Guillain-Barré syndrome; MG, myasthenia gravis; NCV, nerve conduction velocity; NMBA, neuromuscular blocking agent; SNAP, sensory nerve action potential.[23,42]

The most common abnormalities are listed in Table 4–4. Quantitative analysis of motor unit potentials, which requires cooperation by the patient, may be difficult in very weak, confused, and agitated patients. At least three motor nerves (distal latency, amplitude, and conduction velocity) and three sensory nerves (amplitude and conduction velocity), should be studied, followed by needle insertion in multiple muscles.

Rich and associates[43] recently introduced direct stimulation of the muscle in quadriplegic patients with acute myopathy and confirmed the finding in an animal model.[44] The muscle is stimulated with a subdermal electrode with gradually increasing strength

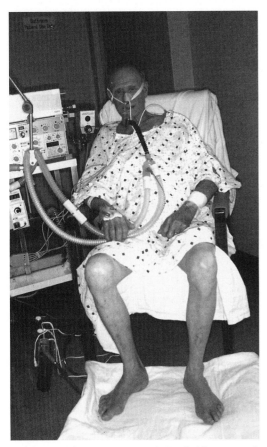

Figure 4–1. A 72-year-old man admitted with severe pulmonary edema received vecuronium for 2 weeks during mechanical ventilation. The patient had generalized muscle weakness (proximal more than distal), and an attempt at weaning had failed. Electrophysiologic studies yielded normal findings. He had full recovery of muscle strength in 3 weeks.

Table 4–5. **Differential Diagnosis of Generalized Weakness in the Intensive Care Unit**

Medication (intravenous corticosteroids combined with NMJ blockers, metronidazole, amiodarone, zidovudine)

Undiagnosed neuromuscular disorder (PM, DM, ALS, GBS, MG, LEMS, acid maltase deficiency, mitochondrial myopathy, muscular dystrophy)

Spinal cord damage (ischemic, compressive hematoma, trauma)

Critical illness (CIP, CIM)

Loss of muscle mass (disuse atrophy, rhabdomyolysis, catabolic state)

Electrolyte disorders (hypokalemia, hypermagnesemia, hypophosphatemia)

Systemic illness (acute porphyria, AIDS, vasculitis neuropathy, endocrine myopathies)

AIDS, acquired immunodeficiency syndrome; ALS, amyotrophic lateral sclerosis; CIM, critical illness myopathy; CIP, critical illness polyneuropathy; DM, dermatomyositis; GBS, Guillain-Barré syndrome; LEMS, Lambert-Eaton myasthenic syndrome; MG, myasthenia gravis; NMJ, neuromuscular junction; PM, polymyositis.

until a twitch is palpable (10 to 100 mA, 0.1 msec, 0.5 Hz). In patients with a critical illness myopathy, muscle was inexcitable, most likely because of inactivation of sodium channels.[45] Abnormal direct muscle stimulation is not found in denervated muscle from polyneuropathy, myasthenia gravis, or motor neuron disease but may be seen in prolonged neuromuscular blockade.

Phrenic nerve stimulation in a patient with diffuse muscle weakness strongly points to a critical illness polyneuropathy if both sides are abnormal. Abnormal blink reflexes are found only in acute or chronic inflammatory polyneuropathies and thus may be helpful in ambiguous cases. F-wave responses are often not tested because of time constraints, but this study may also be useful if it documents delayed responses disproportionate to abnormalities in nerve conduction, suggesting abnormal conduction in the proximal segments of peripheral motor nerves. A waves during F-wave studies may indicate demyelination, but its significance is not established.[46]

CONCLUSIONS

When illness is overwhelming, a fragile clinical condition in itself may seem a biologically plausible reason for weakness. However, a weak patient may have a neuromuscular disorder. Despite lack of prospective studies of critically ill patients with prolonged mechanical ventilation in whom neuromuscular disorders develop, many patients with generalized weakness following sepsis have an axonal polyneuropathy. Prolonged proximal muscle weakness after neuromuscular blockade may be seen relatively frequently without electromyographic abnormalities and with good recovery within weeks. An occasional patient is seen with respiratory failure from a previously undiagnosed neuromuscular disorder. Antibiotics (for example, aminoglycosides, erythromycin) can uncover myasthenia gravis. In other patients, clues in the history may suggest an underlying neuromuscular disorder. Electrodiagnostic tests should include sensory and motor nerve study, direct muscle stimulation, nerve conduction test of the phrenic nerve, and blink responses. Beyond routine examination, muscle or nerve biopsy may be considered in challenging cases. Serum creatine kinase determination and cerebrospinal fluid examination may be helpful in appropriate cases. The differential diagnosis is shown in Table 4–5 ("muscles" is a mnemonic).

REFERENCES

1. Gogia P, Schneider VS, LeBlanc AD, Krebs J, Kasson C, Pientok C. Bed rest effect on extremity muscle torque in healthy men. Arch Phys Med Rehabil 69:1030–1032, 1988.
2. Aurell J, Elmqvist D. Sleep in the surgical intensive care unit: continuous polygraphic recording of sleep in nine patients receiving postoperative care. Br Med J 290:1029–1032, 1985.
3. Leijten FS, De Weerd AW, Poortvliet DC, De Ridder VA, Ulrich C, Harinck-De Weerd JE. Critical illness polyneuropathy in multiple organ dysfunction syndrome and weaning from the ventilator. Intensive Care Med 22:856–861, 1996.
4. Leijten FS, Harinck-de Weerd JE, Poortvliet DC, de Weerd AW. The role of polyneuropathy in motor convalescence after prolonged mechanical ventilation. JAMA 274:1221–1225, 1995.
5. Lacomis D, Petrella JT, Giuliani MJ. Causes of neuromuscular weakness in the intensive care unit: a study of ninety-two patients. Muscle Nerve 21:610–617, 1998.
6. Byrne TN, Benzel EC, Waxman SG (eds). Diseases of the Spine and Spinal Cord. Contemporary Neurology Series 58. Oxford University Press, New York, 2000.
7. Morrison RE, Brown J, Gooding RS. Spinal cord abscess caused by *Listeria monocytogenes*. Arch Neurol 37:243–244, 1980.
8. Chong J, Di Rocco A, Tagliati M, Danisi F, Simpson DM, Atlas SW. MR findings in AIDS-associated myelopathy. Am J Neuroradiol 20:1412–1416, 1999.
9. Di Rocco A. Diseases of the spinal cord in human immunodeficiency virus infection. Semin Neurol 19:151–155, 1999.
10. Hopkins IJ. A new syndrome: poliomyelitis-like illness associated with acute asthma in childhood. Aust Paediatr J 10:273–276, 1974.
11. Shahar EM, Hwang PA, Niesen CE, Murphy EG. Poliomyelitis-like paralysis during recovery from acute bronchial asthma: possible etiology and risk factors. Pediatrics 88:276–279, 1991.
12. Amato AA, Collins MP. Neuropathies associated with malignancy. Semin Neurol 18:125–144, 1998.
13. Bradley WG, Karlsson IJ, Rassol CG. Metronidazole neuropathy. Br Med J 2:610–611, 1977.
14. Eidelberg D, Sotrel A, Vogel H, Walker P, Kleefield J, Crumpacker CS III. Progressive polyradiculopathy in acquired immune deficiency syndrome. Neurology 36:912–916, 1986.
15. So YT, Olney RK. Acute lumbosacral polyradiculopathy in acquired immunodeficiency syndrome: experience in 23 patients. Ann Neurol 35:53–58, 1994.
16. Morgello S, Simpson DM. Multifocal cytomegalovirus demyelinative polyneuropathy associated with AIDS. Muscle Nerve 17:176–182, 1994.
17. Kindler CH, Verotta D, Gray AT, Gropper MA, Yost CS. Additive inhibition of nicotinic acetylcholine receptors by corticosteroids and the neuromuscular blocking drug vecuronium. Anesthesiology 92:821–832, 2000.
18. Argov Z, Mastaglia FL. Drug therapy: disorders of neuromuscular transmission caused by drugs. N Engl J Med 301:409–413, 1979.
19. Engel AG (ed). Myasthenia Gravis and Myasthenic Disorders. Oxford University Press, New York, 1999.
20. Achiron A, Barak Y, Miron S, Sarova-Pinhas I. Immunoglobulin treatment in refractory myasthenia gravis. Muscle Nerve 23:551–555, 2000.
21. Tim RW, Massey JM, Sanders DB. Lambert-Eaton myasthenic syndrome: electrodiagnostic findings and response to treatment. Neurology 54:2176–2178, 2000.
22. Sanders DB, Massey JM, Sanders LL, Edwards LJ. A randomized trial of 3,4-diaminopyridine in Lambert-Eaton myasthenic syndrome. Neurology 54:603–607, 2000.
23. Schaumburg HH, Herskovitz S. The weak child—a cautionary tale. N Engl J Med 342:127–129, 2000.
24. Hirose M, Kaneki M, Sugita H, Yasuhara S, Martyn JA. Immobilization depresses insulin signaling in skeletal muscle. Am J Physiol Endocrinol Metab 279:E1235–E1241, 2000.
25. Danon MJ, Carpenter S. Myopathy with thick filament (myosin) loss following prolonged paralysis with vecuronium during steroid treatment. Muscle Nerve 14:1131–1139, 1991.

26. Gutmann L, Blumenthal D, Schochet SS. Acute type II myofiber atrophy in critical illness. Neurology 46:819–821, 1996.

27. Helliwell TR, Wilkinson A, Griffiths RD, McClelland P, Palmer TE, Bone JM. Muscle fibre atrophy in critically ill patients is associated with the loss of myosin filaments and the presence of lysosomal enzymes and ubiquitin. Neuropathol Appl Neurobiol 24:507–517, 1998.

28. Berger RP, Wadowsky RM. Rhabdomyolysis associated with infection by *Mycoplasma pneumoniae*: a case report. Pediatrics 105:433–436, 2000.

29. Vanholder R, Sever MS, Erek E, Lameire N. Rhabdomyolysis. J Am Soc Nephrol 11:1553–1561, 2000.

30. Lacomis D, Giuliani MJ, Van Cott A, Kramer DJ. Acute myopathy of intensive care: clinical, electromyographic, and pathological aspects. Ann Neurol 40:645–654, 1996.

31. Larsson L, Li X, Edstrom L, et al. Acute quadriplegia and loss of muscle myosin in patients treated with nondepolarizing neuromuscular blocking agents and corticosteroids: mechanisms at the cellular and molecular levels. Crit Care Med 28:34–45, 2000.

32. Leatherman JW, Fluegel WL, David WS, Davies SF, Iber C. Muscle weakness in mechanically ventilated patients with severe asthma. Am J Respir Crit Care Med 153:1686–1690, 1996.

33. Campellone JV, Lacomis D, Kramer DJ, Van Cott AC, Giuliani MJ. Acute myopathy after liver transplantation. Neurology 50:46–53, 1998.

34. Wijdicks EFM, Litchy WJ, Wiesner RH, Krom RA. Neuromuscular complications associated with liver transplantation. Muscle Nerve 19:696–700, 1996.

35. Lacomis D, Zochodne DW, Bird SJ. Critical illness myopathy [editorial]. Muscle Nerve 23:1785–1788, 2000.

36. Pascuzzi RM. Drugs and toxins associated with myopathies. Curr Opin Rheumatol 10:511–520, 1998.

37. Cros D, Palliyath S, DiMauro S, Ramirez C, Shamsnia M, Wizer B. Respiratory failure revealing mitochondrial myopathy in adults. Chest 101:824–828, 1992.

38. Barohn RJ, Clanton T, Sahenk Z, Mendell JR. Recurrent respiratory insufficiency and depressed ventilatory drive complicating mitochondrial myopathies. Neurology 40:103–106, 1990.

39. DeVere R, Bradley WG. Polymyositis: its presentation, morbidity and mortality. Brain 98:637–666, 1975.

40. Dalakas MC, Illa I, Pezeshkpour GH, Laukaitis JP, Cohen B, Griffin JL. Mitochondrial myopathy caused by long-term zidovudine therapy. N Engl J Med 322:1098–1105, 1990.

41. Chalmers AC, Greco CM, Miller RG. Prognosis in AZT myopathy. Neurology 41:1181–1184, 1991.

42. David WS, Roehr CL, Leatherman JW. EMG findings in acute myopathy with status asthmaticus, steroids and paralytics. Clinical and electrophysiologic correlation. Electromyogr Clin Neurophysiol 38:371–376, 1998.

43. Rich MM, Teener JW, Raps EC, Schotland DL, Bird SJ. Muscle is electrically inexcitable in acute quadriplegic myopathy. Neurology 46:731–736, 1996.

44. Rich MM, Pinter MJ, Kraner SD, Barchi RL. Loss of electrical excitability in an animal model of acute quadriplegic myopathy. Ann Neurol 43:171–179, 1998.

45. Rich MM, Pinter MJ. Sodium channel inactivation in an animal model of acute quadriplegic myopathy. Ann Neurol 50:26–33, 2001.

46. Rowin J, Meriggioli MN. Electrodiagnostic significance of supramaximally stimulated A-waves. Muscle Nerve 23:1117–1120, 2000.

Chapter 5

NEUROLOGIC COMPLICATIONS OF INVASIVE PROCEDURES IN THE INTENSIVE CARE UNIT

Advances in procedure technology and ICU apparatus continue, and the indications for invasive hemodynamic monitoring have expanded. Monitoring is a typical line of action in critically ill patients, although practices differ. When neurologic complications occur, they are often curiosities, less commonly iatrogenic (in the true sense of the word) and incidentally related to technical failure of the device. On the surface, the presumption is that neurologic complications of invasive procedures in intensive care units (ICUs) are rare. It is possible, however, that the incidence of procedure-related complications in the ICU is only a crude estimation. Neurologic complications may be very transient, be masked by pharmaceutical agents, or remain undetected. Certain complications, such as mononeuropathies, may be ignored and not tabulated as true complications. Comprehensive studies on complications due to invasive procedures during critical illness are, perhaps understandably, virtually nonexistent. Moses and Kaden[1] published a study of "iatrogenic" neurologic conditions from a prospective series of neurologic consultations at Johns Hopkins Hospital. From this study came the awareness that in one-third of the cases (22% of patients had angiographic studies), neurologic complications could be attributed to invasive diagnostic procedures.

Generally, the categories of complications associated with invasive procedures can be best recapitulated by either reaction to injected material (air or contrast medium) or mobilization of intravascular debris. In some procedures, traumatic damage to vascular or neural structures from needle entry itself is the main cause.

GENERAL CONSIDERATIONS

Neurotoxicity of Radiologic Contrast Agents

Although complications associated with angiography are most likely caused by dislodgment of atherosclerotic debris, there is some evidence that iodinated contrast media are directly involved.[2,3] The pathophysiologic mechanism of neurotoxicity of contrast agents remains unknown.[4] Contrast agents do not enter the brain; therefore, opening of the tight junctions of endothelial cells that maintain the blood–brain barrier is required. However, a number of investigations have documented that repeated injections of contrast agents within several minutes or a major increase in osmolality may predispose the patient to contrast leaks into the brain.[5,6] This explanation is more plausible than "diffuse vasospasm." It has been offered as an alternative explanation in patients with acute confusional states after contrast injection but has not been consistently documented. Conditions well known to facilitate contrast neurotoxicity are shown in Table 5–1. Many complications of contrast studies are related to the underlying hemodynamic condition of the patient—a risk factor that can be avoided.

The clinical manifestations of neurotoxicity are combativeness, acute confusional state with many recognizable elements of delirium, and seizures that are most likely to occur only in patients predisposed because of a seizure disorder. Transient global amnesia or cortical blindness[7] has also been linked to a direct adverse reaction to the contrast agent. All these signs, albeit dramatic in some patients, are transient, and complete recovery is expected within 1 or 2 days.

Treatment of adverse effects of contrast agents is usually focused on management of the systemic allergic manifestations, which include urticaria, angioedema, laryngeal edema, shock, and bronchospasm. Mannitol, at 25%, 1 to 2 g/kg, with the aim to osmotically draw contrast material out, and dexamethasone, a 10 mg bolus intravenously followed by 4 mg intravenously every 6 hr, may be used to reduce the blood–brain barrier permeability.[8] Loading with phenytoin, 20 mg/kg intravenously, should be considered in patients with recurrent seizures. Drainage of cerebrospinal fluid has been recommended in patients with spinal cord injury during abdominal aortography, but the value of this intervention remains controversial. These approaches may be appropriate only in patients who have become stuporous or continue to have seizures. Their use is not justified in the majority of patients who have clinical manifestations for a short time only.

Table 5–1. **Risk Factors for Neurotoxicity of Contrast Agents in Critically Ill Patients**

Previously documented contrast reaction
Hyperthermia
Dehydration
Preexisting renal failure
Congestive heart failure
Prior seizures
Prior ischemic stroke

Cholesterol Embolization

Elderly patients with severe atherosclerosis of the aorta are at risk for cholesterol showers. Difficult catheter manipulation but more commonly multiple arteriographic procedures may precipitate this unusual but often unrecognized entity. The embolic source is the abdominal aorta.[9–12] One provocative study based on retrospective review of pathologic material from patients who died within 6 months of vascular catheterization reported an unexpectedly high incidence of cholesterol embolization (25%). Evidence of embolization to the brain was found in 5% of patients who underwent aortography and in 2% of patients with cardiac catheterization.[13] At autopsy, cholesterol particles are found in various parts of the brain but most often in the middle cerebral artery territory, border zone territories, and caudate nuclei. However, an unselected autopsy series found spontaneous atheroembolism in approximately 2% of the patients, underscoring the possibility of catheterization as a main trigger.[14]

A universal pathogenesis for cholesterol embolization is not known. Arterial trauma during catheter placement may dislodge cholesterol crystals from fractured atheromatous ulcerated plaques and subsequently result in massive showers of embolic material. Occlusion of many small arterioles and capillaries may result in mononuclear cell infiltration, giant cell formation, and, more characteristically, eosinophilic leukocyte infiltration. The location of these cholesterol crystals may depend on the procedure, but no organ is spared.

Frequent targets for cholesterol embolization are the skin, kidney, and pancreas.[12,15,16] The cutaneous manifestations, such as livedo reticularis,[17] acrocyanosis, and purple toes (blue toe syndrome), are important, if not archetypal, initial clinical findings (Plate 5–1). Patients may have only vague complaints of weight loss, headache, myalgias, and fatigue. Symptoms may occur weeks after the procedure, an interval that suggests an immunologic response to the cholesterol emboli. Neurologic manifestations may also appear after relatively long intervals between the clinical presentation and the invasive procedure. In a 1991 well-documented case from Massachusetts General Hospital, a syndrome characterized by headache, tonic–clonic seizure, and encephalopathy occurred 2 months after angiographic examination.[18] The emergence of renal failure and hypertension should be an initial clue to the diagnosis.

Neurologic manifestations of cholesterol embolization are diverse. Muscle weakness masquerading as polymyositis has been confirmed by muscle biopsy showing cholesterol clefts that led to arteritis.[19] A polyneuropathy associated with cholesterol embolization had not been previously recognized as a separate entity in critically ill patients, but in an unconfirmed case report, sural nerve biopsy showed epineural necrotizing arteritis and focal axonal degeneration with cholesterol clefts in vessels of the gastrocnemius muscle.[20] It is thus not certain whether axonal polyneuropathy with cholesterol embolization should become a diagnostic consideration in generalized weakness, particularly when patients are evaluated after multiple endovascular procedures.[20]

Patients with cholesterol embolization may present with retinal hemorrhages. Cholesterol embolus in the retina is usually a pathognomonic clinical sign in a patient with multiorgan involvement but may be absent despite manifestations of peripheral embolization.

Several case reports have also mentioned spinal cord injury, usually in relation to abdominal aortography. The lumbosacral part of the spinal cord is frequently involved, but emboli have been found during postmortem examination in patients who remained asymptomatic during life. Slavin and colleagues[21] found that most patients with spinal cord involvement had multiple organ distribution of emboli.

Besides acute blue toe syndrome and renal failure, the diagnosis remains based on a rather nondescript symptom complex, such as confusion, agitation, and transient hemiparesis. Renal biopsy may demonstrate typical stacked, needle-shaped crystals, but muscle biopsy is the preferred diagnostic test, with a sensitivity of 92%.[13]

The therapeutic options in patients with disseminated cholesterol emboli are limited, and the overall mortality is high.[22] Survival 5 to 8 years after cholesterol embolization, however, has been reported. Management is limited to treatment of hypertension, hemodialysis, and symptomatic treatment of ischemic extremities and perforation of the small intestine and colon. Anticoagulation is hazardous and has even been implicated as a causative factor. Proposed therapies such as vasodilation, lumbar sympathectomy, emergency surgery of the aorta, and corticosteroid administration are unlikely to be effective.

Air Embolism

The risk of cerebral air embolism in patients in the ICU is very low despite the use of multiple lines. Systemic air embolism has been reported as a complication of catheters to measure central venous pressure, subclavian catheters used for parenteral alimentation,[23] arterial catheters, percutaneous aspiration biopsy of the lung,[24] mechanical ventilation with high levels of positive pressure,[25] insufflation for diagnostic procedures, and air bubbles entering the sheath containing the catheter for cardiac ablation[27] (Table 5–2).

Table 5–2. **Potential Causes of Air Embolism in the Intensive Care Unit**

Inadvertent entry through intravenous or intra-arterial catheter*

Extracorporeal bypass pump circuit, incomplete removal of air from heart, carbon dioxide–assisted harvesting of peripheral vein

Insufflation of body cavities (endoscopic or laparoscopic surgery)

Endoscopic retrograde pancreatography

Hemodialysis (catheter and machine)

Chest trauma, lung biopsy

---

*Risk for cerebral embolism is substantial in congenital heart disease (e.g., atrial septal defect); prophylactic filter placement is needed.

Data from Muth and Shank.[26]

The early clinical presentations of systemic air embolism are sensations of dizziness, fear of death, and substernal chest pain.[27,28] Air embolism should be strongly considered when cardiovascular collapse, chest pain, severe dyspnea, or cyanosis suddenly develops in a patient with recent placement of a vascular catheter. Helpful auscultative physical signs are a "millwheel" murmur, sounds resembling the squeezing of a sponge, and wheezing due to acute bronchospasm. A chest radiograph may demonstrate acute pulmonary edema. Air in the heart is seldom seen by echocardiography, probably because air is dispersed or absorbed.

Symptoms of cerebral air embolism include transient or persistent hemiparesis, generalized tonic–clonic seizures, and, more commonly, sudden onset of coma.[28] A computed tomography (CT) scan within 24 hr of the onset of symptoms may directly visualize air bubbles or areas of gyral enhancement. Most lesions associated with air embolization are seen in the distribution of the middle cerebral artery and the anterior cerebral artery.[29–31]

PATHOPHYSIOLOGIC MECHANISMS

An experimental study of the effect of gas emboli on cerebral blood flow demonstrated that a decline in cerebral blood flow could not be readily explained by bubble trapping in arterioles but was perhaps more likely caused by direct gas-induced changes of blood vessels.[32–34]

Cerebral air embolism may occur through a retrograde arterial route in patients with radial artery cannulas[35,36] but is prevented by flush rates of solution from 12 to 15 mL/sec.[36]

Passage of air may occur through a foramen ovale that is physiologically opened by high right atrial pressures, creating a right-to-left shunt. It was present in 40% of 26 reported cases in the literature.[28] A patent foramen ovale may not be a necessary factor,[37] and air emboli may squeeze through the pulmonary capillaries, particularly during conditions of sudden excessive volumes of air.

Prompt treatment of systemic air emboli may decrease the incidence of neurologic sequelae, but mortality and neurologic morbidity remain high. The patient should receive 100% oxygen immediately and be placed in the Trendelenburg and left lateral decubitus position. The central venous pressure catheter may be advanced to the right ventricle for aspiration, which may amount to 50% of the air pocket. Other therapeutic choices in air embolism are optional and without hard documentary evidence. Hyperbaric oxygen therapy reduces the bubble size, but a hyperbaric chamber is not readily available in many institutions. Other recommendations are (*1*) aggressive control of seizures, often with use of barbiturates, (*2*) colloid infusions to counter hemoconcentration, (*3*) avoidance of heparin and corticosteroids, and (*4*) lidocaine in a bolus of 1.5 mg/kg followed by maintenance infusion.[26] Percutaneous aspiration of the right ventricle with a spinal needle may be tried as a last resort. Mortality is higher in patients presenting in coma than in those with hemiparesis only.[28]

NEUROLOGIC COMPLICATIONS ASSOCIATED WITH SPECIFIC PROCEDURES

Although the broad concepts of neurologic complications discussed above apply to many patients, several invasive procedures produce specific neurologic complications, which are reviewed in this section.

Endotracheal Intubation

After extubation, many critically ill patients experience hoarseness, which seldom persists beyond 3 months. Common causes for chronic hoarseness are ulceration and inflammation of the vocal cords, dislocation of the arytenoid cartilages, and vocal polyps, but occasionally direct damage to the recurrent laryngeal nerve produces temporary hoarseness. In a review of the literature, Cavo[38] found that the most likely site of injury (determined by a series of anatomical dissections of the larynx) was the subglottic region. The anterior branch of the recurrent laryngeal nerve, which supplies the adductors of the larynx, probably is compressed between the endotracheal tube cuff and the thyroid cartilage. Most patients fully recover. Proper tube placement at least 5 cm above the carina is quite likely to prevent this uncommon complication. Correct placement can easily be achieved by marking the tube 1.5 cm above the upper end of the cuff.

An unusual complication of endotracheal intubation is partial facial paralysis producing weakness of the orbicularis oris muscle only. Forceful and prolonged digital pressure behind the mandible, applied to prevent airway obstruction from retrograde movement of the tongue, may compress the mandibular branch of the facial nerve against the mandibular bone. The reported cases had an excellent outcome.[39]

Internal Jugular Vein Cannulation

The internal jugular vein is a preferred site for central venous cannulation and pulmonary artery catheterization. Carotid artery puncture, the most frequent complication, occurred in 2% of patients in series of internal jugular vein cannulation alone.[40,41] In a series of 374 internal jugular vein catheterizations, removal of the needle followed by firm pressure over the puncture site did not result in neurologic complications. Ischemic stroke has occasionally been reported after internal jugular vein placement.[41,42] Inadvertent cannulation of the carotid artery for more than 72 hr in one patient resulted in middle cerebral artery territory infarct despite heparinization.[41] Angiography demonstrated a large catheter-enveloping thrombus in the right common carotid artery. This report emphasizes that in patients with puncture of the carotid artery with a large dilating cannula, early surgical exploration and repair are advisable.

Multiple probing attempts may result in peripheral nerve damage. Single case reports have documented Horner's syndrome due to a lesion of the cervical sympathetic chain in proximity to the internal jugular vein.[43] Not infrequently, a consultation is requested for "dilatation" of the opposite eye, but examination in dimmed light reveals failure of the miotic pupil to dilate as a consequence of sympathetic damage[44] (Fig. 5–1). Damage to the vocal cords after bilateral attempts[45] and one startling case of brain stem stroke after use of inappropriate technique and inadvertent vertebral artery puncture[46] have been reported.

An analysis of a prospective study of internal jugular vein cannulation in 66 consecutive critically ill patients revealed no neurologic complications other than one instance of Horner's syndrome.[47] Many of the patients had coagulopathies, multiple probing attempts, and, occasionally, accidental carotid puncture. In the only patient with Horner's syndrome, however, a large neck hematoma was noted, which suggested a compartment syndrome. Needle damage may also cause a carotid dissection.

In patients with a severe coagulopathy or patients in whom insertion is expected to be difficult, Doppler guidance is helpful in localization and may decrease the risk of carotid puncture. Also, after placement of the searching needle or guidewire in the internal jugular vein, the catheter can be connected to a transducer that immediately verifies correct placement. An arterial tracing on the monitor indicates carotid placement and should prompt replacement. This technique should decrease the incidence of ischemic complications that are actually probably related to the introduction of the dilator in the carotid artery, particularly when faulty placement of the catheter is not appreciated.

There is virtually no mention of neurologic complications in patients who require pulmonary artery catheterization.[48,49] In a series of 6245 patients, inadvertent carotid puncture with a 16-gauge catheter in 120 pa-

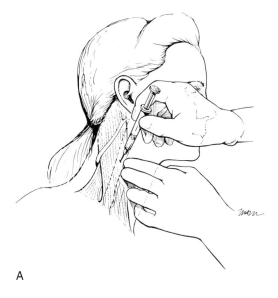

A

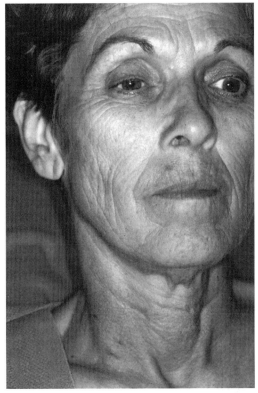

B

Figure 5–1. Horner's syndrome after internal jugular vein cannulation. *A*: Drawing of cannulation of internal jugular vein. *B*: Patient with Horner's syndrome. Note multiple needle probing attempts in the neck. Two-year follow-up revealed some improvement in ptosis alone.

tients (2%) did not result in neurologic complications.[50]

Arterial Cannulation

The prevalence of complications associated with arterial catheters for invasive blood pressure monitoring and blood gas sampling has not been prospectively studied. Radial artery cannulation may be traumatic to peripheral nerves in the vicinity of the puncture site, usually the median nerve. Multiple radial artery punctures and anticoagulation may predispose the patient to nerve damage.[51,52] The superficial cutaneous branches of the radial nerve lie close to the radial artery but are seldom severed after cannulation. Median nerve compression due to hematoma formation around the cannula with extension over the flexor carpi radialis and compression proximal to the transverse carpal ligament is a possible mechanism.[53] Other studies have suggested compression in the carpal tunnel due to prolonged extension of the wrist at the time of splinting to prevent kinking of the catheter.[54]

Persistent paresthesias or pain in areas innervated by the median nerve indicates compression in the carpal tunnel.[54] Motor weakness of the abductor pollicis brevis muscle may occur early. Even after a few weeks, a change in the contour of the thenar may be seen. Exploration is not indicated, because the injuries resolve within 2 months, and only a minority of patients have some residual sensory loss.

Brachial artery cannulation, particularly in patients treated with anticoagulating drugs, may precipitate subfascial hemorrhage leading to a severe median nerve compression syndrome.[55,56] Early recognition of this compression neuropathy is very important, because surgical decompression decreases the chance of permanent sequelae[57,58] (Fig. 5–2). Compression of the median nerve at the level of the elbow (at the lacertus fibrosus, pronator muscle, or fibrous arch of the flexor digitorum superficialis muscle) usually causes pain around the elbow and in the forearm region or produces paresthesias in the fingers. This complication is also recognized by ecchymosis and swelling in the forearm. Clinically, this

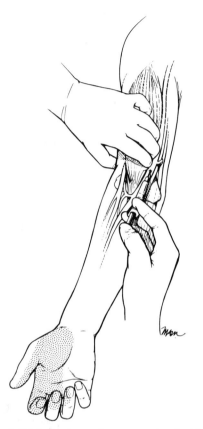

Figure 5–2. Median nerve damage associated with brachial cannulation. Lesion of the median nerve at the elbow produces weakness of the abductor pollicis brevis and flexor digitorum superficialis. Loss of opposition of the thumb may also be seen. As illustrated, sensory loss is indicated in the palm and distal phalanges of the index and middle fingers.

pronator syndrome is diagnosed by tenderness over the median nerve, weak and painful pronation, and weakness and pain at selective testing of the flexor digitorum superficialis muscle.

Cardiac Catheterization

The overall incidence of central nervous system complications in cardiac catheterization is approximately 0.03% to 0.1% but may increase when a transaxillary approach is used. In the Cleveland Clinic series,[59] many complications were caused by embolization into the posterior cerebral circulation. It has been speculated that the transaxillary approach could easily traumatize the vertebral

artery, a less likely hazard in femoral catheterization, because the catheter loops around the aortic arch before entering the coronary ostia.[60] The most frequent clinical manifestations, although still very rare, are listed in Table 5–3.[61]

Cortical blindness from ischemia in the territory of the distal posterior cerebral arteries during cardiac catheterization has been well documented. Patients deny visual loss (Anton's syndrome) and are disoriented or confused but recover, usually completely, within 24 hr.[7,60,62–64]

Transient amnesia after cardiac catheterization has been anecdotally noted.[65] The incidence in angiography is low, with no instances in Hodges' personal series of patients with transient global amnesia.[66] During injection of contrast medium, patients may become agitated, repeatedly asking the same stereotypical questions. Recall of events over preceding days is patchy, and short-term memory is impaired. Typically, the patient has no recollection of the event. Because some sort of Valsalva maneuver is common during the onset of transient global amnesia, it has been speculated that transient blockade of the venous return through the superior vena cava may result in high venous pressure in the cerebral venous system, causing venous ischemia in the mesial temporal lobes.[67] Computed tomographic scan findings have always been normal, but diffusion-weighted magnetic resonance imaging (MRI) has documented increased signal, and thus ischemia, in the splenium of the corpus callosum and left parahippocampal gyrus.[68]

In a 15-year period at the Mayo Clinic, ischemic stroke was documented in 14 patients after cardiac catheterization (0.04% of

Table 5–3. **Neurologic Complications after Cardiac Catheterization**

Acute confusional state with agitation

Transient global amnesia

Cortical blindness

Drowsiness, vivid hallucinations, vertical gaze abnormality (top-of-the-basilar syndrome)

Gait ataxia

Altitudinal hemianopia

Migraine with or without aura

the total number of procedures), most often in the anterior cerebral circulation.[69] All patients except one had ventriculography to assess ejection fraction and wall motion. Half of the patients had acute Q-wave myocardial infarction, and a mural thrombus was found on echocardiography in two patients. These observations superficially suggest a cardioembolic source rather than material thrown off from manipulation damage in the aortic arch. A more recent study documented multiple lesions in symptomatic patients on diffusion-weighted MRI, a finding suggesting emboli showers. Duration of fluoroscopy and severe coronary disease slightly increased the odds of a stroke.[70]

Because the logistics are ideal, patients with an acute ischemic stroke should be eligible for early neuroradiologic intervention. With the recent availability of endovascular procedures and intra-arterial thrombolysis, treatment should be considered when such a patient is in an angiography suite with the sheath in place and 6 hr have not elapsed. However, we recently were successful in mechanically fragmenting a freshly formed embolus that occurred after transmyocardial laser revascularization (Fig. 5–3), which precluded use of thrombolytic agents.[71] The immediate availability of an interventional neu-

roradiology team can make this successful outcome possible.

Cardioversion

Cardioversion is a frequently used procedure in the ICU. A persistent concern is systemic embolization.[72] The risk is remarkably low, even in patients with demonstrated ventricular thrombi. One reported patient tolerated cardioversion without embolization, and echocardiography showed large mobile thrombi.[73] In a study of 454 elective direct-current cardioversions, embolic complications, including peripheral embolism, occurred in 1.3% of the patients. One patient had a fatal ischemic stroke, and the others had "minor visual disturbances."[74] A 1993 study claimed that transesophageal echocardiography can be used to exclude thrombi and obviate anticoagulation,[75] but, not unexpectedly, ischemic stroke in a patient with negative results of transesophageal echocardiographic examination has been reported.[76] The ACUTE (assessment of cardioversion using transesophageal echocardiography) pilot study randomly assigned 62 patients to cardioversion guided by transesophageal echocardiography and found

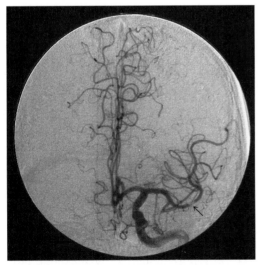
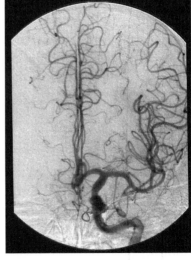

A   B

Figure 5–3. *A*: Initial Towne's projection. Obstructive embolus in the left middle cerebral artery bifurcation (arrow) partly occludes the anterior division and completely occludes the posterior division. *B*: After mechanical fragmentation, flow is restored within both divisions of the middle cerebral artery. (From Wijdicks et al.[71] By permission of the American College of Physicians—American Society of Internal Medicine.)

that successful cardioversion was possible in most patients. No cerebral emboli recurred. The use of transesophageal echocardiography could reduce anticoagulation to 4 weeks instead of the traditional 7 weeks.[77] Postponement of cardioversion was prompted by the documentation of intracardial clots in 13%.[77] Guidance by transesophageal echocardiography may thus select patients for cardioversion, although the practice is not widespread.[78] Moreover, a recent prospective trial found that safety in patients evaluated with transesophageal echocardiography was equal to that with the conventional approach.[79] Embolization remains very uncommon in patients treated with anticoagulation. Whether anticoagulation prevents embolization has not been formally addressed in a randomized trial, and large numbers of patients are required to adequately power such trials.

Anticoagulation beginning at least 2 to 4 weeks before cardioversion is performed remains recommended in patients with a history of cardiogenic embolism, mechanical valve prosthesis, mitral stenosis and documented thrombi on echocardiography, and atrial fibrillation for more than 3 days. In many patients in the ICU who have treatment-refractory arrhythmias of short duration, cardioversion is applied without anticoagulation, and the risk of embolization is very low. Of 702 patients who had cardioversion for recent arrhythmias within 3 days in ICUs at a Mayo Clinic hospital, 1 patient had a pontine infarct immediately after return to sinus rhythm. No peripheral vascular emboli or retinal emboli were noted. Half the patients were receiving anticoagulant therapy (E.F.M. Wijdicks, unpublished observations).

Percutaneous Transluminal Coronary Angioplasty

Indications for percutaneous transluminal coronary angioplasty (PTCA) have been expanded and now include multivessel disease. Immediate PTCA and tissue plasminogen activator therapy for myocardial infarction probably are equally effective in preserving myocardium.[80–82]

Major risks of PTCA are procedure-related myocardial infarction (0.6%) and direct mortality, which can approach 4% in high-risk subsets. The high risks are defined as advanced age, left main coronary artery dilatation, and PTCA for acute myocardial infarction.

Neurologic complications are surprisingly rare.[83] No cerebrovascular complications were mentioned in a series of 6500 PTCA procedures at the Mid America Heart Institute in Kansas City.[84]

Two reports of central nervous system complications also indicated a low incidence (approaching 0.2%) of PTCA-associated stroke or spinal cord injury.[85,86] One study of in-hospital deaths in more than 12,000 patients treated with PTCA found that most were procedure related and that 4% were due to stroke.[87] In many patients, neurologic deficits are transitory and suggest rapid thrombus migration, fragmentation, or possibly air embolus. Fleeting sensory signs, subtle paraphasic errors, sparse verbal output, and mild hemiparesis may not always be recognized or prompt a neurologic consultation, and the reported incidences have to be biased toward more recognizable presentations. The cause of embolization has not been elucidated but again is presumably related to atheromatous or cholesterol embolization from ulcerated plaques in the aortic arch.

Visceral Angiography

Spinal cord damage from visceral angiography has not been reported recently.[88–91] Paraplegia after abdominal aortography has been carefully detailed by Killen and Foster.[91] Their review showed that most patients had complete paralysis of the legs and loss of sphincter control. Motor function returned in slightly more than half the patients. Recovery of motor function was detected as early as 2 days after angiography and as late as 6 months after the procedure. High levels of iodine in the cerebrospinal fluid have been repeatedly found in patients with postangiographic neurologic complications, but the nature of the spinal cord injury remains elusive.[92] Lumbar puncture with immediate substitution of isotonic saline has been recommended, but only one report has been published that claims a sustained beneficial effect with this type of cerebrospinal fluid lavage.[93]

Intra-aortic Balloon Pump

Established indications for counterpulsation devices are intractable cardiac failure after cardiopulmonary bypass and complications of myocardial infarction refractory to pharmacologic therapy.[94] Most complications can be attributed to insertion or removal of the device rather than to its being in place. Two cardiologic series[95,96] with a total of approximately 1500 patients mentioned one ischemic stroke and three patients with femoral nerve neuropathy. Leg ischemia is relatively common after placement (5% to 20%),[97] although necrosis resulting in amputation is seldom seen. Pain in the leg is often reported at the site of insertion, and paresthesias in the cutaneous area of the femoral nerve may also appear transiently. Ischemic neuropathies have been reported in large series and often in patients who required embolectomy after balloon pump removal. Most patients have footdrop and severe pain in the calf, suggesting involvement of branches of the sciatic nerve.

Acute occlusion of a large limb artery may cause an ischemic neuropathy (ischemic monomelic neuropathy).[98–101] This complication is recognized by severe burning pain despite normal blood flow to the affected limb and absence of signs of a compartment syndrome. The electromyographic findings are consistent with loss of motor and sensory nerve axons in the distal part of the tested extremity but may involve conduction block. Conduction block could suggest a reversible injury and prompt replacement of the pump.[102]

Misplacement of the balloon may obstruct the left common carotid artery, and any new onset of aphasia or right hemiparesis should prompt relocation of the device. However, in other patients with ischemic stroke associated with balloon pumps, retrograde embolization may be the operative mechanism. Dissection of the descending aorta also may

contribute, and extension into the left subclavian artery may cause breakup of embolic fragments that subsequently lodge in the left vertebral artery.

A number of well-documented reports have shown that an anterior spinal artery syndrome can occur suddenly in relation to placement of an intra-aortic balloon pump.[103,104] Difficult manipulation on insertion has been implicated, but abrupt paraplegia may occur later, up to 3 days after removal.[105] Aortic dissection occluding the arteries supplying the spinal cord remains the principal causative mechanism in spinal cord infarction in these patients, but occurrence late after insertion may be explained by an expanding intramural hematoma. Alternatively, cholesterol emboli may be responsible for spinal cord infarction after balloon pump insertion. Indeed, cholesterol emboli in radicular arteries were found at autopsy in seven patients with severe atheromatous deposits in the abdominal aorta.[102] As with any other mechanism of spinal cord infarction, outcome is poor.

Ventricular Assist System

Left ventricular assist systems can be expected to become increasingly used to bridge the gap to cardiac transplantation. The inflow tract of the pump is positioned in the left ventricle and the outflow tract in the ascending aorta, with connections to an outside control console. Further technical development may make this console portable, and miniaturized valveless axial pumps are being developed as ventricular assist devices (the costs are very substantial). Experience with the Heartmate (Thermo Cardiosystems, Inc., Woburn, MA) is favorable (average time, 90 days), with a complication rate of 2% to 4% with little or no anticoagulation.[106]

Neurologic complications have been reported in several series, but the University of Pittsburgh series is the most carefully documented experience.[107] This series of 20 patients with implantation devices clearly demonstrated a risk of transient ischemic attack and ischemic strokes with prolonged duration of the device, although transient ischemic attacks were found as early as 6 days after insertion (average, 3 months). Seven of the 20 patients had transient ischemic attack and ischemic stroke, often in the posterior circulation and frequently more than once in the same territory. One patient had a severely disabling stroke, but all others recovered with mild or no residual deficits and underwent successful cardiac transplantation. In our experience, we have frequently noted scattered small infarcts on neuroimaging without a clinical correlate. In the experience from Columbia University, 6 of 233 patients treated with the Heartmate device who were evaluated for more than 500 patient-months had thromboembolic complications, and only 10% of the patients were anticoagulated with warfarin.[108] In a subset monitored with transcranial Doppler ultrasonography, very few patients had high-intensity transient signals indicative of microembolism, confirming the low overall risk.[109] Therefore, despite the initial troubling very high incidence of transient ischemic attack and ischemic strokes, outcome after use of this device and cardiac transplantation seems very satisfactory. Other series have also documented lower incidences of ischemic stroke but with fewer exposure days.[110] Potential mechanisms for ischemic stroke are abnormalities in blood viscosity and activation of thrombotic pathways. One case report pointed to clot formation in the device, which cannot be imaged by ultrasonography because of the metal case.[111] This mechanism of thrombosis within the device may need further study.

Epidural Catheterization and Diagnostic Lumbar Puncture

The results of epidural techniques with use of narcotics to relieve pain after thoracotomy are now quite satisfactory, and this mode of therapy is increasingly used in surgical ICUs. Postoperative analgesia can also be accomplished with lidocaine or bupivacaine administered by rate-controlling infusion pumps. In some instances, patients have prolonged weakness and sensory loss with a burning, prickling feeling. After epidural anesthesia, these symptoms usually disappear within 5 days.

Anticoagulation during epidural catheterization is a major risk factor for epidural spinal hematomas, some of which are devastating.[112–115] Nevertheless, Odoom and Sih[116] reported that there were no neurologic complications in 1,000 epidural anesthetic procedures in patients who were anticoagulated, but their follow-up experience was limited to the hospital stay.

Neurologic complications were not reported in a series of 136 patients who received subcutaneous injection of heparin.[113] However, contributing factors to neurologic complications are heparinization within 1 hr of needle insertion, particularly if traumatic cerebrospinal fluid pours forth in patients with international normalized ratio values outside the therapeutic range and if combinations of antithrombotic agents are used. In exceptional patients, a cutaneous angioma in the dorsal area may indicate a venous angioma in the epidural space.[117] The risk of epidural hematoma during epidural catheterization is decreased in anticoagulated patients when heparin infusion is discontinued 4 to 6 hr before insertion[118,119] and not restarted for at least 1 hr after catheter removal, but no solid scientific data support this common practice.[120] The platelet count is a possible factor, but guidelines for lumbar puncture are less clear. In patients with acute lymphoblastic leukemia, prophylactic platelet transfusion was not required if the platelet count was greater than $10 \times 10^9/L$.[121]

Sudden onset of back pain (coup de poignard, dagger thrust) followed in a few hours by progressive leg weakness is a classic presentation of spinal epidural hematoma, but pain may be absent in patients receiving narcotic agents for postoperative pain control. Emergency laminectomy is not always successful, and paraplegia may remain unchanged even when urgent decompression is done.[122]

A persistent cauda syndrome has been linked to adhesive arachnoiditis, most likely associated with the vehicle of the anesthetic agent. The syndrome of progressive paraparesis is supposedly rare, but occasionally a patient is seen with this complication (Fig. 5–4).

The incidence of epidural infections from catheterization may be higher in critically ill patients treated with immunosuppression or antineoplastic agents, long duration of catheterization, and low-dose anticoagulation. A recent survey from Denmark estimated the incidence to be 1 of 1930 catheters placed for epidural analysis.[123] Epidural abscesses have occurred a few days after placement, and intermittent injections and failure to tunnel the catheter have been implicated as potential risks.[124] (The clinical manifestations and outcome of epidural abscess are discussed in Chapter 6.)

Inadvertent puncture of the dura or, more often, repeated punctures[125] may produce generalized or more frontally located headache on erect position 24 to 72 hr after the procedure. Less common symptoms are nausea, shoulder pain, blurred vision, and abducens palsy, all of which usually resolve within 2 weeks. The incidence of postpuncture headache may indeed be higher in patients who had epidural anesthesia or epidural injections, because larger gauge needles are used than in routine lumbar puncture. A study of 501 patients who had lumbar puncture found that young female patients with low body mass index (weight/height^2) had the highest risk for postlumbar headache.[126] Spontaneous recovery within 1 to 2 weeks is the rule, but in a small percentage, headache is persistently disabling.

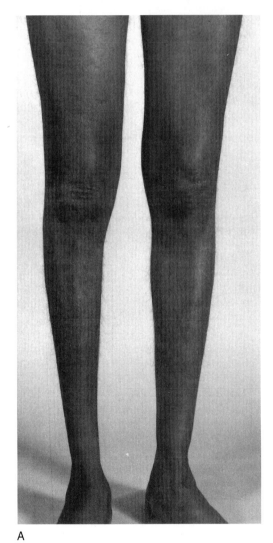
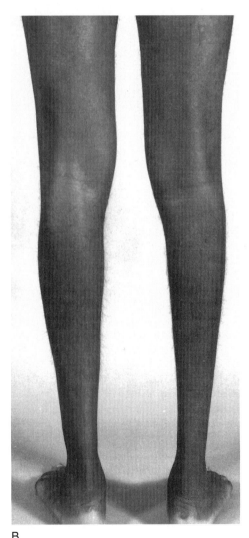

A   B

Figure 5–4. Partially recovered cauda equina syndrome after epidural anesthesia. Note marked atrophy of calves.

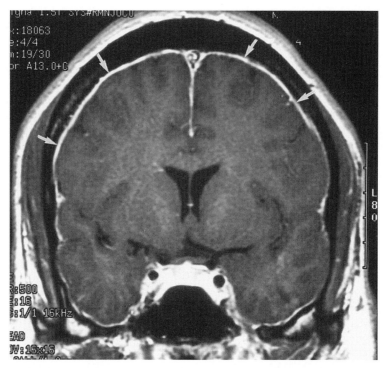

Figure 5–5. Headache associated with cerebrospinal fluid hypotension. Note pachymeningeal enhancement on magnetic resonance image (arrows).

Meningeal enhancement may be seen on MRI in cerebrospinal fluid hypotension (Fig. 5–5) and should not be misinterpreted as evidence of infection.[127,128] It is most likely related to hydrostatic changes in cerebrospinal fluid and diffuse arachnoid cell proliferation.[129] However, meningeal enhancement may be absent.[130] Most patients can be effectively treated with epidural blood patch, orally administered caffeine (300 mg), and liberal fluid intake.

Miscellaneous Complications

A malpositioned chest tube after thoracotomy may be attended by brachial plexus injury.[131] The tube may be pushed up through the pleura and compress the brachial plexus at the root or trunk level. Excruciating upper extremity pain may alert the physician, and withdrawal of the tube immediately relieves pain and results in recovery of motor function. Damage to the intercostal nerve

and long thoracic nerve was mentioned in a review paper on complications of chest tube placement, but documentation was inadequate. Blunt dissection superior to the rib minimizes damage to the neurovascular bundle that is located under the rib.[132] Inadequate technique may result in radiating truncal pain starting at the insertion site.

An intrascalene brachial plexus block is ordinarily used for selective anesthesia in patients scheduled for arteriovenous grafting, particularly those who need dialysis.[133] Complications associated with this procedure include Horner's syndrome, recurrent laryngeal nerve block, and a reversible locked-in syndrome caused by inadvertent injection of a local anesthetic into the intravertebral artery.

Selective pulmonary angiography has been limited to spinal cord ischemia. After injection of contrast material into the fifth intercostal artery, complete cord lesion may occur.[134]

Transient neurologic deficits or visual

field defects, often from carotid sinus massage stimulation during correction of supraventricular tachycardia, have been documented.[135-137] The most impressive case, carefully detailed by Beal and colleagues,[135] showed an embolus in the middle cerebral artery in a patient with severe carotid occlusive disease. A recent prospective study from the Royal Victoria Infirmary found persistent neurologic deficits in 0.1% of patients over 50 years of age but excluded patients with carotid bruits or prior stroke.[138]

Nasogastric tubes have ended in many unwanted locations, and the most spectacular is intracranial placement in patients with basilar skull fracture. Oral insertion, therefore, is the rule in patients with severe head injury and maxillofacial trauma.[139,140]

An unfortunate but probably rare event is ischemic stroke after discontinuation of anticoagulation for ICU procedures associated with a planned biopsy (for example, bronchoscopy). Chronic atrial fibrillation is often the clinical indication for anticoagulation. Whether transesophageal echocardiography before the procedure can reveal which patients are at risk, as discussed with cardioversion, is not known.

CONCLUSIONS

Performing invasive procedures is a common practice in ICUs, and with this performance come complications. As expected, these complications are associated with misplacement of catheters, dislodging of atheromatous material, and hemorrhage.

Neurologic complications pertaining to invasive procedures and assisting devices are ischemic strokes and isolated peripheral nerve damage. The literature on neurologic iatrogenic complications associated with invasive procedures in the ICU is a collection of anecdotes, some truly extreme and out of the ordinary. Neurologic complications indeed may be uncommon, as exemplified by prospective clinical data in a large series of critically ill patients with internal jugular vein catheterization. Despite coagulopathy, multiple probing attempts, and inadvertent carotid puncture, only one patient with Horner's syndrome was found. Likewise, in

cardioversion, another common procedure in the ICU, the incidence of stroke was low. Data on complications from invasive procedures in the ICU are far too preliminary, and therefore preventive measures are not precisely known. Neuroradiologic intervention may be considered if a stroke develops during catheterization, and either thrombolysis or mechanical fragmentation may prevent permanent damage.

REFERENCES

1. Moses H III, Kaden I. Neurologic consultations in a general hospital. Spectrum of iatrogenic disease. Am J Med 81:955–958, 1986.
2. Caillé JM, Allard M. Neurotoxicity of hydrosoluble iodine contrast media. Invest Radiol 23 (Suppl 1): S210–S212, 1988.
3. Lantos G. Cortical blindness due to osmotic disruption of the blood–brain barrier by angiographic contrast material: CT and MRI studies. Neurology 39:567–571, 1989.
4. Rosenberg H. Neurotoxicity of contrast agents [letter]. Anesthesiology 82:1303, 1995.
5. Speck U, Press WR, Mutzel W. Osmolality-related effects of injections into the central nervous system. Invest Radiol 23 (Suppl 1):S114–S117, 1988.
6. Velaj R, Drayer B, Albright R, Fram E. Comparative neurotoxicity of angiographic contrast media. Neurology 35:1290–1298, 1985.
7. Hinchey J, Sweeney PJ. Transient cortical blindness after coronary angiography. Lancet 351:1513–1514, 1998.
8. Ziylan YZ, LeFauconnier JM, Bernard G, Bourre JM. Effect of dexamethasone on transport of alpha-aminoisobutyric acid and sucrose across the blood-brain barrier. J Neurochem 51:1338–1342, 1988.
9. Colt HG, Begg RJ, Saporito JJ, Cooper WM, Shapiro AP. Cholesterol emboli after cardiac catheterization. Eight cases and a review of the literature. Medicine (Baltimore) 67:389–400, 1988.
10. Banning AP, Orr WP, Gribbin B. Cholesterol embolisation. Heart 79:113–114, 1998.
11. Dahlberg PJ, Frecentese DF, Cogbill TH. Cholesterol embolism: experience with 22 histologically proven cases. Surgery 105:737–746, 1989.
12. Rosman HS, Davis TP, Reddy D, Goldstein S. Cholesterol embolization: clinical findings and implications. J Am Coll Cardiol 15:1296–1299, 1990.
13. Fine MJ, Kapoor W, Falanga V. Cholesterol crystal embolization: a review of 221 cases in the English literature. Angiology 38:769–784, 1987.
14. Cross SS. How common is cholesterol embolism? J Clin Pathol 44:859–861, 1991.
15. Case records of the Massachusetts General Hospital (case 24–1998). N Engl J Med 339:329–337, 1998.
16. Meyrier A, Hill GS, Simon P. Ischemic renal dis-

eases: new insights into old entities. Kidney Int 54: 2–13, 1998.

17. Kang K, Botella R, White CR Jr. Subtle clues to the diagnosis of cholesterol embolism. Am J Dermatopathol 18:380–384, 1996.

18. Case records of the Massachusetts General Hospital (case 2–1991). N Engl J Med 324:113–120, 1991.

19. Robinson RJ, Pemberton M, Goddard MJ. Myositis due to cholesterol emboli. Postgrad Med J 69:947–949, 1993.

20. Bendixen BH, Younger DS, Hair LS, et al. Cholesterol emboli neuropathy. Neurology 42:428–430, 1992.

21. Slavin RE, Gonzalez-Vitale JC, Marin OS. Atheromatous emboli to the lumbosacral spinal cord. Stroke 6:411–415, 1975.

22. Geroulakos G, Homer-Vanniasinkam S, Wilkinson A, Galloway I. Cholesterol embolisation. A lethal complication of instrumentation of an aneurysmal aorta: a case report. Int Angiol 16:69–71, 1997.

23. Green HL, Nemir P Jr. Air embolism as a complication during parenteral alimentation. Am J Surg 121:614–616, 1971.

24. Baker BK, Awwad EE. Computed tomography of fatal cerebral air embolism following percutaneous aspiration biopsy of the lung. J Comput Assist Tomogr 12:1082–1083, 1988.

25. Marini JJ, Culver BH. Systemic gas embolism complicating mechanical ventilation in the adult respiratory distress syndrome. Ann Intern Med 110: 699–703, 1989.

26. Muth CM, Shank ES. Gas embolism. N Engl J Med 342:476–482, 2000.

27. Hinkle DA, Raizen DM, McGarvey ML, Liu GT. Cerebral air embolism complicating cardiac ablation procedures. Neurology 56:792–794, 2001.

28. Heckmann JG, Lang CJ, Kindler K, Huk W, Erbguth FJ, Neundorfer B. Neurologic manifestations of cerebral air embolism as a complication of central venous catheterization. Crit Care Med 28: 1621–1625, 2000.

29. Hwang TL, Fremaux R, Sears ES, et al. Confirmation of cerebral air embolism with computerized tomography [letter]. Ann Neurol 13:214–215, 1983.

30. Jensen ME, Lipper MH. CT in iatrogenic cerebral air embolism. Am J Neuroradiol 7:823–827, 1986.

31. Yamaki T, Ando S, Ohta K, Kubota T, Kawasaki K, Hirama M. CT demonstration of massive cerebral air embolism from pulmonary barotrauma due to cardiopulmonary resuscitation. J Comput Assist Tomogr 13:313–315, 1989.

32. Butler BD, Bryan-Brown C, Hills BA. Paradoxical air embolism: transcapillary route [letter]. Crit Care Med 11:837, 1983.

33. Butler BD, Hills BA. The lung as a filter for microbubbles. J Appl Physiol 47:537–543, 1979.

34. Helps SC, Parsons DW, Reilly PL, Gorman DF. The effect of gas emboli on rabbit cerebral blood flow. Stroke 21:94–99, 1990.

35. Chang C, Dughi J, Shitabata P, Johnson G, Coel M, McNamara JJ. Air embolism and the radial arterial line. Crit Care Med 16:141–143, 1988.

36. Lowenstein E, Little JW III, Lo HH. Prevention of cerebral embolization from flushing radial–artery cannulas. N Engl J Med 285:1414–1415, 1971.

37. Marquez J, Sladen A, Gendell H, Boehnke M, Mendelow H. Paradoxical cerebral air embolism without an intracardiac septal defect. Case report. J Neurosurg 55:997–1000, 1981.

38. Cavo JW Jr. True vocal cord paralysis following intubation. Laryngoscope 95:1352–1359, 1985.

39. Fuller JE, Thomas DV. Facial nerve paralysis after general anesthesia. JAMA 162:645, 1956.

40. Briscoe CE, Bushman JA, McDonald WI. Extensive neurological damage after cannulation of internal jugular vein. Br Med J 1:314, 1974.

41. Brown CQ. Inadvertent prolonged cannulation of the carotid artery. Anesth Analg 61:150–152, 1982.

42. Anagnou J. Cerebrovascular accident during percutaneous cannulation of internal jugular vein [letter]. Lancet 2:377–378, 1982.

43. Parikh RK. Horner's syndrome. A complication of percutaneous catheterisation of internal jugular vein. Anaesthesia 27:327–329, 1972.

44. Reddy G, Coombes A, Hubbard AD. Horner's syndrome following internal jugular vein cannulation. Intensive Care Med 24:194–196, 1998.

45. Butsch JL, Butsch WL, Da Rosa JF. Bilateral vocal cord paralysis. A complication of percutaneous cannulation of the internal jugular veins. Arch Surg 111:828, 1976.

46. Sloan MA, Mueller JD, Adelman LS, Caplan LR. Fatal brainstem stroke following internal jugular vein catheterization. Neurology 41:1092–1095, 1991.

47. Garcia EG, Wijdicks EFM, Younge BR. Neurologic complications associated with internal jugular vein cannulation in critically ill patients: a prospective study. Neurology 44:951–952, 1994.

48. Boyd KD, Thomas SJ, Gold J, Boyd AD. A prospective study of complications of pulmonary artery catheterizations in 500 consecutive patients. Chest 84:245–249, 1983.

49. Elliott CG, Zimmerman GA, Clemmer TP. Complications of pulmonary artery catheterization in the care of critically ill patients. A prospective study. Chest 76:647–652, 1979.

50. Shah KB, Rao TL, Laughlin S, El-Etr AA. A review of pulmonary artery catheterization in 6,245 patients. Anesthesiology 61:271–275, 1984.

51. Bedford RF, Wollman H. Complications of percutaneous radial–artery cannulation: an objective prospective study in man. Anesthesiology 38:228–236, 1973.

52. Bonney G. Iatrogenic injuries of nerves. J Bone Joint Surg (Br) 68:9–13, 1986.

53. Marshall G, Edelstein G, Hirshman CA. Median nerve compression following radial arterial puncture. Anesth Analg 59:953–954, 1980.

54. Litler WA. Median nerve palsy—a complication of brachial artery cannulation. Postgrad Med J 52 (Suppl 7):110–113, 1976.

55. Luce EA, Futrell JW, Wilgis EF, Hoopes JE. Compression neuropathy following brachial arterial puncture in anticoagulated patients. J Trauma 16: 717–721, 1976.

56. Macon WL IV, Futrell JW. Median-nerve neuropathy after percutaneous puncture of the brachial artery in patients receiving anticoagulants. N Engl J Med 288:1396, 1973.

57. Dawson DM, Fischer EG. Neurologic complications of cardiac catheterization. Neurology 27: 496–497, 1977.

58. Dawson DM, Krarup C. Perioperative nerve lesions. Arch Neurol 46:1355–1360, 1989.

59. Furlan AJ, Sila CA, Chimowitz MI, Jones SC, Rodman KD. Neurologic complications of cardiac diagnostic procedures, surgery and pharmacotherapy. In: Vinken PJ, Bruyn GW, Klawans HL (eds). Handbook of Clinical Neurology, Vol. 63: Systemic Diseases. Part I. Elsevier Science Publishers, Amsterdam, 1993, pp 175–204.

60. Kosmorsky G, Hanson MR, Tomsak RL. Neuro-ophthalmologic complications of cardiac catheterization. Neurology 38:483–485, 1988.

61. Olivecrona H. Complications of cerebral angiography. Neuroradiology 14:175–181, 1977.

62. Fischer-Williams M, Gottschalk PG, Browell JN. Transient cortical blindness. An unusual complication of coronary angiography. Neurology 20:353–355, 1970.

63. Henzlova MJ, Coghlan HC, Dean LS, Taylor JL. Cortical blindness after left internal mammary artery to left anterior descending coronary artery graft angiography. Cathet Cardiovasc Diagn 15:37–39, 1988.

64. Vik-Mo H, Todnem K, Folling M, Rosland GA. Transient visual disturbance during cardiac catheterization with angiography. Cathet Cardiovasc Diagn 12:1–4, 1986.

65. Shuttleworth EC, Wise GR. Transient global amnesia due to arterial embolism. Arch Neurol 29:340–342, 1973.

66. Hodges JR. Transient amnesia: clinical and neuropsychological aspects. Major Probl Neurol 24:1–161, 1991.

67. Lewis SL. Aetiology of transient global amnesia. Lancet 352:397–399, 1998.

68. Ay H, Furie KL, Yamada K, Koroshetz WJ. Diffusion-weighted MRI characterizes the ischemic lesion in transient global amnesia. Neurology 51:901–903, 1998.

69. Ayas N, Wijdicks EFM. Cardiac catheterization complicated by stroke: 14 patients. Cerebrovasc Dis 5:304–307, 1995.

70. Segel AZ, Abernethy WB, Palacios IF, BeLue R, Redford G. Stroke as a complication of cardiac catheterization: Risk factors and clinical features. Neurology 56:975–977, 2001.

71. Wijdicks EFM, Thielen KR, Reeder GS. Immediate cerebral angiography and mechanical fragmentation of cerebral embolus after percutaneous myocardial revascularization [letter]. Ann Intern Med 132:846–847, 2000.

72. Stein B, Halperin JL, Fuster V. Should patients with atrial fibrillation be anticoagulated prior to and chronically following cardioversion? In: Cheitlin MD (ed). Dilemmas in Clinical Cardiology. FA Davis, Philadelphia, 1990, pp 231–247.

73. Lo YS, Swerdlow CD. Multiple protruding, mobile left ventricular thrombi and risk of embolism after cardioversion [letter]. Chest 97:1023, 1990.

74. Arnold AZ, Mick MJ, Mazurek RP, Loop FD, Trohman RG. Role of prophylactic anticoagulation for direct current cardioversion in patients with atrial fibrillation or atrial flutter. J Am Coll Cardiol 19:851–855, 1992.

75. Manning WJ, Silverman DI, Gordon SP, Krumholz HM, Douglas PS. Cardioversion from atrial fibrillation without prolonged anticoagulation with use of transesophageal echocardiography to exclude the presence of atrial thrombi. N Engl J Med 328:750–755, 1993.

76. Ewy GA. Optimal technique for electrical cardioversion of atrial fibrillation [editorial]. Circulation 86:1645–1647, 1992.

77. Klein AL, Grimm RA, Black IW, et al. Cardioversion guided by transesophageal echocardiography: the ACUTE Pilot Study. A randomized, controlled trial. Assessment of Cardioversion Using Transesophageal Echocardiography. Ann Intern Med 126:200–209, 1997.

78. Murray RD, Goodman AS, Lieber EA, et al. National use of the transesophageal echocardiographic-guided approach to cardioversion for patients in atrial fibrillation. Am J Cardiol 85:239–244, 2000.

79. Klein AL, Grimm RA, Murray RD, et al. Use of transesophageal echocardiography to guide cardioversion in patients with atrial fibrillation. N Engl J Med 344:1411–1420, 2001.

80. Gibbons RJ, Holmes DR, Reeder GS, Bailey KR, Hopfenspirger MR, Gersh BJ. Immediate angioplasty compared with the administration of a thrombolytic agent followed by conservative treatment for myocardial infarction. The Mayo Coronary Care Unit and Catheterization Laboratory Groups. N Engl J Med 328:685–691, 1993.

81. Grines CL, Browne KF, Marco J, et al. A comparison of immediate angioplasty with thrombolytic therapy for acute myocardial infarction. The Primary Angioplasty in Myocardial Infarction Study Group. N Engl J Med 328:673–679, 1993.

82. American College of Emergency Physicians. The role of primary angioplasty in patients presenting with acute myocardial infarction. Ann Emerg Med 35:532–533, 2000.

83. Galbreath C, Salgado ED, Furlan AJ, Hollman J. Central nervous system complications of percutaneous transluminal coronary angioplasty. Stroke 17:616–619, 1986.

84. Hartzler GO, Rutherford BD, McConahay DR, Johnson WL, Giorgi LV. "High-risk" percutaneous transluminal coronary angioplasty. Am J Cardiol 61:33G–37G, 1988.

85. Detre K, Holubkov R, Kelsey S, et al. Percutaneous transluminal coronary angioplasty in 1985–1986 and 1977–1981. The National Heart, Lung, and Blood Institute Registry. N Engl J Med 318:265–270, 1988.

86. Murthy KN, Hubert G, Hess J. Cerebrovascular complications in percutaneous transluminal coronary angioplasty (PTCA) [abstract]. Neurology 42 (Suppl 3):451, 1992.

87. Malenka DJ, O'Rourke D, Miller MA, et al. Cause of in-hospital death in 12,232 consecutive patients undergoing percutaneous transluminal coronary angioplasty. The Northern New England Cardiovascular Disease Study Group. Am Heart J 137:632–638, 1999.

88. Boyarsky S. Paraplegia following translumbar aortography. JAMA 156:599–602, 1954.

89. Efsen F. Spinal cord lesion as a complication of abdominal aortography. Report of 4 cases. Acta Radiol Diagn (Stockh) 4:47–61, 1966.

90. Grossman LA, Kirtley JA. Paraplegia after translumbar aortography. JAMA 166:1035–1037, 1958.

91. Killen DA, Foster JH. Spinal cord injury as a com-

plication of contrast angiography. Surgery 59:969–981, 1966.

92. Mishkin MM, Baum S, Di Chiro G. Emergency treatment of angiography-induced paraplegia and tetraplegia. N Engl J Med 288:1184–1185, 1973.

93. Morariu MA. Transient spastic paraparesis following abdominal aortography: management with cerebrospinal fluid lavage [letter]. Ann Neurol 3: 185; 1978.

94. Maccioli GA, Lucas WJ, Norfleet EA. The intra-aortic balloon pump: a review. J Cardiothorac Anesth 2:365–373, 1988.

95. Grayzel J. Clinical evaluation of the Percor percutaneous intraaortic balloon: cooperative study of 722 cases. Circulation 66 (Suppl 1):I-223–I-226, 1982.

96. Kantrowitz A, Wasfie T, Freed PS, Rubenfire M, Wajszczuk W, Schork MA. Intraaortic balloon pumping 1967 through 1982: analysis of complications in 733 patients. Am J Cardiol 57:976–983, 1986.

97. Honet JC, Wajszczuk WJ, Rubenfire M, Kantrowitz A, Raikes JA. Neurological abnormalities in the leg(s) after use of intraaortic balloon pump: report of six cases. Arch Phys Med Rehabil 56: 346–352, 1975.

98. Lachance DH, Daube JR. Acute peripheral arterial occlusion: electrophysiologic study of 32 cases. Muscle Nerve 14:633–639, 1991.

99. Levin KH. AAEE case report #19: ischemic monomelic neuropathy. Muscle Nerve 12:791–795, 1989.

100. Ugalde V, Rosen BS. Ischemic peripheral neuropathy. Phys Med Rehabil Clin N Am 12:365–380, 2001.

101. Wilbourn AJ, Furlan AJ, Hulley W, Ruschhaupt W. Ischemic monomelic neuropathy. Neurology 33: 447–451, 1983.

102. Kaku DA, Malamut RI, Frey DJ, Parry GJ. Conduction block as an early sign of reversible injury in ischemic monomelic neuropathy. Neurology 43:1126–1130, 1993.

103. Harris RE, Reimer KA, Crain BJ, Becsey DD, Oldham HN Jr. Spinal cord infarction following intraaortic balloon support. Ann Thorac Surg 42: 206–207, 1986.

104. Rose DM, Jacobowitz IJ, Acinapura AJ, Cunningham JN Jr. Paraplegia following percutaneous insertion of an intra-aortic balloon. J Thorac Cardiovasc Surg 87:788–789, 1984.

105. Scott IR, Goiti JJ. Late paraplegia as a consequence of intraaortic balloon pump support. Ann Thorac Surg 40:300–301, 1985.

106. Poirier VL. Worldwide experience with the TCI HeartMate system: issues and future perspective. Thorac Cardiovasc Surg 47 (Suppl 2):316–320, 1999.

107. Eidelman BH, Obrist WD, Wagner WR, Kormos R, Griffith B. Cerebrovascular complications associated with the use of artificial circulatory support services. Neurol Clin 11:463–474, 1993.

108. Slater JP, Rose EA, Levin HR, et al. Low thromboembolic risk without anticoagulation using advanced-design left ventricular assist devices. Ann Thorac Surg 62:1321–1327, 1996.

109. Moazami N, Roberts K, Argenziano M, et al. Asymptomatic microembolism in patients with

long-term ventricular assist support. ASAIO J 43: 177–180, 1997.

110. Mandarino WA, Griffith BP, Kormos RL, et al. Novacor left ventricular assist filling and ejection in the presence of device complications. ASAIO Trans 36:M387–M389, 1990.

111. Li LYJ, Kelkar P, Exconde R, Parry GJ. Fatal cerebral embolic infarctions due to thrombosis of HeartMate left ventricular assist device [abstract]. Ann Neurol 46:480, 1999.

112. Dean WM, Woodside JR. Spinal hematoma compressing cauda equina. Urology 13:575–577, 1979.

113. Dickman CA, Shedd SA, Spetzler RF, Shetter AG, Sonntag VK. Spinal epidural hematoma associated with epidural anesthesia: complications of systemic heparinization in patients receiving peripheral vascular thrombolytic therapy. Anesthesiology 72:947–950, 1990.

114. Gustafsson H, Rutberg H, Bengtsson M. Spinal haematoma following epidural analgesia. Report of a patient with ankylosing spondylitis and a bleeding diathesis. Anaesthesia 43:220–222, 1988.

115. Spurny OM, Rubin S, Wolff JW, Wu WQ. Spinal epidural hematoma during anticoagulant therapy. Arch Intern Med 114:103–107, 1964.

116. Odoom JA, Sih IL. Epidural analgesia and anticoagulant therapy. Experience with one thousand cases of continuous epidurals. Anaesthesia 38: 254–259, 1983.

117. Eastwood DW. Hematoma after epidural anesthesia: relationship of skin and spinal angiomas. Anesth Analg 73:352–354, 1991.

118. Owens EL, Kasten GW, Hessel EA II. Spinal subarachnoid hematoma after lumbar puncture and heparinization: a case report, review of the literature, and discussion of anesthetic implications. Anesth Analg 65:1201–1207, 1986.

119. Ruff RL, Dougherty JH Jr. Complications of lumbar puncture followed by anticoagulation. Stroke 12:879–881, 1981.

120. Horlocker TT, Wedel DJ. Anticoagulants, antiplatelet therapy, and neuraxis blockade. Anesthesiol Clin North Am 10:1–11, 1992.

121. Howard SC, Gajjar A, Ribeiro RC, et al. Safety of lumbar puncture for children with acute lymphoblastic leukemia and thrombocytopenia. JAMA 284:2222–2224, 2000.

122. Rao TL, El-Etr AA. Anticoagulation following placement of epidural and subarachnoid catheters: an evaluation of neurologic sequelae. Anesthesiology 55:618–620, 1981.

123. Wang LP, Hauerberg J, Schmidt JF. Incidence of spinal epidural abscess after epidural analgesia: a national 1-year survey. Anesthesiology 91:1928–1936, 1999.

124. Strong WE. Epidural abscess associated with epidural catheterizatioin: a rare event? Report of two cases with markedly delayed presentation. Anesthesiology 74:943–946, 1991.

125. Seeberger MD, Kaufmann M, Staender S, Schneider M, Scheidegger D. Repeated dural punctures increase the incidence of postdural puncture headache. Anesth Analg 82:302–305, 1996.

126. Kuntz KM, Kokmen E, Stevens JC, Miller P, Offord KP, Ho MM. Post-lumbar puncture headaches: ex-

perience in 501 consecutive procedures. Neurology 42:1884–1887, 1992.

127. Fishman RA, Dillon WP. Dural enhancement and cerebral displacement secondary to intracranial hypotension. Neurology 43:609–611, 1993.

128. Mokri B, Piepgras DG, Miller GM. Syndrome of orthostatic headaches and diffuse pachymeningeal gadolinium enhancement. Mayo Clin Proc 72:400–413, 1997.

129. Mokri B, Parisi JE, Scheithauer BW, Piepgras DG, Miller GM. Meningeal biopsy in intracranial hypotension: meningeal enhancement on MRI. Neurology 45:1801–1807, 1995.

130. Schievink WI, Tourje J. Intracranial hypotension without meningeal enhancement on magnetic resonance imaging. Case report. J Neurosurg 92:475–477, 2000.

131. Mangar D, Kelly DL, Holder DO, Camporesi EM. Brachial plexus compression from a malpositioned chest tube after thoracotomy. Anesthesiology 74:780–782, 1991.

132. Iberti TJ, Stern PM. Chest tube thoracostomy. Crit Care Clin 8:879–895, 1992.

133. Durrani Z, Winnie AP. Brainstem toxicity with reversible locked-in syndrome after intrascalene brachial plexus block. Anesth Analg 72:249–252, 1991.

134. Kardjiev V, Symeonov A, Chankov I. Etiology, pathogenesis, and prevention of spinal cord lesions in selective angiography of the bronchial and intercostal arteries. Radiology 112:81–83, 1974.

135. Beal MF, Park TS, Fisher CM. Cerebral atheromatous embolism following carotid sinus pressure. Arch Neurol 38:310–312, 1981.

136. Calverley JR, Millikan CH. Complications of carotid manipulation. Neurology 11:185–189, 1961.

137. Zeman FD, Siegal S. Monoplegia following carotid sinus pressure in the aged. Am J Med Sci 213:603–607, 1947.

138. Richardson DA, Bexton R, Shaw FE, Steen N, Bond J, Kenny RA. Complications of carotid sinus massage—a prospective series of older patients. Age Ageing 29:413–417, 2000.

139. Bouzarth WF. Intracranial nasogastric tube insertion [editorial]. J Trauma 18:818–819, 1978.

140. Seebacher J, Nozik D, Mathieu A. Inadvertent intracranial introduction of a nasogastric tube, a complication of severe maxillofacial trauma. Anesthesiology 42:100–102, 1975.

Part II

Neurologic Complications in Medical and Surgical Intensive Care Units and Transplantation Units

Chapter 6

NEUROLOGIC MANIFESTATIONS OF BACTERIAL INFECTION AND SEPSIS

Community-acquired bacterial infections evolving into a sepsis syndrome are common reasons for admission to a medical intensive care unit (ICU). The nervous system is part of the cascade of multiorgan failure or is directly damaged by inflammation, septic emboli, or inflammation-related complications. Furthermore, endoscopic procedures, catheter placements, mechanical ventilation, and emergency surgical procedures may be sources for hospital-acquired infections. In susceptible patients, infection may directly involve the central nervous system.

Until neurologists entered ICUs, virtually no mention of the neurologic complications of sepsis and septic shock appeared in leading textbooks of critical care medicine. It is now well recognized that, for example, bacterial infections associated with multiorgan failure may damage peripheral nerves. Less widely appreciated is how profound the systemic effects of sepsis are on the brain.

This chapter focuses on selected disorders associated with bacterial infection, chosen largely because they are potential reasons for neurologic consultation. Many intensive care specialists seek early help with management of bacterial meningitis, epidural abscess, complications of endocarditis, and clostridial syndromes. Infections associated with immunosuppression are discussed in Chapter 18.

BACTERIAL MENINGITIS

Acute bacterial meningitis may occur de novo or in a critical illness. Admissions to medical or surgical ICUs are mostly the result of pneumococcal (*Streptococcus pneumoniae*) meningitis, which remains serious and carries a considerable risk of adverse outcome. Notably, ordinary pneumonia or otitis media predisposes patients to bacterial meningitis. Alcoholics are also more prone to infection with *Listeria monocytogenes* and *Haemophilus influenzae*. Diabetics are more susceptible to Enterobacteriaceae and *Staphylococcus aureus*.

Certain conditions may become infectious sources in the ICU. Potential sources for bacterial meningitis in the uncompromised critically ill host are sinusitis, spinal anesthesia, and traumatic cerebrospinal fluid (CSF) fistula. Bacterial meningitis seldom develops as part of a bacteremia or sepsis syndrome. The risk of meningitis also remains low in fulminant bacteremias. In Mylotte and colleagues' consecutive study[1] of patients with *Staphylococcus aureus* bacteremia, only 1 of 114 episodes was associated with meningitis, and even in this patient staphylococcal endocarditis was found.

Paranasal sinusitis secondary to prolonged nasotracheal intubation is a frequently unrecognized cause of fever. The reported incidence ranges from 2% to 5%, and occurrence may be more common in patients who had emergency intubation.[2] *Staphylococcus epidermidis* and gram-negative organisms predominate in cultures. It is a major source for ventilator-associated pneumonia.[3] Paranasal sinusitis is managed by removal of nasotracheal and nasogastric tubes, leading to clearing of mucopurulent drainage, which can be documented by computed tomography (CT).[4,5] However, without timely management, extension of maxillary sinusitis to the sphenoid sinus has been noted in 25% of cases.[6]

The prevalence of meningitis after diagnostic or therapeutic lumbar puncture and spinal anesthesia is very low.[7–11] Nonetheless, bacterial meningitis after spinal anesthesia is a serious condition because it is frequently associated with *Pseudomonas aeruginosa* and *Staphylococcus aureus*. The patient's skin is obviously an important source, but contaminated needles or hands of the physician who performs the procedure may increase the risk.

Meningitis after basal skull fractures in traumatized patients in the surgical ICU is primarily due to *Streptococcus pneumoniae*, but a trend toward gram-negative organisms has been noted.[12–15] Spontaneous sealing of a CSF fistula is common in basal skull fractures but less frequent in midface fractures. Prophylaxis with antibiotics promotes selection of resistant organisms and is therefore not recommended.[13]

Immunocompromised patients in the ICU are a separate population in whom the major bacterial infections include those caused by *Listeria monocytogenes* and *Nocardia asteroides*. The clinical presentation of these central nervous system infections is discussed in Chapter 18.

Drugs can induce aseptic meningitis[16–18] (Table 6–1), but symptoms usually resolve within 24 hr after administration is discontinued. The most commonly observed form of aseptic meningitis is that associated with muromonab-CD3 (see Chapter 18).

Clinical Features

Because of polypharmacy, the distinctive signs and symptoms of bacterial meningitis may remain unrecognized in critically ill patients. Obviously, neuromuscular blocking drugs can mask the leading clinical signs, such as meningeal irritation, and patients in the ICU may not be able to signal severe headaches. Bacterial meningitis generally is manifested by new-onset high-grade fever, nuchal rigidity, and positive Brudzinski's sign (flexion in hips triggered by flexion of the neck). Nuchal rigidity may be slightly difficult to appreciate in intubated patients, but the modern flexible endotracheal tubes should not greatly confound assessment of neck flexion. Moreover, when present, meningeal irritation is often demonstrated in the first 30° of passive flexion. Diminished level of consciousness is an important initial diagnostic clue in critically ill patients, and conversely, diagnosis is unlikely in a fully alert and attentive patient. In a seminal article on clinical features of bacterial meningitis, only 9 (5%) of 191 patients were fully alert.[19]

Certain microorganisms may be suggested by skin involvement. A maculopapular rash may point to meningitis caused by *Strepto-*

Table 6–1. **Drugs Known to Induce Aseptic Meningitis**

Trimethoprim (sulfamethoxazole)

Ibuprofen

Cytosine arabinoside (high doses)

Carbamazepine

Sulindac

Muromonab-CD3

Isoniazid

coccus pneumoniae or *Staphylococcus aureus* but remains generally nonspecific. Subconjunctival hemorrhages, petechial hemorrhages, and purpura are traditionally linked to meningococcal meningitis.

Focal neurologic signs and papilledema are not seen in the early stages of purulent meningitis but develop during the clinical course in 10% to 20% of patients. Both clinical signs may suggest subdural empyema, intracranial abscess, or cavernous sinus thrombosis. Delayed recognition of maxillary sinusitis may lead to seeding of the meninges, orbital cellulitis, and cavernous sinus thrombosis. Cavernous sinus thrombosis may result in blindness or diplopia due to involvement of cranial nerves III, IV, and VI.[20] Patients in whom sinusitis involves the sphenoid cavity have severe headache, photophobia, and facial paresthesias.

Seizures occur in 20% to 30% of patients with acute bacterial meningitis. Seizures that occur in the course of a few days of antibiotic treatment may indicate an intracranial mass or a hemorrhagic cerebral infarction associated with cerebral venous thrombosis.

Additional Studies

Purulent meningitis is confirmed by examination and culture of the CSF. Frequent sampling of blood is helpful in culturing the organism. Swartz and Dodge[21] demonstrated positive results in 52% of blood cultures but with sensitivity varying by organism (79% in *Haemophilus influenzae* meningitis, 56% in *Streptococcus pneumoniae* meningitis, 33% in *Neisseria meningitidis*, 29% in β-hemolytic streptococcal meningitis, and only 17% in *Staphylococcus aureus*). CSF features of acute bacterial meningitis are cloudy, milky, or turbid appearance and increased opening CSF pressure. Gram's stain frequently demonstrates the microorganism, but the result is negative in approximately 20% of cases. Previous antibiotic treatment can often be implicated in false-negative studies.

Alternative ways to identify bacterial pathogens are available. Cerebrospinal fluid counterimmunoelectrophoresis, CSF latex agglutination, and coagulation tests may detect common bacterial antigens in 70% to 100% of patients and therefore are useful in patients pretreated with antibiotics.

Typically, CSF analysis reveals polymorphonuclear pleocytosis, with leukocyte counts up to 100,000 cells/mm^3; decreased glucose level, to <50% of the serum glucose concentration; and increased protein (more than 100 mg/dL) and lactate values. Very early CSF samples may fail to demonstrate pleocytosis not only in any type of meningitis but also in specific conditions, such as pneumococcal meningitis in asplenic patients and in neutropenia associated with hematologic malignant disease. A traumatic lumbar puncture may confound the interpretation. However, the true leukocyte count can be estimated by subtracting one leukocyte per 700 erythrocytes. A ratio of CSF to serum is probably more reliable.[22] (True leukocytes [CSF] = actual leukocytes [CSF] − leukocytes [serum] × erythrocytes [CSF]/erythrocytes [serum].)

A vexing clinical problem in critically ill patients in whom bacterial meningitis is suspected is whether a CT scan should precede lumbar puncture. Fear of inducing cerebral herniation after lumbar puncture in patients with unrecognized infectious intracranial masses derives from anecdotal reports before the CT scan era. Many neurologists perform lumbar punctures before CT scanning is done, but neuroimaging is warranted in patients with seizures, unequivocal focal signs, or papilledema and in instances of sedation or muscle paralysis hampering neurologic examination. With readily available CT scans and acquisition times of mere minutes, the threshold for performing a CT scan before obtaining CSF should be low. The mortality from delaying antibiotic treatment while organizing and performing CT scanning in bacterial meningitis is 10 to 20 times greater than the risk of complications associated with lumbar puncture.[23] Delay of antibiotic treatment in a patient with bacterial meningitis results in considerably less potential for complete recovery.[24]

Bacterial identification and, more important, the validity of antibiotic-sensitivity testing markedly decrease after the first intravenous treatment with antibiotics. In a study of 78 patients with bacterial meningitis, positive CSF cultures of the most frequent bacteria were found in 43% of those treated with ceftriaxone and in 58% of those treated with ampicillin or chloramphenicol when specimens were obtained after 4 to 12 hr of treatment.[25] Culturing and identification of the infective organism are unlikely to be influenced by antibiotic therapy if CSF is obtained in the first 2 hr. Therefore, intravenous administration of antibiotics should be started, followed by rapid CT imaging and lumbar puncture.

When a CSF leak is suspected, it is important to differentiate among nasal secretion, saliva, and perilymph or endolymph. When the collected fluid is investigated for an extra band of transferrin in the β_2 fraction on protein electrophoresis and levels of glucose are modestly high (50 to 70 mg/dL), a CSF leak is highly likely.

The yield of CT scan in uncomplicated bacterial meningitis is low. In occasional patients, a subdural empyema collection, which may mimic all signs of bacterial meningitis, is detected, but magnetic resonance imaging (MRI) is a much better modality in these complications. The MRI may also detect pus and document inflammation when the meninges are enhanced with gadolinium[26]

(Fig. 6–1A). Fluid-attenuated inversion recovery sequences may detect infarcts due to vasculitis associated with extensive degrees of inflammation[27] (Fig. 6–1B).

Treatment

Rapid CSF sterilization of pathogens is adequately achieved with one of the new third-generation cephalosporins.[28] In patients with a fulminant *Streptococcus pneumoniae* meningitis, penicillin-resistant organisms may be implicated, which should prompt treatment with vancomycin. There is a tendency to add vancomycin preemptively because of the high prevalence of resistant *Streptococcus pneumoniae*. An empirical regimen pending culture and sensitivity results is proposed in Table 6–2. Specific treatment is suggested in Table 6–3. Dexamethasone as an adjunctive therapeutic agent is effective in children, reducing mortality and significantly reducing moderate to severe sensorineural loss, but corresponding data in adults are not yet available.[29] Nonetheless, dexamethasone (10 mg intravenous bolus; 4 mg every 6 hr

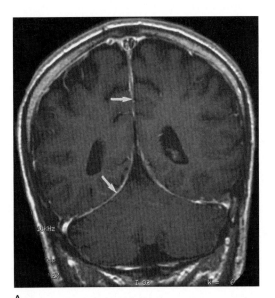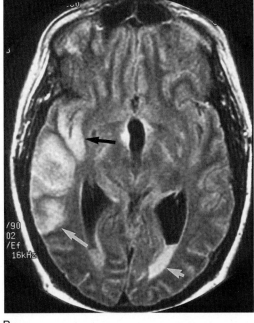

A   B

Figure 6–1. Bacterial meningitis. *A*: Gadolinium enhancement of meninges (arrows). *B*: Middle cerebral artery territorial stroke as a complication (arrows). Note pus in the ventricular compartment (arrowhead).

Table 6–2. **Suggested Empirical Therapy for Bacterial Meningitis in Uncompromised Hosts**

Cefotaxime or	12 g/day IV in divided doses q4h
Ceftriaxone plus	4 g/day IV in divided doses q12h
Vancomycin	2 g/day in divided doses q12h

for 4 days) should be strongly considered in adult patients with fulminant bacterial meningitis.

Outcome

Mortality from bacterial meningitis can be considerable and may approach 22% in patients with pneumococcal meningitis.[30] Elderly patients, as expected, may have higher fatality rates. One study found that mortality (35%) was most frequent in patients with diminished level of consciousness and inadequate (dose, choice, delay) antibiotic therapy.[31] Mortality is particularly high in patients with gram-negative meningitis. Within the first 3 days after onset, brain swelling is seen in 14% of patients and hydrocephalus in 12%[32] and may result in coma. However, failure to awaken after appropriate treatment may be more commonly related to cerebral infarction, sometimes in strategic locations involving the reticular formation connections, such as the thalamus.[27] Outcome in meningitis associated with traumatic CSF leak (almost always caused by *Streptococcus pneumoniae*) is good after treatment with a third-generation cephalosporin, but additional repair of the defect is needed.

SPINAL EPIDURAL ABSCESS

Any infection may set the stage for hematogenous spread to the epidural space.[33,34] Possible causes of epidural abscess are decubitus ulcers, operative wounds, psoas abscess, endocarditis, sinusitis,[35–39] and a postintubation retropharyngeal abscess.[40] The common organism isolated from CSF is *Staphylococcus aureus*. In many patients with spinal

Table 6–3. **Antibiotic Treatment for Bacterial Meningitis**

Organism	Antibiotic	Suggested Dose
Streptococcus pneumoniae	Ceftriaxone or	2–4 g/day IV in divided doses q12h
	Cefotaxime plus	8–12 g/day IV in divided doses q4h
	Vancomycin	2 g/day in divided doses q12h
Neisseria meningitidis	Penicillin G	20–24 million U/day IV in divided doses q4h
	or	
	Ampicillin	12 g/day IV in divided doses q4h
Gram-negative organisms	Ceftriaxone	4 g/day IV in divided doses q12h
	Ceftazidime	6–12 g/day IV in divided doses q8h (for *Pseudomonas aeruginosa* coverage)
Staphylococcus aureus	Nafcillin or	9–12 g/day IV in divided doses q4h
	Oxacillin	9–12 g/day IV in divided doses q4h
Methicillin-resistant *Staphylococcus*	Vancomycin	1 g/day IV in divided doses q12h
Enterobacteriaceae	Ceftriaxone or	4 g/day IV in divided doses q12h
	Cefotaxime	12 g/day IV in divided doses q4h

Data from Cherubin et al.[28] and Tunkel et al.[29]

epidural abscesses, isolation of the organism is possible with blood cultures. However, in up to 40% of patients with a spinal epidural abscess, a source cannot be found.

Clinical Features

Many patients are acutely ill, incoherent, and confused. The deceptive presentation parallels sepsis or any other overwhelming infection with sweating, rigors, tachycardia, and fever. Many patients complain of pain along the spine, which may become associated with limb weakness and paresthesias[39,41] (Table 6–4). The pain is often severe and unresponsive to conventional narcotics. Alternatively, there may be girdle pain from cauda equina compression, or nerve root inflammation may produce severe radicular pain.

Although many initial symptoms and signs may be subtle and difficult to appreciate, a fair number of patients present with spinal tenderness over several vertebrae and weakness, with progression within a few hours to flaccid paraplegia, loss of reflexes, and anesthesia below the level of the lesion (Table 6–4). Most series report clinical deterioration over days, but the clinical course can be more dramatic, with rapid deterioration to complete paraplegia or quadriplegia with no potential for reversal or ambulation, even after emergency laminectomy.

Misdiagnosis of epidural abscesses is common, and disorders that often look confusingly similar besides sepsis are intra-abdominal abscess, pyelonephritis, and cholecystitis.[33,34] The physician should be alert to the diagnosis in an acutely febrile patient without an obvious source for infection and with developing weakness of the extremities.[42]

Table 6–4. Clinical Characteristics of Acute Spinal Epidural Abscess

Signs of systemic infection and fever
Severe back pain or radicular pain
Paraparesis or quadriparesis
Impaired bladder control
Distinctive sensory level

Additional Studies

Magnetic resonance imaging is the most sensitive diagnostic study for identifying epidural abscess[11,43–45] (Fig. 6–2). An epidural mass has an isodense or a hyperintense signal on T1-weighted images and a hyperintense signal on T2 images. Epidural pus and CSF may yield similar signals on MRI, and thus additional gadolinium may be needed to visualize or outline the abscess. The additional presence of osteomyelitis may be helpful in localization. Concomitant osteomyelitis is particularly common in tuberculous abscess.[46] Myelography combined with a CT scan can be used when metallic monitoring devices and infusion pumps in the ICU preclude MRI. In Danner and Hartman's experience,[34] plain CT scanning performed at admission was positive for epidural abscess in only one-third of the

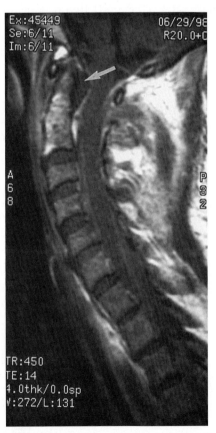

Figure 6–2. Magnetic resonance image of cervical epidural abscess (arrow). Note backward bowing of cord.

patients. Myelography or myelography-CT, however, may enable detection in most cases and may even be more sensitive than MRI in patients with small pus collections and little granulation tissue.

The CSF examination is helpful in patients with pain and fever but without muscle weakness, sensory deficits, sphincter disturbances, or abnormal tendon reflexes. It is, however, more appropriate to delineate the epidural mass by neuroimaging and not risk worsening from lumbar puncture due to CSF hypovolemia. A CSF examination may document pus and frequently demonstrates increased protein concentration, increased neutrophils, usually more than 80 cells/mm³, and disturbed manometric values when a CSF block is present. Frequently, CSF cultures fail to demonstrate the microorganism, and more often the results of blood cultures dictate the mode of antibiotic coverage.

Treatment

Standard management for patients with epidural abscess and neurologic deficits is emergency drainage after surgical exploration followed by antibiotic therapy for 8 weeks. Because *Staphylococcus aureus* is a common pathogen, empirical antibiotic therapy should include a third-generation cephalosporin and a penicillinase-resistant penicillin (vancomycin or nafcillin). Neurosurgeons may prefer additional laminectomy to expose the posteriorly located pockets.

Nonoperative treatment of epidural infection has been suggested in patients without neurologic deficits, and results have been excellent.[47,48] The criteria for conservative medical treatment in patients without neurologic deficits are debatable and perhaps even problematic. However, conservative treatment can be considered in patients with a large epidural abscess involving a considerable length of the vertebral canal, which would necessitate an extensive laminectomy.

Most patients with a localized pocket of epidural pus should be managed surgically to avoid deterioration to complete paraplegia. An analysis from Henry Ford Hospital involving 41 patients identified three factors for poor outcome: age greater than 60 years, thecal sac compression of >50%, and dura-

Table 6–5. Outcome in Spinal Epidural Abscess

Outcome	PATIENTS	
	No.	%
Complete recovery	74	39
Weakness	49	26
Paralysis	41	22
Death	24	13
Total	188	100

Modified from Danner and Hartman.[34] By permission of the University of Chicago Press.

tion of symptoms exceeding 75 hr. When all these factors were present, only 6 of the 41 patients had a good outcome.[49] Outcome is related to the extent of neurologic impairment at presentation and to the duration of the neurologic deficit. Complete recovery is possible in patients with paraplegia or quadriplegia when surgical intervention takes place within 24 hr. Mortality, however, remains at about 15% and is related to delay in appropriate treatment. Outcome in patients with spinal epidural abscess is shown in Table 6–5.

INFECTIVE ENDOCARDITIS

Infective endocarditis is a fairly common reason for admission to a medical or cardiac ICU, and some patients may be quickly transferred to a cardiac surgical unit for the planning of valve replacement. *Streptococcus viridans* is responsible for 60% of cases of endocarditis on native valves. Other bacteria include enterococci (which are very resistant to the bactericidal activity of commonly used antibiotics); *Brucella* organisms (up to 10% of cases reported in Spain and Saudi Arabia); and many other pathogens, such as rickettsiae, *Bartonella* fungi, and chlamydiae. The mean duration before hospitalization is usually 2 months for infection with *Streptococcus viridans* and 2 weeks to 1 month for the more virulent and destructive *Staphylococcus aureus* species.

Nosocomial endocarditis can be a cause of neurologic morbidity in critically ill patients. Hospital-acquired infective endocarditis is usually caused by *Staphylococcus aureus* or coagulase-negative staphylococci and less commonly by streptococci or *Pseudomonas aeruginosa*.[50–53] Many patients have no underlying valvular disease, and damage to the endocardium may be produced by intravascular catheters. The potential dire consequences of pulmonary artery catheterization were addressed in 55 consecutively autopsied patients, of whom 53% had one or more endocardial lesions, including subendocardial hemorrhage and thrombus.[54] These findings were rare in a noncatheterized control population. More frequent iatrogenic portals of entry probably are the genitourinary tract, intratracheal airway, biopsy sites, and surgical wounds.

Central nervous system involvement in infective endocarditis is a highly complex clinical problem.[55] The frequency of neurologic complications varies: 53% in staphylococcal endocarditis, 90% in enteric bacterial infections, and 30% in streptococcal infections. Suspicion should increase when localizing neurologic symptoms appear in a febrile patient.

Clinical Features

The protean clinical manifestations in infective endocarditis require a high degree of awareness, and symptoms may develop insidiously, and the presenting symptoms are typically nonspecific. However, fever occurs in more than 90% of patients. Musculoskeletal manifestations have been noted in 44% of patients, and when they are present, pain, redness, and tenderness can be found in one or more joints. Patients may complain of diffuse myalgias that are usually localized in both the thighs and calves.[56]

The presenting symptoms of endocarditis may be different in several age groups. Tachycardia occurs less often in elderly patients, and the febrile response is significantly lower than in the younger population.[57] A new regurgitation murmur or a preexisting murmur changing in intensity may not be prominent and may even be absent, particularly in patients with right-sided endocarditis. It is useful to search under fingernails or toenails for splinter hemorrhages (Plate 6–1) that represent embolic lesions or

vasculitis. Other helpful clinical features are conjunctival petechiae in the lower eyelid; tender erythematous nodes in the pads of the fingers or toes (Osler's nodes); small, flat, nontender erythematous spots that blanch on pressure (Janeway lesions); and splenomegaly[58–62] (Table 6–6).

Acute infective endocarditis due to *Staphylococcus aureus* bacteremia has a high propensity for life-threatening complications from extensive valve destruction. Left ventricular failure refractory to treatment, abscesses of the annulus of the infected valve, and multiple systemic emboli are accepted indications for valve replacement.[63–65]

The clinical manifestations of prosthetic valve endocarditis differ substantially from those of native valve infective endocarditis.[66,67] The initial presentation is rapid, as opposed to an indolent clinical course, and shock and embolic showers are common. Mortality is high. Prosthetic valve endocarditis may occur early after cardiotomy. Methicillin-resistant *Staphylococcus epidermidis* associated with contaminated operating room equipment, pump-oxygenators, and postoperative wound infections are often implicated. In patients with late-onset prosthetic valve endocarditis, streptococci are the predominant causative agents.

Risk factors for the development of prosthetic valve endocarditis were identified in a series of 2642 patients at Massachusetts Gen-

Table 6–6. **Frequent Symptoms and Signs of Infective Endocarditis**

Signs and Symptoms	Incidence (%)
Cardiac murmur	97
Malaise	94
Fever	86
Anorexia	75
Weight loss	50
Splenomegaly	31
Rales	30
Splinter hemorrhages	28
Petechiae	20
Osler's nodes and Janeway lesions	21

Modified from Von Reyn et al.[62] By permission of the American College of Physicians.

eral Hospital.[68] Recipients of a mechanical prosthesis had a greater early risk of endocarditis than patients who received porcine valves, but the late risk of endocarditis, defined as occurrence 2 months or more after placement, was greater in porcine valves. A greater risk was also evident in patients with multiple valve replacements.

The incidence of transient ischemic attacks and ischemic strokes ranges from 10% to 30%[69] in patients with bacterial endocarditis. Large territory strokes are rare; more frequently, septic emboli occlude small penetrating vessels, causing subcortical in-

farcts, often hemorrhagic (Fig. 6–3). Most ischemic strokes in infective endocarditis occur at presentation, before adequate antimicrobial control. Patients with mitral valve endocarditis and large vegetations are at particular risk for stroke.[70]

Initial Studies

Without previous antibiotic administration, 95% of blood cultures can become positive for the causative microorganism, often already in the first sample. Negative blood cul-

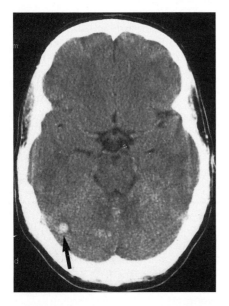
A

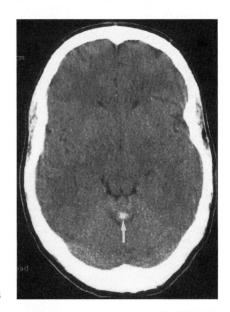
B

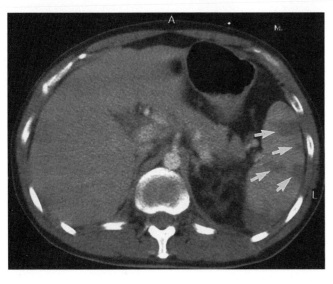
C

Figure 6–3. Computed tomography scans of multiple hemorrhagic embolic infarcts (*A,B*) (arrows) and infarcts in the spleen (*C*) (arrows) in a patient with staphylococcus endocarditis complicated by thrombocytopenia.

tures in patients with infective endocarditis have been reported in 2% to 31% of the patients,[71] and difficult-to-isolate fungal species can be involved in these circumstances. *Legionella* may be the causative agent in prosthetic valve endocarditis; it requires special culture media and can remain undetected in routine studies.[72]

A suggested practical approach is to obtain three separate venous blood cultures on the first day, two more venous blood cultures if these cultures are negative by day 2, and two more venous blood cultures and one arterial blood culture if all cultures are negative on day 3.[73] Laboratory findings may include increased erythrocyte sedimentation rate, increased neutrophil counts, and normochromic, normocytic, or hemolytic anemia. Red cell blood cast and proteinuria may occur as a result of immune complex glomerulonephritis.

Echocardiography is very useful for demonstrating vegetations.[74] The sensitivity for diagnosing infective endocarditis ranges from 80% to 90%, and the specificity is 98%. Transesophageal two-dimensional echocardiography is superior to transthoracic imaging,[75,76] particularly in patients with small vegetations. Echocardiography of prosthetic endocarditis may be more cumbersome because dense echoreflections of the prosthetic valve may overshadow reflections from vegetations. A set of diagnostic criteria that has been validated and recently revised has become known as the "Duke criteria"[77] (Table 6–7).

Management

Theoretically, appropriate antibiotic therapy can eradicate the infection in prosthetic valve endocarditis, but the hemodynamic status usually is greatly compromised. The causes of death are congestive heart failure, septic shock, and cardiac arrest; surgical intervention is often the only option. A recent survey found that operative mortality of

---

Table 6–7. Definition of Infective Endocarditis According to the Proposed Modified Duke Criteria

Definite Infective Endocarditis

Pathologic criteria

Microorganisms demonstrated by culture or histologic examination of a vegetation, a vegetation that has embolized, or an intracardiac abscess specimen; or

Pathologic lesions; vegetation or intracardiac abscess confirmed by histologic examination showing active endocarditis

Clinical criteria

2 major criteria; or
1 major criterion and 3 minor criteria; or
5 minor criteria

Possible Infective Endocarditis

1 major criterion and 1 minor criterion; or
3 minor criteria

Rejected

Firm alternative diagnosis explaining evidence of infective endocarditis; or

Resolution of infective endocarditis syndrome with antibiotic therapy for ≤4 days; or

No pathologic evidence of infective endocarditis at surgery or autopsy with antibiotic therapy for ≤4 days; or

Does not meet criteria for possible infective endocarditis, as above

Major criteria

Blood culture positive for infective endocarditis

Evidence of endocardial involvement

Echocardiogram positive for infective endocarditis

New valvular regurgitation

Minor criteria

Predisposing heart condition or intravenous drug use

Temperature >38°C

Vascular phenomena

Immunologic phenomena

Microbiologic evidence

From Li et al.[77] By permission of the Infectious Diseases Society of America.

7.6% was related to preoperative hemodynamic status.[78]

Use of anticoagulation in native or prosthetic valve endocarditis is controversial. In general, anticoagulants are not indicated in the standard treatment of infective native valve endocarditis. In prosthetic valve endocarditis, anticoagulation should be continued. Valvular lesions are often not propagating clots, and anticoagulation probably does not prevent pieces of vegetation from breaking off. Control of infection alone decreases the risk of embolization. Most cardiovascular surgeons replace the infected valve when infection is not controlled or when multiple emboli occur.

Infective Aneurysms

Septic emboli may lodge in small distal branches and cause inflammatory erosion of the arterial wall. The evolution of cerebral aneurysms is not clear.[79,80] Molinari and colleagues[79] suggested that pulsation against a necrotic wall produces fusiform aneurysms. However, *Staphylococcus aureus* frequently erodes the cerebral artery and may lead to early branch occlusions or small areas of subarachnoid hemorrhage after rupture of sulcal arteries[81,82] (Fig. 6–4).

Mycotic aneurysms may develop in multiple arteries. Those involved are the aorta, cerebral arteries, superior mesenteric artery and branches, and the vessels of the extremities. In a postmortem study from the preantibiotic era, Stengel and Wolferth[83] found more than one aneurysm in 41 of 217 cases (19%). Multiple mycotic aneurysm formation is not unique to certain bacterial species and may occur in 30% of all patients with documented mycotic aneurysms.[84,85] Mycotic aneurysms of the intracranial circulation are often located at distal branches of the middle cerebral artery (Fig. 6–5).

The incidence of ruptured mycotic aneurysm in infective endocarditis varies from 0.6% to 4%.[86–88] Size of the aneurysm probably is not relevant to the risk of rupture.[89] Mortality from ruptured bacterial aneurysm is high (50% to 60%) because rupture produces a large lobar hematoma, often with intraventricular extension, and hydrocephalus.

The clinical presentation of a ruptured mycotic aneurysm is variable and depends on the involved area.[90,91] Patients may have acute thunderclap-like headache followed by a decrease in level of consciousness, aphasia, eye deviation, and hemiparesis. An uncal herniation syndrome may occur within hours of presentation, leading to loss of most

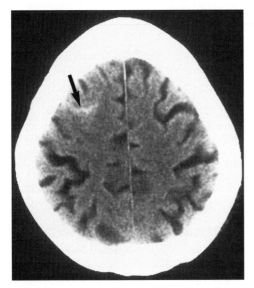
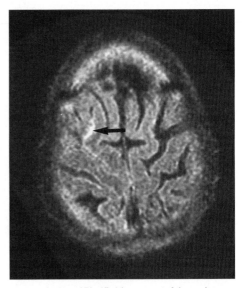

A   B

Figure 6–4. Computed tomography scan (*A*) and magnetic resonance image (*B*) (fluid-attenuated inversion recovery) showing subarachnoid hemorrhage in the sulcus typical in endocarditis (arrows).

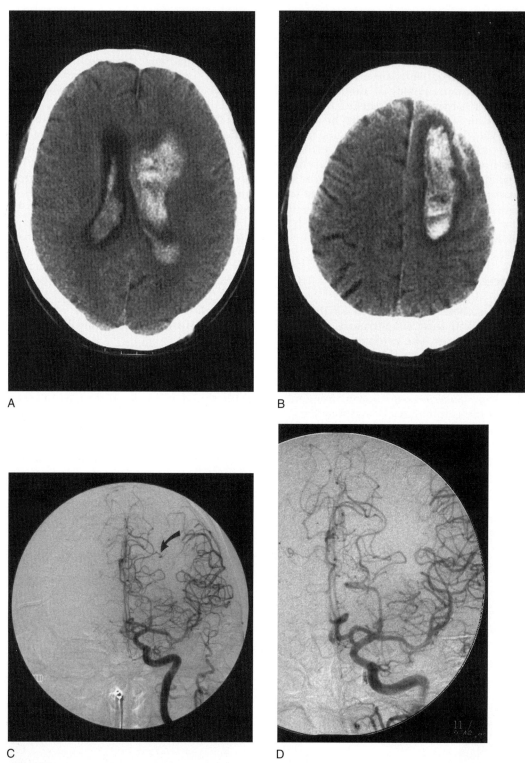

Figure 6–5. Computed tomographic (*A,B*) and angiographic (*C*) views of intracranial hemorrhage and mycotic aneurysm (arrow) inside the hematoma (note displacement of vasculature). After antibiotic treatment, the aneurysm disappeared (*D*).

104

mesencephalon and pontine brain stem reflexes.

Rupture 6 months after antibiotic treatment of endocarditis has been reported.[92] However, in a 1989 study that added 3 cases to the 67 cases of bacterial aneurysm reported in the literature since 1957, late rupture of mycotic aneurysm was rare.[88]

Infective aneurysms are probably more often present in patients with ischemic stroke and infective endocarditis.[87,93] Fundamental problems in the management of infective unruptured aneurysm are that the true incidence of cerebral aneurysms in patients with treated infective endocarditis is not known, although it may be as high as 15%,[94–96] and that no risk factors have been identified that predict rupture.[97–99] Also not entirely known is how many patients have complete disappearance of aneurysms after appropriate antibiotic treatment.[100] Current data suggest that infective aneurysms may disappear in 30% of patients, enlarge in 20%, decrease in size in 20%, increase in number in 15%, and remain unchanged in 15%. Resolution of the aneurysm may take 1 year but is not expected if the size of the lesion is greater than 7 or 8 mm. At the other extreme, patients may have early rupture at any point during the antibiotic therapy, with catastrophic consequences (up to 80% mortality).[101] Monitoring the aneurysms angiographically and trapping those that enlarge, as suggested by Bohmfalk and colleagues,[101] appear reasonable.

A suggested guideline for monitoring patients is presented in Figure 6–6. This guideline is based on indirect evidence and ideally should be tested in a new set of patients. Although both *Staphylococcus aureus* and *Aspergillus* are uncommon causes of endocarditis and difficult to detect, there is a high propensity for cerebral and systemic embolization with these organisms. Thus, evidence of systemic embolization, particularly ultrasonographic evidence of infectious emboli in liver and spleen, should strongly influence the decision to proceed with cerebral angiography to detect mycotic aneurysms. Magnetic resonance angiography or CT angiography can be used to monitor infectious aneurysms.[102,103] A study that analyzed the need for cerebral angiography in infective endocarditis concluded that it should not be routinely performed.[104] This

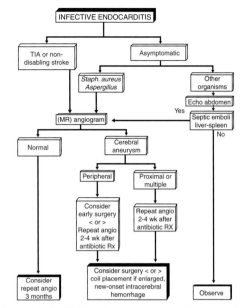

Figure 6–6. Guideline for management of neurologic complications of infective endocarditis. MR, magnetic resonance; Rx, therapy; TIA, transient ischemic attack.

study estimated a low mortality from ruptured mycotic aneurysm (25%) and therefore seriously skewed the data toward a conservative approach.

Peripheral aneurysms of the middle cerebral artery are usually easily excised surgically with very low morbidity and mortality. Proximal aneurysms (often distal to a large first branch) are more difficult to manage and may necessitate temporary occlusion of the vessel. In some patients, additional intracranial bypass grafting is necessary to supply the ischemic area.[105] Surgical clipping of a proximal infective aneurysm is difficult, and the infectious aneurysmal sac may easily break off.[106] Ligation of the arterial segment uninvolved by the process with excision of the aneurysm is another option. Endovascular occlusion with coils alone or combined with clipping may become a promising alternative treatment, and several isolated cases have been reported with good obliteration[107] (Table 6–8 and Fig. 6–7).

This entire proposition is different in patients who need valve replacement after infective endocarditis. Four-vessel angiograms are indicated in patients with mechanical valves who need lifelong anticoagulation.[114,115] When surgery is indicated and a

Table 6–8. Patients with Mycotic Aneurysms Caused by Infective Endocarditis Treated by the Endovascular Approach

Reference	Age (years), Sex	Clinical Presentation	Location	Material	Outcome
Khayata et al., 1993[108]	28, M	Hemorrhage	L PCA, distal	NBCA	Recovered
	44, M	Incidental	R MCA, rolandic branch	Autologous clot	Recovered
	39, M	Hemorrhage	R MCA, M_2; R PCA, calcarine branch	Balloon minicoils	Recovered
Frizzell et al., 1993[107]	44, M	Hemorrhage	L MCA, parietal branch	Coils	Recovered
Utoh et al., 1995[109]	42, M	Hemorrhage	R PCA, P_2	EVAL	Recovered
Katakura et al., 1995[110]	9, M	Hemorrhage	L parieto-occipital; L posterior parietal artery	Coils, NBCA	Recovered
		Enlargement	R anterior parietal artery; R central artery	Coils, NBCA	
Scotti et al., 1996[111]	56, M	Hemorrhage	R MCA, frontal branch	NBCA	Died
	39, F	Hemorrhage	R MCA, angular branch	NBCA	Recovered
Hashimoto et al., 1996[112]	41, M	Incidental	L PCA, P_3	Coils	Recovered
Watanabe et al., 1998[113]	56, M	Hemorrhage	R MCA, M_2; R posterior parietal artery	Coil	Recovered

EVAL, ethylene vinyl alcohol; L, left; MCA, middle cerebral artery; NBCA, N-butyl-cyanoacrylate glue; PCA, posterior cerebral artery; R, right.

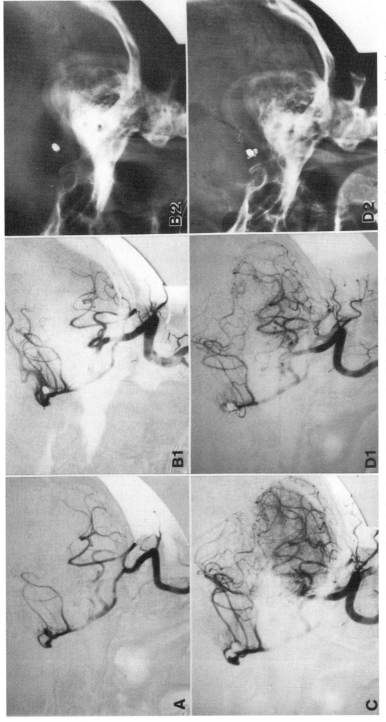

Figure 6-7. In a 45-year-old man with a lobulated mycotic aneurysm involving the distal basilar artery (*A*), platinum coils were inserted in the most worrisome lobule because it was believed to be the source of the bleeding; the other lobule was not amenable to coil occlusion (*B1,B2*). A follow-up angiogram 1 week later demonstrated enlargement of the nontreated lobule of the aneurysm (*C*), which was successfully clipped (*D1,D2*). (Courtesy of Dr. D. A. Nichols.)

mycotic aneurysm has been documented, a bioprosthetic valve is considered by the cardiovascular surgeon not only to obviate long-term anticoagulation but also to better resist recurrent endocarditis. There is no evidence that heparin treatment during cardiopulmonary bypass increases the risk of rupture. Valve replacement in a patient with a recent ischemic stroke may possibly convert it into a hemorrhage. However, in patients with embolic strokes that became hemorrhagic, the data on perioperative risk are conflicting. If possible, most surgeons would like to postpone valve replacement up to 4 weeks after the ictus.[116]

CLOSTRIDIAL SYNDROMES

The two most well-known infections with *Clostridium* species are tetanus and botulism. The neurotoxins producing botulism and tetanus act in different ways. Tetanus neurotoxin binds to the presynaptic membrane of the neuromuscular junction and is transported retroaxonally to the spinal cord. Spinal inhibitory interneurons block neurotransmitter release, leading to spastic paralysis. However, the botulism neurotoxin is at the periphery, causing a flaccid paralysis due to inhibition of acetylcholine release at the neuromuscular junction. Medical and neurologic management of these potentially life-threatening disorders is difficult also, because experience in handling these emergencies typically is absent.

The following sections may assist in management when one is suddenly faced with these disorders. Further details on epidemiology and pathology can be found in infectious disease textbooks or review papers.[117,118] The clostridial infection associated with gas gangrene is a predominantly local muscle infection and is not discussed here.

Botulism

Clostridium botulinum types A, B, and E spores produce a toxin that induces presynaptic inhibition of acetylcholine release. The toxin can be identified in serum or feces by a mouse toxin neutralization test that requires up to 2 days for completion. The clinical

manifestations can be protracted over months but more commonly last for hours to 1 week. Persistent vomiting follows the ingestion of contaminated food, such as frozen or undercooked meat or, more often, home-canned preparations of fruits and vegetables.[119–121] Wound botulism after contamination from soft tissue injury, compound fractures, or intravenous drug abuse is more easily missed because vomiting, abdominal cramps, and diarrhea are absent and wounds may be clean to the naked eye.

The neurologic manifestations follow one another fairly rapidly (Table 6–9). Initially, difficulty with focusing to a near point or diplopia is seen. Dilated pupils with sluggish light response are a sine qua non, often with oculobulbar muscle weakness due to involvement of cranial nerves VI, IX–X, XII, and III (in decreasing order of frequency).[122] Complete bilateral internal ophthalmoplegia without progression to limb weakness has been reported.[123] Ptosis is usually present, whereas dilated pupils may be absent. A typical progression in botulism is prominent ocular signs, dysphagia, and slurred speech, which are followed by diaphragmatic failure and quadriplegia over days.[124] In addition to the descending pattern, preserved tendon reflexes, absent paresthesias, preserved sensory responses, and normal CSF protein concentration may serve to differentiate it from much more frequent Guillain-Barré syndrome.

Autonomic dysfunction is common.[125] Most patients spontaneously mention constipation, orthostatic hypotension, diminished lacrimation, decreased salivation resulting in dry mouth, and urinary retention.[125,126] Rapid, wide swings in blood pressure, such as in tetanus, are not part of the clinical description. Electrodiagnostic testing is diag-

Table 6–9. **Clinical Features of Botulism**

Dilated (sluggish) pupils
Ptosis
Ophthalmoplegia
Facial diplegia
Absent gag reflex
Limb weakness
Hyporeflexia

nostic with normal motor and sensory conduction velocities (differentiating it from Guillain-Barré syndrome), with a gradually decreasing response of the compound muscle action potential to 2 to 3 Hz stimulation in proximal muscles, reduced compound muscle action potential to a supramaximal nerve stimulus, and increased jitter and blocking with single-fiber electromyography.[127,128]

Supportive care with mechanical ventilation is often the only option until the manifestations subside. Most patients have remarkable improvement within 1 month, but in certain cases, prolonged mechanical ventilation has been necessary up to 11 weeks after onset.[129] Improvement can be expected within 2 weeks; therefore, tracheostomy should not be routinely performed in every patient, and one should allow time for spontaneous improvement in pulmonary function measured by vital capacity and maximal inspiratory pressure.

Claims of other therapies have been anecdotal. Guanidine hydrochloride may perhaps improve limb muscle weakness.[130] Polyvalent antitoxin is ineffective once neurologic symptoms are present, and no effect on diaphragmatic muscle strength has been documented. Edrophonium, 10 mg intravenously, may improve the ocular manifestations, muscle weakness, and even diaphragmatic function, but its effect is transient. As an additional therapeutic agent, 4-aminopyridine may be considered, but it has occasionally been associated with seizures. Plasma exchange should be considered, particularly because marked, almost immediate improvement occurred in a patient with wound botulism.[124] Corticosteroids and intravenous immunoglobulin had no measurable effect.

Tetanus

In developed Third World countries, infection with *Clostridium tetani* remains a considerable health problem. In the United States, the incidence is 0.04 per 100,000, and this infection often occurs in elderly persons who have not received a primary series of tetanus toxoid. The incubation period to trismus and reflex spasm varies from several days to months.

The clinical diagnosis of generalized tetanus is made with relative ease because virtually no other disease produces the set of findings consisting of trismus (lockjaw), risus sardonicus (Fig. 6–8), reflex muscle spasm precipitated by touch, laryngospasm, sym-

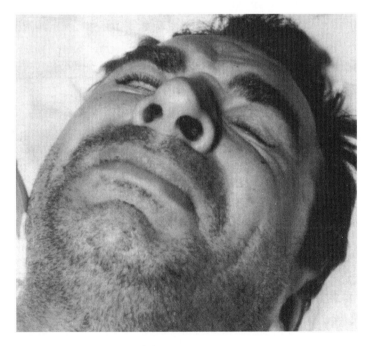

Figure 6–8. Risus sardonicus: Fixed grinning smile from facial musculature contraction. (From Sutter RW, Orenstein WA, Wassilak SG. Tetanus. In: Hoeprich PD, Jordan MC, Ronald AR [eds]. Infectious Diseases: A Treatise of Infectious Processes, 5th ed. JB Lippincott, Philadelphia, 1994, pp 1175–1185. Courtesy of E. Erikson, Karolinska Sjukhuset, Stockholm.)

Table 6–10. **Clinical Features of Tetanus**

Localized or generalized weakness
Stiffness
Difficulty chewing
Trismus
Risus sardonicus
Reflex spasm
Opisthotonos
Laryngospasm
Sympathetic storm

---

pathetic storm, and swiftly developing respiratory failure[117] (Table 6–10). Reflex spasm, besides being extraordinarily painful, may result in often unrecognized instances of tendon rupture, fractures, and rhabdomyolysis. Tetanus is the result of the blocking of inhibitory neurons at the level of the synapse with the alpha motor neuron and loss of inhibition by the intermediolateral cells in the spinal cord. This imbalance causes the excitation and sympathetic storm and can be fatal if not appropriately blunted by muscle-relaxing agents, sedation, and narcotic agents.

Basic management consists of tetanus toxoid (500 to 3000 U), tetanus immune globulin, metronidazole (500 mg every 6 hr), and debridement of the wound, if identified. As mentioned earlier, spiraling respiratory failure may develop in a patient with evolving tetanus. Underdetection may therefore result in delayed intubation and ventilation, which may contribute to aspiration, an important cause of death.[131] Initial management concentrates on neuromuscular blockade with vecuronium or pancuronium, usually guided by a peripheral nerve stimulator (see Chapter 2). Intrathecal injections with baclofen (800 to 1000 μg) are effective and have prevented mechanical ventilation or reduced the time on the ventilator in preliminary studies.[132,133] Dantrolene as an intravenous bolus of 1 mg/kg resolved muscle spasm in a case report, and manifestations of tetanus were milder.[134] Adequate sedation is achieved with midazolam (5 to 15 mg/hr) or lorazepam (50 mg/hr). Magnesium sulfate in doses similar to those in eclampsia

(see Chapter 13) also obviated mechanical ventilation in a recent unconfirmed report. Eight patients from Sri Lanka were treated with a loading dose of 5 g of magnesium sulfate and infusion of 2 g/hr until control of cramps or loss of the patellar reflex. Treatment was successful in all patients within hours.[135]

Dysautonomia remains a challenging management problem, and cardiac arrest is the most common cause of death in most large series.[136] A complete spectrum of bradycardia, sweating, salivation, and rapid swings in blood pressure may be seen. Sudden episodes of tachycardia and hypertension are best muted with a morphine bolus (5 to 30 mg intravenously over 30 min) (Fig. 6–9). Beta-blockers have been linked to sudden cardiac arrest and should be avoided.

Intensive care management has remarkably reduced mortality, but it may reach 13%.[137] Time on the ventilator is often at least 3 to 6 weeks, and, therefore, tracheostomy should be considered early in the disease. Outcome is less favorable in patients who need intubation.

SEPSIS

Sepsis can be divided into that from an identified source of infection and a systemic response to that infection. The genitourinary tract is the most common site of infection, and bacteremia is often initiated by instrumentation of this area. Other common foci are gastrointestinal and respiratory infections, wound infections, burns, pelvic infections, and contaminated intravenous or arterial catheters. Septic shock denotes circulatory collapse that develops as a complication of an overwhelming infection, often related to gram-negative enteric bacteria. *Escherichia coli* (followed by the *Klebsiella–Enterobacter–Serratia* group and *Pseudomonas*) remains the predominant pathogen in septic shock. Cultures of material from the presumed source of infection may be useful, but only 50% of patients with clinical sepsis have positive blood cultures.

The systemic response in sepsis is not circulatory collapse but a hyperdynamic and hypermetabolic reaction. Oxidative metabolism is compromised; therefore, lactate in ar-

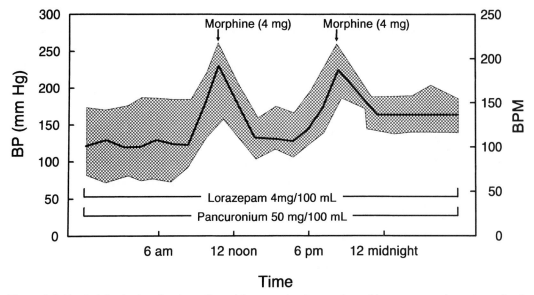

Figure 6–9. Two brief episodes of tachycardia and hypertension in a patient with tetanus are almost immediately muted by intravenous administration of morphine. Inadequate neuromuscular relaxation and sedation or hypovolemia should always be considered as alternative possibilities. Upper boundary of the cross-hatched area is systolic pressure; lower boundary is diastolic pressure. Solid line is heart rate. BP, blood pressure; BPM, beats per minute.

terial blood is increased. This increase has been considered a sign of global decrease in tissue perfusion and is recognized as an indication of poor prognosis. Urinary output is decreased (output less than 30 mL or 0.5 mL/kg for at least 1 hr). Important clinical manifestations are increased cardiac output with low systemic vascular resistance, proteolysis leading to excessive loss of visceral proteins, and increased urinary secretion of nitrogen.

The leukocyte count increases to levels exceeding 20,000 cells/mm³, with a shift to immature polynuclear cells. Decreased platelet counts may reflect disseminated intravascular clotting. Its severity may be determined by host susceptibility.[138]

Sepsis may be followed by rapidly fatal or meandering organ failure. An important complication is the adult respiratory distress syndrome, characterized by severe hypoxemia and increased stiffness of the lungs. The pathologic features of adult respiratory distress syndrome consist of pulmonary capillary congestion, endothelial cell swelling, and microatelectasis followed by fluid leakage, fibrin deposition, and hyaline membranes leading to microvascular destruction.

The transition to multiorgan failure has a poor prognosis and a significant risk of mortality (40% to 80%). Hepatic failure is rapidly followed by progressive renal failure, although the sequence of organ failure may vary greatly. Total body protein catabolism is markedly increased, with rapid loss of skeletal muscle mass, often referred to as "autocannibalism."[139] The American College of Chest Physicians and the Society of Critical Care Medicine Consensus Conference issued a set of definitions[140] (Table 6–11 and Fig. 6–10). The deleterious effects of sepsis on the peripheral and central nervous systems are now well recognized.

PATHOPHYSIOLOGIC MECHANISMS

The categorical definitions of sepsis and septic shock were created to standardize clinical trials, but the artificial grading of clinical responses may be incorrect, theoretical at best, and may not even have application in clinical practice. It has been suggested that after any trigger (for example, infection, trauma, pancreatitis), cytokines (tumor necrosis factor, interleukin-1β, interleukin-6, and interleukin-8)[141] are produced to evoke an inflammatory response

Table 6–11. **Definitions of Sepsis and Organ Failure**

Infection

Microbial phenomenon characterized by an inflammatory response to microorganisms or the invasion of normally sterile host tissue by those organisms

Bacteremia

Viable bacteria in the blood

Systemic Inflammatory Response Syndrome

The systemic inflammatory response to a variety of severe clinical insults. The response is manifested by two or more of the following conditions: (*1*) temperature >38°C or <36°C; (*2*) heart rate >90 beats per minute; (*3*) respiratory rate >20 breaths/min or Pa_{CO_2} <32 mm Hg; and (*4*) leukocyte count >12,000/mm³, <4,000/mm³, or >10% immature (band) forms

Sepsis

The systemic response to infection, manifested by two or more of the following conditions as a result of infection: (*1*) temperature >38°C or <36°C; (*2*) heart rate >90 beats/min; (*3*) respiratory rate >20 breaths/min or Pa_{CO_2} <32 mm Hg; and (*4*) leukocyte count >12,000/mm³, <4,000/mm³, or >10% immature (band) forms

Severe Sepsis

Sepsis associated with organ dysfunction, hypoperfusion, or hypotension. Hypoperfusion and perfusion abnormalities may include, but are not limited to, lactic acidosis, oliguria, and an acute alteration in mental status.

Septic Shock

Sepsis-induced with hypotension despite adequate fluid resuscitation, along with perfusion abnormalities that may include, but are not limited to, lactic acidosis, oliguria, and an acute alteration in mental status. Patients receiving inotropic or vasopressor agents may not be hypotensive at the time that perfusion abnormalities are measured.

Sepsis-induced Hypotension

A systolic blood pressure <90 mm Hg or a reduction of ≥40 mm Hg from baseline in the absence of other causes for hypotension

Multiple Organ Dysfunction Syndrome

Organ function altered in an acutely ill patient in such a way that homeostasis cannot be maintained without intervention

From Bone et al.[140] By permission of the American College of Chest Physicians.

and to prompt defense mechanisms and recruitment of macrophages and platelets.[142]

The initial inflammatory response can be restricted by down-regulating cytokine production (for example, interleukin-4, interleukin-10, interleukin-11, tumor necrosis receptors) to prevent destruction. Failure to mute this response may lead to the next stage, which results in an overwhelming system response, amplification and systemic vasodilatation, depression of myocardial contractility, and other end-organ dysfunction. Many patients die of shock and pulmonary edema. The current conceptional thinking on the development of multiple organ dysfunction is shown in Figure 6–11.

Five stages in the development of multiple organ dysfunction have been proposed, but the time course needs further investigation and refinement. Stage 1 begins at a site of local injury or infection. Proinflammatory mediators are released locally to promote wound healing and to combat foreign organisms or antigens. Anti-inflammatory mediators are then released to down-regulate this process. If the original insult is small and

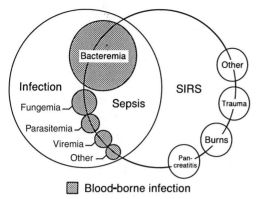

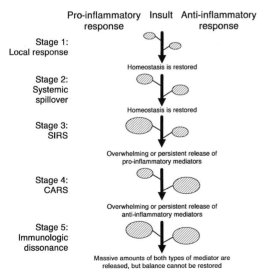

Figure 6–10. Relationship of infection, sepsis, and systemic inflammatory response syndrome (SIRS) to one another (see Table 6–10 for definitions of terms). (From Bone et al.[140] By permission of the American College of Chest Physicians.)

the patient was in good prior health, homeostasis is quickly restored. Stage 2 occurs if local defense mechanisms are insufficient to correct the local injury or eliminate the local infection. Through various mechanisms, proinflammatory mediators are released into the systemic circulation; they recruit additional cells to the local area of injury. Systemic release of anti-inflammatory mediators soon follows; under normal circumstances, these mediators ameliorate the proinflammatory reaction and restore ho-

Figure 6–11. Five stages in the development of multiple organ dysfunction (see text).

meostasis. Stage 3 occurs if the systemic release of proinflammatory mediators is massive or if the anti-inflammatory reaction is insufficient to permit down-regulation. At this stage, most patients have symptoms of systemic inflammatory response syndrome (SIRS) and incipient evidence of multiple organ dysfunction syndrome (MODS). Stage 3 can be represented by excessive systemic levels of anti-inflammatory mediators that develop as a response to a massive proinflammatory response; however, these levels can also develop de novo. Patients with a stage 4 compensatory anti-inflammatory response syndrome (CARS) have marked immunosuppression and thus are at increased risk for infection. If the body can reestablish homeostasis after stage 3 or 4, the patient may survive. Stage 5 is the final stage of MODS. At this stage of immunologic dissonance, the balance between pro- and anti-inflammatory mediators has been lost. Some patients may have persistent, massive inflammation; others may have continuing immunosuppression and secondary infections. Still others may have oscillation between periods of inflammation and immunosuppression.

The spectrum of these responses has been termed "CHAOS": **c**ardiovascular shock, **h**omeostasis, **a**poptosis, **o**rgan dysfunction, and immuno**s**uppression. Future studies are focusing on modulation of the systemic inflammatory response syndrome. Interleukins, transforming growth factor-β, colony-stimulating factors, soluble receptors to tumor necrosis factor, and receptor antagonists to interleukin-1 contribute to and open a more rational approach to clinical trials.[143]

Critical Illness Polyneuropathy

The true prevalence of critical illness polyneuropathy (CIP) in critically ill patients remains unknown, but it probably occurs in 5% to 20% of all patients with severe sepsis and in 50% of all patients remaining in the ICU for more than 2 weeks.[144–149] When electrodiagnostic criteria are used, CIP develops in 58% of patients younger than 75 years who are mechanically ventilated for more than 7 days.[150] Critical illness neuropathy is not invariably associated with sepsis, having been reported in patients with severe burns.[151,152] The initial clinical observations can be credited to Roelofs and associates[153] and Bolton and co-workers[145,154] (who coined the term), although similar observations have been made by others, particularly Op de Coul et al.[147–150] In a comprehensive description by Zochodne and colleagues,[155] 5 patients were seen in a 4-year period and 14 patients in the next 2 years, probably a result of increased recognition of the disorder. After many years of clinical research, no specific cause has yet been found.[155–168]

PATHOPHYSIOLOGIC MECHANISMS

Important findings in CIP are decreased albumin and lymphocyte counts, suggestive of a general nutritional deficit, despite adequate nutrition in all patients. Patients with sepsis frequently have a negative energy balance, but the nutritional status (vitamin or spore elements) in relation to the appearance of CIP has not been adequately assessed. A direct toxic effect or effect of a mediator in the inflammatory response of sepsis directed to the nerve (for example, tumor necrosis factor) is mostly speculative. In a prospective study of sepsis-related critical illness polyneuropathy, Witt and colleagues[156] analyzed predictive factors for CIP and found that time in the ICU, hypoalbuminemia, and relative hyperglycemia significantly correlated with electrophysiologic findings. A specific bacterial pathogen has not emerged, but it may not have been carefully looked for or cultured. Bolton[157] postulated a disturbance of the nerve microvasculation. Increased microvascular permeability due to cytokines, such as tumor necrosis factor, serotonin, or histamine, may increase the toxicity of neuromuscular blocking agents or perhaps antibiotics such as aminoglycosides. Alternative, unproven concepts are impaired transport of axonal proteins, a cytokine-induced direct toxic effect on nerves, and a yet-undefined low-molecular-weight substance.[158–161]

Until recently, "failure to wean" marked the first neurologic consultation.[162] Severe

paradoxical breathing indicative of diaphragmatic and intercostal weakness due to axonal degeneration of the phrenic and intercostal nerves has been noted. It is not entirely clear whether phrenic nerve involvement is the main cause of failure to wean in these patients. Weaning is difficult in any patient after long-term mechanical ventilation, often from inadequate respiratory musculature (disuse atrophy) or more commonly from other contributory factors, such as poor nutrition and chronic lung disease.

On neurologic examination, grimacing may be weak, but other cranial nerves are normal. Ocular signs, swallowing, tongue protrusion, and biting remain normal during the clinical course (Table 6–12). Limb weakness is usually severe, worse distally, with prominent wasting (Plate 6–2). Tendon reflexes are reduced or absent in most patients but may be preserved.[164] Complete quadriplegia is occasionally seen, with sparing of sensation and cranial nerves ("talking heads"). Dysautonomia is conspicuously absent, but specific laboratory studies have not been performed to confirm its absence. Good recovery in months with return of reflexes has been claimed for patients surviving the systemic illness, including the patients seen by the author and associates[165] at Mayo Clinic hospitals. Predictive factors for recovery are not known, but the patient with the most severe quadriplegia may completely recover, to everyone's surprise. Failure to improve, noted in 22% of all 1-year survivors, may be related to severe axonal destruction or superimposed compression neuropathies.[150,165] The disorder may resolve in

Table 6–12. **Clinical Features of Critical Illness Polyneuropathy**

Mild facial weakness
Normal ocular signs
Symmetrical (usually distal) limb weakness
Reduced or absent tendon reflexes
Variable muscle wasting and fasciculations
Diaphragmatic and intercostal weakness
Frequent associated encephalopathy
Normal autonomic function

a stereotypical manner. Improvement occurs first in the upper and proximal lower limbs, successful weaning follows, and later the distal portion of the lower limbs improves.

Most electrophysiologic studies have been done at the peak of severity. Characteristic findings are reduced amplitudes of both compound muscle and sensory nerve action potentials relative to normal conduction velocities, widespread fibrillation potentials, positive sharp waves, and sporadic myotonic or complex repetitive discharges.[144,166] Some electrophysiologic studies have found predominant motor fiber involvement.[167] Results of neuromuscular transmission studies are normal. Phrenic nerve conduction often is bilaterally absent in accordance with the autopsy finding of axonal damage. Needle examination of the external oblique and external intercostal muscles may show evidence of denervation or loss of rhythmic recruitment with breathing. (These findings may have no significance if a recent car-diopulmonary bypass with hypothermia has been performed, which may damage the phrenic nerve [Chapter 15].)

Autopsy and sural nerve biopsy specimens show severe axonal degeneration of peripheral nerves, mostly in the distal segments (Fig. 6–12). Loss of myelinated fibers may be seen, but remyelinization is often absent.[165] Some studies showed occasional mononuclear cells and lipid-laden macrophages, but infiltrates were not recognized in muscle and nerve biopsy specimens.[166,168] Muscle biopsy tissue showed muscle fiber necrosis and type grouping in patients with increased levels of creatine kinase.[166] It should, however, be noted that muscle biopsy specimens from the soleus (often taken at the time of sural nerve biopsy) may not be reliable because of pressure necrosis caused by prolonged immobility. In the most severe of 11 cases of axonal polyneuropathy of critical illness seen at the Mayo Clinic by the author, biopsy tissue taken from iliopsoas muscle

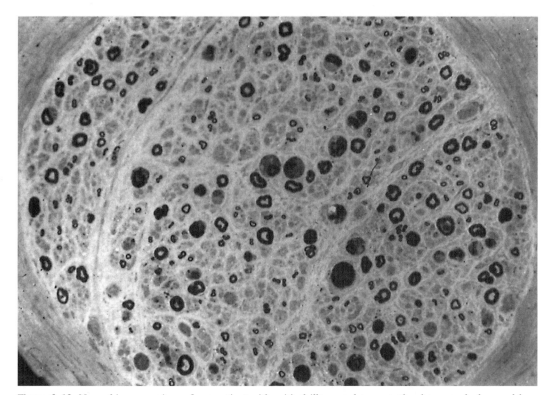

Figure 6–12. Nerve biopsy specimen from patient with critical illness polyneuropathy shows marked axonal loss. Many fibers are undergoing wallerian degeneration.

showed neurogenic changes but also numerous regenerating fibers of similar age, which suggested a monophasic impact to the muscle.

MANAGEMENT

Supportive care remains the only available option and should include passive range of motion with physical therapy, protection of nerve compression sites (particularly ulnar and peroneal nerves), and splinting or braces when patients can support their own weight but are limited by profound distal muscle weakness. Specific therapy is not available. Three patients with CIP treated at our institution with intravenously administered gamma globulin did not have improvement in 2 months.[163] However, a post hoc analysis of a prospective series of 62 patients with sepsis-induced multiorgan failure suggested a possible effect of early (less than 24 hr after diagnosis) intravenous administration of immunoglobulin, indicated by a reduced incidence of CIP.[169] The potential effects of early administration of immunoglobulin should be studied carefully before this very costly therapy is routinely administered to patients with severe sepsis. Plasma exchange or corticosteroids have been used in anecdotal cases but again without dramatic improvement.

Sepsis-Associated Encephalopathy

The term "septic encephalopathy" has not gained universal acceptance or credibility, largely because many clinical manifestations of sepsis can produce brain injury that may reduce level of consciousness. The term "septic encephalopathy" should be discouraged. Labeling the condition "multifactorial" does not help in elucidation of the entity, if it exists at all.[170–173]

CLINICAL FEATURES

The initial clinical manifestations of sepsis are nonspecific. Patients are confused, disoriented, and restless. In the earlier stages, many patients have tachypnea and hyper-ventilation. These may be a result of circulating immunologic mediators on respiratory drive in the brain stem or a result of early lung injury. Therefore, the central nervous system manifestations in early sepsis may be a confusional state or delirium and a direct result of hypercapnia, hypoxemia, hyperthermia, or of all three. Unless marked hypotension or hypoxia develops from rapidly evolving adult respiratory distress syndrome, confusion generally does not progress into coma. Typically, patients are intubated, paralyzed, or sedated and cannot be evaluated properly during management of septic shock and multiple organ failure. Frequently, neurologists are consulted when the acute episode has been mastered and the patient remains unresponsive. At that time, these patients may have survived episodes of severe hypoglycemia, cardiac arrhythmias, diffuse intravascular coagulation, and renal and hepatic failure.

The true incidence and degree of encephalopathy associated with sepsis are not exactly known. Reasons are lack of systematic studies by neurologists and poor characterization of this type of encephalopathy. In a large Veterans Administration study, "septic encephalopathy" was defined as altered mental status as judged by behavioral or cognitive abnormalities.[171] Young and colleagues[172] defined septic encephalopathy as difficulty with attention, recall, and orientation, but these features may be very difficult to accurately assess in very sick patients. In their study, the diagnosis was made in 49 of 69 patients, and 16 were in a coma with less than "nonpurposeful movements to pain."[172] A study from Israel defined septic encephalopathy as "altered mental status" or decrease in Glasgow coma score, and 50% to 70% of the patients were then thought to have encephalopathy due to sepsis.[170] In our retrospective study[173] of 84 patients with surgical sepsis, 14 had decrease in level of consciousness beyond drowsiness and half were unresponsive to pain. Myoclonic jerks and seizures occurred occasionally but were rare. Persistent focal signs were absent.

Many patients with encephalopathy associated with sepsis had severe episodes of hypotension, often managed with increasing doses of inotropic medication. In our study, the contribution of other elements of organ failure (renal, coagulopathy) was not significant in a logistic regression, a strong suggestion that septic encephalopathy is hypoxic–ischemic in origin.[174] Cerebral blood flow is decreased in sepsis, with concordant changes in cerebral oxygen extraction ratios, and severe hypotension may augment the decrease in cerebral perfusion.[175]

Other potential mechanisms for "septic encephalopathy," not thoroughly explored, are disordered amino acid transport similar to that in hepatic encephalopathy[176–178] and primary infection of the central nervous system. Pendlebury and colleagues[179] found a high frequency of microabscesses in the brains of autopsied patients, but this mechanism in the absence of endocarditis seems highly improbable.

DIAGNOSTIC TESTS

The CT scan findings in patients after a bout of severe sepsis have remained normal, but magnetic resonance images are emerging that at least in one recent study showed multiple lesions, indicating cerebritis and abscess.[180] Electroencephalography may document a nonspecific spectrum of abnormalities, including excessive delta waves, triphasic waves, or burst suppression, and these patterns are associated with mortality exceeding 50%.[181] Somatosensory evoked potentials are nonspecific, mainly showing delay of the N_{70} response in more severe cases of encephalopathy with multiorgan failure. Its value for prognostication seems marginal.[182]

A systematic study of neuroimaging and pathology is needed to evaluate this type of encephalopathy. The MRIs of two of our patients with coma after septic shock revealed significant widespread white matter changes indicative of ischemia in watershed zones and also hyperintensities in the putamen and globus pallidus (a consequence of parenteral nutrition).

CONCLUSIONS

Allowing the pathogen in sepsis to induce a massive inflammatory response greatly decreases the chances of survival, and early recognition and intervention, if possible, are paramount. Vigorous efforts to define sepsis and systemic inflammatory syndrome continue. Underlying these discussions of definition is the attempt to develop adequate and cost-effective therapies for a frequently fatal disease.

The focus, however, has widened, and more insights into neurologic complications of sepsis have been gained. Major deficiencies in our understanding of the two main manifestations, sepsis-associated encephalopathy and critical illness polyneuropathy, remain. Coma or considerable change in cognitive function during or after sepsis predicts poor outcome. In many of these patients, hypoxic–ischemic insult may be a major contender. In other patients with a decrease in responsiveness, the findings can be caused by the effects of disseminated intravascular coagulation, multiple intracranial hemorrhages (Chapter 11), multiple embolic strokes, or, very unusually, cerebral abscesses.

Critical care physicians and cardiovascular surgeons frequently call in neurologists for patients with endocarditis. No data validate one approach over another, but the increased risk of mycotic aneurysm in patients with transient ischemic attacks, nondisabling stroke, or endocarditis from *Staphylococcus aureus* or *Aspergillus* dictates a more aggressive approach. This consists of follow-up with MRI and angiography and possible surgical intervention or coil placement when the aneurysm is still present or has enlarged after a course of antibiotic therapy.

REFERENCES

1. Mylotte JM, McDermott C, Spooner JA. Prospective study of 114 consecutive episodes of *Staphylococcus aureus* bacteremia. Rev Infect Dis 9:891–907, 1987.
2. Deutschman CS, Wilton P, Sinow J, Dibbell D Jr, Konstantinides FN, Cerra FB. Paranasal sinusitis associated with nasotracheal intubation: a frequently unrecognized and treatable source of sepsis. Crit Care Med 14:111–114, 1986.
3. Holzapfel L, Chastang C, Demingeon G, Bohe J, Piralla B, Coupry A. A randomized study assessing the systematic search for maxillary sinusitis in nasotracheally mechanically ventilated patients. Influence of nosocomial maxillary sinusitis on the

occurrence of ventilator-associated pneumonia. Am J Respir Crit Care Med 159:695–701, 1999.

4. Carter BL, Bankoff MS, Fisk JD. Computed tomographic detection of sinusitis reponsible for intracranial and extracranial infections. Radiology 147:739–742, 1983.

5. Eustis HS, Mafee MF, Walton C, Mondonca J. MR imaging and CT of orbital infections and complications in acute rhinosinusitis. Radiol Clin North Am 36:1165–1183, 1998.

6. Lew D, Southwick FS, Montgomery WW, Weber AL, Baker AS. Sphenoid sinusitis. A review of 30 cases. N Engl J Med 309:1149–1154, 1983.

7. Kilpatrick ME, Girgis NI. Meningitis—a complication of spinal anesthesia. Anesth Analg 62:513–515, 1983.

8. Lanska DJ, Lanska MJ, Selman WR. Meningitis following spinal puncture in a patient with a CSF leak. Neurology 39:306–307, 1989.

9. Lee JJ, Parry H. Bacterial meningitis following spinal anaesthesia for caesarean section. Br J Anaesth 66:383–386, 1991.

10. Bouhemad B, Dounas M, Mercier FJ, Benhamou D. Bacterial meningitis following combined spinal-epidural analgesia for labour. Anesthesia 33:292–295, 1998.

11. Teman AJ. Spinal epidural abscess. Early detection with gadolinium magnetic resonance imaging. Arch Neurol 49:743–746, 1992.

12. Denning DW, Gill SS. *Neisseria lactamica* meningitis following skull trauma. Rev Infect Dis 13:216–218, 1991.

13. Choi D, Spann R. Traumatic cerebrospinal fluid leakage: risk factors and the use of prophylactic antibiotics. Br J Neurosurg 10:571–575, 1996.

14. Bernal-Sprekelsen M, Bleda-Vazquez C, Carrau RL. Ascending meningitis secondary to traumatic cerebrospinal fluid leaks. Am J Rhinol 14:257–259, 2000.

15. Ignelzi RJ, VanderArk GD. Analysis of the treatment of basilar skull fractures with and without antibiotics. J Neurosurg 43:721–726, 1975.

16. Gordon MF, Allon M, Coyle PK. Drug-induced meningitis. Neurology 40:163–164, 1990.

17. Hoppmann RA, Peden JG, Ober SK. Central nervous system side effects of nonsteroidal anti-inflammatory drugs. Aseptic meningitis, psychosis, and cognitive dysfunction. Arch Intern Med 151:1309–1313, 1991.

18. Joffe AM, Farley JD, Linden D, Goldsand G. Trimethoprim-sulfamethoxazole-associated aseptic meningitis: case reports and review of the literature. Am J Med 87:332–338, 1989.

19. Carpenter RR, Petersdorf RG. The clinical spectrum of bacterial meningitis. Am J Med 33:262–275, 1962.

20. Gallagher RM, Gross CW, Phillips CD. Suppurative intracranial complications of sinusitis. Laryngoscope 108:1635–1642, 1998.

21. Swartz MN, Dodge PR. Bacterial meningitis—a review of selected aspects. 1. General clinical features, special problems and unusual meningeal reactions mimicking bacterial meningitis. N Engl J Med 272:779–787, 1965.

22. Conly JM, Ronald AR. Cerebrospinal fluid as a diagnostic body fluid. Am J Med 75 (Special Issue 1B):102–108, 1983.

23. Archer BD. Computed tomography before lumbar puncture in acute meningitis: a review of the risks and benefits. Can Med Assoc J 148:961–965, 1993.

24. Talan DA, Hoffman JR, Yoshikawa TT, Overturf GD. Role of empiric parenteral antibiotics prior to lumbar puncture in suspected bacterial meningitis: state of the art. Rev Infect Dis 10:365–376, 1988.

25. del Rio MA, Chrane D, Shelton S, McCracken GH Jr, Nelson JD. Ceftriaxone versus ampicillin and chloramphenicol for treatment of bacterial meningitis in children. Lancet 1:1241–1244, 1983.

26. Chang KH, Han MH, Roh JK, Kim IO, Han MC, Kim CW. Gd-DTPA-enhanced MR imaging of the brain in patients with meningitis: comparison with CT. AJNR Am J Neuroradiol 11:69–76, 1990.

27. Vernino S, Wijdicks EFM, McGough PF. Coma in fulminant pneumococcal meningitis: new MRI observations. Neurology 51:1200–1202, 1998.

28. Cherubin CE, Eng RH, Norrby R, Modai J, Humberg G, Overturf G. Penetration of newer cephalosporins into cerebrospinal fluid. Rev Infect Dis 11:526–548, 1989.

29. Tunkel AR, Wispelwey B, Scheld WM. Bacterial meningitis: recent advances in pathophysiology and treatment. Ann Intern Med 112:610–623, 1990.

30. Geiseler PJ, Nelson KE, Levin S, Reddi KT, Moses VK. Community-acquired purulent meningitis: a review of 1,316 cases during the antibiotic era, 1954–1976. Rev Infect Dis 2:725–745, 1980.

31. Behrman RE, Meyers BR, Mendelson MH, Sacks HS, Hirschman SZ. Central nervous system infections in the elderly. Arch Intern Med 149:1596–1599, 1989.

32. Pfister HW, Feiden W, Einhaupl KM. Spectrum of complications during bacterial meningitis in adults. Results of a prospective clinical study. Arch Neurol 50:575–581, 1993.

33. Baker AS, Ojemann RG, Swartz MN, Richardson EP Jr. Spinal epidural abscess. N Engl J Med 293:463–468, 1975.

34. Danner RL, Hartman BJ. Update on spinal epidural abscess: 35 cases and review of the literature. Rev Infect Dis 9:265–274, 1987.

35. Akalan N, Ozgen T. Infection as a cause of spinal cord compression: a review of 36 spinal epidural abscess cases. Acta Neurochir (Wien) 142:17–23, 2000.

36. Clark R, Carlisle JT, Valainis GT. *Streptococcus pneumoniae* endocarditis presenting as an epidural abscess. Rev Infect Dis 11:338–340, 1989.

37. Harries-Jones R, Hernandez-Bronchud M, Anslow P, Davies CJ. Meningitis and spinal subdural empyema as a complication of sinusitis [letter]. J Neurol Neurosurg Psychiatry 53:441, 1990.

38. Kaufman DM, Kaplan JG, Litman N. Infectious agents in spinal epidural abscesses. Neurology 30:844–850, 1980.

39. Verner EF, Musher DM. Spinal epidural abscess. Med Clin North Am 69:375–384, 1985.

40. Kricun R, Shoemaker EI, Chovanes GI, Stephens HW. Epidural abscess of the cervical spine: MR findings in five cases. AJR Am J Roentgenol 158:1145–1149, 1992.

41. Lasker BR, Harter DH. Cervical epidural abscess. Neurology 37:1747–1753, 1987.

42. Mackenzie AR, Laing RB, Smith CC, Kaar GF, Smith FW. Spinal epidural abscess: the importance of early diagnosis and treatment. J Neurol Neurosurg Psychiatry 65:209–212, 1998.

43. Angtuaco EJC, McConnell JR, Chadduck WM, Flanigan S. MR imaging of spinal epidural sepsis. AJNR Am J Neuroradiol 8:879–883, 1987.

44. Post MJ, Quencer RM, Montalvo BM, Katz BH, Eismont FJ, Green BA. Spinal infection: evaluation with MR imaging and intraoperative US. Radiology 169:765–771, 1988.

45. Erntell M, Holtas S, Norlin K, Dahlquist E, Nilsson-Ehle I. Magnetic resonance imaging in the diagnosis of spinal epidural abscess. Scand J Infect Dis 20:323–327, 1988.

46. Nussbaum ES, Rockswold GL, Bergman TA, Erickson DL, Seljeskog EL. Spinal tuberculosis: a diagnostic and management challenge. J Neurosurg 83:243–247, 1995.

47. Leys D, Lesoin F, Viaud C, et al. Decreased morbidity from acute bacterial spinal epidural abscesses using computed tomography and nonsurgical treatment in selected patients. Ann Neurol 17:350–355, 1985.

48. Mampalam TJ, Rosegay H, Andrews BT, Rosenblum ML, Pitts LH. Nonoperative treatment of spinal epidural infections. J Neurosurg 71:208–210, 1989.

49. Khanna RK, Malik GM, Rock JP, Rosenblum ML. Spinal epidural abscess: evaluation of factors influencing outcome. Neurosurgery 39:958–964, 1996.

50. Griffin MR, Wilson WR, Edwards WD, O'Fallon WM, Kurland LT. Infective endocarditis. Olmsted County, Minnesota, 1950 through 1981. JAMA 254:1199–1202, 1985.

51. Naggar CZ, Forgacs P. Infective endocarditis: a challenging disease. Med Clin North Am 70:1279–1294, 1986.

52. Powderly WG, Stanley SL Jr, Medoff G. Pneumococcal endocarditis: report of a series and review of the literature. Rev Infect Dis 8:786–791, 1986.

53. Terpenning MS, Buggy BP, Kauffman CA. Hospital-acquired infective endocarditis. Arch Intern Med 148:1601–1603, 1988.

54. Rowley KM, Clubb KS, Smith GJ, Cabin HS. Right-sided infective endocarditis as a consequence of flow-directed pulmonary–artery catheterization. A clinicopathological study of 55 autopsied patients. N Engl J Med 311:1152–1156, 1984.

55. Dean RH, Waterhouse G, Meacham PW, Weaver FA, O'Neil JA Jr. Mycotic embolism and embolomycotic aneurysms. Neglected lessons of the past. Ann Surg 204:300–307, 1986.

56. Churchill MA Jr, Geraci JE, Hunder GG. Musculoskeletal manifestations of bacterial endocarditis. Ann Intern Med 87:754–759, 1977.

57. Terpenning MS, Buggy BP, Kauffman CA. Infective endocarditis: Clinical features in young and elderly patients. Am J Med 83:626–634, 1987.

58. Case records of the Massachusetts General Hospital (case 7–1988). N Engl J Med 318:427–440, 1988.

59. Case records of the Massachusetts General Hospital (case 14-1990). N Engl J Med 322:988–999, 1990.

60. Hermans PE. The clinical manifestations of infective endocarditis. Mayo Clin Proc 57:15–21, 1982.

61. Jones HR Jr, Siekert RG, Geraci JE. Neurologic manifestations of bacterial endocarditis. Ann Intern Med 71:21–28, 1969.

62. Von Reyn CF, Levy BS, Arbeit RD, Friedland G, Crumpacker CS. Infective endocarditis: an analysis based on strict case definitions. Ann Intern Med 94:505–518, 1981.

63. David TE, Bos J, Christakis GT, Brofman PR, Wong D, Feindel CM. Heart valve operations in patients with active infective endocarditis. Ann Thorac Surg 49:701–705, 1990.

64. Dreyfus G, Serraf A, Jebara VA, et al. Valve repair in acute endocarditis. Ann Thorac Surg 49:706–711, 1990.

65. Weinstein L. Life-threatening complications of infective endocarditis and their management. Arch Intern Med 146:953–957, 1986.

66. Dalen JE. Valvular heart disease, infected valves and prosthetic heart valves. Am J Cardiol 65:29C–31C, 1990.

67. Davenport J, Hart RG. Prosthetic valve endocarditis 1976–1987. Antibiotics, anticoagulation, and stroke. Stroke 21:993–999, 1990.

68. Calderwood SB, Swinski LA, Waternaux CM, Karchmer AW, Buckley MJ. Risk factors for the development of prosthetic valve endocarditis. Circulation 72:31–37, 1985.

69. Pruitt AA, Rubin RH, Karchmer AW, Duncan GW. Neurologic complications of bacterial endocarditis. Medicine (Baltimore) 57:329–343, 1978.

70. Cabell CH, Pond KK, Peterson GE, et al. The risk of stroke and death in patients with aortic and mitral valve endocarditis. Am Heart J 142:75–80, 2001.

71. Van Scoy RE. Culture-negative endocarditis. Mayo Clin Proc 57:149–154, 1982.

72. Tompkins LS, Roessler BJ, Redd SC, Markowitz LE, Cohen ML. *Legionella* prosthetic-valve endocarditis. N Engl J Med 318:530–535, 1988.

73. Tunkel AR, Kaye D. Endocarditis with negative blood cultures [editorial]. N Engl J Med 326:1215–1217, 1992.

74. O'Brien JT, Geiser EA. Infective endocarditis and echocardiography. Am Heart J 108:386–394, 1984.

75. Roe MT, Abramson MA, Li J, et al. Clinical information determines the impact of transesophageal echocardiography on the diagnosis of infective endocarditis by the Duke criteria. Am Heart J 139:945–951, 2000.

76. Erbel R, Rohmann S, Drexler M, et al. Improved diagnostic value of echocardiography in patients with infective endocarditis by transesophageal approach. A prospective study. Eur Heart J 9:43–53, 1988.

77. Li JS, Sexton DJ, Mick N, et al. Proposed modifications to the Duke criteria for the diagnosis of infective endocarditis. Clin Infect Dis 30:633–638, 2000.

78. Alexiou C, Langley SM, Stafford H, Lowes JA, Livesey SA, Monro JL. Surgery for active culture-positive endocarditis: determinants of early and late outcome. Ann Thorac Surg 69:1448–1454, 2000.

79. Molinari GF, Smith L, Goldstein MN, Satran R.

Pathogenesis of cerebral mycotic aneurysms. Neurology 23:325–332, 1973.

80. Morawetz RB, Karp RB. Evolution and resolution of intracranial bacterial (mycotic) aneurysms. Neurosurgery 15:43–49, 1984.

81. Vincent FM, Zimmerman JE, Auer TC, Martin DB. Subarachnoid hemorrhage—the initial manifestation of bacterial endocarditis. Report of a case with negative arteriography and computed tomography. Neurosurgery 7:488–490, 1980.

82. Krapf H, Skalej M, Voigt K. Subarachnoid hemorrhage due to septic embolic infarction in infective endocarditis. Cerebrovasc Dis 9:182–184, 1999.

83. Stengel A, Wolferth CC. Mycotic (bacterial) aneurysms of intravascular origin. Arch Intern Med 31:527–554, 1923.

84. Frazee JG, Cahan LD, Winter J. Bacterial intracranial aneurysms. J Neurosurg 53:633–641, 1980.

85. Trevisani MF, Ricci MA, Michaels RM, Meyer KK. Multiple mesenteric aneurysms complicating subacute bacterial endocarditis. Arch Surg 122:823–824, 1987.

86. Delahaye JP, Poncet P, Malquarti V, Beaune J, Gare JP, Mann JM. Cerebrovascular accidents in infective endocarditis: role of anticoagulation. Eur Heart J 11:1074–1078, 1990.

87. Salgado AV, Furlan AJ, Keys TF. Mycotic aneurysm, subarachnoid hemorrhage, and indications for cerebral angiography in infective endocarditis. Stroke 18:1057–1060, 1987.

88. Salgado AV, Furlan AJ, Keys TF, Nichols TR, Beck GJ. Neurologic complications of endocarditis: a 12-year experience. Neurology 39:173–178, 1989.

89. Calopa M, Rubio F, Aguilar M, Peres J. Giant basilar aneurysm in the course of subacute bacterial endocarditis. Stroke 21:1625–1627, 1990.

90. Bullock R, Van Dellen JR. Rupture of bacterial intracranial aneurysms following replacement of cardiac valves. Surg Neurol 17:9–11, 1982.

91. Venger BH, Aldama AE. Mycotic vasculitis with repeated intracranial aneurysmal hemorrhage. Case report. J Neurosurg 69:775–779, 1988.

92. Bamford J, Hodges J, Warlow C. Late rupture of a mycotic aneurysm after "cure" of bacterial endocarditis. J Neurol 233:51–53, 1986.

93. Roberts G, Allcutt D, Farrell M. Embolic bacterial aneurysm of the basilar artery: case report. Br J Neurosurg 12:440–444, 1998.

94. Brust JC, Dickinson PC, Hughes JE, Holtzman RN. The diagnosis and treatment of cerebral mycotic aneurysms. Ann Neurol 27:238–246, 1990.

95. Jones HR Jr, Siekert RG. Neurological manifestations of infective endocarditis. Review of clinical and therapeutic challenges. Brain 112:1295–1315, 1989.

96. Kanter MC, Hart RG. Cerebral mycotic aneurysms are rare in infective endocarditis [letter]. Ann Neurol 28:590–591, 1990.

97. Hart RG, Kagan-Hallet K, Joerns SE. Mechanisms of intracranial hemorrhage in infective endocarditis. Stroke 18:1048–1056, 1987.

98. Le Cam B, Guivarch G, Boles JM, Garre M, Cartier F. Neurologic complications in a group of 86 bacterial endocarditis. Eur Heart J 5 (Suppl C):97–100, 1984.

99. Leipzig TJ, Brown FD. Treatment of mycotic aneurysms. Surg Neurol 23:403–407, 1985.

100. Moskowitz MA, Rosenbaum AE, Tyler HR. Angiographically monitored resolution of cerebral mycotic aneurysms. Neurology 24:1103–1108, 1974.

101. Bohmfalk GL, Story JL, Wissinger JP, Brown WE Jr. Bacterial intracranial aneurysm. J Neurosurg 48:369–382, 1978.

102. Ahmadi J, Tung H, Giannotta SL, Destian S. Monitoring of infectious intracranial aneurysms by sequential computed tomographic/magnetic resonance imaging studies. Neurosurgery 32:45–49, 1993.

103. Kim SJ, Lee JY, Kim TH, et al. Imaging of the neurological complications of infective endocarditis. Neuroradiology 40:109–113, 1998.

104. van der Meulen JH, Weststrate W, van Gijn J, Habbema JD. Is cerebral angiography indicated in infective endocarditis? Stroke 23:1662–1667, 1992.

105. Day AL. Extracranial–intracranial bypass grafting in the surgical treatment of bacterial aneurysms: report of two cases. Neurosurgery 9:583–588, 1981.

106. Ojemann RG, Heros RC, Crowell RM. Surgical Management of Cerebrovascular Disease, 2nd ed. Williams & Wilkins, Baltimore, 1988, pp 337–346.

107. Frizzell RT, Vitek JJ, Hill DL, Fisher WS III. Treatment of a bacterial (mycotic) intracranial aneurysm using an endovascular approach. Neurosurgery 32:852–854, 1993.

108. Khayata MH, Aymard A, Casasco A, Herbreteau D, Woimant F, Merland JJ. Selective endovascular techniques in the treatment of cerebral mycotic aneurysms. Report of three cases. J Neurosurg 78:661–665, 1993.

109. Utoh J, Miyauchi Y, Goto H, Obayashi H, Hirata T. Endovascular approach for an intracranial mycotic aneurysm associated with infective endocarditis. J Thorac Cardiovasc Surg 110:557–559, 1995.

110. Katakura K, Kayama T, Kondo R, et al. A case of multiple cerebral mycotic aneurysms treated with endovascular surgery. No Shinkei Geka 23:1127–1132, 1995.

111. Scotti G, Li MH, Righi C, Simionato F, Rocca A. Endovascular treatment of bacterial intracranial aneurysms. Neuroradiology 38:186–189, 1996.

112. Hashimoto T, Hyodo A, Matsumaru Y, Sato H, Nose T. Cerebral mycotic aneurysm treated with endovascular surgery: a case report. Rinsho Hoshasen 41:677–680, 1996.

113. Watanabe A, Hirano K, Ishii R. Cerebral mycotic aneurysm treated with endovascular occlusion—case report. Neurol Med Chir (Tokyo) 38:657–660, 1998.

114. Stein PD, Kantrowitz A. Antithrombotic therapy in mechanical and biological prosthetic heart valves and saphenous vein bypass grafts. Chest 95 (Suppl):S107–S117, 1989.

115. Opal SM. The uncertain value of the definition for SIRS. Systemic inflammatory response syndrome [editorial]. Chest 113:1442–1443, 1998.

116. Gillinov AM, Shah RV, Curtis WE, et al. Valve replacement in patients with endocarditis and acute neurologic deficit. Ann Thorac Surg 61:1125–1129, 1996.

117. Bleck TP. Tetanus. In Scheld WM, Whitley RL, Du-

rack DT (eds). Infections of the Central Nervous System. Raven Press, New York, 1991, pp 603–624.

118. Mandell GL, Douglas RG, Bennett JE. Principles and Practice of Infectious Diseases, 3rd ed. Churchill Livingstone, New York, 1990.

119. Cherington M. Botulism. Ten-year experience. Arch Neurol 30:432–437, 1974.

120. Hughes JM, Blumenthal JR, Merson MH, Lombard GL, Dowell VR Jr, Gangarosa EJ. Clinical features of types A and B food-borne botulism. Ann Intern Med 95:442–445, 1981.

121. Wainwright RB, Heyward WL, Middaugh JP, Hatheway CL, Harpster AP, Bender TR. Foodborne botulism in Alaska, 1947–1985: epidemiology and clinical findings. J Infect Dis 157:1158–1162, 1988.

122. Terranova W, Palumbo JN, Breman JG. Ocular findings in botulism type B. JAMA 241:475–477, 1979.

123. Ehrenreich H, Garner CG, Witt TN. Complete bilateral internal ophthalmoplegia as sole clinical sign of botulism: confirmation of diagnosis by single fibre electromyography. J Neurol 236:243–245, 1989.

124. Rapoport S, Watkins PB. Descending paralysis resulting from occult wound botulism. Ann Neurol 16:359–361, 1984.

125. Vita G, Girlanda P, Puglisi RM, Marabello L, Messina C. Cardiovascular-reflex testing and single-fiber electromyography in botulism. A longitudinal study. Arch Neurol 44:202–206, 1987.

126. Jenzer G, Mumenthaler M, Ludin HP, Robert F. Autonomic dysfunction in botulism B: a clinical report. Neurology 25:150–153, 1975.

127. Maselli RA, Bakshi N. AAEM case report 16. Botulism. American Association of Electrodiagnostic Medicine. Muscle Nerve 23:1137–1144, 2000.

128. Cherington M. Clinical spectrum of botulism. Muscle Nerve 21:701–710, 1998.

129. Lewis SW, Pierson DJ, Cary JM, Hudson LD. Prolonged respiratory paralysis in wound botulism. Chest 75:59–61, 1979.

130. Kaplan JE, Davis LE, Narayan V, Koster J, Katzenstein D. Botulism, type A, and treatment with guanidine. Ann Neurol 6:69–71, 1979.

131. Trujillo MJ, Castillo A, España JV, Guevara P, Eganez H. Tetanus in the adult: intensive care and management experience with 233 cases. Crit Care Med 8:419–423, 1980.

132. Saissy JM, Demaziere J, Vitris M, et al. Treatment of severe tetanus by intrathecal injections of baclofen without artificial ventilation. Intensive Care Med 18:241–244, 1992.

133. Engrand N, Guerot E, Rouamba A, Vilain G. The efficacy of intrathecal baclofen in severe tetanus. Anesthesiology 90:1773–1776, 1999.

134. Tidyman M, Prichard JG, Deamer RL, Mac N. Adjunctive use of dantrolene in severe tetanus. Anesth Analg 64:538–540, 1985.

135. Attygalle D, Rodrigo N. Magnesium sulphate for control of spasms in severe tetanus. Can we avoid sedation and artificial ventilation? Anaesthesia 52:956–962, 1997.

136. Hsu SS, Groleau G. Tetanus in the emergency department: a current review. J Emerg Med 20:357–365, 2001.

137. Kanchanapongkul J. Tetanus in adults: a review of 85 cases at Chon Buri Hospital. J Med Assoc Thai 84:494–499, 2001.

138. Faust SN, Heyderman RS, Levin M. Coagulation in severe sepsis: a central role for thrombomodulin and activated protein C. Crit Care Med 29:S62–S68, 2001.

139. Cerra FB, Siegel JH, Coleman B, Border JR, McMenamy RR. Septic autocannibalism. A failure of exogenous nutritional support. Ann Surg 192:570–580, 1980.

140. Bone RC, Balk RA, Cerra FB, et al. Definitions for sepsis and organ failure and guidelines for the use of innovative therapies in sepsis. The ACCP/SCCM Consensus Conference Committee. American College of Chest Physicians/Society of Critical Care Medicine. Chest 101:1644–1655, 1992.

141. Blackwell TS, Christman JW. Sepsis and cytokines: current status. Br J Anaesth 77:110–117, 1996.

142. Bone RC. Immunologic dissonance: a continuing evolution in our understanding of the systemic inflammatory response syndrome (SIRS) and the multiple organ dysfunction syndrome (MODS). Ann Intern Med 125:680–687, 1996.

143. Koch T. Origin and mediators involved in sepsis and the systemic inflammatory response syndrome. Kidney Int 53 (Suppl 64):S66–S69, 1998.

144. Bolton CF. Electrophysiologic studies of critically ill patients. Muscle Nerve 10:129–135, 1987.

145. Bolton CF, Laverty DA, Brown JD, Witt NJ, Hahn AF, Sibbald WJ. Critically ill polyneuropathy: electrophysiological studies and differentiation from Guillain-Barré syndrome. J Neurol Neurosurg Psychiatry 49:563–573, 1986.

146. Bolton CF, Breuer AC. Critical illness polyneuropathy. Muscle Nerve 22:419–424, 1999.

147. Lycklama À, Nijeholt J, Troost J. Critical illness polyneuropathy. In: Vinken PJ, Bruyn GW, Klawans HL (eds). Handbook of Clinical Neurology, Vol. 51: Neuropathies. Elsevier Science Publishers, Amsterdam, 1987, pp 575–585.

148. Op de Coul AA, Lambregts PC, Koeman J, van Puyenbroek MJ, Ter Laak HJ, Gabreels-Festen AA. Neuromuscular complications in patients given Pavulon (pancuronium bromide) during artificial ventilation. Clin Neurol Neurosurg 87:17–22, 1985.

149. Berek K, Margreiter J, Willeit J, Berek A, Schmutzhard E, Mutz NJ. Polyneuropathies in critically ill patients: a prospective evaluation. Intensive Care Med 22:849–855, 1996.

150. Leijten FS, Harinck-de Weerd JE, Poortvliet DC, de Weerd AW. The role of polyneuropathy in motor convalescence after prolonged mechanical ventilation. JAMA 274:1221–1225, 1995.

151. Anastakis DJ, Peters WJ, Lee KC. Severe peripheral burn polyneuropathy: a case report. Burns Incl Therm Inj 13:232–235, 1987.

152. Carver N, Logan A. Critically ill polyneuropathy associated with burns: a case report. Burns 15:179–180, 1989.

153. Roelofs RI, Cerra F, Bielka N, Rosenberg L, Delaney J. Prolonged respiratory insufficiency due to acute motor neuropathy: a new syndrome? [abstract]. Neurology 33 (Suppl 2):240, 1983.

154. Bolton CF, Gilbert JJ, Hahn AF, Sibbald WJ.

Polyneuropathy in critically ill patients. J Neurol Neurosurg Psychiatry 47:1223–1231, 1984.

155. Zochodne DW, Bolton CF, Wells GA, et al. Critical illness polyneuropathy: a complication of sepsis and multiple organ failure. Brain 110:819–841, 1987.

156. Witt NJ, Zochodne DW, Bolton CF, et al. Peripheral nerve function in sepsis and multiple organ failure. Chest 99:176–184, 1991.

157. Bolton CF. Sepsis and the systemic inflammatory response syndrome: neuromuscular manifestations. Crit Care Med 24:1408–1416, 1996.

158. Waldhausen E, Mingers B, Lippers P, Keser G. Critical illness polyneuropathy due to parenteral nutrition [letter]. Intensive Care Med 23:922–923, 1997.

159. Marino PL, Millili JJ. Possible role of dietary lipids in critical illness polyneuropathy [letter]. Intensive Care Med 24:87, 1998.

160. Druschky A, Herkert M, Radespiel-Troger M, et al. Critical illness polyneuropathy: clinical findings and cell culture assay of neurotoxicity assessed by a prospective study. Intensive Care Med 27:686–693, 2001.

161. Verheul GA, de Jongh-Leuvenink J, Op de Coul AA, van Landeghem AA, van Puyenbroek MJ. Tumor necrosis factor and interleukin-6 in critical illness polyneuropathy. Clin Neurol Neurosurg 96:300–304, 1994.

162. Covert CR, Brodie SB, Zimmerman JE. Weaning failure due to acute neuromuscular disease. Crit Care Med 14:307–308, 1986.

163. Wijdicks EF, Fulgham JR. Failure of high dose intravenous immunoglobulins to alter the clinical course of critical illness polyneuropathy. Muscle Nerve 17:1494–1495, 1994.

164. Hund EF, Fogel W, Krieger D, DeGeorgia M, Hacke W. Critical illness polyneuropathy: clinical findings and outcomes of a frequent cause of neuromuscular weaning failure. Crit Care Med 24:1328–1333, 1996.

165. Wijdicks EFM, Litchy WJ, Harrison BA, Gracey DR. The clinical spectrum of critical illness polyneuropathy. Mayo Clin Proc 69:955–959, 1994.

166. Zifko UA, Zipko HT, Bolton CF. Clinical and electrophysiological findings in critical illness polyneuropathy. J Neurol Sci 159:186–193, 1998.

167. Hund E, Genzwurker H, Bohrer H, Jakob H, Thiele R, Hacke W. Predominant involvement of motor fibres in patients with critical illness polyneuropathy. Br J Anaesth 78:274–278, 1997.

168. Latronico N, Fenzi F, Recupero D, et al. Critical illness myopathy and neuropathy. Lancet 347:1579–1582, 1996.

169. Mohr M, Englisch L, Roth A, Burchardi H, Zielmann S. Effects of early treatment with immunoglobulin on critical illness polyneuropathy following multiple organ failure and gram-negative sepsis. Intensive Care Med 23:1144–1149, 1997.

170. Eidelman LA, Putterman D, Putterman C, Sprung CL. The spectrum of septic encephalopathy. Definitions, etiologies, and mortalities. JAMA 275:470–473, 1996.

171. Sprung CL, Peduzzi PN, Shatney CH, et al. Impact of encephalopathy on mortality in the sepsis syndrome. The Veterans Administration Systemic Sepsis Cooperative Study Group. Crit Care Med 18:801–806, 1990.

172. Young GB, Bolton CF, Austin TW, Archibald YM, Gonder J, Wells GA. The encephalopathy associated with septic illness. Clin Invest Med 13:297–304, 1990.

173. Wijdicks EFM, Stevens M. The role of hypotension in septic encephalopathy following surgical procedures. Arch Neurol 49:653–656, 1992.

174. Adams JH, Brierley JB, Connor RC, Treip CS. The effects of systemic hypotension upon the human brain. Clinical and neuropathological observations in 11 cases. Brain 89:235–268, 1966.

175. Bowton DL, Bertels NH, Prough DS, Stump DA. Cerebral blood flow is reduced in patients with sepsis syndrome. Crit Care Med 17:399–403, 1989.

176. Freund HR, Ryan JA Jr, Fischer JE. Amino acid derangements in patients with sepsis: treatment with branched chain amino acid rich infusions. Ann Surg 188:423–430, 1978.

177. Naylor CD, O'Rourke K, Detsky AS, Baker JP. Parenteral nutrition with branched-chain amino acids in hepatic encephalopathy. A meta-analysis. Gastroenterology 97:1033–1042, 1989.

178. Takezawa J, Taenaka N, Nishijima MK, et al. Amino acids and thiobarbituric acid reactive substances in cerebrospinal fluid and plasma of patients with septic encephalopathy. Crit Care Med 11:876–879, 1983.

179. Pendlebury WW, Perl DP, Karibo RM, McQuillen JB. Disseminated microabscesses of the central nervous system [abstract]. Neurology 33 (Suppl 2):223, 1983.

180. Hollinger P, Zurcher R, Schroth G, Mattle HP. Diffusion magnetic resonance imaging findings in cerebritis and brain abscesses in a patient with septic encephalopathy. J Neurol 247:232–234, 2000.

181. Young GB, Bolton CF, Archibald YM, Austin TW, Wells GA. The electroencephalogram in sepsis-associated encephalopathy. J Clin Neurophysiol 9:145–152, 1992.

182. Zauner C, Gendo A, Kramer L, Kranz A, Grimm G, Madl C. Metabolic encephalopathy in critically ill patients suffering from septic or nonseptic multiple organ failure. Crit Care Med 28:1310–1315, 2000.

Chapter 7

NEUROLOGIC COMPLICATIONS OF CARDIAC ARREST

The mortality and morbidity associated with cardiopulmonary resuscitation remain a major public health problem. Rapid defibrillation and intensive care admission may affect survival and the probability of intact neurologic function.[1,2] Survivors of out-of-hospital arrest continue to overburden intensive care units (ICUs), and the neurologist plays a central role in assessment of coma. Cardiac arrest in critically ill patients is an even more disquieting event and devastating for some.[3,4] Cardiopulmonary resuscitation (CPR) during downward spiraling shock, sepsis, or cardiac failure may be considered futile to many intensive care specialists.

Outcome may vary by unit and age, but there is no doubt about the importance of ischemic brain injury in affecting outcome.[1–4] The critical role of anoxic–ischemic encephalopathy in survival has been confirmed in many studies, and this recognition has led to a revival of research into mechanisms and a search for treatments. Although pathologic studies have indicated a potential

window for reversing global tissue ischemia and salvaging neurons in the first hours, pharmacologic intervention in two major randomized trials of CPR did not improve outcome.[5,6]

It is not uncommon for many individuals to remain comatose on the day of resuscitation. These fortunate survivors may indeed have a good chance to recover to their premorbid state if they overcome the systemic complications in the first week.[7] However, the number of patients who survive is proportionally small because of recurrent cardiac arrest[5,6,8–11] (Fig. 7–1).

This chapter introduces the current knowledge of resuscitation medicine and incorporates the most common manifestations of resuscitation-associated encephalopathy.

GENERAL CONSIDERATIONS IN RESUSCITATION MEDICINE

In recent years, the American Heart Association has achieved a consensus that CPR should be divided into two phases: basic life support and advanced cardiac life support.[12] The steps of basic life support in resuscitation are airway control, breathing, and circulation support. Although there are many unanswered questions about the dynamics of chest compression, the effects on cerebral blood flow have been extensively studied in animal models. Alternative modes of chest compression with additional abdominal compression may increase carotid blood flow, but as yet no clinical studies or animal

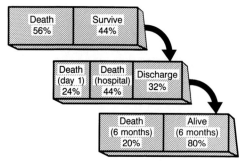

Figure 7–1. Estimated outcome of patients after cardiac resuscitation.

experiments have demonstrated improved outcome.

The traditional explanation that compression of the heart between the sternum and the vertebral column results in forceful emptying of the cardiac chambers during upstroke is an oversimplification. Angiographic and echocardiographic studies have shown that chest compression sets in motion an increase in intrathoracic pressure that causes blood to flow from the lung passively through the left side of the heart. However, the marked increase of carotid perfusion pressures to 30% of normal values (rather than the usual 5%) during simultaneous abdominal compression–ventilation CPR underscored the fact that the thoracic pump is responsible for blood flow during chest compression.[13,14] This finding resulted in the development of alternatives to standard CPR, including the use of circumferential thoracic binders and continuous use of interposed abdominal counterpressure. As expected, only open-chest cardiac massage may correct cerebral blood flow to prearrest levels, but this physiologically superior method has not resulted in a better neurologic outcome than that with any form of closed chest CPR. A recent study with a compression–decompression device showed marginal improvement in neurologic outcome.[15]

The current focus in resuscitation research is use of cardiopulmonary bypass, particularly in patients with severe left ventricular failure. Cardiopulmonary bypass may have a role in the distribution of potential salvaging agents as well. Conversely, cardiopulmonary bypass may increase the risk of air and particulate emboli, which may exacerbate ischemic damage.

These new methods have been summarized under the colorful title "ultra advanced life support."[16] Included are minimally invasive direct cardiac massage by a plunger-like device introduced through a small opening and improved cerebral flow by aortic balloon catheters. Further comprehensive discussions of this subject, with the major focus on anesthesia management, can be found in two reviews.[17,18]

Following a successful cardiac resuscitation, postresuscitation multiorgan failure may emerge.[19] A significant proportion of deaths is caused by recurrent cardiac arrest (approximately 22%), refractory dysrhythmias often ventricular in origin, and irreversible cardiogenic shock. Important prognostic factors for cardiac failure and arrhythmias are history of remote myocardial infarction, prior congestive heart failure, and previous cardiac arrest from ventricular fibrillation not caused by an acute transmural infarction. The most common deleterious effects of resuscitation are summarized in Table 7–1.

Studies of the neurologic damage in cardiac arrest have focused on reperfusion injury of the brain. This concept has been convincingly demonstrated in animal experiments, but data in humans are sparse and

Table 7–1. **Effects after Cardiac Resuscitation**

Neurologic
Postanoxic–ischemic encephalopathy
Ischemic myelopathy
Cerebral infarct in arterial watershed zone

Cardiac
Left ventricular failure
Dysrhythmias
Pulmonary edema and acute respiratory distress syndrome

Distant
Acute tubular necrosis
Traumatic liver damage
Ischemic colon and sepsis
Fractured ribs, pneumothorax, and bone marrow embolus

Data from Kaye and Bircher.[17]

conflicting. When ischemia is brief, the brain parenchyma has the ability to recover almost immediately. The exact critical time threshold for reperfusion damage is not known, but injury presumably begins after circulation arrest of more than 5 min.

Three phases of cerebral blood flow have been recognized. The first phase after cardiac arrest is probably best characterized by an initial moderate hyperemia during resumption of circulation. This phenomenon lasts for 10 to 20 min and most likely is not uniformly distributed in the brain, but it is followed by a considerable decrease in blood flow, up to 50% of normal. This second phase is tentatively explained by vasospasm, glial edema, or microcirculatory plugs. The third phase of changes in cerebral blood flow after resuscitation is less well defined. Baseline values may return, or cerebral blood flow may progressively deteriorate to very low levels. This hypothesis is supported by studies[20–22] that showed more extensive ischemic neuronal necrosis in comatose patients who survived longer after comparable times of cardiac arrest than in patients who died earlier. This observation may suggest that ischemic injury is not permanent from the outset and in fact may progress in the first hours after resuscitation. If this concept is true, the ideal time to administer pharmacologic agents is in the early hours of the hyperemia episode.

Thus, clinical investigators have advocated the use of hemodilution with dextran, anticoagulation, or blood pressure support to overcome microcirculatory arrest in the phase after hyperemia. In a randomized trial, high doses of epinephrine and norepinephrine did not improve neurologic outcome.[23] In addition, a cerebral blood flow study using xenon Xe 133 showed no marked differences between patients who regained consciousness and patients who remained comatose. Despite adequate blood pressure, postischemic hypoperfusion occurred in all patients immediately after CPR, and perfusion further declined in the subsequent hours.[24]

Future research may be more tailored toward restoration of the metabolic changes induced by free radical damage, abnormal calcium shifts, and release of excitatory neurotransmitters. Improvement in field resuscitation and administration of drugs at the site may be beneficial, but preliminary results are discouraging.

POSTRESUSCITATION ENCEPHALOPATHY

The hallmark of global ischemia is neuronal loss in border zone frontoparietal cortex, insular cortex, putamen, hippocampus, and end folium. The location and degree of damage are unpredictable, and early autopsies may not document hippocampal damage. In severe cases, subcortical gray matter, including thalamus and basal ganglia, cerebellar Purkinje's cells, and even nuclei of the brain stem, may become necrotic. Bilateral boundary zone infarcts are usually hemorrhagic at postmortem examination and are probably related to reperfusion. This condition has been collectively referred to as "anoxic–ischemic encephalopathy." In clinical practice, it is difficult to single out anoxia as a trigger, and its injurious effect may be much less than previously appreciated. "Postresuscitation encephalopathy" may be a more appropriate term.

Clinical Features

Postresuscitation encephalopathy may come in different guises. Neurologic examination may document many intriguing subtleties, some of which have prognostic value. Generally, the approach is to assess the Glasgow coma scale, pupil responses to light, eye position and movement, and myoclonic jerks, all of which are key features in prognostication.

Findings in large cohorts of patients following cardiac arrest who have detailed neurologic assessment show that the initial degree of motor responsiveness may point to a potential for recovery.[25,26] Certainly, outcome is quite favorable when, immediately after resuscitation, the patient moans and strongly fends off a painful stimulus. Conversely, lack of a motor response to noxious stimulus in the first post-arrest hours does not necessarily imply that neurologic impairment is inevitable, and up to 22% of the

Table 7–2. **Recovery of Independent Function after Initial Absence of Motor Responses**

Prospective series	Patients	NO MOTOR RESPONSE TO PAIN		NONRESPONDING PATIENTS WITH INDEPENDENT RECOVERY	
		No.	%	No.	%
Earnest et al., 1979[7]	117	89	76	0	0
Snyder et al., 1980[27]	63	18	29	4	22
Levy et al., 1985[25]	210	102	49	4	4
BRCT I, 1986[5]	262	162	62	26	16

BRCT, Brain Resuscitation Clinical Trial.

patients have recovered (Table 7–2). Patients who awaken on the day of cardiac arrest gradually progress from an amnesic and dazed state to complete attention, perception, and self-awareness.

However, a profound amnesic syndrome has been reported that may persist for months.[28,29] It has been suggested that preferential ischemic hippocampal injury is responsible for this partial memory disorder. This syndrome is uncommon and occurs in patients who have been comatose for at least 24 hr after resuscitation and not when coma is short-lived.[28,29] The immediate presence of localizing responses is the best evidence that the duration of anoxia has been brief.[27] Long duration of circulatory arrest results in a more profound insult and may be apparent by the documentation of abnormal extensor or flexor response or flaccidity in the arms and legs.

Patients with a more severe anoxic–ischemic insult usually remain comatose on the day of resuscitation but recover in the following days. The mean time to awakening (defined as the ability to follow commands or comprehensible speech) was 3 days in a large study that focused primarily on recovery from coma.[30] The longest period before awakening occurred was 100 days. In our series, 17 of 20 patients with postanoxic coma awoke within 24 hr after arrest.[31] The remaining three patients gradually awoke within 5 days.

Some improvement in level of consciousness, albeit indistinct, is typical over time. A persistent vegetative state is fortunately uncommon. However, further deterioration to stupor after initial improvement has been reported but is very uncommon. Plum and colleagues[32] found extensive hemispheric white matter demyelination without pathologic evidence of edema in these patients, who had progression to coma and died after an asymptomatic interval (4 to 14 days). Early ambulation preceded deterioration and suggested relative hypotension as a possible trigger. Ginsberg[33] suggested that any metabolic derangement, such as hypoglycemia, hyponatremia, marked hypoxemia, or labile blood pressure, may be present. After an ischemic episode, the white matter could have become vulnerable to metabolic changes or changes in cerebral perfusion pressure, and any additional challenge would lead to severe damage. It remains a very unusual clinical entity after cardiac resuscitation and is more commonly seen in patients with carbon monoxide inhalation (Chapter 16).

Localizing neurologic signs are uncommon but may arise from lesions in arterial border zone territories. Bibrachial paralysis may be found in some patients after cardiac arrest.[34] (This syndrome has been termed "man-in-the-barrel syndrome,"[35] but one should take care not to mistake a brisk triple flexion response and absent motor response in the arms for this syndrome.) As expected, many patient cohorts with adequate neurologic examination have highlighted the dire consequences of abnormal brain stem reflexes.[25,36]

During or immediately after resuscitative efforts, the pupil diameter widens and light responses are abolished within a few minutes after cardiac standstill. Initial pupillary dilatation gives way to moderate constriction after return of spontaneous circulation.[37,38] A prospective study of pupil size and light response during CPR pointed out several types of pupil responses.[39] Dilated, fixed pupils were more frequently associated with asystole than with electromechanical dissociation or ventricular fibrillation. Successful cardiac resuscitation with good neurologic recovery more often occurred in patients with persistently contracted pupils from the onset or in patients who had initial dilatation of pupils followed by contraction. Fixed, dilated pupils throughout the resuscitation procedure indicated a poor chance of success. It remains questionable whether knowledge of these pupil variables is of importance in clinical practice, and resuscitative efforts probably should not be gauged by it.

Corneal reflexes are absent in approximately one-third of comatose patients at the initial examination but reappear soon. The general clinical impression is that early loss of corneal reflexes together with ophthalmoplegia is a strong predictor of poor outcome, but often other brain stem reflexes are absent. In Levy and colleagues' study,[25] 3 of 71 patients who lacked early corneal reflexes remarkably recovered. However, there appears little hope for patients who have sustained upward gaze.[40] In these patients, horizontal eye movement remains full, although periodic alternating gaze deviation (or ping-pong) may occur transiently. The neuropathologic counterpart consists of diffuse severe cerebellar and cortical changes, but the upper midbrain is normal.

In a study of 15 comatose patients with sustained upward gaze after cardiac arrest or shock, 2 patients "awakened," but 1 patient died later in the hospital and the other remained in a vegetative state.[40] Upward gaze can occur immediately after resuscitation (Fig. 7–2), generally resolves within 2 weeks, but may persist for 2 months. Also, myoclonic facial jerks or generalized myoclonic jerks may produce brief opening of eyelids with repetitive upward jerking of both globes.

Persistent downward gaze is nonlocalizing and less common but also most likely reflects global bihemispheric injury.[41] Ocular dipping has been described in coma after cardiac arrest,[42] although it may also occur in other encephalopathies, as described and illustrated in Chapter 1. In ocular dipping, both eyes conjugately move downward, sometimes completely obscuring the pupil beneath the lower eyelid, remain in a resting downward position for several seconds, and then rapidly return to their primary position.[42] Pathologic examination of these patients revealed, in addition to diffuse cortical damage, bilateral basal ganglia and thalamic lesions. The prognostic significance of ocular dipping remains uncertain because complete neurologic recovery may occur. It should be differentiated from ocular bobbing, which is strongly associated with intrapontine and cerebellar lesions[43,44] (Chapter 1).

Various reports have documented seizures in comatose survivors. The clinical manifestations of seizures are not adequately detailed in all major reports on cardiac resuscitation, in part because they are not directly witnessed by physicians (see Chapter 3). In

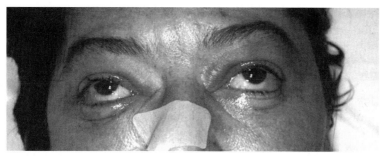

Figure 7–2. Upward gaze persisting until fatal recurrent cardiac arrhythmia in comatose patient after cardiopulmonary resuscitation.

some patients, it is possible that spontaneous decerebrate posturing or shivering during or immediately after cardiac massage probably has been interpreted as a seizure. The reported frequency of clinical seizures after cardiac resuscitation has ranged from 9% to 50%.

Generalized tonic–clonic seizures are infrequent and may be linked to multiple doses of lidocaine during resuscitation. Snyder and colleagues[45] noted that some patients have frequent rhythmic, rapid, low-amplitude limb movements called "shivering." The mechanism of these abnormal movements, mostly evident in the immediate aftermath of resuscitation, remains obscure, but shivering movements may be associated with hypothermia or use of anesthetic agents. It is perhaps more important, however, to recognize that single tonic–clonic seizures, focal seizures, and shivers have no prognostic value.

Of greater concern is myoclonic status epilepticus. Myoclonus often involves the facial musculature, the limbs, and the axial muscles.[46–48] These rapid, repetitive, brief jerks can be elicited by hand clap, pressure to the nail beds, insertion of central catheters, or tracheal suctioning, but in the first hours after CPR, there may be unrelenting spontaneous jerking. Generalized myoclonus is common during resuscitative measures and is very often seen in patients with a sudden decrease in blood pressure from decreased cardiac output. (This relationship of myoclonic jerks and hypotension may be similar to that of convulsions during vasovagal collapse, a situation presumed to be caused by diminished cortical inhibition.)

Myoclonic status epilepticus in comatose patients strongly indicates diffuse cortical damage. A pathologic study in comatose patients with therapy-resistant myoclonus status epilepticus demonstrated marked ischemic cell damage in the neocortex, hippocampus, and dentate nucleus and widespread central gray matter damage in the spinal cord.[49] Myoclonic status epilepticus in comatose survivors from cardiac arrest should be considered an agonal phenomenon. The evidence comes from several series, including ours of 107 comatose survivors of out-of-hospital arrest in which 40 patients had generalized

repetitive and often sound-sensitive myoclonus involving the limbs and face.[31] Frequently, mechanical ventilation and gas exchange were hampered by either vigorous movements or involvement of the diaphragm. None of these patients awakened or survived, whereas in a comparable group of comatose patients without myoclonus, one-fourth awakened in the first days after resuscitation.

Additional laboratory tests are also supportive of a major injury to the brain. Comatose patients with myoclonic status epilepticus more commonly have burst suppression (Fig. 7–3) or alpha coma patterns on electroencephalograms, cerebral edema or watershed infarcts on computed tomography (CT) scan, and more extensive cortical damage in postmortem histologic sections (Table 7–3).

Two recent reports[50,51] questioned the sweeping statement that myoclonic status epilepticus is indicative of a poor outcome on the basis of several survivors. In all these patients, high doses of sedative agents confounded examination. Nonetheless, it should be emphasized that myoclonus status epilepticus following asphyxia or any other profound anoxia may not necessarily indicate a poor prognosis, because long-term outcome data are not available. Suffice it to say that additional laboratory confirmation of severe brain damage (burst suppression on electroencephalograms, abnormal somatosensory evoked potentials, magnetic resonance imaging [MRI] or CT evidence of widespread infarction) should be documented when intensive care support is withdrawn before 3 days of observation.

Myoclonic status epilepticus should be differentiated from isolated myoclonic jerk, other types of seizures, and an action myoclonus of Lance-Adams. Lance-Adams syndrome frequently follows respiratory arrest and becomes evident after awakening (Chapter 19).

Brain death is seldom encountered after successful restoration of circulation. In our series, 5 of 107 patients fulfilled the clinical criteria for brain death.[31] All these patients were admitted with loss of most brain stem reflexes and quickly lost the ability to trigger the respirator. Persistent vegetative state (Chapter 1)

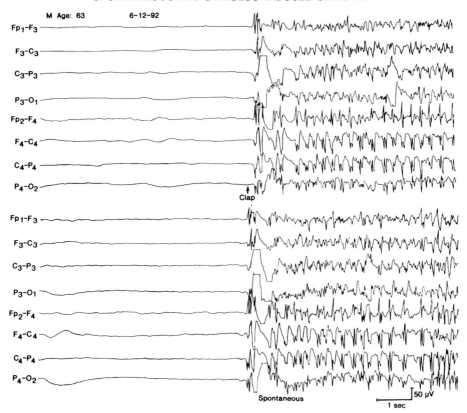

SPONTANEOUS AND STIMULUS-INDUCED SEIZURES

Figure 7–3. Electroencephalographic recording of spontaneous and sound-sensitive burst suppression in a comatose patient with severe generalized myoclonic status epilepticus.

is an uncommon outcome category and occurs in fewer than 5% of patients. After extubation, these patients are mute or occasionally groan. Generalized paratonia is common. Brisk corneomandibular, palmomental, and snout reflexes appear within a few days.

PATHOPHYSIOLOGIC MECHANISMS

The pathways to neuronal damage precipitated by an acute no-flow state can only be broadly characterized, because only some of the premises are rooted in facts. Elucidation of current concepts may lead to potential pharmacologic targets.

Ischemia remains a key factor in brain injury, and hypoxia, if any, in cardiac arrest may aggravate the damage. Studies in lab-oratory animals have failed to document brain necrosis from pure hypoxia unless Pa_{O_2} approaches 25 mm Hg. Hypoxic injury may cause temporary synaptic dysfunction, with a significant potential for regeneration, and it is clinically reflected in many cases with recovery from asphyxia-associated coma.[52–54]

The primary determinant in ischemic brain injury is exposure to excitatory transmitted glutamate, which activates N-methyl-D-aspartate (NMDA) receptors and α-amino-3-hydroxy-5-methyl-4-isoxazole propionic acid (AMPA) receptors.[55] Glutamate bombardment opens calcium and sodium channels, and catastrophic enzymatic processes and cell death follow.[56,57]

Ischemic injury may cause frank necrosis or apoptosis. Apoptosis results in digestion

Table 7–3. **Clinical, Electroencephalographic, and Computed Tomographic Findings in 107 Comatose Survivors of Cardiac Arrest**

Feature	MYOCLONIC STATUS (n = 40)		NO MYOCLONIC STATUS (n = 67)	
	No.	%	No.	%
Cranial Nerve Deficits				
Fixed pupils	5	13	9	13
No corneal reflexes	1	3	0	0
No oculocephalic responses	2	5	0	0
Motor Response				
None	34	85	43	64
Posturing	6	15	11	16
Flexion	0	0	13	19
EEG Findings				
Burst suppression	33	83	5	7
Polyspiked waves	3	8	2	3
PLEDs	0	0	4	6
Alpha coma	3	8	2	3
Diffuse slowing	1	3	44	66
Not done	0	0	10	15
CT Scan				
Cerebral infarcts	6 ⎤		1 ⎤	
Cerebral edema	6 ⎦	41	3 ⎦	10
Normal	17		38	
Not done	11		25	
Outcome				
Awakened	0	0	20	30
Poor outcome or death	40	100	52	78
Good outcome	0	0	15	22

CT, computed tomography; EEG, electroencephalographic; PLED, periodic lateralized epileptiform discharge. (From Wijdicks et al.[31] By permission of the American Neurological Association.)

of DNA from the action of endonucleases in the cell and seems to be induced by activation of a genetic program. No inflammatory response occurs, and the biochemical execution may be quick and unstoppable (similar to leaves falling off a tree). In addition, activation of caspases, a family of aspartate-specific cysteine proteases, represents an irreversible event in the apoptotic process. Ischemia may trigger both processes simultaneously, but more important, blocking excitotoxicity may enhance apoptosis. More recent insights point toward a possible role for zinc neurotoxicity due to direct influx into the cell. The current state of thinking is eloquently summarized by Lee and associates[58] and reproduced in Figure 7–4.

Laboratory Investigations

Many clinicians think that further diagnostic assessment of postresuscitation encephalopathy provides little information for prognostication and thus adds nothing more to a detailed neurologic examination over time. Only a few reports in the resuscitation literature have described CT scan findings in coma, probably because transport to the

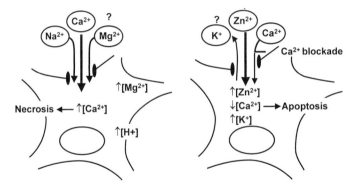

Figure 7–4. *Left*: Calcium influx: increased intracellular calcium and Mg^{2+} entry and Na^{2+} entry leading to acute excitotoxic neuronal swelling and cell death are facilitated by a decrease in intracellular pH. *Right*: Reduction of intracellular calcium and potassium efflux favors apoptosis because excessive Zn^{2+} remains to contribute to apoptosis. (Modified from Lee et al.[58] By permission of Macmillan magazines.)

radiology suite is usually deferred in patients who have frequent arrhythmias, sudden decreases in blood pressure, and need for specific modes of ventilation. The most common early abnormal CT finding is effacement of sulci from edema.[59] Decrease in the cortical gray matter density from edema, resulting in loss of contrast difference between gray and white matter and obliteration of basal cisterns, is unusual and is more common in patients who fulfill or almost fulfill the clinical criteria for brain death.[60] Bird and colleagues[61] convincingly showed that this phenomenon of loss of contrast difference of gray and white matter can be explained by venous distention of the deep white matter veins. Drainage of these veins into subependymal veins is obstructed as a result of a transient increase in intracranial pressure.

The CT scans in comatose patients after CPR may also show watershed infarcts, bilateral thalamic hypodensities, and, due to susceptibility, cerebellar infarction and swelling (Fig. 7–5). The CT scan findings are usually normal after resuscitation, but these abnormalities may become more apparent in the next days. Cortical necrosis may be demonstrated on CT with high intravenous doses of contrast material, but its value in prognostication is unknown.[62] Brain swelling and cerebral infarcts on CT scan predict a poor outcome. None of our patients with abnormal findings on CT scans awakened.[31]

Magnetic resonance imaging is problematic because of transport, anesthetic coverage during image acquisition, and availability. Serial MRI may demonstrate high-signal-intensity lesions in the cortex compatible with laminar necrosis and white matter lesions from watershed infarcts.[63,64] In a study of MRI findings in 52 patients with cardiac arrest, 25% had cortical infarcts, 14% had cortical watershed infarcts, 21% had deep cerebral infarcts, and 4% had deep watershed infarcts. One-fourth of the patients had normal findings on MRI scans. Comparison with controls showed that only deep cerebral infarcts were significantly more common. In this study, abnormal MRI findings did not predict functional outcome.[65]

In our experience, diffusion-weighted and fluid-attenuated inversion recovery MRI has been a very helpful confirmatory investigation, certainly in instances in which the family is unable to accept the prognosis on the basis of the clinical examination alone. Abnormalities on MRI can be widespread, and the study can document cortical necrosis, edema, and involvement of the basal ganglia and thalamus[66] (Fig. 7–6). None of our patients with abnormal fluid-attenuated inversion recovery MRI findings involving cortical structures improved beyond a vegetative state. Because none of these patients had other clinical or electroencephalographic (EEG) prognosticators of poor outcome, MRI may have a role in indicating outcome for these patients. If these preliminary observations are confirmed, the cost of a single MRI may offset the mounting costs of unnecessary prolonged intensive care of a crippled comatose survivor.

The value of EEG recording in prognostication, although unresolved, is most likely limited. Many EEG patterns in postresuscitation coma have been described, but only some are strong indicators of poor outcome.[67–75]

Widespread theta or delta waves, some-

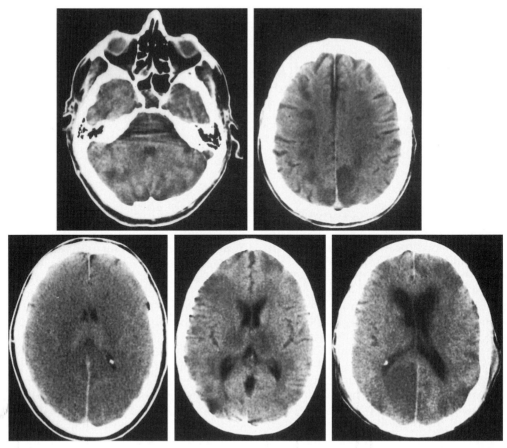

Figure 7–5. Computed tomography scan patterns in comatose patients and myoclonic status epilepticus. *Top row* (one patient): Multiple hypodensities in the cerebellum, cortex, and white matter. *Bottom row* (three patients): *Left*: Cerebral edema evidenced by loss of white–gray matter differentiation and loss of sulci. *Center*: Watershed infarcts with bilateral hypodensities in the thalamus. *Right*: Multiple small and large territory cortical infarcts. (From Wijdicks et al.[31] By permission of the American Neurological Association.)

times with clear asymmetries between the activities of both hemispheres, are common findings, and some patients have prominent superimposed isolated sharp waves and spikes. Attention has been drawn to EEG rhythms of alpha frequency (alpha pattern coma).[69,76–78] Alpha-pattern coma denotes rhythmic activity that emerges more prominently over the anterior or middle regions and is unreactive to auditory, noxious, or photic stimuli. This pattern is seen in the first days after cardiac arrest and can be later replaced by slow delta–theta wave patterns.[69,77,78] Occasionally, this alpha pattern changes into low-voltage theta and beta waves. Electro-oculographic potentials indicative of slow, pendular eye movements re-

sembling the first stages of sleep may be recorded. Alpha coma may also alternate with burst suppression patterns.[31] Generally, it has been accepted that outcome is poor in patients with EEG characteristics of alpha coma, but one report pointed out that the prognosis of patients with alpha coma was not worse than that of other patients with similar depths of coma.[78] Reactivity of the alpha coma pattern (change in voltage or frequency after pain) may favor the potential for awakening.[79]

Other well-organized EEG patterns are spindle coma (activity resembling slow-wave sleep), burst–suppression patterns (common in myoclonus), and rhythmic discharges of synchronous sharp waves. Status

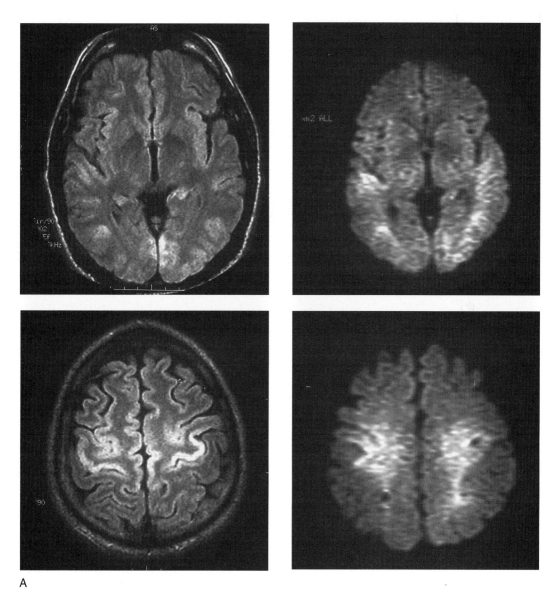

A

Figure 7–6. (*A*) Axial fluid-attenuated inversion recovery (FLAIR) magnetic resonance images (*upper* and *lower left*) show widespread T2-weighted signal abnormalities throughout the cortex of both cerebral hemispheres. Diffusion-weighted images (*upper* and *lower right*) show high-intensity signals at these locations. None of the patients with these abnormalities awakened. (*Continued*)

epilepticus patterns may be found on EEG in postresuscitation coma. Close observation may reveal subtle jerking of jaw and eyelids accompanied by continuous or episodic spike-and-wave activity with occasional sharp transients. These patterns may occur without any other clinical signs of seizures. Status epilepticus on EEG in coma after cardiac arrest is often also resistant to therapy[80,81] and probably also should be considered a marker

of severe brain damage. There are no convincing series of patients after cardiac arrest with status epilepticus or burst–suppression patterns on EEG in whom treatment with antiepileptic drugs has resulted in awakening or even improved the level of consciousness.

The difficulties of interpreting conventional EEGs have been overcome by the introduction of compressed spectral array, but

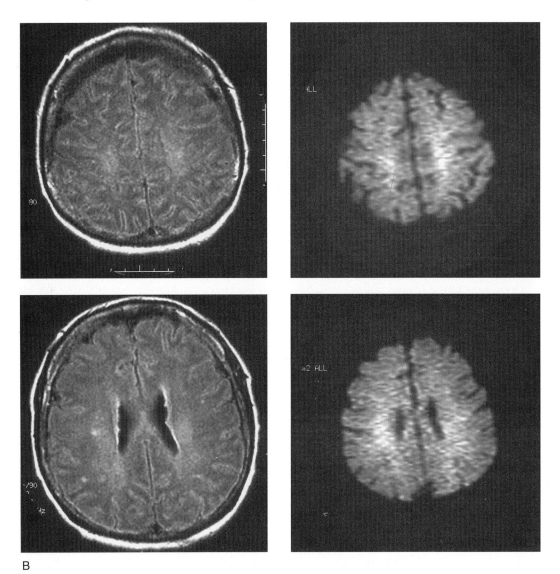

B

Figure 7–6. (*Continued*) (*B*) Axial FLAIR images (*upper* and *lower left*) show cerebral edema with effacement of sulci and T2-weighted signal abnormalities in the white matter. Corresponding diffusion-weighted images (*upper* and *lower right*) show abnormalities only in the white matter. None of these patients recovered. (*Continued*)

this technique may not be available to everyone.[82] A preliminary study in 18 survivors of cardiopulmonary arrest classified the taped data into four groups and found that virtually all patients survived with patterns consisting of predominance of either delta frequency with various amounts of theta activity or theta and alpha frequencies with various amounts of delta activity.[83] However, prolonged EEG recording in the ICU is consid-erably limited by pharmaceutical agents and artifacts.

Because somatosensory evoked potentials are generally not influenced by medication, they are a much more promising modality (Fig. 7–7). Very high doses of propofol and midazolam, however, can reduce the evoked amplitude. A fairly consistent prognostic rule seems to have emerged. Brunko and Zegers de Beyl[84] showed in 50 consecutive

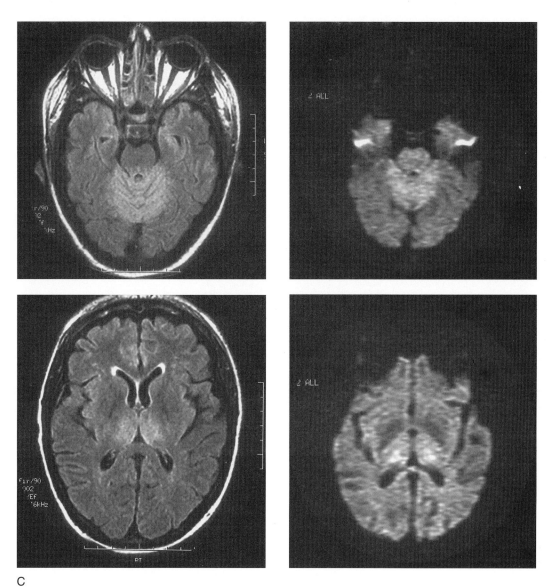

C

Figure 7–6. (*Continued*) (*C*) Axial FLAIR images (*upper* and *lower left*) at the level of the superior cerebellum and thalamus show symmetrical T2-weighted signal abnormalities. The diffusion-weighted sequence (*upper* and *lower right*) at the same level shows abnormalities at the same locations. The patients recovered without major neurologic deficit. (*A* and *B* from Wijdicks et al.[66] By permission of the American Society of Neuroradiology.)

patients that lack of cortical bilateral short-latency N_{19}–P_{22} waves along with retention of identifiable cervical response was associated with a persistent vegetative state or death. All patients were studied within 8 hr after arrest, and serial studies did not show recovery of any cortical component in the first 2 weeks. Widespread anoxic–ischemic damage of cortex, thalamus, and cerebellum has been found in autopsy in patients without cortical evoked responses. Patients with preserved cortical somatosensory evoked potentials have the potential to recover (cortical evoked response is retained in approximately two-thirds of the patients), and prediction of outcome is not clear. A recent study in 216 patients with hypoxic–ischemic coma found that 42% of somatosensory

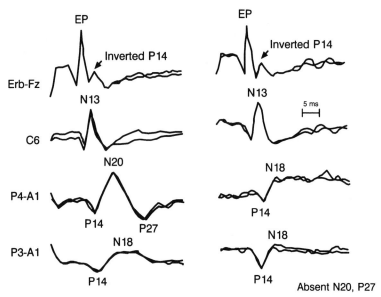

Figure 7–7. Somatosensory evoked potential (EP) in comatose patient (best motor response on admission was extensor posturing to pain) with absent cortical responses (N20 and P27). *Left,* Normal reference. The response is seen at Erb, at the cervical spine, and at the scalp. The last two responses (left and right) reflect the pathway between the cervicomedullary junction and the primary sensory cortex. *Right,* Comatose patient with absent scalp potentials after resuscitation.

evoked potential recordings were abnormal, and all 86 patients died without awakening from coma.[85] These findings were presaged in an earlier study that also claimed that long-latency evoked potentials (the third negative cortical peak N_{70}, seen after changing the band-pass filter) may have additional prognostic value in patients with retained cortical (short-latency) response.[86] These long-latency sensory evoked potentials probably are generated by thalamocortical and intercortical connections and may disappear in a stepwise fashion while the short-term potentials remain visible. Lack of the N_{70} peak or significant delay differentiated favorable from poor outcome, but recognition of this peak (and its delay) may be very difficult.[86] Motor evoked responses may, however, have additional prognostic value, particularly in patients with preserved cortical somatosensory evoked potential responses.

There has also been considerable interest in finding a useful chemical marker to discriminate between patients who will recover and patients who will never awaken.[87–92] After an ischemic global insult to the brain, the abundantly present cytosolic enzymes leak into the cerebrospinal fluid. Peaks in brain-type (BB) creatine kinase isoenzyme (CK_1)

levels in the cerebrospinal fluid may suggest massive ischemic tissue injury.[93] A preliminary study found a significant association between an increase in CK_1 in the cerebrospinal fluid and histologic damage at autopsy.[93] In another study, measurement of CK_1 in the cerebrospinal fluid had a positive predictive value of 93% for persistent coma.[48] However, serum CK_1 levels did not correlate with outcome. Recent experience with 52 comatose patients at the University of Washington in Seattle found that cerebrospinal fluid creatine kinase BB ≥ 205 U/L or bilateral absence of scalp potentials on somatosensory evoked potential recordings (or both) predicted failure to awaken with a sensitivity of 69% and a specificity of 100%.[94]

Analysis of neuron-specific enolase measured in the cerebrospinal fluid within 24 hr after cardiac arrest was also highly specific in detecting patients who remained comatose. All patients with neuron-specific enolase values >24 ng/mL (controls, 6.4 ± 0.5 ng/mL) remained unconscious and died (positive predictive value, 100%; negative predictive value, 89%).[87] However, both neuron-specific enolase and S-100 protein, a calcium-binding protein found in the brain, may leak in serum after brain cell damage. A recent study in 56 patients suggested that serum levels of neuron-specific enolase are highly predictive when measured 3 days after resuscitation (cutoff value of 16.4 μg/L) but may have only confirmatory value at that time.[95] The predictive serum values with different cutoff points shown in Table 7–4 suggest that these may be valuable adjunctive tests.

To summarize, the reliability of clinical examination alone for prognosis remains unchallenged. Additional laboratory tests are emerging quickly but are difficult to perform (for example, MRI), are not always available in time (somatosensory evoked potentials), or are less than perfect in prediction (EEG). Preliminary experience with serum and cerebrospinal fluid markers is very promising. Measurement is only helpful if clinical findings confirm a poor outlook.

TREATMENT AND SUPPORTIVE CARE

Very little is known about the merits of current management strategies of cerebral protection in resuscitation survivors. The emphasis has shifted to neuroprotective therapy, and several treatment trials have been performed with no[5] or extremely meager[6] benefit. There are no definitive guidelines for basic management in comatose survivors.

Basic Management

Because no drugs effectively reduce the impact of anoxia and ischemia to the brain, management is tailored to minimize secondary brain damage. Many patients have underlying myocardial infarction with arrhythmias and hypotension. Conversely, transient increases in systolic arterial blood pressure are common after resuscitation. Hypertension is not a reflection of increased intracranial pressure but more often is associated with administration of epinephrine. In time, blood pressures level off, and aggressive treatment with agents that have a relatively long duration of action may decrease cerebral perfusion pressure in areas devoid of autoregulation.

The basic form of standard CPR has been extended by inclusion of a third phase, cerebral resuscitation, mainly through the pioneering efforts of the Brain Resuscitation Clinical Trial study group.[5,6] Although the importance of implementation of standard guidelines for cerebral protection is recognized, its effect on outcome is not established. The data from controlled clinical trials comparing the cerebral resuscitation protocol with and without a cerebral protection agent did not settle the issue of how to additionally manage these patients. Separating the results of the cerebral resuscitation regimen did not document a far better outcome than expected in this compromised patient population.[5,6]

Safar and Bircher's guidelines consist of

Table 7–4. Serum Markers for Poor Outcome in Comatose Patients after Cardiac Arrest

Reference	No. of Patients	Substance	Cutoff Value (μg/L)	PPV (%)	NPV (%)
Roine et al., 1989[87]	75	NSE	17	89	79
Fogel et al., 1997[89]	43	NSE	33	100	78
Rosén et al., 1998[90]*	41	S-100	0.2	71	85
Martens et al., 1998[91]	64	S-100	0.7	95	63
		NSE	20	86	65
Böttiger et al., 2001[92]	66	S-100	0.2	87	100

NPV, negative predictive value; NSE, neuron-specific enolase; PPV, positive predictive value; S-100, astroglial protein.

Positive predictive value is the probability that poor outcome exists when the value is attained; negative predictive value is the probability that good outcome is possible with a value lower than the cutoff value.

*Survival only.

induction of mild hypertension (mean arterial pressure, 120 to 140 mm Hg) for 1 to 5 min with or without plasma volume expansion with Ringer's solution or dextran 40 in doses of 40 mL/kg.[17,18] These guidelines have a certain relevance because they reflect the observations in animal models, but their clinical value has not been proven in randomized studies. Moreover, a 1992 study of high doses of epinephrine used in out-of-hospital arrest did not show improved neurologic outcome.[96]

An additional argument for increasing baseline mean arterial blood pressure is absent autoregulation. Also, autoregulation is right-shifted after resuscitation associated with hypoxic–ischemic damage. Thus, in general, pharmaceutical agents that reduce blood pressure even further need to be withdrawn.[97]

Hyperglycemia has been associated with worse outcome in survivors of cardiac arrest.[98] Ischemic tissue lactate may increase in hyperglycemic patients, but whether maintaining normoglycemia attenuates the anoxic–ischemic damage after resuscitation is unknown.[99,100] The understanding, based on a canine study, has been that dextrose solutions should not be used, because they may greatly increase blood glucose levels after resuscitation and profoundly increase morbidity and mortality.[101] However, in a randomized study of 5% dextrose or isotonic saline infused in patients with cardiac arrest by paramedics in Seattle, no significant differences in outcome were found.[102] The significance of hyperglycemia in postresuscitation brain damage needs further investigation, and it may be an epiphenomenon after all.

Finally, a small clinical trial of moderate hypothermia (33°C for 24 hr) with ice packs and neuromuscular blocking agents to prevent shivering found a significant increase in number of patients with good outcome.[11,103] This result should prompt the planning of further prospective studies.

Use of antiepileptic agents has repeatedly failed to reduce the frequency of myoclonic jerks. Therefore, treatment should focus on temporary use of neuromuscular blocking agents mainly to eliminate a dreadful sight to family members. Our preliminary experience also suggests a possible role for propofol (20 to 40 μg/kg per minute). The decision to withdraw support should be strongly influenced by the presence of myoclonic status epilepticus, certainly when other laboratory test results point in the same direction. Patients with myoclonic status epilepticus have a very high probability of death. Survivors have been reported, but in this clinical situation, none without devastating disability.

Intracranial Pressure Monitoring

The use of intracranial pressure monitoring and its subsequent management after CPR are not well established.[104] It is reasonable to assume that after a considerable insult, some brain swelling may occur as well as an increase in intracranial pressure. Frequent suctioning for pulmonary secretions, agitation in patients who are fighting the respirator, and positive end-expiratory pressure >10 cm H_2O are additional factors that may further increase intracranial pressure. It is usually prudent to use muscle relaxants and sedatives in these agitated patients.

The practice of monitoring intracranial pressure in postanoxic coma may have very little justification. Only a limited number of monitored patients have been reported, and intracranial pressure did not appear to be of primary importance. A study of six patients with intracranial pressure monitoring showed that none with a Glasgow coma scale score of 3 or 4 had values above 20 mm Hg, except one patient with seizures.[104] We have occasionally used fiberoptic intracranial monitors in young comatose resuscitated patients with progressive sulcal effacement on CT scan after severe anoxic insults but have not found significant increased intracranial pressure readings. The dilemma of intracranial pressure monitoring in near-drowning is of similar proportion (Chapter 16).

Specific Treatment

Many enthusiastic reports of possibly effective treatments in animal studies have been published, but the results of clinical controlled trials have been disappointing thus far. A prospective investigator will readily recognize that one of the major drawbacks in controlled, randomized trials in this category of patients is that mortality within the first month is very high in comatose survivors, and an effect, if any, may be difficult to demonstrate. Nevertheless, most randomized studies conducted thus far had sufficient power to detect improvement in disability of at least 20%.[5,6]

The efficacy of thiopental loading has been studied in a randomized, blinded clinical trial. The mechanism of action for thiopental in postresuscitation coma has not been satisfactorily clarified but probably is derived from a decrease in cerebral metabolic rate or a decrease in cerebral edema. The studied patients had no purposeful motor response to pain after adequate systemic circulation was reestablished and were randomly allocated to a thiopental loading dose of 30 mg/kg given intravenously within 10 to 50 min. A large percentage of the patients had cardiac arrest outside the hospital. Thiopental loading had no benefit.[5] In addition, use of thiopental in high doses resulted in severe hypotension, and many patients needed vasopressors.

Corticosteroids have not been formally tested in a clinical trial, but in a post hoc analysis of the Brain Resuscitation Clinical Trial I, glucocorticoid administration in the first 8 hr after arrest had no effect.[105] In this study, use of steroids was left to the clinician in charge, and as a surprising result, approximately 70% of enrolled patients received steroids.

To circumvent the long delay between out-of-hospital cardiac arrest and treatment, intravenous administration of nimodipine was begun in ambulances.[106] Unfortunately, immediate treatment with calcium channel blockers did not significantly change the prognosis for victims of out-of-hospital ventricular fibrillation. However, there was an important trend toward higher 1-year survival and good recovery rates in patients treated after a delay of at least 10 minutes from the time of cardiac arrest. In addition, recurrent ventricular fibrillation was significantly lower in the nimodipine-treated group. Unfortunately, an analysis of the Brain Resuscitation Clinical Trial II (lidoflazine intravenously) did not show marked differences in outcome.[6]

CONCLUSIONS

At one end of the spectrum of events is the devastation of postresuscitation encephalopathy. One is often forced to conclude that recovery cannot be expected.

Detailed examination of the comatose patient after successful resuscitation remains the mainstay of assessment. Light-fixed pupils and myoclonus status epilepticus on the first day invariably predict very poor outcome (death in most cases). Approximately one-third of patients have one or both of these distinguishing features. Additional examination of somatosensory evoked potentials may demonstrate absent cortical evoked responses, a finding that may place another 10% to 20% of patients in the grim-outcome category. A CT scan or MRI of the brain, which may show multiple cerebral infarcts or cerebral edema in an occasional patient, may add prognostic value, as may cerebrospinal fluid creatine kinase BB fraction exceeding 205 U/L. The prognostic value of EEG remains unconvincing, except perhaps in patients with burst–suppression patterns. When these poor prognostic signs are combined (in roughly 40% of patients), one may make a strong case for do-not-resuscitate orders or withdrawal of life-prolonging treatment after a detailed discussion with family members. These patients do not have much of a chance to recover to any functionally productive level.

Supportive care consists of adequate volume replacement and blood pressure stabilization and normothermia. Intracranial pressure monitoring is not likely of benefit. Specific drugs, such as thiopental, nimodipine, lidoflazine, and corticosteroids, have shown no effect on outcome.

REFERENCES

1. Zoch TW, Desbiens NA, DeStefano F, Stueland DT, Layde PM. Short- and long-term survival after cardiopulmonary resuscitation. Arch Intern Med 160: 1969–1973, 2000.

2. Eisenberg MS, Mengert TJ. Primary care: cardiac resuscitation. N Engl J Med 344:1304–1313, 2001.

3. Landry FJ, Parker JM, Phillips YY. Outcome of cardiopulmonary resuscitation in the intensive care setting. Arch Intern Med 152:2305–2308, 1992.

4. Peterson MW, Geist LJ, Schwartz DA, Konicek S, Moseley PL. Outcome after cardiopulmonary resuscitation in a medical intensive care unit. Chest 100:168–174, 1991.

5. Brain Resuscitation Clinical Trial I Study Group. Randomized clinical study of thiopental loading in comatose survivors of cardiac arrest. N Engl J Med 314:397–403, 1986.

6. Brain Resuscitation Clinical Trial II Study Group. A randomized clinical study of a calcium-entry blocker (lidoflazine) in the treatment of comatose survivors of cardiac arrest. N Engl J Med 324:1225–1231, 1991.

7. Earnest MP, Breckinridge JC, Yarnell PR, Oliva PB. Quality of survival after out-of-hospital cardiac arrest: predictive value of early neurologic evaluation. Neurology 29:56–60, 1979.

8. Bedell SE, Delbanco TL, Cook EF, Epstein FH. Survival after cardiopulmonary resuscitation in the hospital. N Engl J Med 309:569–576, 1983.

9. Murphy DJ, Murray AM, Robinson BE, Campion EW. Outcomes of cardiopulmonary resuscitation in the elderly. Ann Intern Med 111:199–205, 1989.

10. Myerburg RJ, Conde CA, Sung RJ, et al. Clinical, electrophysiologic and hemodynamic profile of patients resuscitated from prehospital cardiac arrest. Am J Med 68:568–576, 1980.

11. Bernard SA, Jones BM, Horne MK. Clinical trial of induced hypothermia in comatose survivors of out-of-hospital cardiac arrest. Ann Emerg Med 30:146–153, 1997.

12. Thel MC, O'Connor CM. Cardiopulmonary resuscitation: historical perspective to recent investigations. Am Heart J 137:39–48, 1999.

13. Niemann JT, Rosborough JP, Hausknecht M, Garner D, Criley JM. Pressure-synchronized cineangiography during experimental cardiopulmonary resuscitation. Circulation 64:985–991, 1981.

14. Werner JA, Greene HL, Janko CL, Cobb LA. Visualization of cardiac valve motion in man during external chest compression using two-dimensional echocardiography. Implications regarding the mechanism of blood flow. Circulation 63:1417–1421, 1981.

15. Plaisance P, Adnet F, Vicaut E, et al. Benefit of active compression–decompression cardiopulmonary resuscitation as a prehospital advanced cardiac life support. A randomized multicenter study. Circulation 95:955–961, 1997.

16. Tisherman SA, Vandevelde K, Safar P, et al. Future directions for resuscitation research. V. Ultra-advanced life support. Resuscitation 34:281–293, 1997.

17. Kaye W, Bircher NG (eds). Cardiopulmonary Resuscitation. Clinics in Critical Care Medicine, Vol. 16. Churchill Livingstone, New York, 1989.

18. Safar P. On the future of reanimatology. Acad Emerg Med 7:75–89, 2000.

19. Bass E. Cardiopulmonary arrest. Pathophysiology and neurologic complications. Ann Intern Med 103:920–927, 1985.

20. Petito CK, Feldmann E, Pulsinelli WA, Plum F. Delayed hippocampal damage in humans following cardiorespiratory arrest. Neurology 37:1281–1286, 1987.

21. Petito CK, Pulsinelli WA. Sequential development of reversible and irreversible neuronal damage following cerebral ischemia. J Neuropathol Exp Neurol 43:141–153, 1984.

22. Pulsinelli WA, Brierley JB, Plum F. Temporal profile of neuronal damage in a model of transient forebrain ischemia. Ann Neurol 11:491–498, 1982.

23. Callaham M, Madsen CD, Barton CW, Saunders CE, Pointer J. A randomized clinical trial of high-dose epinephrine and norepinephrine vs standard-dose epinephrine in prehospital cardiac arrest. JAMA 268:2667–2672, 1992.

24. Safar P, Grenvik A, Abramson NS, Bircher NG (eds). Reversibility of clinical death: symposium on resuscitation research. Crit Care Med 16:919–1084, 1988.

25. Levy DE, Caronna JJ, Singer BH, Lapinski RH, Frydman H, Plum F. Predicting outcome from hypoxic-ischemic coma. JAMA 253:1420–1426, 1985.

26. Mullie A, Verstringe P, Buylaert W, et al. Predictive value of Glasgow coma score for awakening after out-of-hospital cardiac arrest. Cerebral Resuscitation Study Group of the Belgian Society for Intensive Care. Lancet 1:137–140, 1988.

27. Snyder BD, Loewenson RB, Gumnit RJ, Hauser WA, Leppik IE, Ramirez-Lassepas M. Neurologic prognosis after cardiopulmonary arrest: II. Level of consciousness. Neurology 30:52–58, 1980.

28. Volpe BT, Herscovitch P, Raichle ME. PET evaluation of patients with amnesia after cardiac arrest [abstract]. Stroke 15:196, 1984.

29. Volpe BT, Holtzman JD, Hirst W. Further characterization of patients with amnesia after cardiac arrest: preserved recognition memory. Neurology 36:408–411, 1986.

30. Longstreth WT Jr, Diehr P, Inui TS. Prediction of awakening after out-of-hospital cardiac arrest. N Engl J Med 308:1378–1382, 1983.

31. Wijdicks EFM, Parisi JE, Sharbrough FW. Prognostic value of myoclonus status in comatose survivors of cardiac arrest. Ann Neurol 35:239–243, 1994.

32. Plum F, Posner JB, Hain RF. Delayed neurological deterioration after anoxia. Arch Intern Med 110:56–63, 1962.

33. Ginsberg MD. Delayed neurological deterioration following hypoxia. Adv Neurol 26:21–44, 1979.

34. Sage JI, Van Uitert RL. Man-in-the-barrel syndrome. Neurology 36:1102–1103, 1986.

35. Delavelle J, Lalanne B, Megret M. Man-in-the barrel syndrome: first CT images. Neuroradiology 29:501, 1987.

36. Snyder BD, Gumnit RJ, Leppik IE, Hauser WA, Loewenson RB, Ramirez-Lassepas M. Neurologic prognosis after cardiopulmonary arrest: IV. Brainstem reflexes. Neurology 31:1092–1097, 1981.

37. Jordanov J, Ruben H. Reliability of pupillary changes as a clinical sign of hypoxia. Lancet 2:915–917, 1967.

38. Kapp J, Paulson G. Pupillary changes induced by circulatory arrest. Neurology 16:225–229, 1966.

39. Steen-Hansen JE, Hansen NN, Vaagenes P, Schreiner B. Pupil size and light reactivity during cardiopulmonary resuscitation: A clinical study. Crit Care Med 16:69–70, 1988.

40. Keane JR. Sustained upgaze in coma. Ann Neurol 9:409–412, 1981.

41. Johkura K, Komiyama A, Kuroiwa Y. Sustained downgaze in coma after cardiac arrest [letter to the editor]. J Neurol Neurosurg Psychiatry 71: 278–279, 2001.

42. Ropper AH. Ocular dipping in anoxic coma. Arch Neurol 38:297–299, 1981.

43. Fisher CM. Ocular bobbing. Arch Neurol 11:543–546, 1964.

44. Fisher CM. The neurological examination of the comatose patient. Acta Neurol Scand 45 (Suppl): 1–56, 1969.

45. Snyder BD, Hauser WA, Loewenson RB, Leppik IE, Ramirez-Lassepas M, Gumnit RJ. Neurologic prognosis after cardiopulmonary arrest: III. Seizure activity. Neurology 30:1292–1297, 1980.

46. Jumao-as A, Brenner RP. Myoclonic status epilepticus: a clinical and electroencephalographic study. Neurology 40:1199–1202, 1990.

47. Krumholz A, Stern BJ, Weiss HD. Outcome from coma after cardiopulmonary resuscitation: relation to seizures and myoclonus. Neurology 38: 401–405, 1988.

48. Vaagenes P, Kjekshus J, Torvik A. The relationship between cerebrospinal fluid creatine kinase and morphologic changes in the brain after transient cardiac arrest. Circulation 61:1194–1199, 1980.

49. Young GB, Gilbert JJ, Zochodne DW. The significance of myoclonic status epilepticus in postanoxic coma. Neurology 40:1843–1848, 1990.

50. Morris HR, Howard RS, Brown P. Early myoclonic status and outcome after cardiorespiratory arrest. J Neurol Neurosurg Psychiatry 64:267–268, 1998.

51. Arnoldus EP, Lammers GJ. Postanoxic coma: good recovery despite myoclonus status. Ann Neurol 38:697–698, 1995.

52. Pearigen P, Gwinn R, Simon RP. The effects in vivo of hypoxia on brain injury. Brain Res 725:184–191, 1996.

53. Miyamoto O, Auer RN. Hypoxia, hyperoxia, ischemia, and brain necrosis. Neurology 54:362–371, 2000.

54. Simon RP. Hypoxia versus ischemia. Neurology 52:7–8, 1999.

55. Pulsinelli W. Excitotoxic damage in global ischemia. Adv Neurol 71:61–62, 1996.

56. Dubinsky JM, Rothman SM. Intracellular calcium concentrations during "chemical hypoxia" and excitotoxic neuronal injury. J Neurosci 11:2545–2551, 1991.

57. Roettger V, Lipton P. Mechanism of glutamate release from rat hippocampal slices during in vitro ischemia. Neuroscience 75:677–685, 1996.

58. Lee JM, Zipfel GJ, Choi DW. The changing landscape of ischaemic brain injury mechanisms. Nature 399 (Suppl):A7–A14, 1999.

59. Morimoto Y, Kemmotsu O, Kitami K, Matsubara I, Tedo I. Acute brain swelling after out-of-hospital cardiac arrest: pathogenesis and outcome. Crit Care Med 21:104–110, 1993.

60. Kjos BO, Brant-Zawadski M, Young RG. Early CT findings of global central nervous system hypoperfusion. AJR Am J Roentgenol 141:1227–1232, 1983.

61. Bird CR, Drayer BP, Gilles FH. Pathophysiology of "reverse" edema in global cerebral ischemia. AJNR Am J Neuroradiol 10:95–98, 1989.

62. Liwnicz BJ, Mouradian MD, Ball JB Jr. Intense brain cortical enhancement on CT in laminar necrosis verified by biopsy. AJNR Am J Neuroradiol 8:157–159, 1987.

63. Sawada H, Udaka F, Seriu N, Shindou K, Kameyama M, Tsujimura M. MRI demonstration of cortical laminar necrosis and delayed white matter injury in anoxic encephalopathy. Neuroradiology 32:319–321, 1990.

64. Takahashi S, Higano S, Ishii K, et al. Hypoxic brain damage: cortical laminar necrosis and delayed changes in white matter at sequential MR imaging. Radiology 189:449–456, 1993.

65. Roine RO, Raininko R, Erkinjuntti T, Ylikoski A, Kaste M. Magnetic resonance imaging findings associated with cardiac arrest. Stroke 24:1005–1014, 1993.

66. Wijdicks EFM, Campeau NG, Miller GM. MR imaging in comatose survivors of cardiac resuscitation. AJNR Am J Neuroradiol 22:1561–1565, 2001.

67. Binnie CD, Prior PF, Lloyd DS, Scott DF, Margerison JH. Electroencephalographic prediction of fatal anoxic brain damage after resuscitation from cardiac arrest. Br Med J 4:265–268, 1970.

68. Britt CW Jr. Nontraumatic "spindle coma": clinical, EEG, and prognostic features. Neurology 31: 393–397, 1981.

69. Grindal AB, Suter C, Martinez AJ. Alpha-pattern coma: 24 cases with 9 survivors. Ann Neurol 1: 371–377, 1977.

70. Jørgensen EO, Malchow-Møller A. Natural history of global and critical brain ischaemia. Part I: EEG and neurological signs during the first year after cardiopulmonary resuscitation in patients subsequently regaining consciousness. Resuscitation 9:133–153, 1981.

71. Jørgensen EO, Malchow-Møller A. Natural history of global and critical brain ischaemia. Part II: EEG and neurological signs in patients remaining unconscious after cardiopulmonary resuscitation. Resuscitation 9:155–174, 1981.

72. Jørgensen EO, Malchow-Møller A. Natural history of global and critical brain ischaemia. Part III: Cerebral prognostic signs after cardiopulmonary resuscitation. Cerebral recovery course and rate during the first year after global and critical ischaemia monitored and predicted by EEG and neurological signs. Resuscitation 9:175–188, 1981.

73. Moss J, Rockoff M. EEG monitoring during cardiac arrest and resuscitation. JAMA 244:2750–2751, 1980.

74. Sørensen K, Thomassen A, Wernberg M. Prognostic significance of alpha frequency EEG rhythm in coma after cardiac arrest. J Neurol Neurosurg Psychiatry 41:840–842, 1978.

75. Thomassen A, Sorensen K, Wernberg M. The prognostic value of EEG in coma survivors after cardiac arrest. Acta Anaesthesiol Scand 22:483–490, 1978.

76. Obeso JA, Iragui MI, Marti-Masso JF, et al. Neu-

rophysiological assessment of alpha pattern coma. J Neurol Neurosurg Psychiatry 43:63–67, 1980.

77. Vignaendra V, Wilkus RJ, Copass MK, Chatrian GE. Electroencephalographic rhythms of alpha frequency in comatose patients after cardiopulmonary arrest. Neurology 24:582–588, 1974.

78. Westmoreland BF, Klass DW, Sharbrough FW, Reagan TJ. Alpha-coma. Electroencephalographic, clinical, pathologic, and etiologic correlations. Arch Neurol 32:713–718, 1975.

79. Kaplan PW, Genoud D, Ho TW, Jallon P. Etiology, neurologic correlations, and prognosis in alpha coma. Clin Neurophysiol 110:205–213, 1999.

80. Lowenstein DH, Aminoff MJ. Clinical and EEG features of status epilepticus in comatose patients. Neurology 42:100–104, 1992.

81. Simon RP, Aminoff MJ. Electrographic status epilepticus in fatal anoxic coma. Ann Neurol 20:351–355, 1986.

82. Cant BR, Shaw NA. Monitoring by compressed spectral array in prolonged coma. Neurology 34:35–39, 1984.

83. Morillo LE, Tulloch JW, Gumnit RJ, Snyder BD. Compressed spectral array patterns following cardiopulmonary arrest. A preliminary report. Arch Neurol 40:287–289, 1983.

84. Brunko E, Zegers de Beyl D. Prognostic value of early cortical somatosensory evoked potentials after resuscitation from cardiac arrest. Electroencephalogr Clin Neurophysiol 66:15–24, 1987.

85. Madl C, Kramer L, Yeganehfar W, et al. Detection of nontraumatic comatose patients with no benefit of intensive care treatment by recording of sensory evoked potentials. Arch Neurol 53:512–516, 1996.

86. Madl C, Grimm G, Kramer L, et al. Early prediction of individual outcome after cardiopulmonary resuscitation. Lancet 341:855–858, 1993.

87. Roine RO, Somer H, Kaste M, Viinikka L, Karonen SL. Neurological outcome after out-of-hospital cardiac arrest. Prediction by cerebrospinal fluid enzyme analysis. Arch Neurol 46:753–756, 1989.

88. Scarna H, Delafosse B, Steinberg R, et al. Neuron-specific enolase as a marker of neuronal lesions during various comas in man. Neurochem Int 4:405–411, 1982.

89. Fogel W, Krieger D, Veith M, et al. Serum neuron-specific enolase as early predictor of outcome after cardiac arrest. Crit Care Med 25:1133–1138, 1997.

90. Rosén H, Rosengren L, Herlitz J, Blomstrand C. Increased serum levels of the S-100 protein are associated with hypoxic brain damage after cardiac arrest. Stroke 29:473–477, 1998.

91. Martens P, Raabe A, Johnsson P. Serum S-100 and neuron-specific enolase for prediction of regaining consciousness after global cerebral ischemia. Stroke 29:2363–2366, 1998.

92. Böttiger BW, Möbes S, Glätzer R, et al. Astroglial protein S-100 is an early and sensitive marker of hypoxic brain damage and outcome after cardiac arrest in humans. Circulation 103:2694–2698, 2001.

93. Vaagenes P, Safar P, Diven W, et al. Brain enzyme levels in CSF after cardiac arrest and resuscitation in dogs: markers of damage and predictors of outcome. J Cereb Blood Flow Metab 8:262–275, 1988.

94. Sherman AL, Tirschwell DL, Micklesen PJ, Longstreth WT Jr, Robinson LR. Somatosensory potentials, CSF creatine kinase BB activity, and awakening after cardiac arrest. Neurology 54:889–894, 2000.

95. Schoerkhuber W, Kittler H, Sterz F, et al. Time course of serum neuron-specific enolase: a predictor of neurological outcome in patients resuscitated from cardiac arrest. Stroke 30:1598–1603, 1999.

96. Brown CG, Martin DR, Pepe PE, et al. A comparison of standard-dose and high-dose epinephrine in cardiac arrest outside the hospital. The Multicenter High-Dose Epinephrine Study Group. N Engl J Med 327:1051–1055, 1992.

97. Sundgreen C, Larsen FS, Herzog TM, Knudsen GM, Boesgaard S, Aldershvile J. Autoregulation of cerebral blood flow in patients resuscitated from cardiac arrest. Stroke 32:128–132, 2001.

98. Mullner M, Sterz F, Binder M, Schreiber W, Deimel A, Laggner AN. Blood glucose concentration after cardiopulmonary resuscitation influences functional neurological recovery in human cardiac arrest survivors. J Cereb Blood Flow Metab 17:430–436, 1997.

99. Kushner M, Nencini P, Reivich M, et al. Relation of hyperglycemia early in ischemic brain infarction to cerebral anatomy, metabolism, and clinical outcome. Ann Neurol 28:129–135, 1990.

100. Longstreth WT Jr, Inui TS. High blood glucose level on hospital admission and poor neurological recovery after cardiac arrest. Ann Neurol 15:59–63, 1984.

101. D'Alecy LG, Lundy EF, Barton KJ, Zelenock GB. Dextrose containing intravenous fluid impairs outcome and increases death after eight minutes of cardiac arrest and resuscitation in dogs. Surgery 100:505–511, 1986.

102. Longstreth WT Jr, Copass MK, Dennis LK, Rauch-Matthews ME, Stark MS, Cobb LA. Intravenous glucose after out-of-hospital cardiopulmonary arrest: a community-based randomized trial. Neurology 43:2534–2541, 1993.

103. Zeiner A, Holzer M, Sterz F, et al. Mild resuscitative hypothermia to improve neurological outcome after cardiac arrest: a clinical feasibility trial. Stroke 31:86–94, 2000.

104. Sakabe T, Tateishi A, Miyauchi Y, et al. Intracranial pressure following cardiopulmonary resuscitation. Intensive Care Med 13:256–259, 1987.

105. Jastremski M, Sutton-Tyrrell K, Vaagenes P, Abramson N, Heiselman D, Safar P. Glucocorticoid treatment does not improve neurological recovery following cardiac arrest. Brain Resuscitation Clinical Trial I Study Group. JAMA 262:3427–3430, 1989.

106. Roine RO, Kaste M, Kinnunen A, Nikki P, Sarna S, Kajaste S. Nimodipine after resuscitation from out-of-hospital ventricular fibrillation. A placebo-controlled, double-blind, randomized trial. JAMA 264:3171–3177, 1990.

NEUROLOGIC MANIFESTATIONS OF ACID–BASE DERANGEMENTS, ELECTROLYTE DISORDERS, AND ENDOCRINE CRISES

Critically ill patients, by nature of their illness, display a gamut of homeostatic imbalances. These aberrations are not always consequential, and overlapping or simultaneously mounting physiologic disturbances do not in all instances explain the neurologic features at the bedside. What the ultimate clinical response will be in any given patient with any degree of acute metabolic crisis is virtually impossible to predict.

Be that as it may, the clinical spectrum associated with acute metabolic or endocrine derangements ranges from transient and subtle neurologic manifestations to alarming, irreversible damage to the central nervous system. Because several electrolyte and acid–base abnormalities are encountered so regularly, they deserve specific discussion. In this chapter, the salient events and representative clinical manifestations are selected to guide clinicians in their differential diagnosis, and the extent of the disorder on the nervous system is clarified.

ACID–BASE DISORDERS

Acid–base disorders are common in the intensive care unit (ICU), but unless there is an acute change in arterial pH, neurologic manifestations are absent. Many buffer systems in the body assist in maintaining a constant pH, primarily as a result of a balance between carbon dioxide (P_{CO_2}) and serum bicarbonate. Either component can become abnormal, resulting in a compensatory response by respiratory or renal control systems. The characteristic features of primary

143

Table 8–1. **Characteristic Features of Simple Acid–Base Disorders**

Type of Disorder	pH	Pa_{CO_2}	HCO_3^-
Metabolic acidosis	Decreased	Decreased*	Decreased
Metabolic alkalosis	Increased	Increased*	Increased
Respiratory acidosis	Decreased	Increased	Increased
Respiratory alkalosis	Increased	Decreased	Decreased

*Compensatory change.

From Shapiro JI, Kaehny WD. Pathogenesis and management of metabolic acidosis and alkalosis. In: Schrier RW (ed). Renal and Electrolyte Disorders, 5th ed. Lippincott-Raven, Philadelphia, 1997, pp 130–171. By permission of the publisher.

acid–base disturbances are presented in Table 8–1. The interpretation of mixed acid–base conditions is complex and beyond the scope of this chapter.

Passive distribution of the H^+ and HCO_3^- ions between blood and cerebrospinal fluid (CSF) usually produces a steady state. When challenged, the acid–base state of CSF changes significantly,[1,2] and as a rule, the acute changes in serum pH and P_{CO_2} are similar in CSF. Whether changes in CSF in acid–base disorders reflect clinical signs is unknown. Experimental studies have clearly demonstrated that changes in intracellular brain pH are probably more relevant,[1,3] although the complex mechanisms of the buffering capacity of the brain have not been completely understood.

In acute respiratory acidosis with persistent hypercapnia, CSF pH returns to normal within several hours after the induced change.[1,3] In respiratory alkalosis, identical compensation occurs but probably also as a result of cerebral vasoconstriction leading to increased anaerobic metabolism and lactate production, which may in turn produce an effective decrease in CSF bicarbonate.[4]

Counterbalancing changes can also be expected in metabolic acidosis and alkalosis. Even paradoxical reduction of CSF pH from bicarbonate treatment in these patients may occur, caused by equilibration of carbon dioxide between blood and CSF and poor diffusion of bicarbonate from blood to CSF.[1,3,5]

Respiratory Acidosis

In this acid–base disorder, hypercapnia is the primary abnormality.[6] Parenchymal lung in-

jury is a major cause of respiratory acidosis. Abnormal diaphragm function from a neuromuscular disorder as a direct cause of respiratory acidosis is seldom seen outside neurologic ICUs. Occasionally, hypoventilation producing respiratory acidosis is a presenting symptom of a previously undiagnosed motor neuron disease or myopathy, a result of prolonged blockade of the neuromuscular junction, a manifestation of critical illness neuropathy, or a consequence of a cervical spinal lesion due to trauma. Common causes of respiratory acidosis in medical and surgical ICUs are summarized in Table 8–2.

The clinical manifestations of respiratory acidosis are related to the degree of hypercapnia. Few patients presumably have all the symptoms, and patients who chronically retain carbon dioxide may have none at all. Indeed, patients with profound hypercapnia (Pa_{CO_2} values of 175 mm Hg) and crystal clear mentation have been reported.[7,8]

Table 8–2. **Common Causes of Respiratory Acidosis**

Airway obstruction (mucus plug, aspiration of vomit, foreign body)

Pulmonary abnormalities (flail chest, pneumothorax, pneumonia, smoke inhalation, adult respiratory distress syndrome)

Neuromuscular disorders (Guillain-Barré syndrome, spinal cord lesion at or above C3, amyotrophic lateral sclerosis, myasthenia gravis, botulism)

Narcotic or sedative agents

Most patients with hypercapnia are fatigued from the increased work of breathing. Many patients fall asleep exhausted when hypoxemia is relieved.[7] As hypercapnia worsens, patients become irritable, and coarse multifocal twitches and asterixis develop. Tremors may be seen, but these can also be from repeated doses of β-adrenergic agents such as albuterol to treat the underlying disease. Overdose of these agents may cause a fine tremor, evident only with outstretched hands or when magnified by a card placed on the outstretched fingers. Headaches that are worse at night or early in the morning are typical of chronic hypercapnia and are not common in acute cases.[9,10] Papilledema has been noted in patients with acute pulmonary disorders, but the mechanism—cerebral vasodilatation causing increased cerebral blood flow or increased venous pressure from "backup pressure" formed in the chest cage—is not entirely clear.

Profound carbon dioxide narcosis may eventually occur; earlier reports mentioned seizures and coma without motor responses.[11] Recovery is less common in hypercapnic patients who reach such a state, presumably also because of the concomitant effect of severe shock associated with extremely high P_{CO_2} levels, and death may soon follow.

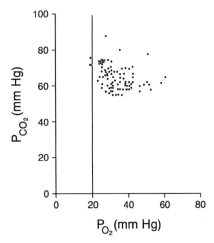

Figure 8–1. Distribution of arterial oxygen and carbon dioxide values in patients with severe respiratory failure but without any therapeutic intervention at the time of measurement. (Modified from McNicol MW, Campbell EJM. Severity of respiratory failure: arterial blood-gases in untreated patients [letter to the editor]. Lancet 1: 336–338, 1965. By permission of the journal.)

PATHOPHYSIOLOGIC MECHANISMS

The association of pulmonary encephalopathy and hypercapnia is mysterious and complex. "Supercarbia," a term coined by Nunn,[12] is most often seen in patients with chronic obstructive pulmonary disease when they are given 100% oxygen. In fact, P_{CO_2} seldom rises above 80 mm Hg in severely hypoxic patients with acute exacerbations of chronic respiratory disease, and a dramatic increase in P_{CO_2} has been attributed to uncontrolled administration of oxygen (Fig. 8–1).

Aubier and co-workers[13] studied the changes in arterial blood gases and minute ventilation in patients with previously diagnosed chronic obstructive pulmonary disease and recent acute respiratory failure (Fig. 8–2). After administration of oxygen,

hypoxemia drive was reduced, as measured by a significant decrease in both components of minute ventilation (tidal volume and frequency). However, in these patients with chronic obstructive pulmonary disease, the increase in P_{CO_2} can also be explained in part by aggravation of the al-

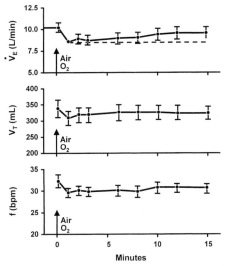

Figure 8–2. Time course of changes in ventilation ($\dot{V}_E$), tidal volume (V_T), and respiratory frequency (f) after oxygen administration. (From Aubier et al.[13] By permission of the American Lung Association.)

ready existing impairment of gas exchange during inhalation of 100% oxygen. Return to baseline minute ventilation was observed over time, most likely from increased Pa_{CO_2} and acidosis, which stimulate the carotid body and aortic chemoreceptors in a manner analogous to previous hypoxemic stimulation.

In patients with long-standing retention of carbon dioxide (from hypoventilation due to marked wasted ventilation associated with pulmonary tissue destruction), one can conclude that removal of the stimulus by oxygen therapy eliminates the drive, reduces ventilation, and intensifies hypercapnia. This potential sequence has made some physicians reluctant to give oxygen to patients with severe pulmonary disease.

Nonetheless, hypoxemia accompanying carbon dioxide retention must be treated, because insufficient oxygen delivery is dangerous to the heart. Rapid reduction of Pa_{CO_2} most likely is not needed, and the physiologic targets probably can be set higher ("permissive hypercapnia"). Mechanical ventilation and correction of hypoxemia are needed in many of these patients with acute respiratory failure.

Respiratory Alkalosis

In the ICU, alveolar hyperventilation is typically observed as a response to hypoxia or metabolic acidosis or is associated with a specific illness from an almost inexhaustible list of disorders (Table 8–3). Respiratory alkalo-

Table 8–3. Common Causes of Respiratory Alkalosis

Mechanical ventilation
Pulmonary disorders
Adult respiratory distress syndrome
Pulmonary emboli
Chronic obstructive pulmonary disease
Anxiety, postoperative pain
Sepsis syndrome (early)
Liver failure
Salicylate overdose
Thyroid hormone excess
Central neurogenic hyperventilation

sis may point to liver disease (hepatic cirrhosis) from increased pulmonary shunting and increased arterial ammonia. Spontaneous hyperventilation may frequently occur after major surgery and is largely determined by postoperative delirium or pain. Other common causes are early sepsis but also inappropriate ventilation settings. Respiratory alkalosis without obvious cause and with maintained oxygenation is an occasional incentive leading to a request for a neurologic consultation to address the possibility of primary central neurogenic hyperventilation. Respiratory alkalosis is profound in sustained neurogenic hyperventilation. If central hyperventilation is present, the disorder is a consequence of a midbrain or pontine lesion and can be associated with pontine hemorrhages, embolus to the basilar artery, and progressive brain herniation from a hemispheric lesion. Other signs localizing the lesion to the brain stem are present (Chapter 1). Most of these manifestations are brief. In head injury, periodic hyperventilation may occur with tachycardia, fever, and sweating and is related to sympathetic storms (Chapter 17).

Brain lesions only rarely cause central neurogenic hyperventilation.[14–17] For unknown reasons, the incidence of primary cerebral lymphoma in patients with central neurogenic hyperventilation appears to be high.[14–16] The responsible lesion is in the pons, and sustained hyperventilation leads to severe respiratory alkalosis, often with pH values greater than 7.60 mm Hg. The patient cannot inhibit respiratory drive, and carbon dioxide rebreathing augments the patient's need to breathe and increases the respiratory rate.[16] Infiltration of tumor, whether lymphoma or astrocytoma, presumably destroys the inhibiting descending neurons from the pons to the medullary respiratory center. Lactate production from the tumor, another possibility, is discounted by several studies as a major trigger. The respiratory rate can be reduced by an intravenous bolus of morphine (5 mg), which may produce reduction for up to 1 day, but sustained reduction of the respiratory rate can be accomplished with methadone, 5 mg every 8 hr.[17]

Typical symptoms of respiratory alkalosis are lightheadedness and perhaps drowsiness

Table 8–4. **Common Causes of Metabolic Acidosis**

Elevated Anion Gap	Normal Anion Gap
Renal failure	Diarrhea
Ketoacidosis	Hyperalimentation
Lactic acidosis	Hypoaldosteronism

but not a consistent decrease in level of consciousness. Tetanic cramps may occur but are rare. Respiratory alkalosis may reduce the threshold for seizures in patients with previous stroke or seizure disorder.

Metabolic Acidosis

The neurologic manifestations of metabolic acidosis with a normal anion gap (difference between unmeasured anions and cations in serum) are attributed either to cardiovascular collapse or to associated electrolyte disorders (discussed in separate sections) (Table 8–4). In ICUs, lactate acidosis is frequently seen with sepsis, cardiogenic shock, and multiorgan failure but can be due to thiamine deficiency or a series of tonic–clonic seizures (Chapter 3).

Metabolic Alkalosis

Metabolic alkalosis is generally associated with volume contraction;[18] causes are listed in Table 8–5. Paresthesias and muscle cramping may be early signs of systemic alkalemia, but metabolic alkalosis more characteristi-

Table 8–5. **Common Causes of Metabolic Alkalosis**

Volume chloride depletion
Diuretic therapy
Endocrine disorders
   Cushing's disease
   Primary aldosteronism
Massive blood transfusion

cally gradually decreases the level of consciousness and, as the condition worsens, leads to tonic–clonic seizures. Hypocalcemia has been implicated as a predisposing factor for seizures in this situation, but the relation is very weak.

ELECTROLYTE DISORDERS

Electrolyte derangements are common to nearly all patients with critical illness. Sodium abnormalities are often prevalent in critically ill patients. The concentration of sodium in serum reflects the extracellular fluid osmolality and often not the total sodium content in the body. Many electrolyte disorders directly produce central nervous system symptoms, but in some unfortunate cases, symptoms can be attributed to adverse effects of treatment. This situation is exemplified by the potential ravages of acute demyelination in the brain after rapid correction of severe hyponatremia.

PATHOPHYSIOLOGIC MECHANISMS

The most pertinent challenges to the brain adaptive capacity are disturbances of body fluid osmolality (Fig. 8–3). Although hyponatremia and hypernatremia are common clinical problems, the hypo-osmolar or hyperosmolar state rather than the electrolyte abnormality itself is the cause of neurologic manifestations. Thus, conditions that produce pseudohyponatremia are not symptomatic except possibly when they result from severe hyperglycemia.

In acute dilutional hyponatremia associated with hypo-osmolality, brain swelling occurs from water gain due to the osmotic gradient. It is corrected within hours by cellular loss of sodium, potassium, chloride, and water (rapid adaptation). The hypo-osmolar state is corrected gradually (within days) through loss of so-called osmolytes. These extruded "idiogenic osmols" are solutes such as glutamate, glutamine, taurine, and *myo*-inositol, but the transcription of genes coding for activation of transporters takes time (slow adaptation process). The brain adaptation to hyperosmolality is not the reverse, but in acute

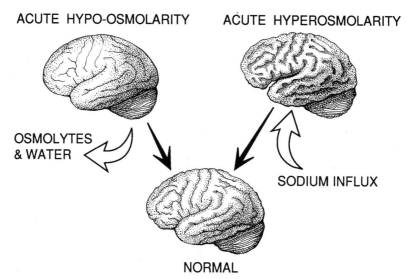

Figure 8–3. Brain adaptation in acute changes of osmolarity.

hyperosmolality, rapid electrolyte accumulation from CSF, plasma, and extracellular fluid results in correction of intracellular brain water.[19–21]

Hyponatremia

In hospital-based studies, hyponatremia is the most frequent electrolyte disorder. The syndrome of inappropriate secretion of antidiuretic hormone (SIADH) is often implicated, but in 30% of the patients, hyponatremia can be attributed to hyperglycemia, severe renal failure, or potentially preventable excessive administration of free water.[22] In other hospital series, depending on whether the studied population was medical or surgical, a high incidence of congestive heart failure and hypovolemia associated with diuretic therapy was found in hyponatremic patients. Hyponatremia is associated with decreased, increased, or normal volume of extracellular fluid. Decreased volume of extracellular fluid may be due to renal or extrarenal sodium loss, such as that from vomiting or diarrhea. The potential causes of hyponatremia in critically ill patients are shown in Table 8–6.

The early neurologic manifestations of hyponatremia are nonspecific and can easily be overlooked. Although many patients may initially have headache, nausea, and vomiting, an acute confusional state, delirium, or profound drowsiness emerges.[23,24] A consistent and reproducible clinical symptom in hyponatremia is progressive impaired responsiveness when serum sodium values rapidly decline to 125 mEq/L. With advancing hyponatremia, the depression of

Table 8–6. Common Causes of Hyponatremia

Decreased Extracellular Volume
Diuretics (thiazide)
Hypoadrenalism
Hypovolemic state (gastrointestinal, skin, or renal loss: diarrhea, sweating, fluid sequestration in "third space")

Normal Extracellular Volume
Syndrome of inappropriate antidiuretic hormone
Postoperative fluid overload (gastrointestinal and cardiovascular procedures)
Hypothyroidism
Iatrogenic hypotonic fluid loading

Increased Extracellular Volume
Congestive heart failure
Cirrhosis
Nephrotic syndrome

consciousness progresses substantially, punctuated by generalized tonic–clonic seizures. Nonconvulsive status epilepticus or a prolonged ictal state after a cluster of generalized tonic–clonic seizures may complicate the interpretation of the level of consciousness (see Chapter 3). Patients with rapidly developing hyponatremia (to values <110 mEq/L) become unresponsive and may display pathologic motor responses from developing brain edema. Seizures in patients with hyponatremia may suggest a higher probability of poor outcome, but in many patients, the underlying condition that led to hyponatremia or control of brain edema is the main determinant of poor outcome.

As a rule, symptoms are more likely to occur if hyponatremia develops acutely than if it occurs over a longer period. Pertinent signs and symptoms of hyponatremia do not occur until plasma sodium concentration is <125 mmol/L, but irritability, restlessness, and confusion can occur at higher levels in patients who have a rapid decrease in sodium levels. It should be emphasized that some patients have severe muscle cramps. Hyponatremia may result in very severe generalized cramps in limbs and abdominal muscles. Hemiparesis from hyponatremia alone has been reported in older literature in a few case reports, with complete resolution after correction but without neuroimaging correlation.

In the past decade, three possible neurologic syndromes associated with acute hyponatremia have emerged, each with specific clinical features.

CENTRAL PONTINE MYELINOLYSIS

The name "central pontine myelinolysis" (CPM), first coined by Adams and colleagues,[25] implies that demyelination is at the base of the pons, but later descriptions noted occasional extension into the tegmentum.[26] Focal areas of myelinolysis may be additionally present in the thalamus and putamen.[27]

Central pontine myelinolysis is a clinical entity that is frequently linked to treatment, particularly rapid correction of severe hyponatremia.[28–53] However, CPM is associated with severe debilitating disease, such as systemic advanced cancer or chronic alcoholism. It has also been described in patients with major osmolality fluctuations, such as severely burned patients[35] and patients who have had liver transplantation, and in patients with an almost extinct disease, Reye's syndrome (after mannitol therapy).

The clinical manifestations of CPM can be diverse, but pseudobulbar palsy, facial weakness, inability to swallow or speak, and quadriplegia are prominent.[36,37] Quadriplegia may be more pronounced in the arms in some patients; in others, asymmetries or hemiparesis is evident. Clinically, differentiation from an evolving basilar artery occlusion can be difficult, but the circumstances of recent sodium correction should point to this disorder. Moreover, the central location in the pons precludes neuro-ophthalmologic signs except in patients with extension of demyelination beyond its central localization. In these more extensive forms, nystagmus, abducens palsy, miosis, and limitation of conjugate eye movement in the horizontal direction are noted. In extreme examples, CPM may be manifested by a locked-in syndrome with, as expected, only blinking and vertical eye movements as a means of communication.[52]

Central pontine myelinolysis may not be manifested clinically by neurologic symptoms other than behavioral changes, although emotional lability, such as crying, can be linked to pseudobulbar palsy. Restless behavior, irritability, and catatonia may be the sole initial presentation of CPM.[27,40]

In addition, CPM characteristically has been difficult to diagnose after liver transplantation.[41,42,52] Many patients are drowsy, often because of increased ammonia from slowly improving graft function, renal failure, and other acute electrolyte derangements. In the Mayo Clinic series, the prevalence of CPM after orthotopic liver transplantation was 1%. All patients affected had impaired levels of consciousness alone and no typical pseudobulbar signs.[41] If magnetic resonance imaging (MRI) of the brain is not performed, the diagnosis can be missed and may become apparent only at postmortem examination or when pseudobulbar palsy and quadriparesis become evident during rehabilitation from surgery.

Extrapontine lesions may occur simultaneously but are manifested differently. On the basis of autopsy material, it is estimated that approximately 10% of patients with CPM have extrapontine lesions,[27] usually found in the caudate nucleus, putamen, lateral thalamus, and lateral geniculate nucleus.

Delayed onset of parkinsonism—3 weeks to 5 months after rapid correction of hyponatremia and subsequent clinical diagnosis of CPM—has been described.[27,43-47]

Computed tomography (CT) scanning with detailed views of the pons may yield clearly distinctive abnormalities, but MRI has facilitated the diagnosis of CPM ante mortem and has carefully characterized the disorder. A symmetrical oval or round area on T1- or T2-weighted images is found (Fig. 8–4A,D), but lesions in the base of the pons may also be trident or bat shaped because horizontal tracts are preferentially involved and vertical tracts are spared (Fig. 8–4B,C).

Magnetic resonance imaging may reveal bilateral thalamic involvement of the lateral and centromedian nucleus, typical in extrapontine myelinolysis and differentiating it from the bilateral paramedian thalamic infarctions.[48,49] It may be 2 weeks before lesions appear on MRI.[50]

Follow-up MRI may show resolution of the T1 hypointensity, presumably as a result of diminished edema in the area of demyelination. The extrapontine manifestations resolve first.[51] Gradual recovery to virtually normal neurologic function is possible, even in patients with a locked-in syndrome.[52] No correlation exists between persistent MRI findings and subsequent potential for recovery. Bulbar dysfunction and spastic quadriparesis remain sources of impairment for many patients.[53] Many of the reported patients in whom CPM developed after liver transplantation did poorly.[41]

POSTOPERATIVE HYPONATREMIA SYNDROME IN YOUNG HEALTHY WOMEN

A fulminant neurologic disorder associated with severe (and probably unrecognized) hyponatremia has been specifically linked to elective surgery.[54,55] The condition is rare, because in the first defining retrospective survey, 15 women were seen in 15 medical centers in 10 years.[54] Two days after surgery, patients had generalized tonic–clonic seizures followed within 1 hr by respiratory arrest. In many of the patients, serum sodium levels were not routinely measured postoperatively, and the nonspecific signs of early brain swelling, such as nausea, vomiting, and headache, were not recognized as such. At the time of deterioration and resuscitation, plasma sodium values decreased greatly, to at least <110 mmol/L.

Many of the original 15 patients had fixed, dilated pupils after resuscitation; four patients died, and nine patients remained in a vegetative state. The remaining two patients, who survived with moderate deficits, had been treated immediately after the first seizure. A CT scan in these patients may show brain edema with obliteration of sulci and basal cisterns. Autopsy demonstrated "demyelination" in addition to cerebral edema. It has been assumed that brain swelling may have caused the respiratory arrest from compression of the medulla through brain herniation.

An intriguing feature of this syndrome is the female preponderance. Most reported patients are healthy women undergoing abdominal, gynecologic, cosmetic, or other mostly relatively minor elective procedures. This syndrome of postoperative hyponatremia in women with cerebral edema has been tentatively linked to sodium–potassium–adenosinetriphosphatase pump dysfunction, because sex differences in this pump have been found in animal studies.

Postoperative severe hyponatremia with respiratory arrest has also been documented in patients with transurethral prostatectomy, usually associated with bladder irrigation. Nevertheless, in many male patients, the outcome is good despite seizures.[55] Hyponatremia can be severe in post-transurethral prostatectomy, but serum osmolality is quite high from bladder absorption of hypertonic glycine, frequently used as an irrigant. Rapid excretion of the glycine by the kidney restores plasma osmolality, and it is important to make this distinction rather than superficially attribute sex differences to complications of hyponatremia.

How hyponatremia can develop in these patients and not in many others is not entirely clear, but in the reported cases, large volumes of free water had been administered. In addition, in the first postoperative hours,

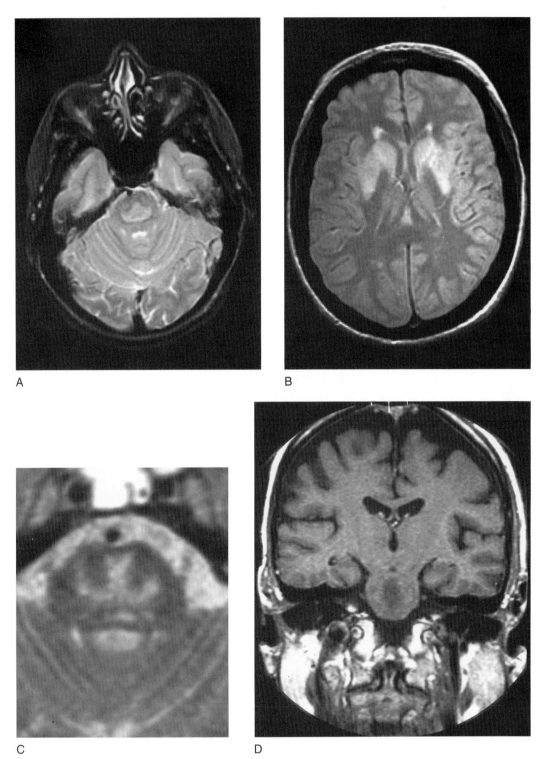

Figure 8–4. Magnetic resonance images of lesions due to central pontine myelinolysis. *A:* Batlike central pontine lesion. *B:* Lesions in caudate nucleus and putamen bilaterally. *C:* Typical trident shape in central pontine myelinolysis. *D:* Oval punched-out abnormality in the pons.

151

many patients may have self-administered morphine for pain control. Repeated doses of morphine may cause vomiting and, together with extensive fluid administration in the immediate postoperative course, may lead to rapidly evolving hyponatremia.

A review of all postoperative respiratory and cardiac arrests in women during 1976 to 1992 in Rochester, Minnesota, was negative for associated severe hyponatremia.[56] In this period, 1498 of 290,815 women (0.5%) who had surgical procedures experienced postoperative cardiac or respiratory arrest. In none of these patients was severe hyponatremia of <125 mmol/L found. New-onset postoperative seizures occurred in three elderly patients with hyponatremia, but all had hyponatremia associated with a severe life-threatening illness. Since this survey, we still have not encountered any convincing case at the Mayo Clinic. The true prevalence of this disorder needs to be further determined, but our data convince us that the entity is extremely uncommon.

A variant syndrome of central diabetes mellitus and insipidus, reported in 1990, is controversial.[57] After seizures and respiratory arrest, decorticate posturing was soon followed by loss of virtually all brain stem reflexes. Whether this clinical syndrome represents a new entity or, much more likely, simply reflects systemic manifestations in patients who became brain dead from severe cerebral edema after prolonged resuscitation remains unresolved. Transtentorial herniation and ischemic infarcts of pituitary lobes and the hypothalamus were found and tentatively linked to clinical findings of diabetes mellitus and insipidus, but both these abnormalities alone are also compatible with brain death or with brain-swelling–induced compression of the diencephalon against the clivus, resulting in hypothalamic infarcts or severing of the pituitary stalk.

Confirmation of this controversial finding of young female susceptibility to acute osmotic stress was also sought in animal experiments. Initial claims in rat studies by Arief and investigators[58] that seemed to support a female proclivity to hyponatremia-induced brain injury were not confirmed in a subsequent study. Brain adaptation to acute hyponatremia in prepubescent rats was similar to that in older rats.[58,59]

OSMOTIC DEMYELINATION SYNDROME

Although directly related to the correction of hyponatremia, this well-described clinical phenomenon remains an enigma.[60,61] In their report on eight patients treated over a 5-year period at two institutions, Sterns and associates[62–64] postulated that myelinolytic lesions in the deep cortical cell layers and in the pons result from iatrogenic rapid correction of hyponatremia. Possible etiologic considerations are the "grid" phenomenon, suggesting strangulation of myelinated fibers by surrounding edema in the pons, and "osmotic endothelial injury," which implies that rapid osmotic changes of endothelial cells in the gray matter may release myelotoxic factors.

A 1991 experimental study, however, offered a novel hypothesis based on the finding that lost osmoles are not rapidly replaced when needed.[65] Loss of osmoles in hyponatremia treated with rapid infusion of hypertonic saline is offset not by an accumulation of osmoles in the brain but by electrolyte reaccumulation and as a consequence a much slower increase in osmoles. The absence of osmole protection and increased high ionic strength may be harmful to protein interactions in oligodendrocytes. Whether this explanation is sufficient to explain this syndrome has not yet been unarguably shown.

The clinical features of this syndrome tend to be stereotypical. After correction of severe hyponatremia with hypertonic saline, patients awake without any major appreciable deficit only to have gradual deterioration 2 to 3 days later. After rapid correction of serum sodium deficiency, patients significantly improve in level of consciousness but continue to complain of throbbing headaches and nausea. New-onset vomiting and seizures mark the beginning of a lapse into an unresponsive coma, occasionally with a fatal course. Some clinical features (but not the pathologic findings) may be reminiscent of delayed postresuscitation encephalopathy, as reported by Plum and co-workers[66] (see Chapter 7).

Pathologic data for these patients are scarce, but one carefully documented case report noted multifocal demyelination without any evidence of massive brain edema.[60]

This rare syndrome may be considered a variant of CPM and thus may occur less frequently if hyponatremia is prudently managed.

TREATMENT OF ACUTE SEVERE HYPONATREMIA

Many guidelines for intervention in acute hyponatremia have been proposed,[30,67–69] but trials in human subjects are lacking. Readers are referred to many excellent reviews on this subject.[30,67,70–72]

The clinical dilemma, if the concept of Arieff[54] is accepted, is that acute severe hyponatremia may, in predisposed patients, be associated with severe brain edema resulting in irreversible herniation. On the other hand, rapid correction (>24 mmol/L a day) may result in CPM or osmotic demyelination syndrome. Most experts refute rapid correction methods and aim at a gradual increase in plasma sodium.

Treatment of acute severe hyponatremia should depend on whether symptoms are present. In the vast majority of patients, fluid overload causes hyponatremia, but other triggers should be identified and corrected.

It may be prudent to increase the serum sodium concentration to values of 125 mmol/L with 3% hypertonic saline. Additional furosemide or any other loop diuretic may be appropriate to decrease excess free water, but the initial diuretic response may be unpredictable and may lead to unexpected higher sodium values.

Treatment of symptomatic hyponatremia is typically begun with 3% hypertonic saline. Knowledge of the treatment protocol is important for the consulting neurologist in judging, in any one patient, the possible risk of CPM (Table 8–7). Using the formula by Androgué and Madias in Table 8–7 may be helpful. For example, the correction in a female patient (body weight 60 kg) with a hypotonic hyponatremia of 100 mmol/L, with use of 3% hypertonic saline, is $513 - 100/0.5 \times 60 \times 1 = 13.3$ mmol/L. Thus, 1 L of 3% hypertonic saline (assuming a closed system and no substantial additional renal losses by mannitol or furosemide) will increase the serum sodium concentration with 13.3 mmol/L. The infusion rate depends on the presence of symptoms (brain edema) but sodium increase should remain within 1 mmol/L per hour. Thus, an increase by

Table 8–7. Formula for Use in Managing Hyponatremia and Characteristics of Infusates

FORMULA*		CLINICAL USE	
Change in Serum Na$^+$ = $\dfrac{\text{Infusate Na}^+ - \text{Serum Na}^+}{\text{Total Body Water} + 1}$		Estimate Effect of 1 L of any Infusate on Serum Na$^+$	
Infusate		Infusate Na$^+$ (mmol/L)	Extracellular-Fluid Distribution (%)
5% sodium chloride in water		855	100
3% sodium chloride in water		513	100
0.9% sodium chloride in water		154	100
Ringer's lactate solution		130	97
0.45% sodium chloride in water		77	73
0.2% sodium chloride in 5% dextrose in water		34	55
5% dextrose in water		0	40

*The numerator in the formula is a simplification of the expression (infusate Na$^+$ − serum Na$^+$) × 1 L, with the value yielded by the equation in mmole/L. The estimated total body water (in liters) is calculated as a fraction of body weight. The fraction is 0.6 in children; 0.6 and 0.5 in nonelderly men and women, respectively; and 0.5 and 0.45 in elderly men and women, respectively. Normally, extracellular and intracellular fluids account for 40% and 60% of total body water, respectively.

Modified from Adrogué and Madias.[71] By permission of the Massachusetts Medical Society.

3 mmol/L over 3 hr would require 3/13.3, or 0.23, liter of hypertonic saline or 230/3, or 77 mL per hour.[71] When hyponatremia has been corrected to approximately 130 mmol, the patient can be treated with fluid restriction only and infusion can be discontinued. Plasma sodium concentration should be checked every hour to prevent rapid correction and, more important, "overcorrection" to values above 140 mEq/L. Patients who do not have improvement and who continue to have seizures should be given a phenytoin load rather than a rapid increase in the rate of sodium administration. Another approach is use of vasopressin antagonists, and preliminary experience shows a rapid correction of hyponatremia. This treatment should not be used until its safety has been demonstrated.[73]

Patients may benefit from a short course of dexamethasone (for example, 4 mg given four times a day) when sodium correction is unexpectedly rapid. Data in rats suggest that demyelination can be prevented with high doses of corticosteroids.[74]

Acute parkinsonism from CPM responds to levodopa substitution. Generalized dystonia or predominant orolingual dystonia and athetosis may respond to trihexyphenidyl (maximum of 40 mg/day) or tiapride (maximum of 900 mg/day).[46,47] Excellent response with recovery to the point of independent life was anecdotally reported in a patient treated with thyrotropin-releasing hormone injections after plasma exchange (5 to 14 exchanges),[75] but spontaneous recovery from CPM is well known.

Hypernatremia

Patients are susceptible to hypernatremia when there is no access to water.[76,77] No access to water is countered by renal concentrating mechanisms and is followed by a sensation of thirst. Hypernatremia is usually the result of water depletion in excess of sodium, but hypernatremia can occur in states of euvolemia or hypervolemia. Common causes of increased total body sodium are excess administration of hypertonic sodium bicarbonate to correct metabolic acidosis, malfunction of the dialysate-proportioning system during hemodialysis, and seawater drowning.

Table 8–8. Common Causes of Hypernatremia

Net water loss
Increased insensible fluid loss
  Fever
  Respiratory infection
  Burns
Osmotic diarrhea (lactulose); osmotic diuresis
Allergenic diabetes insipidus
Head injury, brain death
Massive brain swelling
Nephrogenic diabetes insipidus
  Lithium
  Demeclocycline
  Amphotericin
  Methoxyflurane
  Cisplatin
Hypertonic sodium gain
  Sodium bicarbonate
  Dialysis fluids
  Seawater ingestion

Another common cause is sustained infusion of large volumes of isotonic sodium chloride in patients with hypotonic fluid loss or shock. The most frequently encountered causes of hypernatremia in the ICU are listed in Table 8–8. Failure to replace insensible losses from the skin and respiratory tract is the most common cause of hypernatremia in ICUs.

CLINICAL FEATURES

A fair degree of concordance exists between the clinical manifestations of hypernatremia and the extracellular fluid deficit. Although hypernatremia has its greatest effect on the central nervous system, other features immediately suggest a hyperosmolar state. Signs of extracellular volume depletion are dehydration, skin tenting, dry mucous membranes, and tachycardia. These signs are less obvious in elderly patients. Most patients are drowsy, but periods of diminished arousability may be interspersed with periods of restlessness and confusion. In many elderly patients, a mild degree of Alzheimer's disease or vascular dementia may be unmasked or aggravated by hypernatremia. Focal motor signs do not occur, and if present, a stroke with dehydration is a more likely explanation than the converse. Generalized tonic–clonic seizures are unusual, even in patients with marked increase in sodium levels (>160 mmol/L). Asterixis and myoclonus have been described but are generally seen in patients who also have hepatic encephalopathy. Other very infrequent clinical manifestations are rigidity, tremor, myoclonus, and chorea.[23,78]

As dehydration and hypernatremia become severe, patients become unresponsive. The clinical course may be fulminant in postoperative patients or patients in whom hemodialysis is associated with technical problems.

Arieff and Carroll's study[79] on hyperglycemia and hypernatremia showed that most patients remained alert when plasma osmolality remained under 350 mosm/kg. Progressive drowsiness occurred beyond this critical value. Usually, however, there is a marked overlap between the degree of hypernatremia and the degree of coma.

Hypernatremia may not significantly increase the probability of neurologic sequelae. Although permanent cognitive changes, attentional deficits, and poor memory are common in patients who survive severe hypernatremia, the underlying clinical condition truly determines outcome and morbidity.[80,81] Mortality from severe hypernatremia (>160 mmol/L) can be 70% in susceptible patients. Recovery in patients who remain alert at peak sodium values is common.

TREATMENT

The ideal rate of fluid resuscitation in hypernatremic patients is not known but may depend in part on the rate at which hypernatremia develops. Fatal cerebral edema, often accompanied by grand mal seizures, occurred in patients within 24 hr after acute hypernatremia had been corrected. As in hyponatremia, overly rapid correction may be hazardous, but clinical evidence is lacking. In hypovolemic patients, intravascular volume should be replaced with isotonic saline or colloids, and a reduction of 1 to 2 mEq/L of sodium per hour may be prudent.[81] Hypernatremia may reoccur if the underlying systemic disease is not corrected and administration of triggering drugs is not discontinued.

Hypokalemia

Most critically ill patients seem to have hypokalemia at some stage in their clinical course, and often there is more than one reason for potassium deficiency. Common causes for hypokalemia are gastrointestinal or from skin losses or drugs (Table 8–9). Nasogastric suctioning can cause extracellular fluid volume deficits that result in increased serum concentration of aldosterone, which in turn results in increased renal excretion of potassium and thus hypokalemia. The development of metabolic alkalosis from nasogastric suctioning may also cause an increase in renal potassium excretion. Muscle weakness is the only neurologic manifestation in profound hypokalemia.

MYOPATHY

Potassium loss reduces excitable tissue such as muscle by increasing the threshold for initiation of the action potential; depletion of glycogen stores or rhabdomyolysis may be the main cause of muscle weakness. Potassium depletion from any cause may lead to

Table 8–9. **Common Causes of Hypokalemia**

Gastrointestinal
Vomiting
Fistula
Nasogastric suction

Skin Losses
Profound sweating
Burns

Drugs
Loop or thiazide diuretics
Amphotericin B
β-adrenergic agents (e.g., albuterol inhalant)
Insulin
Penicillin derivatives

Neoplastic Disorders
Acute leukemia
Primary hyperaldosteronism

Metabolic Disorders
Hypocalcemia
Hypomagnesemia
Metabolic alkalosis

severe muscle weakness and, in its extreme form, to quadriplegia and respiratory failure. Neurologic manifestations are inevitable with plasma potassium concentrations of <2 mEq/L, but many patients with potassium losses remain symptom-free. When the serum potassium level decreases (<3 mEq/L), total body potassium stores most likely are significantly depleted and electrocardiographic changes are often seen. Prominent U waves, ST segment changes, dampened T wave, and, more important, atrial and ventricular arrhythmias are typical findings.

Muscle weakness usually progresses over several days in the ICU. Proximal leg, neck, and trunk muscle weakness is an early sign. Many patients cannot sit without help or lift their head from the pillow.[82] Aching pain in the back and larger proximal fleshy muscles is common. Muscle cramps, nocturnal myoclonus, and symptoms mimicking restless leg syndrome may become extremely disruptive at night and result in additional fatigue and exhaustion. In exceptional cases, hypokalemia may be associated with rapidly ascending weakness and respiratory failure suggesting Guillain-Barré syndrome, but hallmarks of this disorder, such as tingling, areflexia, and cranial nerve deficits, are absent. Distal muscles seldom become prominently involved, but if they do, they recover first after correction of hypokalemia. Ventilatory failure, difficulty swallowing secretions, and slurred speech have been described, but as mentioned previously, usually the electrocardiographic abnormalities and progressive weakness have already prompted rapid correction.

Most patients with severe hypokalemia have a mild degree of rhabdomyolysis. The mechanism of rhabdomyolysis in severe hypokalemia is not known. Rhabdomyolysis (see Chapter 4) is not significant enough to result in its classic manifestations with compartment syndromes or acute tubular necrosis. Widespread muscle pain that may have started in the calves is present. Muscles are firmly swollen and extremely tender to touch. Many patients complain of intensifying pain with movement. Creatine kinase levels are increased, but the marked surge in value may be short and thus missed in a random sample. Muscle biopsies in a few reported cases have not led to new insight into the pathologic mechanisms. The specimens show vacuolization of T tubules, nonspecific necrosis, type II fiber atrophy, and phagocytosis and regeneration.[83] Correction of hypokalemia results in marked improvement in a few weeks, as it does in patients with abnormal muscle biopsy findings.

TREATMENT

Correction in patients with severe hypokalemia is usually at a maximum rate of 10 to 20 mEq/hr. An infusion rate exceeding 20 mEq/hr may result in potentially life-threatening heart block and should in general be avoided, including in patients with severe muscle pain. Patients may have a relapse of proximal weakness after potassium correction, usually from rapid entry of potassium into depleted cells. Therefore, the potassium correction should be continued until most of the weakness has resolved. Permanent weakness has not been described after intravenous correction of potassium concentration.

Hyperkalemia

Increased plasma potassium levels may alter the electrical excitability of nerve and muscle membranes, usually when the concentration reaches 7 mEq/L. Muscle weakness has been explained by potassium-triggered sustained depolarization. This state results in sodium channel inactivation, and despite intact synaptic transmission, the motor end plate and muscle cell membrane remain inexcitable.

Hyperkalemia is common in medical ICUs because a disproportionately large number of the patients have renal failure.

Hyperkalemia has also been anecdotally described in patients on cardiac bypass. In these patients, increased plasma potassium may be induced by washout of ischemic underperfused areas during the body's bypass period or may be caused by rewarming after hypothermia. Most commonly, hyperkalemia is encountered in patients with renal or adrenal failure. Hypoadrenalism is the most common adrenal disorder resulting in

Table 8–10. Common Causes of Hyperkalemia

Pseudohyperkalemia
Renal disorders
Hypoadrenalism
Pharmacologic agents
  Potassium-sparing diuretics
  Angiotensin-converting enzyme inhibitors
  Cyclosporine
  Succinylcholine
Diabetic ketoacidosis
Multiple blood transfusions

hyperkalemia, is potentially life threatening, and can be overlooked for some time in the ICU. Certain drugs, often those that impair renal function, may increase potassium levels (Table 8–10).

Other causes are pseudohyperkalemia from hemolysis during venipuncture, pseudohyperkalemia associated with severe thrombocytosis or leukocytosis, and hyperkalemia associated with succinylcholine use.

CLINICAL FEATURES

The pathophysiologic consequences of hyperkalemia (potassium concentrations >7.5 mEq/L) are predominantly cardiac. Cardiac conduction abnormalities can lead to widening of the PR interval and QRS complex, but initial changes are a peaking, narrowed T wave and a shortened QT interval. Ventricular fibrillation may occur.

The relationship between hyperkalemia and cardiac manifestations is not always clear, particularly when the increase in potassium concentration is gradual. Neurologic manifestations may precede cardiac manifestations. Neurologic manifestations may become more evident than cardiac manifestations in patients who have hypercalcemia, which may protect the heart from dysrhythmias.

Similar to hypokalemia, hyperkalemia may result in proximal leg weakness with inability to lift the legs from the bed.[84–86] Percussion myotonia can be demonstrated in some patients. Burning dysesthesias without objective sensory loss are very common, also suggesting peripheral nerve involvement rather than primary muscular disease. When hyperkalemia is not appreciated, the condition may worsen to quadriplegia and respiratory failure. Transient diplopia has been ascribed to myotonia in the internal and external ocular muscles. Facial and pharyngeal muscles may be affected; otherwise, cranial nerve deficits are uncommon. Some patients may have generalized myotonia in the forearms, hands, and calves.

TREATMENT AND OUTCOME

In life-threatening hyperkalemia, efforts should be directed at all levels—that is, stabilization of the heart with calcium carbonate, increasing potassium influx with insulin and glucose or bicarbonate, and elimination of total body potassium stores with cation-exchange resins or dialysis if necessary. In less critical situations, efforts should be directed at correcting the underlying cause, eliminating potassium sources, and increasing potassium excretion (for example, by cation-exchange resins, diuretics, or dialysis). All patients recover from weakness within 1 to 4 hr after treatment; lack of recovery suggests other causes.

Hypophosphatemia

The true incidence of severe phosphorus depletion in the ICU is not known, but this patient population is certainly predisposed. Critically ill patients have an increased need of phosphate. Most instances of depletion are associated with long-term antacid therapy, hemodialysis, hyperalimentation with phosphate-poor solutions, and sepsis[87–94] (Table 8–11). In 10% to 20% of patients, the cause of hypophosphatemia is unknown. In patients with severe burns, profound hypophosphatemia often occurs in the recovery phase, presumably from increased anabolism during healing. Mild asymptomatic hypophosphatemia may occur in patients with respiratory alkalosis either from mechanical ventilation with relatively large tidal volumes or from spontaneous hyperventilation. In other patients, hypophosphatemia

Table 8–11. **Common Causes of Hypophosphatemia**

Malabsorption syndrome (bypass surgery)
Prolonged vomiting or gastric suction
Gram-negative and gram-positive sepsis
Hepatic failure
Burns
Chronic alcoholism
Pharmacologic agents
    Catecholamines
    Thiazide diuretics
    Antacids

may become more profound after glucose infusion, particularly in those who are starved and emaciated.

The neurologic manifestations can be realistically expected only when serum phosphate levels are below 1 mg/dL.[92] For seizures and profound neuromuscular manifestations to occur, a substantial decrease below 0.5 mg/dL must take place.[92]

ACUTE FLACCID AREFLEXIC PARALYSIS

A salient feature of this generally uncommon condition is its rapid onset and progression. Usually within 1 day, perioral paresthesias are followed by virtually complete quadriplegia, ptosis, and difficulty swallowing. Sensory ataxia may occur. This dramatic progression of symptoms is seldom seen in ICUs staffed by physicians aware of the dangers of suboptimal supplementation of phosphate in these patients.

A probably much more common manifestation of severe hypophosphatemia is diaphragmatic weakness associated with proximal muscle weakness.[95–97] Diaphragmatic failure associated with hypophosphatemia results in an inability to be weaned from the ventilator. In patients with chronic pulmonary disease and any medical or surgical critical illness, hypophosphatemia may markedly contribute to the already high propensity for weaning failure. Phosphorus has been shown to improve inspiratory pressures and therefore may optimize the clinical conditions for weaning from the ventilator.

HYPOPHOSPHATEMIC ENCEPHALOPATHY

An incompletely delineated encephalopathy associated with phosphorus depletion has been described.[93,94] Severe hypophosphatemia may be associated with combative behavior, acute confusional state, seizures, and coma. Tremor, ataxia, nystagmus, and bilateral abducens paresis have been noted, closely mimicking Wernicke's encephalopathy. Many other clinical manifestations have been reported, including asterixis, tremors, ataxia, and pseudobulbar palsy, but many of these lapidary descriptions have not been confirmed by neurologists. In addition, changes in level of consciousness in these unusual cases reported in the literature are more likely to be associated with marked hypoxia from alveolar hypoventilation caused by diaphragmatic weakness.

TREATMENT

In the vast majority of the patients, oral phosphate supplementation is preferred and can be easily achieved by increasing milk products in the diet or by adding standard oral preparations. In severe cases, intravenous phosphate supplementation at a dose of 2 mg/kg every 6 hr is appropriate.[98,99] The neurologic findings completely resolve when the serum phosphate concentration returns to values above 1.5 mg/dL.

Hyperphosphatemia

A small rise in serum phosphate concentration is sufficient to cause a decrease in serum ionized calcium. Therefore, an increase in serum phosphate results in clinical manifestations from hypocalcemia. Hyperphosphatemia may affect many organs, but deposition of amorphous calcium phosphate usually occurs in chronic conditions. Acute hyperphosphatemia is invariably associated with acute hypocalcemia, which may be severe enough to cause tetanic cramps.

Hypomagnesemia

Magnesium depletion is common in the ICU from loss of gastrointestinal fluid, prolonged

Table 8–12. **Common Causes of Hypomagnesemia**

Parenteral nutrition

Acute pancreatitis

Bowel surgery

Renal disorders

  Acute tubular necrosis

  Postdiuretic-phase renal transplantation

Endocrine disorders

  Hypoparathyroidism

  Hyperaldosteronism

Pharmacologic agents

  Antibiotic combinations

  Antineoplastic drugs

parenteral nutrition, or abdominal surgical procedures associated with depleted magnesium stores[100–103] (Table 8–12).

CLINICAL FEATURES

The frequent association of magnesium deficiency with hypocalcemia, hypokalemia, and alkalosis markedly confounds its clinical manifestations. In addition, magnesium administration alone often results in correction of other laboratory abnormalities. The biochemical significance of hypomagnesemia, therefore, remains somewhat obscure.

Magnesium deficiency readily induces muscular twitching, myoclonus, startle responses, and postural tremor.[104] Trousseau's and Chvostek's signs, carpopedal spasm, and, rarely, tetany have also been reported but these are most characteristic of hypocalcemia. In many afflicted patients, brief periods of anxiety and fear, dilated pupils, sweating, tachycardia, hostile behavior, and hallucinations develop, associated in some with downbeat nystagmus[105] and ataxia. Unrecognized severe hypomagnesemia may predispose to tonic–clonic seizures.

TREATMENT

Hypomagnesemia, defined as a plasma level of <1.7 mg/dL, should be treated immediately, especially in patients with seizures, although threshold levels are generally <1 mEq/L. Magnesium sulfate in a dose of 2 g of a 10% solution should be administered over a 2-min period and be followed by infusion of 12 g in 1 L of fluid over a 12-hr period. A more prudent schedule in patients with less urgent manifestations is intramuscular injection with 1 g of magnesium sulfate every 4 hr.

Hypermagnesemia

At the neuromuscular junction, magnesium competes with calcium and displaces it from its target site. As a result, release of acetylcholine and, to a large extent, the excitability of the muscle membrane decrease. Its effects on the central nervous system are less well characterized but may be related to stabilization of the synaptic membrane, which leads to decreased excitability.

Most commonly, hypermagnesemia occurs with the use of magnesium-containing antacids and laxatives in patients with renal failure or in eclamptic mothers[106] (Table 8–13) (Chapter 13). Clinical features generally appear when serum magnesium levels exceed 4 mg/dL. Magnesium levels reaching 12 mg/dL almost certainly result in severe weakness and areflexia.

The typical neurologic manifestations of magnesium excess are usually not present in clinical conditions without exogenous intake of magnesium. Chronic renal failure, lithium therapy, hypothyroidism, hyperparathyroidism with renal disease, and pheochromocytoma may all cause a patient to be susceptible to increases of serum magnesium, but in these instances, transmission block of the neuromuscular junction is generally not clinically relevant.

Table 8–13. **Common Causes of Hypermagnesemia**

Exogenous magnesium intake

  Antacids

  Eclampsia treatment

Hemodialysis with high magnesium content

Rhabdomyolysis

Endocrine disorders

Acute diabetic ketoacidosis

CLINICAL FEATURES

Increasing plasma levels of magnesium lead to nausea, vomiting, cutaneous flushing, and dry mouth. A decrease in tendon reflexes is typical. In some patients, progression of limb weakness is rapid and bifacial weakness occurs. Extraocular and oropharyngeal muscles become involved, and some patients may become "locked in." Decreased level of consciousness is not a feature of hypermagnesemia.

TREATMENT

Gradual improvement over days can be expected when no further magnesium or magnesium-containing substances are administered. In severe cases with heart block, calcium gluconate (10 mL of a 10% solution) reverses hypermagnesemia. Occasionally, patients do not recover completely, and they may have underlying myasthenic syndromes.[107]

Hypocalcemia

Hypocalcemia signifies a poor prognosis in patients who are critically ill. Causes frequently encountered in the ICU are outlined in Table 8–14.[108,109] Approximately half the total serum calcium is protein bound, primarily by albumin. Differences in serum albumin concentration and state of hydration may cause variations in serum total calcium concentration.[110] The effect of albumin can be corrected by use of the fol-

lowing formula: adjusted measured serum calcium = serum calcium + 0.8 (4 − serum albumin). A decrease in the concentration of serum albumin by 1 g/dL produces a decrease in total serum calcium from 0.8 to 1 mg/dL, but the ionized fraction of calcium remains unchanged. Hypocalcemia associated with hypoalbuminemia does not cause symptoms because the ionized fraction remains similar.

CLINICAL FEATURES

Signs and symptoms of hypocalcemia have been well characterized, but many patients may be asymptomatic and it is only a reflection of severity of illness.[111–115] Paresthesias in the hands and feet and around the lips are early signs but almost certainly go unnoticed in critically ill patients. Muscle cramps, carpopedal spasm, and laryngeal stridor may follow as hypocalcemia progresses. Plantar flexion of the toes, arching of the feet, and contraction of calf muscles may also be cardinal signs.

Chvostek's sign is frequently found, and this typical sign in hypocalcemia is elicited by tapping three fingers over the branches of the facial nerve anterior to the external auditory meatus. A positive response is indicated by twitching of all ipsilateral facial muscles (lip at angle of mouth, nasal bridge, and lateral angle of eye), although there may be a graded response. Twitching of the mouth alone should not be interpreted as diagnostic, because it may occur in 25% of normal patients.[116] Latent tetany may also be demonstrated when a blood pressure cuff on one arm is inflated above the systolic blood pressure (Trousseau's sign) for at least 5 min.[117] Flexion of the fingers and adduction of the thumb produce a carpopedal spasm, or main d'accoucheur (obstetrician's hand).

Tonic–clonic seizures occur when serum calcium concentration is <3 mEq/L. In occasional cases, focal or nonconvulsive status epilepticus may develop. Seizures stop after correction of hypocalcemia, but grand mal seizures may evolve into convulsive status epilepticus. Prolonged coma from hypocalcemia seldom occurs; if it does, it is usually the result of anoxia associated with laryngeal stridor or poorly controlled status epilepticus.

Table 8–14. **Common Causes of Hypocalcemia**

Hypoalbuminemia
Gram-negative sepsis
Acute pancreatitis
Fat embolism
Severe crush injury
Thyroid surgery (hypoparathyroidism)
Pharmacologic agents
   Chemotherapy
   Pentamidine and foscarnet
   Antiepileptic drugs

TREATMENT

Hypocalcemia can be promptly corrected by a 2-hr intravenous infusion with 20 to 40 mL of a 10% solution of calcium gluconate followed by oral administration of calcium, 5 g/day. Muscle spasm, however, may persist for several hours after normalization of the calcium concentration. Virtually no patient has major neurologic sequelae after treatment.

Hypercalcemia

Hypercalcemia may result from primary hyperparathyroidism and malignant disease with or without metastasis. Neurologic manifestations are nonspecific and are usually found in patients with significant dehydration. Findings include marked drowsiness and impaired concentration, which occasionally progress to coma. Many patients recover after general measures have been taken to correct dehydration.

ENDOCRINE EMERGENCIES

Patients with acute endocrine disturbances are often gravely ill, clinical manifestations are dramatic, and neurologic manifestations are common. At the other end of the spectrum, stressors in the ICU, whether major surgical procedures or infection, may challenge the endocrine axis.

Nonketotic Hyperosmolar State

The physiologic changes in nonketotic hyperosmolar state (NKHS) are predominantly hyperglycemia with no or only minimal ketosis and extreme dehydration, reflected in greatly increased plasma osmolality. Type II diabetes has been undiagnosed at the time of presentation in one-third of patients with NKHS. In other patients with type II diabetes, intercurrent infection and failure to achieve adequate hydration trigger the derangement.

Nonketotic hyperosmolar state can occur as a complication of any bacterial infection or septic shock, extensive burns, acute pancreatitis, hyperalimentation, use of corticosteroids, and peritoneal dialysis (Table

Table 8–15. Precipitants of Hyperosmolar Hyperglycemic Nonketotic State

Drugs
Thiazide diuretics
Phenytoin
β-adrenergic blocking agents
Corticosteroids

Hypovolemia
Severe burns
Gastrointestinal hemorrhage

Infection
Gram-negative sepsis
Pneumonia

Stroke
Middle cerebral artery occlusion
Cerebral hematoma
Subarachnoid hemorrhage

Miscellaneous
Myocardial infarction
Pulmonary embolus
Hyperalimentation

8–15). However, postoperative NKHS is very common, and, in fact, most patients with NKHS are seen in surgical ICUs.[118,119] This disorder can be triggered by drugs with a known hyperglycemic effect (for example, furosemide, dopamine) or by fever in the first days after major surgical procedures. Seki[119] found that, on average, NKHS occurred on the sixth day after coronary bypass (range, 3 to 10 days). Meticulous attention to early clinical signs and frequent serum glucose determinations may prevent patients with type II diabetes mellitus from lapsing into this potentially fatal complication.

CLINICAL FEATURES

The classic features of NKHS consist of decrease in level of consciousness, progressive slipping into deep coma, and barely apparent motor responses to pain. Nonketotic hyperglycemic coma occurs with a sixfold to tenfold increase in serum glucose. Occasionally, focal signs or focal seizures are the presenting indications.[120–123] In its most acute form, the syndrome can be manifested by refractory status epilepticus. Focal neurologic signs that lead admitting physicians to believe that their patients have had a stroke are aphasia, hemiparesis, and visual field defects, which have been reported in one-third of patients. Focal neurologic signs are found virtually only in the nonketotic hyperosmolar state and are commonly absent in other metabolic derangements. The phenomenon is difficult to explain, but previous silent strokes, particularly in these patients with major cerebrovascular risk factors, may become more apparent during hyperglycemia. Transient bilateral Babinski's signs, muscle twitching, and tonic eye deviation may also occur. In patients with less severe hyperglycemia, focal seizures may dominate the clinical picture. A review of 158 patients noted seizures in about one-fourth of the patients with NKHS and focal motor seizures in 19%. Epilepsia partialis continua, however, generally occurs in patients with a preexisting structural lesion, usually as a result of an earlier ischemic stroke.[124] Unusual types of focal epilepsy, including stereotypical movements, speech arrest, and flashing colored lights,[125] have also been described in patients with nonketotic hyperglycemia. Uncommon manifestations are opsoclonus–myoclonus,[126] choreoathetosis, hemiballismus, and posture-induced seizures (clonic and brief jerking movements triggered by active or passive change in head or arm position).[127] The MRI studies in these patients documented transient T2 signal changes in the putamen or caudate nucleus.[110]

Neurologic signs and the degree of decrease in the level of consciousness appear to have a better correlation with plasma osmolality (Fig. 8–5) and serum sodium level than with absolute serum glucose concentration.[79,128]

In patients with nonketotic hyperosmolar states, hyponatremia often occurs because increased osmotic pressure from hyperglycemia shifts fluid from cells into the extracellular fluid space. Despite hyponatremia, a hyperosmolar state exists, and efforts should be directed to correcting the hyperosmolar–hyperglycemic state and not the hyponatremia per se.

The corrected serum sodium value (a decrease of 2.4 mEq/L in sodium concentration per 100 mg/dL increase in glucose

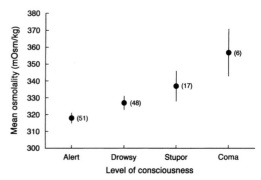

Figure 8–5. Serum osmolality and its relation to mental status in 122 patients with ketoacidosis. Numbers in parentheses indicate patients. (From Kitabchi AE, Fisher JN. Insulin therapy of diabetic ketoacidosis: physiologic versus pharmacologic doses of insulin and their routes of administration. In: Brownlee M [ed]. Handbook of Diabetes Mellitus, Vol. 5: Current and Future Therapies. Garland STPM Press, New York, 1981, pp 95–149. By permission of Garland Publishing.)

concentration) is better than the "1.6" correction factor.[129] Patients with hyponatremia but normal corrected serum sodium concentrations, increased plasma osmolality, and hyperglycemia usually do not have neurologic signs, because dehydration is limited. On the other hand, patients with a normal, low, or high serum sodium level but a high corrected serum sodium value who are in a hyperglycemic and hyperosmolar state may have a severely depressed consciousness.

TREATMENT

Nonketotic hyperosmolar coma is associated with hypovolemia, which explains hyperglycemia (euvolemia would result in increased secretion of glucose and prevent high concentration in the blood). A crucial element in the treatment of nonketotic hyperosmolar coma is rehydration with isotonic saline to establish adequate filling of the intravascular compartment. Insulin therapy can be withheld because of (unproven) concerns that the combination with rehydration will induce cerebral edema.

Outcome in nonketotic hyperosmolar coma is generally determined by early recognition and proper measures. Whether aggressive correction of the hyperosmolality results in secondary insults to the brain is not supported by clinical data. Also, virtually no long-term outcome data are available on patients who survive the insult.[128] With one-third of the outcomes fatal in most medical and surgical series, mortality remains unacceptably high. The most common cause of death is the underlying disease that triggered coma.

Diabetic Ketoacidotic Coma

The hallmarks of this disorder are severe hyperglycemia, ketoacidosis, and hyperosmolarity. Frequently, patients are known to have type I (juvenile-onset) diabetes, whereas nonketotic hyperosmolar coma more often occurs in type II diabetes. Ketoacidotic coma, however, may be a presenting feature of diabetes mellitus.

Hyperosmolarity may be less prominent in ketoacidosis than in the nonketotic state, but again degree of drowsiness may be more proportional to the severity of dehydration (Fig. 8–5). A large retrospective study of 287 episodes of diabetic ketoacidosis found only a weak correlation between H^+ concentrations and the degree of coma and confirmed the clinical impression that many diabetic patients with severe metabolic acidosis are alert.[130]

Focal signs are extremely uncommon in ketoacidotic coma and should suggest an underlying structural cause. Fulminant bacterial meningitis should be considered in any patient with diabetic coma unresponsive to fluid resuscitation (see Chapter 6).

Only general guidelines to treatment of diabetic ketoacidotic coma can be given because randomized trials are lacking. Most experts in this field favor infusion with saline, 100 to 150 mmol/L in the first 12 hr and 50 to 70 mmol/L thereafter.[131] A small randomized study on the effect of additional bicarbonate infusion showed no advantage in patients with an initial pH of 6.9 to 7.1.[132] A study comparing different regimens of insulin therapy concluded that intravenous infusion of insulin (low doses), saline, and dextrose, with the addition of bicarbonate only if the pH was <7.1, was superior to other regimens.[133] Use of colloid in an attempt to restore the circulating volume is not supported by any controlled trial and is not without risk and expense.[134]

Most patients survive the metabolic derangement without any significant residual deficit. Cerebral edema during treatment of diabetic ketoacidosis is a rare but nearly uniformly fatal complication.[135,136] The occurrence of massive cerebral edema, mostly in children and adolescents, is unpredictable, and patients at high risk have not been identified.[137,138]

The clinical presentation of cerebral edema associated with treatment of diabetic acidosis is striking. After initial biochemical and clinical improvement, the patient rapidly slips back into coma with spontaneous extensor posturing, soon followed by fixed and dilated pupils. The clinical criteria for brain death are present within 1 to 2 hr in patients with massive cerebral edema. Increased muscle tone, gegenhalten, or focal seizures may herald the drowsiness. Papilledema may be present but only in patients with progression to brain death due to massive bihemispheric swelling acutely increasing intracranial pressure. The classic stages of transtentorial herniation are usually not present, and most patients have sudden respiratory arrest and immediate loss of brain stem reflexes.

Treatment with mannitol, fluid restriction, and corticosteroids is unsuccessful in most cases, but rapid initiation of mannitol (2 g/kg of body weight) and fluid restriction (1.3 L/m^2 per 24 hr) occasionally salvages patients. Clinical deterioration may occur up to 24 hr after initiation of therapy. Favorable outcome has been reported, but many patients may have residual severe cognitive deficits and ataxia.

Computed tomography scanning may demonstrate signs of cerebral edema, marked by decrease in size of the lateral ventricles and obliteration of the ambient cisterns. Two serial CT scan studies showed that brain swelling (defined as decreased size of ventricles or cisterns) was present before treatment, was largely unchanged after 6 to 8 hr of treatment, and resolved significantly a week after treatment.[139,140] Fatal cerebral edema, however, did not occur. Hoffman and associates[139] therefore raised the possibility that fatal edema during treatment may be merely a progression of an already initiated physiologic process. Patients who survive brain edema, however, may remain disabled by infarcts in the distribution of the anterior cerebral artery and thalamic perforating arteries due to mechanical compression or stretch from acute downward displacement of the brain stem from edema. These infarcts can be documented by CT.[141]

PATHOPHYSIOLOGIC MECHANISMS

Two major hypotheses have emerged over the years. Cerebral edema may be explained in terms of idiogenic osmoles that serve to protect the brain from shrinkage at the time of profound dehydration. Unfortunately, these molecules may slowly dissipate, and their unwanted presence may consequently lead to brain edema when fluid infusion rapidly results in a hypoosmotic state. However, this hypothesis lacks good support, because no correlation could be found with any of the following treatment modes or biochemical factors: excessive hypotonic fluid replacement, serum sodium values, osmolality, and insulin protocols. Others have suggested that a Na^+/H^+ exchanger may be involved.[142] This hypothesis would indeed support the pretreatment subclinical presence of cerebral edema and temporal relation with insulin and fluid treatment.

This Na^+/H^+ exchanger can be activated by insulin, as convincingly demonstrated in other tissues (for example, muscle).[143] This activation results in sodium influx into the cells and brain swelling. There may be a rationale for Na^+/H^+ exchanger inhibitors such as amiloride (which, on the basis of molecular properties, should be able to cross the blood–brain barrier),[142] but clinical and experimental studies have not yet been performed.

A recent study in children suggested that brain ischemia followed by edema has a role because of the significant association with hypocapnia (vasoconstriction) and high initial serum urea nitrogen concentrations (dehydration). Bicarbonate therapy may additionally reduce cerebrospinal fluid partial pressure of oxygen and exacerbate vasoconstriction.[144]

Hypoglycemia

In most patients in the hospital or ICU, a hypoglycemic episode is a consequence of treatment with insulin. In others, inadequate management of parenteral nutrition can be held responsible for symptomatic episodes of hypoglycemia.[145]

Use of beta-blockers may generate hypoglycemia in insulin-treated diabetic patients but, more importantly, may also mask typical symptoms of hypoglycemia, such as tachycardia, sweating, and tremor.[146] These symptoms of hyperepinephrinemia may theoretically also go unnoticed in heavily sedated patients in the ICU. Other triggering events for significant hypoglycemia are fulminant hepatic failure, sepsis, and drugs with stimulating effects on insulin[56] (Table 8–16).

The symptoms of hypoglycemia are produced by an adrenergic reaction and include pallor, sweating, tachycardia, sensation of hunger, anxiety, and palpitations. (The author is aware of several instances in which these events were misinterpreted as ICU psychosis.)

Neurologic symptoms cannot be predicted from blood glucose levels, but the depth of coma may have some correlation with the degree of hypoglycemia. Surprisingly, some patients with severe biochemical hypoglycemia are fully awake or only mildly disoriented. When hypoglycemia develops slowly, blurred vision and slurred speech are prominent.[145,146] Patients who become comatose quickly awaken after intravenous administration of glucose but may remain unconscious after prolonged hypoglycemic coma or after a concomitant tonic–clonic seizure. Seizures in hypoglycemia may occur in diabetic patients with previous strokes and

Table 8–16. **Causes of Hypoglycemia in the Intensive Care Unit**

Sepsis

Hepatic failure

Drugs
  Insulin
  Ouabain
  β-adrenergic blocking agents
  Pentamidine

Alimentary
  Postprandial after gastrectomy
  Discontinuing total parenteral alimentation

Table 8–17. **Neurologic Manifestations of Hypoglycemia**

Presenting Symptom	No.
Coma or stupor	55
Behavioral changes	38
Drowsiness	10
Dizziness, tremor	10
Seizures	9
Sudden hemiparesis	3

From Malouf and Brust.[145] By permission of the American Neurological Association.

rapid shifts in blood glucose concentration. In probably the largest series of patients with symptomatic hypoglycemia admitted to an emergency room, 9 of 125 visits were associated with seizures, usually tonic–clonic, but most patients had a seizure disorder or alcohol dependency. The neurologic manifestations of hypoglycemia are summarized in Table 8–17.

The principal signs and symptoms of hypoglycemia are behavior changes marked by confusion, vacant stare, or, in the extreme situation, unresponsiveness to pain stimuli. Marked chorioathetosis with facial grimacing at the time of hypoglycemia has been reported.[148] Transient hemiplegia has been associated with severe hypoglycemia.[147] Normalization of blood glucose concentration results in resolution of hemiplegia within minutes.

Episodes of hypoglycemia are treated with glucose in the range of 25 to 50 mL of 50% solution, and further deterioration should be prevented, often with simple measures. Severe hypoglycemic reactions may also be treated with glucagon. As alluded to earlier, most patients recover completely. The delay in recognition and the duration of coma probably determine neurologic sequelae. Patients with hypoglycemic coma of long duration (estimated to be from 4 to 6 hr) have a great chance of persistent vegetative state or severe disabling cerebellar signs.[149]

Many patients in whom autopsy was performed after prolonged hypoglycemic coma had selective neuronal vulnerability consisting of damage in the hippocampus, striatum, substantia nigra, and, particularly, the cerebellum.[150–152] Associated hypotension or marked hypoxia from gastric aspiration or hypoventilation in patients with prolonged hypoglycemia may be a confounding factor. Damage in the hippocampus may now be recognized on MRI (Fig. 8–6).

Thyroid Storm

An endocrine disorder of major importance is sudden thyrotoxicosis. Thyroid storm frequently occurs in patients with incomplete control but may be the first presentation of thyroid imbalance.[153] The key clinical features (Table 8–18) are hyperthermia, tachycardia, and delirium.[154] Early in the course, patients may be anxious, nervous, and overreactive. Marked psychiatric symptoms with vivid visual and acoustic hallucinations are occasionally present.[155,156] Untreated patients lapse into coma and may have extensor posturing or pathologic flexion responses, prominent pyramidal signs with profound spasticity, pathologic brain stem reflexes, bilateral clonus, and Babinski's signs.[157]

Elderly patients may display a distinctive

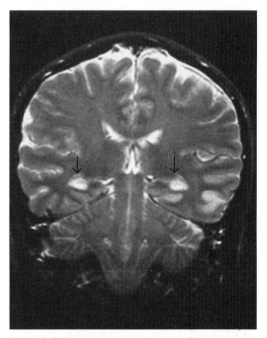

Figure 8–6. Magnetic resonance image, T2-weighted, of severe hippocampal damage (arrows) after severe hypoglycemia. (Courtesy of Dr. B. F. Boeve.)

Table 8–18. Clinical Features of Thyroid Storm

Hyperthermia
New-onset tachyarrhythmias
Jaundice
Delirium, stupor, coma
Proptosis, ophthalmoplegia
Pyramidal signs
Tremor, myoclonic jerks
Brisk tendon reflexes

---

clinical syndrome of apathetic thyrotoxicosis (patients who "quietly and peacefully sink into coma and die an absolutely relaxed death").[158] Other distinctive features of apathetic thyrotoxicosis are profound blepharoptosis (but no proptosis) and proximal myopathy. Patients with severe thyrotoxicosis more often have periorbital puffiness and proptosis, which may be more prominent unilaterally. Hyperthermia (often >39.5°C) with excessive sweating and moist skin is a rather specific symptom. Multinodular thyromegaly is another frequent finding but may be absent in 10% of the patients.

Hyperthyroidism may be accompanied by acute thyrotoxic myopathy.[159] This entity is characterized by rapid muscular weakness associated with diaphragmatic failure, but unfortunately, accurate documentation is scarce. To complicate matters further, thyrotoxicosis may be associated with myasthenia gravis and familial periodic paralysis. Thyrotoxic storm may also result in rhabdomyolysis.

Prompt treatment with propylthiouracil, propranolol, and corticosteroids results in a favorable outcome. Excess circulating thyroid hormone may also be removed by plasma exchange or peritoneal dialysis. Emergency thyroid surgery may be indicated in patients with thyroid storm not controlled by these measures. Fatal outcome may be a consequence of irreversible congestive heart failure, extreme dehydration, and hypoglycemia, but many patients survive.

Hashimoto's Encephalopathy

A fascinating neurologic disorder has been linked to autoimmune thyroiditis (Hashimoto's encephalopathy). The antithyroid antibody titers, particularly those of the antithyroid peroxidase antibodies, are elevated. Thyroid-stimulating hormone, but not thyroid hormone, is usually markedly increased, although hypothyroidism may evolve later. Confusional state, myoclonus, hallucinations, and a panoply of psychiatric manifestations should point to the possibility of this rare disorder.

Magnetic resonance imaging may document a diffuse leukoencephalopathy (Fig. 8–7), but findings may be normal in florid cases. Slowing of the electroencephalographic pattern interrupted by focal epileptiform abnormalities has been repeatedly documented but without specific characteristics. One autopsy study documented a vasculitic infiltrate in venules, suggesting vasculitis. Response to intravenous administration of 1 g of methylprednisolone for 5 days followed by 60 mg of prednisone is remarkable.[160–165] A more recent patient example stressed a prompt response with plasma exchange after an unsatisfactory result with intravenous immunoglobulin or corticosteroids.[166]

Myxedema Coma

The encephalopathy of hypothyroidism can be expected in patients with previously treated thyroid disease but may also develop from new-onset autoimmune thyroiditis. Other important triggers are bacterial infections, trauma, and recent thyroid surgery. Anesthesia, barbiturates, phenothiazines, and, in particular, imipramine may result in exacerbation of myxedema.[167] Exposure to cold is a well-recognized trigger, and one should be alert for a thyroid disorder in comatose patients during the winter season.

In patients with myxedema coma, the clinical characteristics are those of metabolic encephalopathy, with seizures and multifocal myoclonus. Tapping of muscles frequently leaves a transient local swelling that resembles myotonia. Tendon reflexes are diminished and may have a prolonged recovery phase. The typical features of hypothyroidism in patients with myxedema coma are usually present: dry, rough skin and yellow discoloration, puffy face and eyelids (Plates 8–1 and 8–2), and loss of outer eyebrows.

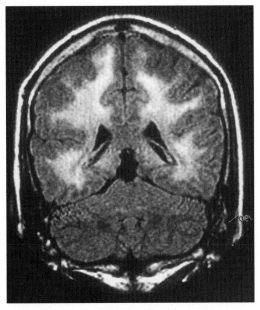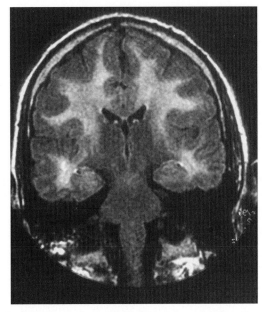

Figure 8–7. Leukoencephalopathy by magnetic resonance imaging in a patient with Hashimoto's encephalopathy.

Most patients hypoventilate and are cyanotic.[168] Hypothermia and bradycardia may also be the predominant findings.

It is important to recognize that associated metabolic factors, such as hypoglycemia, hyponatremia, and hypercalcemia, may cause coma.

Aggressive treatment of myxedema includes mechanical ventilation, fluid resuscitation in patients with hypotension, and parenteral administration of thyroxine (500 μg, intravenous push).[169] Addison's disease may coexist; therefore, many patients need additional hydrocortisone (100 mg intravenously). Conversely, hypothyroidism is not uncommon in Addison's disease, and after corticosteroid therapy, abnormal results of the thyroid-stimulating hormone test may normalize.

Hypothermia usually responds rapidly to correction of thyroxine and triiodothyronine levels. Except in patients with severe hypothermia, additional support other than blankets is not necessary. Heating blankets, however, may worsen shock.

Outcome of myxedema coma can be good. Hylander and Rosenqvist[170] analyzed factors associated with fatal outcome and concluded that old age, initial hypothermia, shock, and excessive hormone doses of triiodothyronine to correct hypothyroid state predicted poor outcome.

Adrenal Crisis

Acute adrenal insufficiency (Addison's disease) is a potential problem in any ICU. Adrenal crisis typically occurs in patients previously treated with corticosteroids in whom the dose was not increased during intervals of stress. Sepsis, recent major surgery, or use of drugs that interfere with hepatic biosynthesis or with the peripheral action of corticosteroids (for example, ketoconazole, barbiturates, phenytoin, spironolactone) may predispose patients to Addison's disease.

Addison's disease is manifested by rapidly evolving shock and dehydration. Laboratory diagnosis reveals a plasma cortisol value of <15 μg/L, but the triad of hyponatremia, hyperglycemia, and hyperkalemia is also supportive. Many patients complain of migratory myalgias and weakness, and flexion pseudocontractures of the knees and hips are often present.[171] Pain may occur in any weak muscle, but the thigh muscles are particularly tender. Creatine kinase concentration may reach extremely high values and decrease after substitution. Electromyographic examination of affected muscles may show myopathic features with short duration and low-amplitude potentials.

Alternatively, weakness in an addisonian crisis may be associated with hyperkalemic myopathy[86] with flaccid tetraplegia or, in exceptional cases, with a Guillain-Barré-like syndrome.[172–174] The clinical features of Addison's disease are listed in Table 8–19.[175] Hyperpigmentation in scars, in mucous membranes, and along the gingival margin is a leading sign but may not be present.

The encephalopathy of adrenal insufficiency may have features of profound perceptual impairment, with lethargy progressing to coma. Bilateral papilledema has been described but only in association with pathologically demonstrated cerebral edema. Cerebral edema has been reported as a presenting feature of Addison's disease.[176] In patients with severe electrolyte abnormalities and profound hypotension, "encephalopathie addisonienne," a term introduced by Klippel in 1899, may be difficult to diagnose.

Substitution of cortisol by corticosteroids (for example, hydrocortisone, 300 mg/day intravenously) and replacement of sodium and water deficit and electrolytes are the mainstays of treating the addisonian crisis. Outcome in most patients is good if the underlying cause is recognized and appropriately treated.

CONCLUSIONS

Rather than annoy the intensive care specialist with terms such as "multifactorial" and "toxic–metabolic," consulted neurologists must have a clear idea of how each of the various disturbances may produce an effect on the nervous system.

The correlation between neurologic features and acid–base derangements or severe electrolyte disorders is based on the first, rapid sign of recovery when the abnormality is being corrected. Electrolyte abnormalities are prevalent in critical illness. In principle, to produce neurologic symptoms, electrolyte abnormalities have to be severe, with substantial deviation from normal values but often also with a shift in a very short time span. However, patients can remain asymptomatic.

The most common hospital- and ICU-associated electrolyte abnormality is hyponatremia. Causes in the postoperative period, in which hyponatremia is frequent, are morphine use that leads to vomiting in susceptible patients, water retention, and liberal use of fluids often given to overcome postoperative oliguria. Severe, unrecognized hyponatremia may cause seizures, respiratory arrest, and vegetative state or progression to brain death, particularly in young women. The condition is fortunately extremely rare. In many other patients, a single seizure or decrease in level of consciousness is seen. Although considerable debate has centered on the speed of correction, and some investigators insist that the issue is currently unresolved, many believe that correction of severe hyponatremia should be carefully orchestrated and gradual to prevent demyelination. An important practical consideration is that overcorrection to values above 140 mEq/L may be a contributory cause of central pontine myelinolysis. One guideline is to correct the plasma sodium concentration to a value above 125 mmol/L with 3% hypertonic saline administered at 0.5 mL/kg per hour. Other electrolyte abnormalities (potassium, phosphate, calcium, and magnesium) produce limb weakness, diaphragm weakness

Table 8–19. **Major Symptoms and Signs of Addison's Disease in 100 Patients**

Findings	Patients (%)
Weakness and fatigability	100
Weight loss	100
Hyperpigmentation	92
Hypotension	88
Hyponatremia	88
Hyperkalemia	64
Gastrointestinal symptoms	56
Postural dizziness	12
Muscle and joint pains	6
Hypercalcemia	6
Vitiligo	4

From Nerup.[175] By permission of Acta Endocrinologica.

(hypophosphatemia alone), tetanic cramps, or occasional tonic–clonic seizures.

Endocrine crises are often perplexing not only in the initial presentation but also in the neurologic sequelae of biochemical correction. If recognition is delayed, hyperglycemic or hypoglycemic coma may cause severe cognitive defects. Cerebral edema after treatment of diabetic ketoacidosis, most often in children and young adults, is a fatal complication. Aggressive management of cerebral edema with conventional therapy may save an occasional patient but often at the expense of persistent disability. Hypothyroid coma or thyroid storm can be suspected by changes in skin color and heart rate and, in patients with hyperthyroidism, by proptosis and conjunctival injection. Hashimoto's thyroiditis may be considered in unexplained psychiatric behavior, leukoencephalopathy, and increased antibody titers, but the disorder is rare and very difficult to diagnose. Addison's disease may cause weakness, but the laboratory features of hyponatremia, hyperglycemia, and hyperkalemia are usually detected and corrected in the ICU before progression to marked encephalopathy and coma.

REFERENCES

1. Arieff AI, Kerian A, Massry SG, DeLima J. Intracellular pH of brain: alterations in acute respiratory acidosis and alkalosis. Am J Physiol 230:804–812, 1976.
2. Posner JB, Swanson AG, Plum F. Acid–base balance in cerebrospinal fluid. Arch Neurol 12:479–496, 1965.
3. Arieff AI. Acid–base balance in specialized tissues: central nervous system. In Seldin DW, Giebisch G (eds). The Regulation of Acid–base Balance. Raven Press, New York, 1989, pp 107–121.
4. Hornbein TF, Pavlin EG. Distribution of H^+ and HCO_3 minus between CSF and blood during respiratory alkalosis in dogs. Am J Physiol 228:1149–1154, 1975.
5. Pavlin EG, Hornbein TTF. Distribution of H^+ and HCO_3 minus between CSF and blood during metabolic alkalosis in dogs. Am J Physiol 228:1141–1144, 1975.
6. Preuss HG. Fundamentals of clinical acid–base evaluation. Clin Lab Med 13:103–116, 1993.
7. Caroll GC, Rothenberg DM. Carbon dioxide narcosis. Pathological or "pathillogical"? Chest 102:986–988, 1992.
8. Meissner HH, Franklin C. Extreme hypercapnia in a fully alert patient. Chest 102:1298–1299, 1992.
9. Austen FK, Carmichael MW, Adams RD. Neuro-

logic manifestations of chronic pulmonary insufficiency. N Engl J Med 257:579–590, 1957.
10. Faden A. Encephalopathy following treatment of chronic pulmonary failure. Neurology 26:337–339, 1976.
11. Sieker HO, Hickam JB. Carbon dioxide intoxication: the clinical syndrome, its etiology and management with particular reference to the use of mechanical respirators. Medicine (Baltimore) 35:389–423, 1956.
12. Lumb A. Nunn's Applied Respiratory Physiology, 5th ed. Butterworth-Heinemann, Oxford, 2000.
13. Aubier M, Murciano D, Milic-Emili J, et al. Effects of the administration of O_2 on ventilation and blood gases in patients with chronic obstructive pulmonary disease during acute respiratory failure. Am Rev Respir Dis 122:747–754, 1980.
14. Pauzner R, Mouallem M, Sadeh M, Tadmor R, Farfel Z. High incidence of primary cerebral lymphoma in tumor-induced central neurogenic hyperventilation. Arch Neurol 46:510–512, 1989.
15. Siderowf AD, Balcer LJ, Kenyon LC, Nei M, Raps EC, Galetta SL. Central neurogenic hyperventilation in an awake patient with a pontine glioma. Neurology 46:1160–1162, 1996.
16. Shibata Y, Meguro K, Narushima K, Shibuya F, Doi M, Kikuchi Y. Malignant lymphoma of the central nervous system presenting with central neurogenic hyperventilation. J Neurosurg 76:696–700, 1992.
17. Jaeckle KA, Digre KB, Jones CR, Bailey PL, McMahill PC. Central neurogenic hyperventilation: pharmacologic intervention with morphine sulfate and correlative analysis of respiratory, sleep, and ocular motor dysfunction. Neurology 40:1715–1720, 1990.
18. Perez GO, Oster JR, Rogers A. Acid–base disturbances in gastrointestinal disease. Dig Dis Sci 32:1033–1043, 1987.
19. Lien YH, Shapiro JI, Chan L. Effects of hypernatremia on organic brain osmoles. J Clin Invest 85:1427–1435, 1990.
20. Lien YH, Shapiro JI, Chan L. Study of brain electrolytes and organic osmoles during correction of chronic hyponatremia. Implications for the pathogenesis of central pontine myelinolysis. J Clin Invest 88:303–309, 1991.
21. Kumar S, Berl T. Sodium. Lancet 352:220–228, 1998.
22. Anderson RJ, Chung HM, Kluge R, Schrier RW. Hyponatremia: a prospective analysis of its epidemiology and the pathogenetic role of vasopressin. Ann Intern Med 102:164–168, 1985.
23. Arieff AI, Guisado R. Effects on the central nervous system of hypernatremic and hyponatremic states. Kidney Int 10:104–116, 1976.
24. Arieff AI, Llach F, Massry SG. Neurological manifestations and morbidity of hyponatremia: correlation with brain water and electrolytes. Medicine (Baltimore) 55:121–129, 1976.
25. Adams RD, Victor M, Mancall EL. Central pontine myelinolysis: a hitherto undescribed disease occurring in alcoholic and malnourished patients. Arch Neurol Psychiatry 81:154–172, 1959.
26. Endo Y, Oda M, Hara M. Central pontine myelinolysis. A study of 37 cases in 1,000 consecutive

autopsies. Acta Neuropathol (Berl) 53:145–153, 1981.

27. Chalela J, Kattah J. Catatonia due to central pontine and extrapontine myelinolysis: case report. J Neurol Neurosurg Psychiatry 67:692–693, 1999.

28. Ayus JC, Krothapalli RK, Arieff AI. Changing concepts in treatment of severe symptomatic hyponatremia. Rapid correction and possible relation to central pontine myelinolysis. Am J Med 78:897–902, 1985.

29. Ayus JC, Olivero JJ, Frommer JP. Rapid correction of severe hyponatremia with intravenous hypertonic saline solution. Am J Med 72:43–48, 1982.

30. Berl T. Treating hyponatremia: damned if we do and damned if we don't. Kidney Int 37:1006–1018, 1990.

31. Brunner JE, Redmond JM, Haggar AM, Kruger DF, Elias SB. Central pontine myelinolysis and pontine lesions after rapid correction of hyponatremia: a prospective magnetic resonance imaging study. Ann Neurol 27:61–66, 1990.

32. Cluitmans FH, Meinders AE. Management of severe hyponatremia: rapid or slow correction? Am J Med 88:161–166, 1990.

33. Laureno R. Central pontine myelinolysis following rapid correction of hyponatremia. Ann Neurol 13:232–242, 1983.

34. Illowsky BP, Laureno R. Encephalopathy and myelinolysis after rapid correction of hyponatraemia. Brain 110:855–867, 1987.

35. McKee AC, Winkelman MD, Banker BQ. Central pontine myelinolysis in severely burned patients: relationship to serum hyperosmolality. Neurology 38:1211–1217, 1988.

36. Goebel HH, Zur PH. Central pontine myelinolysis. A clinical and pathological study of 10 cases. Brain 95:495–504, 1972.

37. Messert B, Orrison WW, Hawkins MJ, Quaglieri CE. Central pontine myelinolysis. Considerations on etiology, diagnosis, and treatment. Neurology 29:147–160, 1979.

38. Gross P, Reimann D, Neidel J, et al. The treatment of severe hyponatremia. Kidney Int Suppl 64: S6–S11, 1998.

39. Oster JR, Singer I. Hyponatremia, hyposmolality, and hypotonicity: tables and fables. Arch Intern Med 159:333–336, 1999.

40. Price BH, Mesulam MM. Behavioral manifestations of central pontine myelinolysis. Arch Neurol 44:671–673, 1987.

41. Wijdicks EFM, Blue PR, Steers JL, Wiesner RH. Central pontine myelinolysis with stupor alone after orthotopic liver transplantation. Liver Transplant Surg 2:14–16, 1996.

42. Estol CJ, Faris AA, Martinez AJ, Ahdab-Barmada M. Central pontine myelinolysis after liver transplantation. Neurology 39:493–498, 1989.

43. Maraganore DM, Folger WN, Swanson JW, Ahlskog JE. Movement disorders as sequelae of central pontine myelinolysis: report of three cases. Mov Disord 7:142–148, 1992.

44. Tinker R, Anderson MG, Anand P, Kermode A, Harding AE. Pontine myelinolysis presenting with acute parkinsonism as a sequel of corrected hyponatraemia. J Neurol Neurosurg Psychiatry 53: 87–88, 1990.

45. Tison FX, Ferrer X, Julien J. Delayed onset movement disorders as a complication of central pontine myelinolysis. Mov Disord 6:171–173, 1991.

46. Tomita I, Satoh H, Satoh A, Seto M, Tsujihata M, Yoshimura T. Extrapontine myelinolysis presenting with parkinsonism as a sequel of rapid correction of hyponatraemia. J Neurol Neurosurg Psychiatry 62:422–423, 1997.

47. Seiser A, Schwarz S, Aichinger-Steiner MM, Funk G, Schnider P, Brainin M. Parkinsonism and dystonia in central pontine and extrapontine myelinolysis. J Neurol Neurosurg Psychiatry 65:119–121, 1998.

48. Miller GM, Baker HL Jr, Okazaki H, Whisnant JP. Central pontine myelinolysis and its imitators: MR findings. Radiology 168:795–802, 1988.

49. Moriwaka F, Tashior K, Maruo Y, Nomura M, Hamada K, Kashiwaba T. MR imaging of pontine and extrapontine myelinolysis. J Comput Assist Tomogr 12:446–449, 1988.

50. Kumar SR, Mone AP, Gray LC, Troost BT. Central pontine myelinolysis: delayed changes on neuroimaging. J Neuroimaging 10:169–172, 2000.

51. Ho VB, Fitz CR, Yoder CC, Geyer CA. Resolving MR features in osmotic myelinolysis (central pontine and extrapontine myelinolysis). AJNR Am J Neuroradiol 14:163–167, 1993.

52. Fryer JP, Fortier MV, Metrakos P, et al. Central pontine myelinolysis and cyclosporine neurotoxicity following liver transplantation. Transplantation 61:658–661, 1996.

53. Laureno R, Karp BI. Myelinolysis after correction of hyponatremia. Ann Intern Med 126:57–62, 1997.

54. Arieff AI. Hyponatremia, convulsions, respiratory arrest, and permanent brain damage after elective surgery in healthy women. N Engl J Med 314: 1529–1535, 1986.

55. Ayus JC, Wheeler JM, Arieff AI. Postoperative hyponatremic encephalopathy in menstruant women. Ann Intern Med 117:891–897, 1992.

56. Ben-Ami H, Nagachandran P, Mendelson A, Edoute Y. Drug-induced hypoglycemic coma in 102 diabetic patients. Arch Intern Med 159:281–284, 1999.

57. Fraser CL, Arieff AI. Fatal central diabetes mellitus and insipidus resulting from untreated hyponatremia: a new syndrome. Ann Intern Med 112: 113–119, 1990.

58. Arieff AI, Kozniewska E, Roberts TP, Vexler ZS, Ayus JC, Kucharczyk J. Age, gender, and vasopressin affect survival and brain adaptation in rats with metabolic encephalopathy. Am J Physiol 268: R1143–R1152, 1995.

59. Silver SM, Schroeder BM, Bernstein P, Sterns RH. Brain adaptation to acute hyponatremia in young rats. Am J Physiol 276:R1595–R1599, 1999.

60. Clifford DB, Gado MH, Levy BK. Osmotic demyelination syndrome. Lack of pathologic and radiologic imaging correlation. Arch Neurol 46: 343–347, 1989.

61. Kleinschmidt-DeMasters BK, Norenberg MD. Rapid correction of hyponatremia causes demyelination: relation to central pontine myelinolysis. Science 211:1068–1070, 1981.

62. Sterns RH. Neurological deterioration following

treatment for hyponatremia. Am J Kidney Dis 13: 434–437, 1989.

63. Sterns RH, Riggs JE, Schochet SS Jr. Osmotic demyelination syndrome following correction of hyponatremia. N Engl J Med 314:1535–1542, 1986.

64. Sterns RH, Thomas DJ, Herndon RM. Brain dehydration and neurologic deterioration after rapid correction of hyponatremia. Kidney Int 35:69–75, 1989.

65. Verbalis JG, Gullans SR. Hyponatremia causes large sustained reductions in brain content of multiple organic osmolytes in rats. Brain Res 567:274–282, 1991.

66. Plum F, Posner JB, Hain RF. Delayed neurological deterioration after anoxia. Arch Intern Med 110: 18–25, 1962.

67. Narins RG. Therapy of hyponatremia: does haste make waste? N Engl J Med 314:1573–1575, 1986.

68. Norenberg MD, Leslie KO, Robertson AS. Association between rise in serum sodium and central pontine myelinolysis. Ann Neurol 11:128–135, 1982.

69. Sterns RH. Severe symptomatic hyponatremia: treatment and outcome. A study of 64 cases. Ann Intern Med 107:656–664, 1987.

70. Laureno R, Karp BI. Pontine and extrapontine myelinolysis following rapid correction of hyponatraemia. Lancet 1:1439–1441, 1988.

71. Adrogué HJ, Madias NE. Hyponatremia. N Engl J Med 342:1581–1589, 2000.

72. Gross P. Correction of hyponatremia. Semin Nephrol 21:269–272, 2001.

73. Decaux G. Difference in solute excretion during correction of hyponatremic patients with cirrhosis or syndrome of inappropriate secretion of antidiuretic hormone by oral vasopressin V2 receptor antagonist VPA-985. J Lab Clin Med 138:18–21, 2001.

74. Oh MS, Choi KC, Uribarri J, Sher J, Rao C, Carroll HJ. Prevention of myelinolysis in rats by dexamethasone or colchicine. Am J Nephrol 10: 158–161, 1990.

75. Bibl D, Lampl C, Gabriel C, Jungling G, Brock H, Kostler G. Treatment of central pontine myelinolysis with therapeutic plasmapheresis. Lancet 353:1155, 1999.

76. Mahowald JM, Himmelstein DU. Hypernatremia in the elderly: relation to infection and mortality. J Am Geriatr Soc 29:177–180, 1981.

77. Palevsky PM, Bhagrath R, Greenberg A. Hypernatremia in hospitalized patients. Ann Intern Med 124:197–203, 1996.

78. Sparacio RR, Anziska B, Schutta HS. Hypernatremia and chorea. A report of two cases. Neurology 26:46–50, 1976.

79. Arieff AI, Carroll HJ. Nonketotic hyperosmolar coma with hyperglycemia: clinical features, pathophysiology, renal function, acid–base balance, plasma-cerebrospinal fluid equilibria and the effects of therapy in 37 cases. Medicine (Baltimore) 51:73–94, 1972.

80. Morris-Jones PH, Houston IB, Evans RC. Prognosis of the neurological complications of acute hypernatraemia. Lancet 2:1385–1389, 1967.

81. Adrogué HJ, Madias NE. Hypernatremia. N Engl J Med 342:1493–1499, 2000.

82. Manary MJ, Keating JP, Hirshberg GE. Quadri- paresis due to potassium depletion. Crit Care Med 14:750–752, 1986.

83. Comi G, Testa D, Cornelio F, Comola M, Canal N. Potassium depletion myopathy: a clinical and morphological study of six cases. Muscle Nerve 8:17–21, 1985.

84. Brady HR, Goldberg H, Lunski C, Uldall PR. Dialysis-induced hyperkalaemia presenting as profound muscle weakness. Int J Artif Organs 11: 43–44, 1988.

85. Layzer RB. Neuromuscular Manifestations of Systemic Disease. FA Davis, Philadelphia, 1985.

86. Pollen RH, Williams RH. Hyperkalemic neuromyopathy in Addison's disease. N Engl J Med 263: 273–278, 1960.

87. Betro MG, Pain RW. Hypophosphataemia and hyperphosphataemia in a hospital population. Br Med J 1:273–276, 1972.

88. Anonymous. Postoperative hypophosphatemia: a multifactorial problem. Nutr Rev 47:111–116, 1989.

89. Hayek ME, Eisenberg PG. Severe hypophosphatemia following the institution of enteral feedings. Arch Surg 124:1325–1328, 1989.

90. Juan D, Elrazak MA. Hypophosphatemia in hospitalized patients. JAMA 242:163–164, 1979.

91. King AL, Sica DA, Miller G, Pierpaoli S. Severe hypophosphatemia in a general hospital population. South Med J 80:831–835, 1987.

92. Knochel JP. Neuromuscular manifestations of electrolyte disorders. Am J Med 72:521–535, 1982.

93. Larsson L, Rebel K, Sorbo B. Severe hypophosphatemia—a hospital survey. Acta Med Scand 214: 221–223, 1983.

94. Silvis SE, DiBartolomeo AG, Aaker HM. Hypophosphatemia and neurological changes secondary to oral caloric intake: a variant of hyperalimentation syndrome. Am J Gastroenterol 73: 215–222, 1980.

95. Gravelyn TR, Brophy N, Siegert C, Peters-Golden M. Hypophosphatemia-associated respiratory muscle weakness in a general inpatient population. Am J Med 84:870–876, 1988.

96. Hasselstrom L, Wimberley PD, Nielsen VG. Hypophosphatemia and acute respiratory failure in a diabetic patient. Intensive Care Med 12:429–431, 1986.

97. Rie MA. Hypophosphatemia and diaphragmatic contractility [letter]. N Engl J Med 314:519–520, 1986.

98. Lentz RD, Brown DM, Kjellstrand CM. Treatment of severe hypophosphatemia. Ann Intern Med 89:941–944, 1978.

99. Vannatta JB, Whang R, Papper S. Efficacy of intravenous phosphorus therapy in the severely hypophosphatemic patient. Arch Intern Med 141: 885–887, 1981.

100. Barton CH, Vaziri ND, Martin DC, Choi S, Alikhani S. Hypomagnesemia and renal magnesium wasting in renal transplant recipients receiving cyclosporine. Am J Med 83:693–699, 1987.

101. Chernow B, Bamberger S, Stoiko M, et al. Hypomagnesemia in patients in postoperative intensive care. Chest 95:391–397, 1989.

102. June CH, Thompson CB, Kennedy MS, Nims J, Thomas ED. Profound hypomagnesemia and re-

nal magnesium wasting associated with the use of cyclosporine for marrow transplantation. Transplantation 39:620–624, 1985.

103. Kes P, Reiner Z. Symptomatic hypomagnesemia associated with gentamicin therapy. Magnes Trace Elem 9:54–60, 1990.

104. Kingston ME, Al-Siba'I MB, Skooge WC. Clinical manifestations of hypomagnesemia. Crit Care Med 14:950–954, 1986.

105. Saul RF, Selhorst JB. Downbeat nystagmus with magnesium depletion. Arch Neurol 38:650–652, 1981.

106. Swift TR. Weakness from magnesium-containing cathartics: electrophysiologic studies. Muscle Nerve 2:295–298, 1979.

107. Bashuk RG, Krendel DA. Myasthenia gravis presenting as weakness after magnesium administration. Muscle Nerve 13:708–712, 1990.

108. Falk SA, Birken EA, Baran DT. Temporary postthyroidectomy hypocalcemia. Arch Otolaryngol Head Neck Surg 114:168–174, 1988.

109. Michie W, Duncan T, Hamer-Hodges DW, et al. Mechanism of hypocalcaemia after thyroidectomy for thyrotoxicosis. Lancet 1:508–514, 1971.

110. Lai PH, Tien RD, Chang MH, et al. Choreaballismus with nonketotic hyperglycemia in primary diabetes mellitus. AJNR Am J Neuroradiol 17:1057–1064, 1996.

111. Fonseca OA, Calverley JR. Neurological manifestations of hypoparathyroidism. Arch Intern Med 120:202–206, 1967.

112. Frame B. Neuromuscular manifestations of parathyroid disease. In: Vinken PJ, Bruyn GW (eds). Handbook of Clinical Neurology, Vol. 27. North-Holland Publishing, Amsterdam, 1976, pp 283–320.

113. Gotta AH. Tetany and epilepsy. Arch Neurol Psychiatry 66:714–721, 1951.

114. Rose GA, Vas CJ. Neurological complications and electroencephalographic changes in hypoparathyroidism. Acta Neurol Scand 42:537–550, 1966.

115. Zivin JR, Gooley T, Zager RA, Ryan MJ. Hypocalcemia: a pervasive metabolic abnormality in the critically ill. Am J Kidney Dis 37:689–698, 2001.

116. Hoffman E. The Chvostek sign: a clinical study. Am J Surg 96:33–37, 1958.

117. Lewis T. Trousseau's phenomenon in tetany. Clin Sci 4:361–364, 1942.

118. Ellison DA, Forman DT. Transient hyperglycemia during abdominal aortic surgery. Clin Chem 36:815–817, 1990.

119. Seki S. Clinical features of hyperosmolar hyperglycemic nonketotic diabetic coma associated with cardiac operations. J Thorac Cardiovasc Surg 91:867–873, 1986.

120. Grant C, Warlow C. Focal epilepsy in diabetic nonketotic hyperglycaemia. Br Med J 290:1204–1205, 1985.

121. Guisado R, Arieff AI. Neurologic manifestations of diabetic comas: correlation with biochemical alterations in the brain. Metabolism 24:665–679, 1975.

122. Khardori R, Soler NG. Hyperosmolar hyperglycemic nonketotic syndrome. Report of 22 cases and brief review. Am J Med 77:899–904, 1984.

123. MacDonald JT, Brown DR. Acute hemiparesis in juvenile insulin-dependent diabetes mellitus (JIDDM). Neurology 29:893–896, 1979.

124. Singh BM, Strobos RJ. Epilepsia partialis continua associated with nonketotic hyperglycemia: clinical and biochemical profile of 21 patients. Ann Neurol 8:155–160, 1980.

125. Harden CL, Rosenbaum DH, Daras M. Hyperglycemia presenting with occipital seizures. Epilepsia 32:215–220, 1991.

126. Matsumura K, Sonoh M, Tamaoka A, Sakuta M. Syndrome of opsoclonus–myoclonus in hyperosmolar nonketotic coma. Ann Neurol 18:623–624, 1985.

127. Rector WG Jr, Herlong HF, Moses H III. Nonketotic hyperglycemia appearing as choreoathetosis or ballism. Arch Intern Med 142:154–155, 1982.

128. Kitabchi AE, Murphy MB. Diabetic ketoacidosis and hyperosmolar hyperglycemic nonketotic coma. Med Clin North Am 72:1545–1563, 1988.

129. Hillier TA, Abbott RD, Barrett EJ. Hyponatremia: evaluating the correction factor for hyperglycemia. Am J Med 106:399–403, 1999.

130. Rosival V. The influence of blood hydrogen ion concentration on the level of consciousness in diabetic ketoacidosis. Ann Clin Res 19:23–25, 1987.

131. Harris GD, Fiordalisi I, Finberg L. Safe management of diabetic ketoacidemia. J Pediatr 113:65–68, 1988.

132. Morris LR, Murphy MB, Kitabchi AE. Bicarbonate therapy in severe diabetic ketoacidosis. Ann Intern Med 105:836–840, 1986.

133. Jos J, Oberkampf B, Couprie C, Paclot C, Bougneres P. Comparison of 2 modes of treatment of diabetic ketoacidosis in children [in French]. Arch Fr Pediatr 45:15–19, 1988.

134. Hillman K. Fluid resuscitation in diabetic emergencies—a reappraisal. Intensive Care Med 13:4–8, 1987.

135. Clements RS Jr, Blumenthal SA, Morrison AD, Winegrad AI. Increased cerebrospinal-fluid pressure during treatment of diabetic ketosis. Lancet 2:671–675, 1971.

136. Duck SC, Weldon VV, Pagliara AS, Haymond MW. Cerebral edema complicating therapy for diabetic ketoacidosis. Diabetes 25:111–115, 1976.

137. Duck SC, Wyatt DT. Factors associated with brain herniation in the treatment of diabetic ketoacidosis. J Pediatr 113:10–14, 1988.

138. Garre M, Boles JM, Garo B, Mabin D. Cerebral oedema in diabetic ketoacidosis: do we use too much insulin? [letter]. Lancet 1:220, 1986.

139. Hoffman WH, Steinhart CM, el Gammal T, Steele S, Cuadrado AR, Morse PK. Cranial CT in children and adolescents with diabetic ketoacidosis. AJNR Am J Neuroradiol 9:733–739, 1988.

140. Krane EJ, Rockoff MA, Wallman JK, Wolfsdorf JI. Subclinical brain swelling in children during treatment of diabetic ketoacidosis. N Engl J Med 312:1147–1151, 1985.

141. Shrier DA, Shibata DK, Wang HZ, Numaguchi Y, Powers JM. Central brain herniation secondary to juvenile diabetic ketoacidosis. AJNR Am J Neuroradiol 20:1885–1888, 1999.

142. Van der Meulen JA, Klip A, Grinstein S. Possible

mechanism for cerebral oedema in diabetic ketoacidosis. Lancet 2:306–308, 1987.

143. Klip A, Ramlal T, Cragoe EJ Jr. Insulin-induced cytoplasmic alkalinization and glucose transport in muscle cells. Am J Physiol 250:C720–C728, 1986.

144. Glaser N, Barnett P, McCaslin I, et al. Risk factors for cerebral edema in children with diabetic ketoacidosis. N Engl J Med 344:264–269, 2001.

145. Malouf R, Brust JC. Hypoglycemia: causes, neurological manifestations, and outcome. Ann Neurol 17:421–430, 1985.

146. Heller SR, Macdonald IA, Herbert M, Tattersall RB. Influence of sympathetic nervous system on hypoglycaemic warning symptoms. Lancet 2:359–363, 1987.

147. Montgomery BM, Pinner CA. Transient hypoglycemic hemiplegia. Arch Intern Med 114:680–684, 1964.

148. Newman RP, Kinkel WR. Paroxysmal choreoathetosis due to hypoglycemia. Arch Neurol 41:341–342, 1984.

149. Agardh CD, Rosen I, Ryding E. Persistent vegetative state with high cerebral blood flow following profound hypoglycemia. Ann Neurol 14:482–486, 1983.

150. Auer RN. Progress review: hypoglycemic brain damage. Stroke 17:699–708, 1986.

151. Simon RP, Meldrum BS, Schmidley JW, Swan JH, Chapman AG. Mechanisms of selective vulnerability: hypoglycemia. Cerebrovasc Dis 15:13–24, 1987.

152. Fujioka M, Okuchi K, Hiramatsu K-I, Sakaki T, Sakaguchi S, Ishii Y. Specific changes in human brain after hypoglycemic injury. Stroke 28:584–587, 1997.

153. Bennett MH, Wainwright AP. Acute thyroid crisis on induction of anaesthesia. Anaesthesia 44:28–30, 1989.

154. Gavin LA. Thyroid crises. Med Clin North Am 75:179–193, 1991.

155. Leigh H, Kramer SI. The psychiatric manifestations of endocrine disease. Adv Intern Med 29:413–445, 1984.

156. Logothetis J. Neurologic and muscular manifestations of hyperthyroidism. Arch Neurol 5:533–544, 1961.

157. Newcomer J, Haire W, Hartman CR. Coma and thyrotoxicosis. Ann Neurol 14:689–690, 1983.

158. Thomas FB, Mazzaferri EL, Skillman TG. Apathetic thyrotoxicosis: a distinctive clinical and laboratory entity. Ann Intern Med 72:679–685, 1970.

159. Hashizume K. Severe myopathy in patients with thyrotoxicosis. Ann Intern Med 39:442–443, 2000.

160. Brain L, Jellinek EH, Ball K. Hashimoto's disease and encephalopathy. Lancet 2:512–514, 1966.

161. Henchey R, Cibula J, Helveston W, Malone J, Gilmore RL. Electroencephalographic findings in Hashimoto's encephalopathy. Neurology 45:977–981, 1995.

162. Bohnen NI, Parnell KJ, Harper CM. Reversible MRI findings in a patient with Hashimoto's encephalopathy. Neurology 49:246–247, 1997.

163. Garrard P, Hodges JR, De Vries PJ, et al. Hashimoto's encephalopathy presenting as "myxoedematous madness." J Neurol Neurosurg Psychiatry 68:102–103, 2000.

164. Nolte KW, Unbehaun A, Sieker H, Kloss TM, Paulus W. Hashimoto encephalopathy: a brainstem vasculitis? Neurology 54:769–770, 2000.

165. McCabe DJ, Burke T, Connolly S, Hutchinson M. Amnesic syndrome with bilateral mesial temporal lobe involvement in Hashimoto's encephalopathy. Neurology 54:737–739, 2000.

166. Boers PM, Colebatch JG. Hashimoto's encephalopathy responding to plasmapheresis [letter]. J Neurol Neurosurg Psychiatry 70:132, 2001.

167. Lindberger K. Myxoedema coma. Acta Med Scand 198:87–90, 1975.

168. Rajagopal KR, Abbrecht PH, Derderian SS, et al. Obstructive sleep apnea in hypothyroidism. Ann Intern Med 101:491–494, 1984.

169. Cook DM, Boyle PJ. Rapid reversal of myxedema madness with triiodothyronine. Ann Intern Med 104:893–894, 1986.

170. Hylander B, Rosenqvist U. Treatment of myxoedema coma—factors associated with fatal outcome. Acta Endocrinol (Copenh) 108:65–71, 1985.

171. Ebinger G, Six R, Bruyland M, Somers G. Flexion contractures: a forgotten symptom in Addison's disease and hypopituitarism. Lancet 2:858, 1986.

172. Abbas DH, Schlagenhauff RE, Strong HE. Polyradiculoneuropathy in Addison's disease. Case report and review of literature. Neurology 27:494–495, 1977.

173. Calabrese LH, White CS. Musculoskeletal manifestations of Addison's disease. Arthritis Rheum 22:558, 1979.

174. Mor F, Green P, Wysenbeek AJ. Myopathy in Addison's disease. Ann Rheum Dis 46:81–83, 1987.

175. Nerup J. Addison's disease—clinical studies. A report of 108 cases. Acta Endocrinol (Copenh) 76:127–141, 1974.

176. Geenen C, Tein I, Ehrlich RM. Addison's disease presenting with cerebral edema. Can J Neurol Sci 23:141–144, 1996.

Chapter 9

NEUROLOGIC COMPLICATIONS OF ACUTE RENAL DISEASE

Patients can be distinguished by renal involvement during any critical illness, such as sepsis, hypovolemic shock, major endocrine disturbances, and rhabdomyolysis. Renal failure in an intensive care unit (ICU) after surgery has been recognized as a major cause of morbidity, and postoperative hemodynamic instability has an important role in pathogenesis. Temporarily, replacement of renal function may be needed through use of hemodialysis or peritoneal dialysis, but oliguric acute renal failure is a major cause of death in the ICU.[1]

In this chapter, the neurologic manifestations of acute renal failure are discussed in relation to the most common clinical problems seen in critically ill patients and to those that may pose difficulty in assessment during consultation in ICUs. Hypertensive encephalopathy is included in this chapter because of its interrelation with acute renal failure. Hypertension as a manifestation of eclampsia, albeit with characteristics similar to those of other causes, is discussed in Chapter 13 on pregnancy-associated neurologic illness, but its management is distinctly different.

UREMIC ENCEPHALOPATHY

The recognition of uremic encephalopathy is not trivial, because in many ICUs, its signs and symptoms are usually an indication to initiate hemodialysis. The clinical features of uremic encephalopathy range from asterixis to profound drowsiness, but usually manifestations are typical of any metabolic encephalopathy. Its clinical features may be few or many, subtle or startling.

Instinctively, acute uremia may seem the main problem in uremic encephalopathy, but other systemic derangements may predominantly contribute to the clinical signs. For example, in some patients, marked hypotension may result in both acute renal failure and brain injury, but improvement of renal function may not coincide with awakening. Drugs administered daily may suddenly reach toxic levels in acute renal failure, and electrolyte disturbances associated with renal failure may also cause clinical signs closely mimicking uremic encephalopathy (Table 9–1). Even so, the clinical signs of uremic encephalopathy are distinct in

Table 9–1. **Systemic Abnormalities in Acute Renal Failure That May Confound Signs of Uremic Encephalopathy**

Prolonged hypotension

Hyponatremia

Hypocalcemia

Metabolic alkalosis

Drug toxicity (penicillin, cephalosporins, digoxin)[2–4]

many ways and can be set apart from these confounding conditions.

PATHOPHYSIOLOGIC MECHANISMS

Urea crosses the blood–brain barrier through endothelial cells of brain capillaries, but tight junctions, absent fenestrae, and lack of pinocytosis hinder transport, and its diffusion is much slower than that of water.[5] Urea itself cannot be accounted for alone in the genesis of encephalopathy, because urea and creatinine levels are not related to the degree of impairment of consciousness or even emergence of asterixis and myoclonus.[6]

Accumulation of various other substances may be implicated, particularly because they have mimicked uremic encephalopathy in animal models. Proposed substances include purines, organic phosphates, oxalate, ascorbic acid, beta$_2$-microglobulin guanidosuccinic acid, and hippuric acid.[7] In addition, compounds with a molecular weight between 300 and 12,000 Da ("middle molecules," with a molecular weight higher than urea and creatinine but lower than myoglobulin), such as parathyroid hormone, peptides, glucuronate conjugates, and microglobulin, have been considered. These organic acids increase the permeability of the blood–brain barrier, impair cellular transport mechanisms, or decrease γ-aminobutyric acid (GABA) levels.[7]

Parathyroid hormone has been suggested in the pathogenesis because of a recently discovered increase in intracellular calcium linking parathyroid hormone

with uremic encephalopathy, but this indirect evidence is far from convincing.[8,9]

Clinical Features

Gradual but progressive drowsiness, multifocal myoclonus, and asterixis are collectively recognized as signs and symptoms of uremic encephalopathy, but none is pathognomonic for the disorder.[10–13] Each patient reacts differently to the consequences of severe and abrupt reduction of renal function. However, if rapidly progressive renal failure is associated with severe uremia, it should produce clinical signs of an encephalopathy. Uremic encephalopathy usually is signaled by impaired wakefulness. Other patients, however, appear alert but are easily distracted and act blasé about their often critical condition. Perseveration and failure to sustain attention to a simple task are early signs of uremic encephalopathy, but in other patients, early manifestations are predominant explosive panic spells, aggressive behavior, restlessness, disorganized and rambling speech, and hallucinatory symptoms.[14] Untreated uremic encephalopathy progresses to coma with frontal release signs and other pathologic motor responses.

Localizing signs are uncommon, and thus a dense hemiplegia generally points to structural central nervous system damage, typically a lobar or subdural hematoma. In exceptional patients, slurred speech with irregular pitch and loudness is evident. The characteristics of this dysarthria may falsely suggest drug intoxication, certainly when observed in a patient with a sudden reduction in glomerular filtration rate. Asterixis of the tongue may also impair speech.

Abnormal limb movements are common in patients with metabolic encephalopathy associated with acute renal failure. Carpopedal spasm may occur in patients with associated hypocalcemia, although it seldom evolves to a true Trousseau's sign (see Chapter 8). Multifocal myoclonus is frequent in uremic encephalopathy,[15] and its incidence is probably higher in uremic encephalopathy than in other encephalopathies. Myoclonus can be identified by repetitive jerks or shock-like involuntary movements involving many muscles.[16]

Action tremor is a common involuntary movement in uremia. Posture exacerbates the amplitude of the tremor, which may also increase at the end of a requested task, such as the finger-to-nose test. Asterixis is a well-appreciated clinical sign. It appears predominantly in drowsy patients and can be elicited by asking the patient to hold out the arms or by hip flexion-abduction.[17,18] Limb asterixis may be combined with bursts of arrhythmic movements (1/sec) in the face and tongue muscles and brought on by puckering of the lips, sustained baring of the teeth, and protrusion of the tongue (Fig. 9–1).

Asterixis has been fully characterized by electromyography, although its origin remains unknown. Shahani and Young[17] showed in a study of 70 patients with asterixis of various types that lapses of posture appeared as silent periods of 50 to 200 msec in tonically active muscles. When lapses are frequent and pauses short, asterixis may mimic a high-frequency tremor. Although common in dialysis units, asterixis is not characteristic of uremic encephalopathy and may also be seen in hepatic encephalopathy and severe hypercapnia. It is important to emphasize that unilateral asterixis typically occurs in structural brain lesions, mainly in the thalamus or putamen, and is commonly due to stroke.[19]

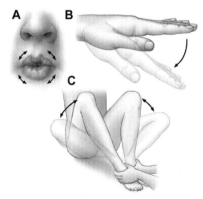

Figure 9–1. Asterixis. *A:* Puckering of the lips may produce bursts of arrhythmic movements. *B:* Sudden shocklike flexion in wrist, fingers, and thumb when patient is asked to hold out the arms. *C:* Flexion in the hip and abduction with 60° between the legs produce rapid jerking movement.[18]

Laboratory Tests

As expected in most patients with uremic encephalopathy, computed tomography (CT) scans are normal, but because of a coagulopathy, a subacute or chronic subdural hematoma can be seen. Spontaneous subdural hematomas can occur in patients with renal failure and autosomal dominant polycystic kidney disease.[20] Also, in a well-documented case report, severe white matter hypodensities on CT scan not associated with hypertension were found and appeared to be reversible after dialysis.[21]

Electroencephalographic (EEG) findings in uremic patients are nonspecific but may demonstrate shift of spectral power into the delta frequencies. The EEG may reflect the degree of drowsiness, and serial recordings may show progression in disorganization, intermittent bursts of semiarrhythmic slow waves, and periodic epileptiform abnormalities, all without clinical evidence of seizures. Triphasic waves are seen (Chapter 1), but they are more common in hepatic failure and may disappear when theta or delta slowing becomes more perceptible. If the objective of EEG recording is to exclude seizures or nonconvulsive status epilepticus in obtunded uremic patients, it should be emphasized that bilateral spike and wave abnormalities can be expected in 14% of patients with chronic renal failure.[22] However, EEG recordings in the ICU may be confounded by other metabolic or pharmacologic factors and thus limited in clinical usefulness.

Cerebrospinal fluid examinations have shown that most patients with uremic encephalopathy have increased protein values between 80 and 100 mg. Pleocytosis (from 7 to 600 leukocytes/mm³) may be found in half of patients with uremic encephalopathy.[23] In addition, neurologists evaluating patients with uremic encephalopathy for possible meningitis need to be aware of the relatively frequent occurrence of nonspecific neck stiffness in uremia and of the risk of bleeding from uremia-induced platelet dysfunction after lumbar puncture. Administration of large doses of cryoprecipitate or desmopressin acetate shortens bleeding time in preparation for lumbar puncture.

Treatment

Hemodialysis has reduced the mortality from acute renal failure, and resolution of clinical signs of uremic encephalopathy can be expected. Overall mortality from acute renal failure, however, remains between 20% and 72% but obviously is determined by the number of associated systemic complications.[24] Outcome of uremic encephalopathy is further discussed in Chapter 19.

DIALYSIS DYSEQUILIBRIUM SYNDROME

The dysequilibrium syndrome of hemodialysis is fortunately rare, and therefore its diagnosis requires exclusion of conditions that may simulate this entity. Moreover, the dysequilibrium syndrome seldom appears with all its clinical features. Its presentation with only a few pertinent clinical signs is now more common. Predisposing factors for dysequilibrium syndrome have been identified, and the risk is proportionally increased if blood urea nitrogen values are initially high, dialysis is rapid, and large surface membranes are used. The dysequilibrium syndrome appears at the end of a dialysis procedure and is virtually at all times associated with the first treatment.[25] Clinical presentation is commonly abrupt, but onset may be insidious (Table 9–2).

Clinical Features

Restlessness, agitation, and combative behavior are followed by headache, promi-

Table 9–2. **Associated Factors and Potential Causes of Dysequilibrium Syndrome**

Hyponatremia

Hypo-osmolality

Hyperphosphatemia

Rapid dialysis (450–500 mL/min)

Large dialysis membrane

Surface area >1 m^2 and initially high blood urea nitrogen value

nently bifrontal, throbbing, and more severe in a reclining position. Myoclonic jerks in proximal muscles and cramps are occasionally reported as early signs. Acute cortical blindness may become apparent during dialysis. Denial of visual loss may make recognition even more difficult.[26] Monocular blindness from an anterior ischemic optic neuropathy has been described but is more often associated with an episode of marked hypotension.[27]

If the syndrome is not recognized, the time course of clinical presentation is rapid. Many patients lapse into coma with extensor posturing, frequently preceded by one or two generalized tonic–clonic seizures. Therapeutic measures are unsuccessful when patients become comatose from extensive brain swelling, and many die within a few hours after onset. A CT scan may demonstrate slit-like ventricles, effacement of sulci, and obliteration of ambient cisterns, and autopsy studies have indeed confirmed massive swelling of white matter without evidence of border-zone infarction or intracranial hemorrhage.

Variants of the dysequilibrium syndrome, however, are well known by nephrologists in dialysis units. Hemodialyzed patients may have clinical signs indicative but not characteristic of dysequilibrium syndrome. These mild clinical signs of headache,[28] restlessness, and tremor in extremities subside after the procedure but may again occur when hemodialysis is repeated. Usually, these symptoms disappear after a few sessions and very frequently after adjustment of the rate and fluid composition of dialysis.

Another rare condition is so-called hard water syndrome. The predominant causes are hypercalcemia and hypermagnesemia from failure of a water treatment process in locations with a high content of calcium and magnesium in the water. Characterized by lethargy, headache, dysarthria, seizures, hallucinations, and burning sensations of the skin, the syndrome has some similarities with the classic dysequilibrium syndrome. Most patients are confused, display vivid hallucinations, and have considerable muscle weakness. Acute intoxication with aluminum or other trace materials (copper, zinc) from tubing lines may also occur, but only a

Table 9–3. Differential Diagnosis of Dysequilibrium Syndrome

Hypoxic–ischemic encephalopathy (associated with severe hypotension)[31]

Air embolism

Subdural hematoma[32–34]

Hypernatremia

Hyponatremia

Wernicke's encephalopathy[35,36]

Hypoglycemia associated with beta-blockade

few well-documented cases have been reported.[29,30]

Various other disorders (largely anecdotal) may superficially resemble dysequilibrium syndrome but are decidedly rare (Table 9–3). The incidence of stroke in patients with maintenance hemodialysis is 9%, most commonly hypertension-associated ganglionic–thalamic hemorrhage. In a study of 1064 patients receiving long-standing dialysis, use of heparin was not identified as a risk factor.[37]

Biochemical changes may mimic dysequilibrium syndrome and are usually a result of technical errors. Hyponatremia is noted when plasma is allowed to equilibrate with hypotonic dialysis fluid. Several other potential causes of hyponatremia have been described, but the most frequent is failure to connect the concentrate container or failure to test the dialysate before the start of the procedure. The resulting hypo-osmolar hypervolemia may cause marked hemolysis that is associated with shock. Seizures are frequent.

PATHOPHYSIOLOGIC MECHANISMS

Brain swelling has been established as the entity responsible for the dominant manifestations of the dysequilibrium syndrome, but its pathogenesis is open to question. Two opposing views exist, each with considerable scientific arguments but also with some degree of common ground.

In the "reverse urea" hypothesis introduced by Pappius and associates[38] and confirmed by Silver and associates,[39–41] a significant urea gradient between blood and brain after dialysis results in water influx to the brain. In normal circumstances, urea diffuses more slowly than water across the blood–brain barrier; thus, when blood urea is rapidly increased, an osmotic difference is created, resulting in water extraction from the brain. Reversing this gradient with dialysis results in a higher brain-to-plasma urea concentration, and this phenomenon causes brain edema. It thus can be corrected by adding urea or mannitol or by increasing the sodium concentrate of the dialysate. In dialyzed uremic rats, plasma urea decreased by 53% but brain edema decreased by 13%, resulting in urea retention in the brain.[39]

The "idiogenic osmole" hypothesis developed by Arieff[42,43] argues that the urea concentrates in the brain are not high enough to account for the increase in brain water. Brain swelling, in their view, is promoted by formation of idiogenic osmoles, possibly organic acids formed during rapid dialysis, leading to an increase in brain osmolality and water influx. Direct measurements of brain osmolality showed an increase in brain osmolality that cannot be explained by the sum of urea and electrolyte concentrations, suggesting a new formation of osmotically active particles (osmoles). Formation of organic osmoles in the brain during osmotic stress has been documented, but whether they formed after dialysis remains unknown.

The controversy seemed to have been resolved by a diffusion-weighted magnetic resonance imaging (MRI) study in nephrectomized rats receiving dialysis.[44] By measuring brain water, this technique discriminated between increase of the extracellular volume (increase in the apparent diffusion coefficient) and increase of the intracellular volume (decrease in the apparent diffusion coefficient). The study showed an increase in the apparent diffusion coefficient compatible with interstitial edema and thus consistent with the reverse urea gradient explanation. None of these changes in this experimental study were found when dialysis was used with a urea bath.

Treatment

To prevent recurrence of dysequilibrium syndrome, the addition of hyperosmotic or hyperoncotic solute, such as glycerol or mannitol, or the substitution of sodium bicarbonate for sodium lactate in the dialysate has been suggested.[43] Headache alone may be treated by changing the acetate in the dialysate.

Whether postdialysis cerebral edema occurs subclinically is unclear, but one CT and EEG study showed no appreciable changes in brain density and ventricular size or change in background EEG in asymptomatic patients.[45] Therefore, increase of slow wave activity with delta-wave burst and early loss of posterior alpha rhythm may indicate the potential for dysequilibrium in selected patients.[46,47] Monitoring patients with EEG recordings is probably worthwhile if dysequilibrium syndrome is suspected, and abnormalities should lead to preventive measures, such as shortened and more frequent hemodialyses.

Prophylactic administration of antiepileptic drugs is generally not indicated, usually because seizures are related to concomitant hyponatremia and do not recur after normalization of serum sodium. Intravenous phenytoin loading is indicated only in patients with recurrent seizures. One session of hemodialysis or 24 hr of continuous ambulatory peritoneal dialysis should not influence the therapeutic window of phenytoin.[48]

HYPERTENSIVE ENCEPHALOPATHY

There is conclusive evidence that the incidence of hypertensive encephalopathy has declined over the years but remains higher among African-Americans and the elderly.[49,50] Certainly, improved surveillance and aggressive drug treatment have resulted in a much lower incidence, but improved definition of the clinical entity should be considered a factor as well.

For many reasons, critically ill patients have a sudden significant increase in systolic blood pressure, but an encephalopathy develops in only a small proportion of patients. Sudden withdrawal of antihypertensive treatment in patients with long-standing hypertension is probably the most frequent cause (Table 9–4), followed by acute parenchymal renal disease. Drug-induced causes of hypertensive encephalopathy have been reported in single cases and are often without any warning.[51] In addition, cases associated with erythropoietin treatment are continuously reported.[52,53] Hypertension may occur in up to 70% of patients treated with recombinant human erythropoietin. It may be the result of increased blood viscosity and platelet activation releasing thromboxane and other vasoconstrictors.[54] Postoperative causes of hypertension, such as cross-clamping of the aorta in coronary artery bypass surgery, renal vascularization, heart transplantation, and carotid endarterectomy, have been well recognized, but many anesthesiologists anticipate these surges in blood pressure and correct them promptly. A systematic pathologic examination of hypertensive encephalopathy by Chester and associates[55] in the late 1970s remains the most informative study to date.

The most common vascular change in hypertensive encephalopathy is fibrinoid necrosis of arterioles in virtually any target organ besides the brain. Patients with long-lasting hypertension may have additional hyalinization and medial hypertrophy. Many arterioles may show obliteration caused by fibrin thrombi, with recanalization in some. Microscopic examination often reveals miliary infarction in the brain and occasionally petechial hemorrhages.[56]

Table 9–4. Causes of Hypertensive Encephalopathy in the Intensive Care Unit

Withdrawal of antihypertensive drugs

Erythropoietin

Acute parenchymal renal disease

Renovascular disease

Major thermal burns

Eclampsia

Aortic dissection

Systemic vasculitis

Pheochromocytoma, Cushing's syndrome, or renin-producing tumor

Generally, the vascular and intravascular changes in patients with hypertensive encephalopathy probably should be considered to be a direct result of endothelial damage, platelet aggregation, release of platelet factors and thromboxane, increased blood viscosity, and, finally, microangiopathic hemolytic anemia and intravascular coagulation. Cerebral edema is absent in most autopsy cases, including patients with increased cerebrospinal fluid pressure and papilledema.

PATHOPHYSIOLOGIC MECHANISMS

Earlier explanations of hypertensive encephalopathy are probably too simple.[51,57] They include the breakthrough concept (forced dilation of cerebral blood vessels, causing disruption of the blood–brain barrier, increase in cerebral blood flow, leakage of plasma proteins, and resultant focal or generalized edema). A second but less likely theory is the overregulation concept, which assumes that exaggerated vasoconstriction of arterioles results in cerebral ischemia.[58,59] Studies with single-photon emission scan indicating regional hyperperfusion support the existence of a vasodilatory mechanism.[60] Cerebrovascular vasodilatation is therefore due to failure of autoregulation at such high blood pressures. Vascular permeability increases, and comparative lack of sympathetic innervation in the posterior circulation may account for the proclivity for posterior lesions, such as those in the occipital lobe.

In most patients with clinical signs of hypertensive encephalopathy, diastolic blood pressure is significantly increased (>120 mm Hg). Equally important in the definition of hypertensive crisis is whether there is end organ damage. Outcome in patients with hypertensive encephalopathy is generally not determined by the degree of focal brain edema but depends on acute congestive heart failure, pulmonary edema, acute anuria requiring emergency dialysis, and microangiopathic hemolytic anemia.

The pathophysiologic trigger of target organ involvement other than the brain has

not been clarified, but arteries are alternately constricted and dilated (sausage string), often with endothelial damage and overlying platelet thrombi. Platelet-derived growth factors eventually lead to vascular proliferation of smooth muscle cells and further narrowing of vessels.

Patients with a sudden increase in blood pressure have signs of left ventricular failure manifested by paroxysmal dyspnea at night, wheezing, or sustained orthopnea. In extreme conditions, the patient may look pale, slightly cyanotic, cold, and sweaty. In the most advanced cases, severe pulmonary edema may occur.

Coincident with left ventricular failure is the potential for renal failure. Renal failure associated with hypertensive encephalopathy is typically defined as a twofold or greater increase in blood urea nitrogen or creatinine concentration. Proteinuria, microscopic hematuria, and red cell casts can be expected with urinalysis. Peripheral blood smears may show target cells and schistocytes. These indicators of microangiographic hemolytic anemia are common in patients with acute renal failure.

Clinical Features

The manifestations of hypertensive encephalopathy are typified by severe, throbbing, generalized headache associated with vomiting and nausea, decreased level of consciousness, transient neurologic signs, and seizures.[61] The severity of the headache in hypertensive encephalopathy is not related to the systolic or diastolic blood pressure level. Headaches in hypertensive encephalopathy are seldom continuous over the day, more often consisting of brief waves of throbbing, generalized occipital or facial pain. Very frequently, coughing or straining triggers a pulsating headache. Headache in patients with malignant hypertension may be extremely intense. A temporal profile with a split-second onset (thunderclap headache) should raise the clinical suspicion of a subarachnoid or cerebellar hemorrhage resulting in hypertension rather than the converse, but we have noted this headache onset as a first presentation of hypertensive encephalopathy.[62] The mechanism of headaches in malignant hypertension is not known. Sudden increases in blood pressure may result in dilatation of intracranial arteries or displacement of pain-sensitive intracranial structures at the base of the skull.

Another characteristic clinical feature is clouding of consciousness. In the accelerated phase of hypertension, an acute confusional state may occur.

Common in patients with hypertensive encephalopathy are visual disturbances. Blurred vision (reported in 20% to 50% of patients) is the most frequent complaint. Some patients have cortical blindness accompanied by vivid visual hallucinations.[63,64] Loss of color vision at the ictus or as a permanent sequela of malignant hypertensive crisis has been reported in exceptional cases. Some patients have visual perseveration[65] or visual manifestations from seizures.[66]

Papilledema is a frequent presenting feature of hypertensive encephalopathy, varying from early disc hyperemia to impressively engorged retinal veins with multiple splinter hemorrhages and obliterated optic cups. The diagnosis of hypertensive encephalopathy becomes problematic without this finding, but it may be absent even in patients with typical MRI abnormalities of T2 hyperintensities in the occipital lobe. Malignant hypertensive crisis frequently occurs in patients with long-standing hypertension; therefore, some papilledema may be part of a widespread retinopathy with soft exudates, gray discoloration of the retina, epithelial necrosis with serous detachment of the retina, and dilated and tortuous arterioles. Papilledema can present with prominent bilateral obscurations. These brief periods of blindness usually occur in patients with rapidly progressive papilledema. Obscurations may appear several times a day and are common immediately after a change in posture. Some of these episodes may last minutes, but again with complete resolution of symptoms. Generally, outcome is favorable after control of blood pressure. Effective control of hypertension results in resolution of papilledema in 6 to 8 weeks. However, blurred disc margins and abnormalities of the peripapillary retinal nerve fiber may remain for months.[67] Peripheral facial palsy is a well-documented early presentation of malignant hypertension. The condition, tentatively linked to hemorrhage within the facial canal, is more frequent in children and young adults and resolves completely.[68]

Localizing findings such as hemiparesis and aphasia are uncommon manifestations and should point to an underlying stroke. Two prospective series reported conflicting results.[57,69] In a study from Harlem Hospital Center, 10 of 34 patients with an initial admission diagnosis of malignant hypertension had lateralizing signs, but they were associated with cerebral infarction.[57] In contrast, a Scandinavian study reported focal signs in 23% of 64 patients with admission diastolic blood pressures of 135 mm Hg or more.[69] Most patients had permanent limb weakness after treatment of blood pressure, but clinical details and imaging study findings were not given.

Generalized tonic–clonic seizures may accompany hypertensive encephalopathy. Myoclonus and asterixis are not features of hypertensive encephalopathy except in patients who have marked uremia and need dialysis.

Neuroimaging

Both CT scanning and MRI can be very helpful in the evaluation of hypertensive encephalopathy. A fairly consistent abnormal finding is diffuse or focal areas of lucency with diminished attenuation values, most frequently in the parietal and occipital white matter (posterior reversible encephalopathy syndrome, or PRES).[21,70–72] Some patients may have generalized diffuse hypodensity of the white matter, which most likely reflects cerebral edema. Cortical effacement may also be present in the acute stage.[73]

Most reports with serial MRI studies demonstrate reversal of white matter edema,[74,75] but residual hypodensity in the centrum semiovale may remain. Although the degree of encephalopathy is not closely related to the degree of white matter disease on CT scan, many patients with marked papilledema, seizures, and acute confusional state have white matter abnormalities on CT scan. Usually, MRI images are consistent with the CT scan patterns. The MRI demonstrates increased T2 signals in the bilateral occipital lobes or at the parieto-occipital junction and superior frontal lobes[76] (Fig. 9–2). T2-

weighted images on MRI may also preferentially show abnormalities in the pons, including reversible edema,[77,78] the cerebellum, and the basal ganglia. In some patients, compression of the fourth ventricle may cause obstructive hydrocephalus, which may resolve within 24 hr after blood pressure control, precluding ventricular draining.[79]

Treatment

Irrespective of what triggered the event, early aggressive treatment of hypertensive encephalopathy limits the progression of the cascade of events and increases the chances of satisfactory outcome. Current recommendations are summarized in Table 9–5.[80–82] Labetalol (a nonselective β-blocker and postsynaptic α_1-blocker) is a good initial choice and is less likely to cause overshooting to hypotension. A decrease in systemic vascular resistance is prominent, but no change in cardiac output occurs. Treatment with nitroprusside, a potent vasodilator, is more complex. An angiotensin-converting enzyme inhibitor, such as enalaprilat, may be useful, and hypotension is uncommon. It is contraindicated, however, in pregnancy and in patients with renal artery stenosis. Another successful drug is fenoldopam, a dopamine D_1-like receptor agonist. The goal is to reduce the mean arterial blood pressure by 20% within a few hours. This target value is crucial, because cerebral blood flow autoregulatory limits are altered in patients with long-standing hypertension. These changes result in a shift of both lower and upper limits toward higher pressures. Decreasing blood pressure more than 25% of the baseline value may result in failure of the brain to maintain unchanged metabolism through extraction of more oxygen from the blood and thus in ischemia.

Single seizures are usually not treated with antiepileptic drugs. A loading dose of phenytoin may be used to cover the first days during recovery from the clinical manifestations

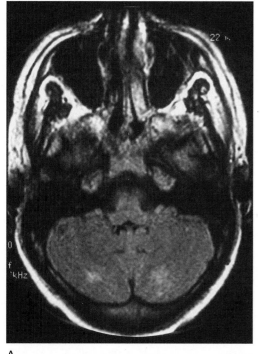
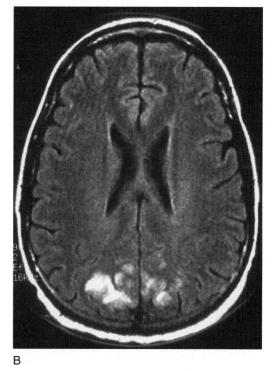

A   B

Figure 9–2. Magnetic resonance imaging patterns of hypertensive encephalopathy. *A*: Cerebellar lesions. *B*: Areas of hyperintensity in occipital lobes (T2-weighted image).

Table 9–5. **Emergency Treatment of Hypertensive Encephalopathy**

Drug	Dosage
Labetalol hydrochloride	20–80 mg by IV bolus every 10 min or 2 mg/min by IV infusion
Sodium nitroprusside	0.3–10 μg/kg/min IV; maximal dose in 10 min
Enalaprilat	1.25 mg IV over 5 min every 6 hr; maximum of 5 mg every 6 hr
Fenoldopam	0.1 μg/kg/min; maximum of 1.6 μg/kg/min

Data from Gifford,[81] Calhoun and Oparil,[80] Varon and Marik,[49] and Vaughan and Delanty.[50]

of hypertensive encephalopathy. In patients with eclampsia, magnesium sulfate (therapeutic level of magnesium, 2 to 3 mmol/L) is preferred and is more successful in seizure management than phenytoin or diazepam[83] (for details, see Chapter 13).

Therapeutic options are limited for brain edema, if present at all. Mannitol may be given to patients who remain stuporous and have CT scan evidence of white matter hypodensity with effacement of the ambient cisterns despite normalization of blood pressure. However, mannitol may be contraindicated in patients with acute renal failure. Intracranial pressure monitoring may be considered, but its value is unknown.[84]

NEUROMUSCULAR DISORDERS

Neuromuscular involvement is inevitable in patients with long-standing renal failure but may take weeks to months to become prevalent. In the ICU, generalized weakness associated with acute renal failure is very often due to muscle involvement. Weakness from polyneuropathy is found in chronic renal disease but also appears in patients who require admission to an ICU for management of decompensated renal function. Considerable information has accumulated about polyneuropathies and mononeuropathies in renal failure, and a comprehensive account can be found in Bolton and Young's monograph.[85]

Myopathy

The catabolic state in acute renal failure may produce muscle weakness, particularly when nutritional needs are not met. Muscle mass vanishes if patients with acute renal failure do not receive adequate caloric intake (up to 50 kcal/kg per day). Loss of muscle mass alone may be a sufficient explanation for "weakness." Nevertheless, in patients with chronic renal failure, maintenance hemodialysis, and osteomalacia, proximal weakness from myopathy is well recognized. Often it is documented on electromyography by motor unit potentials with reduced duration and amplitude together with large numbers of polyphasic potentials. Muscle fiber degeneration in myopathy associated with chronic renal failure is at times evident only by electron microscopic examination.[86] Abnormalities in vitamin D metabolism or aluminum may contribute, but the pathways to muscle damage have not been elucidated. Electrolyte abnormalities from acute renal failure are virtually never severe enough to produce muscle weakness but could contribute when neuromuscular blocking agents have been used. A prospective study identified hypermagnesemia and renal failure as important factors in the otherwise poorly understood post-vecuronium paralysis syndrome[87] (see Chapter 4).

Muscle cramps also may occur during hemodialysis, often late during dialysis. Rapid fluid removal or hypo-osmolality may be implicated, and significant relief can be achieved with a hypertonic (50%) dextrose intravenous injection or hypertonic saline infusion.[88–90]

Polyneuropathy of Renal Disease

Polyneuropathy is seen in approximately 60% of patients with renal disease, but this number is largely derived from series with patients receiving hemodialysis regularly.[6,85,91–94] A fully developed motor and sensory polyneuropathy is not expected in patients with mild renal failure that does not (yet) necessitate hemodialysis. A relation with plasma creatinine level has been reported, and moderate-to-severe mixed polyneuropathy can indeed be observed in patients with creatinine levels above 6 mg/dL. Below this level, the incidence of severe polyneuropathy is low, although many patients have loss of vibration sense and lack of ankle reflexes. Polyneuropathy is not seen in patients with new-onset acute renal failure, but when it is present, systemic vasculitis must be strongly considered as an underlying mechanism (see Chapter 12).

The pathologic basis of uremic polyneuropathy is axonal degeneration with secondary demyelination from accumulation of toxins such as molecules of medium molecular weight. (For an extensive discussion of the so-called middle molecule hypothesis, see the review by Bolton and Young.[85]) Other researchers continue to question primary axonal damage and favor the hypothesis that both axons and Schwann cells are targets.[95]

Electrodiagnostic studies in patients with uremic polyneuropathy largely show reduction of the amplitudes of muscle and sensory compound action potential, reflecting axonal damage. Conduction in sural nerves is invariably lost. Nielsen[96] found a statistically significant relation between creatinine clearance and motor nerve conduction of the peroneal nerve. The course of uremic neuropathy as measured by motor conduction velocity is variable, and most patients have relatively constant values over years or gradual improvement after dialysis or renal transplantation. In Bolton's series,[97] occasional transient worsening in nerve conduction velocity was seen in patients with intercurrent illness.

Most patients at presentation have predominantly sensory symptoms with hypoesthesia to light touch and pinprick in a sock-like distribution and loss of ankle reflexes.[85,91] Vibratory thresholds increase later, and distal motor weakness worsens to the point of inability to stand and walk unsupported. An acute, fulminant, severe motor polyneuropathy has been repeatedly reported, and the rapid clinical course, sometimes a month after first dialysis,[98–101] results in a bedbound state. The condition closely mimics Guillain-Barré syndrome but is not associated with ophthalmoplegia, severe dysautonomia, or need for mechanical ventilation. In reported patients, renal failure is stable, and no association with rapid worsening of kidney function is found. This unusual clinical course of uremic polyneuropathy has been estimated to occur in 0.6% of dialyzed patients.[95]

Outcome from fulminant uremic neuropathy is unpredictable but a satisfactory outcome with independent mobility after dialysis has been reported. In a 1993 series of patients, improvement was seen after more frequent use of dialysis.[101] In others, however, severe muscle wasting and severe footdrop remained, despite hemodialysis and renal transplantation, after years of follow-up.[95,99]

Generally, uremic polyneuropathy may progress to different degrees of severity, but most patients, whether receiving long-term hemodialysis or peritoneal dialysis, have signs of mild polyneuropathy. Renal transplantation results in improvement both clinically and electrophysiologically, often striking in severe cases and commonly within weeks of transplantation.[96,102]

In most patients with renal failure, the course is more indolent. Tingling in the legs is frequently the first complaint, but burning pain is rare. Paradoxical heat sensation (low temperature evokes the sensation of high temperature) and pruritus occur commonly.[103] Restless legs and nocturnal cramps are common and disrupt sleep. Nocturnal cramps in the calf muscles are painful and often occur in the first few hours of sleep. Restless legs are equally common in patients with early uremic polyneuropathy, and these prickling and crawling sensations are only transiently relieved by movement. These symptoms can be relieved with clonazepam, 2 mg at night; carbamazepine, 300 to 1000 mg daily; bromocriptine, 7.5 mg; carbidopa-levodopa, 25 to 100 mg; or verapamil, 120 mg.[104–109] When pain predominates in uremic polyneuropathy, imipramine or amitriptyline, 25 to 75 mg/day, or tramadol, 50 mg every 6 hr to a maximum of 400 mg/day; gabapentin, up to 3600 mg/day; and carbamazepine, up to 600 mg/day, can be recommended.[110]

Whether clinically significant autonomic neuropathy is present is controversial.[111] The causes of hypotension after dialysis may include excessive ultrafiltration or acute hypovolemia from hemorrhage. Nevertheless, reduced baroreceptor sensitivity was found in one study that used Valsalva's maneuver and the amyl nitrite test. Other studies have shown normal adrenergic responses[88,112] and normal responses to physiologic testing with Valsalva's maneuver, head-up tilt, cold pressor test, and sustained hand grip.[113,114]

Mononeuropathies

Acute mononeuropathies in patients with renal failure are rare. Most mononeuropathies are associated with placement of temporary catheters or long-term use of arteriovenous shunts.[115] A potential complication from temporary access procedures in patients requiring hemodialysis is a retroperitoneal hematoma. Perforation of the iliac vein during insertion of a catheter through the femoral vein results in acute flank or abdominal pain and femoral neuropathy.[116] (Diagnosis and management of psoas hematoma are discussed in Chapter 11.)

The most common neuropathy in patients receiving long-term dialysis is carpal tunnel syndrome.[117–119] It occurs in both sexes with equal incidences and appears at any time, but only after several years of dialysis. The incidence of carpal tunnel syndrome is virtually the same in patients with peritoneal dialysis. Carpal tunnel syndrome is most commonly caused by amyloid deposition from increased serum levels of β_2-microglobulin.[120,121] Regular electrodiagnostic studies are necessary in dialyzed patients, because the results of sectioning of the flexor retinaculum in these patients are disappointing once both motor and sensory symptoms have been present for more than 2 years.[122–124] This outcome undoubtedly reflects concomitant uremic neuropathy. Therefore, early surgery in patients with sensory symptoms is recommended; only then may it prevent loss of hand function.[123,124]

Upper arm (brachial artery, antecubital vein) shunts may cause multiple brachial mononeuropathies, particularly in patients with diabetes. Shunt ligation leads to improvement.[125]

CONCLUSIONS

Neurologists do not routinely see patients with uremic encephalopathy or hypertensive encephalopathy. Rapid favorable response to dialysis or antihypertensive treatment does not strongly impel internists to call in a neurologist. Both encephalopathies are characterized clinically by confusion and clouding of consciousness. In uremic encephalopathy, asterixis and tremor (although nonspecific) are frequent; in hypertensive encephalopathy, papilledema, cortical blindness, or seizures predominate. Magnetic resonance imaging has shown a characteristic picture of posterior encephalopathy. Hemodialyzed patients may have problems that occur during hemodialysis, such as headache, restlessness, and tremor, that become progressively less frequent with following sessions. These symptoms are much more common than those of a typical dysequilibrium syndrome. Dialyzed patients have a low proclivity for this entity, which is linked to rapid dialysis and large dialysis membranes.

Neuromuscular manifestations of renal failure are usually long-term effects. Restless legs with discomfort that is difficult to manage are a common manifestation of uremic polyneuropathy. Remarkable improvement in polyneuropathy has occurred after renal transplantation, noticeable within weeks in some patients.

REFERENCES

1. de Mendonca A, Vincent JL, Suter PM, et al. Acute renal failure in the ICU: risk factors and outcome

evaluated by the SOFA score. Intensive Care Med 26:915–921, 2000.

2. Geyer J, Hoffler D, Demers HG, Niemeyer R. Cephalosporin-induced encephalopathy in uremic patients [letter]. Nephron 48:237, 1988.

3. Josse S, Godin M, Fillastre JP. Cefazolin-induced encephalopathy in a uraemic patient [letter]. Nephron 45:72, 1987.

4. Pascual J, Liano F, Ortuno J. Cefotaxime-induced encephalopathy in an uremic patient [letter]. Nephron 54:92, 1990.

5. Cserr HF, Fenstermacher JD, Rall DP. Comparative aspects of brain barrier systems for nonelectrolytes. Am J Physiol 234:R52–R60, 1978.

6. Asbury AK, Victor M, Adams RD. Uremic polyneuropathy. Arch Neurol 8:413–428, 1963.

7. Vanholder R, De Smet R, Hsu C, Vogeleere P, Ringoir S. Uremic toxicity: the middle molecule hypothesis revisited. Semin Nephrol 14:205–218, 1994.

8. Parfitt AM. The hyperparathyroidism of chronic renal failure: a disorder of growth. Kidney Int 52: 3–9, 1997.

9. Moe SM, Sprague SM. Uremic encephalopathy. Clin Nephrol 42:251–256, 1994.

10. Biasioli S, D'Andrea G, Feriani M, et al. Uremic encephalopathy: an updating. Clin Nephrol 25: 57–63, 1986.

11. Lockwood AH. Metabolic encephalopathies: opportunities and challenges. J Cereb Blood Flow Metab 7:523–526, 1987.

12. Lockwood AH. Neurologic complications of renal disease. Neurol Clin 7:617–627, 1989.

13. Mahoney CA, Arieff AI. Uremic encephalopathies: clinical, biochemical, and experimental features. Am J Kidney Dis 2:324–336, 1982.

14. Locke S, Merrill JP, Tyler HR. Neurologic complications of acute uremia. Arch Intern Med 108: 519–530, 1961.

15. Stark RJ. Reversible myoclonus with uraemia. Br Med J 282:1119–1120, 1981.

16. Chadwick D, French AT. Uraemic myoclonus: an example of reticular reflex myoclonus? J Neurol Neurosurg Psychiatry 42:52–55, 1979.

17. Shahani BT, Young RR. Asterixis—a disorder of the neural mechanisms underlying sustained muscle contraction. In: Shahani M (ed). The Motor System—Neurophysiology and Muscle Mechanisms; Proceedings of a Satellite Symposium to the XXVIth International Congress of Physiology Held in India 1974. Elsevier Scientific Publishing, Amsterdam, 1976, pp 301–316.

18. Noda S, Ito H, Umezaki H, Minato S. Hip flexion-abduction to elicit asterixis in unresponsive patients. Ann Neurol 18:96–97, 1985.

19. Tatu L, Moulin T, Martin V, et al. Unilateral asterixis and focal brain lesions. 12 cases [in French]. Rev Neurol (Paris) 152:121–127, 1996.

20. Wijdicks EFM, Torres VE, Schievink WI. Chronic subdural hematoma in autosomal dominant polycystic kidney disease. Am J Kidney Dis 35:40–43, 2000.

21. Komatsu Y, Shinohara A, Kukita C, Nose T, Maki Y. Reversible CT changes in uremic encephalopathy [letter]. AJNR Am J Neuroradiol 9:215–216, 1988.

22. Hughes JR. Correlations between EEG and chemical changes in uremia. Electroencephalogr Clin Neurophysiol 48:583–594, 1980.

23. Madonick MJ, Berke K, Schiffer I. Pleocytosis and meningeal signs in uremia: report on sixty-two cases. Arch Neurol Psychiatry 64:431–436, 1950.

24. Bullock ML, Umen AJ, Finkelstein M, Keane WF. The assessment of risk factors in 462 patients with acute renal failure. Am J Kidney Dis 5:97–103, 1985.

25. Levin R. Dialysis disequilibrium syndrome [letter]. West J Med 152:77, 1990.

26. Moel DI, Kwun YA. Cortical blindness as a complication of hemodialysis. J Pediatr 93:890–891, 1978.

27. Servilla KS, Groggel GC. Anterior ischemic optic neuropathy as a complication of hemodialysis. Am J Kidney Dis 8:61–63, 1986.

28. Bana DS, Yap AU, Graham JR. Headache during hemodialysis. Headache 12:1–14, 1972.

29. Bakir AA, Hryhorczuk DO, Berman E, Dunea G. Acute fatal hyperalbuminemic encephalopathy in undialyzed and recently dialyzed uremic patients. ASAIO Trans 32:171–176, 1986.

30. Campistol JM, Cases A, Botey A, Revert A. Acute aluminum encephalopathy in an uremic patient. Nephron 51:103–106, 1989.

31. Harris RD, Campbell JK, Howard FM, Woods JE, Anderson CF, Sayre GP. Neurovascular complications of dialysis and transplantation. Stroke 5:725–729, 1974.

32. Bechar M, Lakke JP, van der Hem GK, Beks JW, Penning L. Subdural hematoma during long-term hemodialysis. Arch Neurol 26:513–516, 1972.

33. Kopitnik TA Jr, de Andrade R Jr, Gold MA, Nugent GR. Pressure changes within a chronic subdural hematoma during hemodialysis. Surg Neurol 32:289–293, 1989.

34. Leonard A, Shapiro FL. Subdural hematoma in regularly hemodialyzed patients. Ann Intern Med 82:650–658, 1975.

35. Descombes E, Dessibourg CA, Fellay G. Acute encephalopathy due to thiamine deficiency (Wernicke's encephalopathy) in a chronic hemodialyzed patient: a case report. Clin Nephrol 35:171–175, 1991.

36. Faris AA. Wernicke's encephalopathy in uremia. Neurology 22:1293–1297, 1972.

37. Kawamura M, Fijimoto S, Hisanaga S, Yamamoto Y, Eto T. Incidence, outcome, and risk factors of cerebrovascular events in patients undergoing maintenance hemodialysis. Am J Kidney Dis 31: 991–996, 1998.

38. Pappius HM, Oh JH, Dossetor JB. The effects of rapid hemodialysis on brain tissues and cerebrospinal fluid of dogs. Can J Physiol Pharmacol 45: 129–147, 1967.

39. Silver SM. Cerebral edema after rapid dialysis is not caused by an increase in brain organic osmolytes. J Am Soc Nephrol 6:1600–1606, 1995.

40. Silver SM, Sterns RH, Halperin ML. Brain swelling after dialysis: old urea or new osmoles? Am J Kidney Dis 28:1–13, 1996.

41. Silver SM. Cerebral edema after hemodialysis: the "reverse urea effect" lives. Int J Artif Organs 21: 247–250, 1998.

42. Arieff AI, Massry SG, Barrientos A, Kleeman CR. Brain water and electrolyte metabolism in uremia: effects of slow and rapid hemodialysis. Kidney Int 4:177–187, 1973.

43. Arieff AI. More on the dialysis disequilibrium syndrome. West J Med 151:74–76, 1989.

44. Galons JP, Trouard T, Gmitro AF, Lien YH. Hemodialysis increases apparent diffusion coefficient of brain water in nephrectomized rats measured by isotropic diffusion-weighted magnetic resonance imaging. J Clin Invest 98:750–755, 1996.

45. Basile C, Miller JD, Koles ZJ, Grace M, Ulan RA. The effects of dialysis on brain water and EEG in stable chronic uremia. Am J Kidney Dis 9:462–469, 1987.

46. Hampl H, Klopp HW, Michels N, et al. Electroencephalogram investigations of the disequilibrium syndrome during bicarbonate and acetate dialysis. Proc Eur Dial Transplant Assoc 19:351–359, 1983.

47. Noriega-Sanchez A, Martinez-Maldonado M, Haiffe RM. Clinical and electroencephalographic changes in progressive uremic encephalopathy. Neurology 28:667–669, 1978.

48. Steele WH, Lawrence JR, Elliott HL, Whiting B. Alterations of phenytoin protein binding with in vivo haemodialysis in dialysis encephalopathy. Eur J Clin Pharmacol 15:69–71, 1979.

49. Varon J, Marik PE. The diagnosis and management of hypertensive crises. Chest 118:214–227, 2000.

50. Vaughan CJ, Delanty N. Hypertensive emergencies. Lancet 356:411–417, 2000.

51. Houston MC. Pathophysiology, clinical aspects, and treatment of hypertensive crises. Prog Cardiovasc Dis 32:99–148, 1989.

52. Buckner FS, Eschbach JW, Haley NR, Davidson RC, Adamson JW. Hypertension following erythropoietin therapy in anemic hemodialysis patients. Am J Hypertens 3:947–955, 1990.

53. Edmunds ME, Walls J, Tucker B, et al. Seizures in haemodialysis patients treated with recombinant human erythropoietin. Nephrol Dial Transplant 4:1065–1069, 1989.

54. Delanty N, Vaughan C, Frucht S, Stubgen P. Erythropoietin-associated hypertensive posterior leukoencephalopathy. Neurology 49:686–689, 1997.

55. Chester EM, Agamanolis DP, Banker BQ, Victor M. Hypertensive encephalopathy: a clinicopathologic study of 20 cases. Neurology 28:928–939, 1978.

56. Hudson AJ, Hyland HH. Hypertensive cerebrovascular disease: a clinical and pathologic review of 100 cases. Ann Intern Med 49:1049–1072, 1958.

57. Healton EB, Brust JC, Feinfeld DA, Thomson GE. Hypertensive encephalopathy and the neurologic manifestations of malignant hypertension. Neurology 32:127–132, 1982.

58. Strandgaard S, Paulson OB. Cerebral blood flow and its pathophysiology in hypertension. Am J Hypertens 2:486–492, 1989.

59. Tamaki K, Sadoshima S, Baumbach GL, Iadecola C, Reis DJ, Heistad DD. Evidence that disruption of the blood–brain barrier precedes reduction in cerebral blood flow in hypertensive encephalopathy. Hypertension 6 (Suppl I):I-75–I-81, 1984.

60. Schwartz RB, Jones KM, Kalina P, et al. Hypertensive encephalopathy: findings on CT, MR imaging, and SPECT imaging in 14 cases. AJR Am J Roentgenol 159:379–383, 1992.

61. Ziegler DK, Zosa A, Zileli T. Hypertensive encephalopathy. Arch Neurol 12:472–478, 1965.

62. Tang-Wai DF, Phan TG, Wijdicks EFM. Hypertensive encephalopathy presenting with thunderclap headache. Headache 41:198–200, 2001.

63. Jellinek EH, Painter M, Prineas J, Russell RR. Hypertensive encephalopathy with cortical disorders of vision. Q J Med 33:239–256, 1964.

64. Liebowitz HA, Hall PE. Cortical blindness as a complication of eclampsia. Ann Emerg Med 13:365–367, 1984.

65. Dinsdale HB. Hypertensive encephalopathy. Neurol Clin 1:3–16, 1983.

66. Bakshi R, Bates VE, Mechtler LL, Kinkel PR, Kinkel WR. Occipital lobe seizures as the major clinical manifestation of reversible posterior leukoencephalopathy syndrome: magnetic resonance imaging findings. Epilepsia 39:295–299, 1998.

67. Walsh FB. Walsh and Hoyt's Clinical Neuro-Ophthalmology, Vol. 1, 4th ed. Miller NR (ed). Williams & Wilkins, Baltimore, 1982, pp 175–211.

68. Siegler RL, Brewer ED, Corneli HM, Thompson JA. Hypertension first seen as facial paralysis: case reports and review of the literature. Pediatrics 87:387–389, 1991.

69. Krogsgaard AR, McNair A, Hilden T, Nielsen PE. Reversibility of cerebral symptoms in severe hypertension in relation to acute antihypertensive therapy. Danish Multicenter Study. Acta Med Scand 220:25–31, 1986.

70. Jespersen CM, Rasmussen D, Hennild V. Focal intracerebral oedema in hypertensive encephalopathy visualized by computerized tomographic scan. J Intern Med 225:349–350, 1989.

71. Rail DL, Perkin GD. Computerized tomographic appearance of hypertensive encephalopathy. Arch Neurol 37:310–311, 1980.

72. Weingarten L, Barbut D, Filippi C, Zimmerman RD. Acute hypertensive encephalopathy: findings on spin-echo and gradient-echo MR imaging. AJR Am J Roentgenol 162:665–670, 1994.

73. Fisher M, Maister B, Jacobs R. Hypertensive encephalopathy: diffuse reversible white matter CT abnormalities. Ann Neurol 18:268–270, 1985.

74. Gibby WA, Stecker MM, Goldberg HI, et al. Reversal of white matter edema in hypertensive encephalopathy [letter]. AJNR Am J Neuroradiol 10 (Suppl 5):S78, 1989.

75. Hauser RA, Lacey DM, Knight MR. Hypertensive encephalopathy. Magnetic resonance imaging demonstration of reversible cortical and white matter lesions. Arch Neurol 45:1078–1083, 1988.

76. Hinchey J, Chaves C, Appignani B, et al. A reversible posterior leukoencephalopathy syndrome. N Engl J Med 334:494–500, 1996.

77. Drees C, Alkotob L, Hall PM, Krieger D. Reversible pontine edema in hypertension. Neurology 56:659, 2001.

78. de Seze J, Mastain B, Stojkovic T, et al. Unusual MR findings of the brain stem in arterial hypertension. AJNR Am J Neuroradiol 21:391–394, 2000.

79. Wang MC, Escott EJ, Breeze RE. Posterior fossa swelling and hydrocephalus resulting from hypertensive encephalopathy: case report and review of the literature. Neurosurgery 44:1325–1327, 1999.

80. Calhoun DA, Oparil S. Treatment of hypertensive crisis. N Engl J Med 323:1177–1183, 1990.

81. Gifford RW Jr. Management of hypertensive crises. JAMA 266:829–835, 1991.

82. Rubenstein EB, Escalante C. Hypertensive crisis. Crit Care Clin 5:477–495, 1989.

83. Cunningham FG, Lindheimer MD. Hypertension in pregnancy. N Engl J Med 326:927–932, 1992.

84. Griswold WR, Viney J, Mendoza SA, James HE. Intracranial pressure monitoring in severe hypertensive encephalopathy. Crit Care Med 9:573–576, 1981.

85. Bolton CF, Young GB. Neurological Complications of Renal Disease. Butterworths, Boston, 1990.

86. Layzer RB. Neuromuscular Manifestations of Systemic Disease. Contemporary Neurology Series, Vol. 25. FA Davis, Philadelphia, 1985.

87. Segredo V, Caldwell JE, Matthay MA, Sharma ML, Gruenke LD, Miller RD. Persistent paralysis in critically ill patients after long-term administration of vecuronium. N Engl J Med 327:524–528, 1992.

88. Nakashima Y, Fouad FM, Nakamoto S, Textor SC, Bravo EL, Tarazi RC. Localization of autonomic nervous system dysfunction in dialysis patients. Am J Nephrol 7:375–381, 1987.

89. Neal CR, Resnikoff E, Unger AM. Treatment of dialysis-related muscle cramps with hypertonic dextrose. Arch Intern Med 141:171–173, 1981.

90. Sherman RA, Goodling KA, Eisinger RP. Acute therapy of hemodialysis-related muscle cramps. Am J Kidney Dis 2:287–288, 1982.

91. Bazzi C, Pagani S, Sorgato G, Albonico G, Fellin G, D'Amico G. Uremic polyneuropathy: a clinical and electrophysiological study in 135 short- and long-term hemodialyzed patients. Clin Nephrol 35:176–181, 1991.

92. Dyck PJ, Johnson WJ, Lambert EH, O'Brien PC. Segmental demyelination secondary to axonal degeneration in uremic neuropathy. Mayo Clin Proc 46:400–431, 1971.

93. Jennekens FG, Mees EJ, van der Most van Spijk D. Clinical aspects of uraemic polyneuropathy. Nephron 8:414–426, 1971.

94. Nielsen VK. The peripheral nerve function in chronic renal failure. I. Clinical symptoms and signs. Acta Med Scand 190:105–111, 1971.

95. Said G, Boudier L, Selva J, Zingraff J, Drueke T. Different patterns of uremic polyneuropathy: clinicopathologic study. Neurology 33:567–574, 1983.

96. Nielsen VK. The peripheral nerve function in chronic renal failure. VIII. Recovery after renal transplantation. Clinical aspects. Acta Med Scand 195:163–170, 1974.

97. Bolton CF. Peripheral neuropathies associated with chronic renal failure. Can J Neurol Sci 7:89–96, 1980.

98. Lynch PG, Yuill GM, Nicholson JA. Acute polyneuropathy complicating chronic renal failure. Nephron 8:278–288, 1971.

99. McGonigle RJ, Bewick M, Weston MJ, Parsons V. Progressive, predominantly motor, uraemic neuropathy. Acta Neurol Scand 71:379–384, 1985.

100. Meyrier A, Fardeau M, Richet G. Acute asymmetrical neuritis associated with rapid ultrafiltration dialysis. Br Med J 2:252–254, 1972.

101. Ropper AH. Accelerated neuropathy of renal failure. Arch Neurol 50:536–539, 1993.

102. Bolton CF, Baltzan MA, Baltzan RB. Effects of renal transplantation on uremic neuropathy. A clinical and electrophysiologic study. N Engl J Med 284:1170–1175, 1971.

103. Yosipovitch G, Yarnitsky D, Mermelstein V, et al. Paradoxical heat sensation in uremic polyneuropathy. Muscle Nerve 18:768–771, 1995.

104. Baltodano N, Gallo BV, Weidler DJ. Verapamil vs quinine in recumbent nocturnal leg cramps in the elderly. Arch Intern Med 148:1969–1970, 1988.

105. Brodeur C, Montplaisir J, Godbout R, Marinier R. Treatment of restless legs syndrome and periodic movements during sleep with L-dopa: a double-blind, controlled study. Neurology 38:1845–1848, 1988.

106. Trenkwalder C, Stiasny K, Pollmacher T, et al. L-dopa therapy of uremic and idiopathic restless legs syndrome: a double-blind, crossover trial. Sleep 18:681–688, 1995.

107. Telstad W, Sørensen Ø, Larsen S, Lillevold PE, Stensrud P, Nyberg-Hansen R. Treatment of the restless legs syndrome with carbamazepine: a double blind study. Br Med J [Clin Res] 288:444–446, 1984.

108. von Scheele C. Levodopa in restless legs. Lancet 2:426–427, 1986.

109. Walters AS, Hening WA, Chokroverty S. Review and videotape recognition of idiopathic restless legs syndrome. Mov Disord 6:105–110, 1991.

110. Sindrup SH, Jensen TS. Pharmacologic treatment of pain in polyneuropathy. Neurology 55:915–920, 2000.

111. Vita G, Messina C, Savica V, Bellinghieri G. Uraemic autonomic neuropathy. J Auton Nerv Syst 30 (Suppl):S179–S184, 1990.

112. Faber MD, Dumler F, Zasuwa GA, Levin NW. Relationship between sympathetic dysfunction and hemodialysis instability. ASAIO Trans 33:280–285, 1987.

113. Davies IB, Mathias CJ, Sudera D, Sever PS. Agonist regulation of alpha-adrenergic receptor responses in man. J Cardiovasc Pharmacol 4 (Suppl 1):S139–S144, 1982.

114. Naik RB, Mathias CJ, Wilson CA, Reid JL, Warren DJ. Cardiovascular and autonomic reflexes in haemodialysis patients. Clin Sci (Colch) 60:165–170, 1981.

115. Bolton CF, Driedger AA, Lindsay RM. Ischaemic neuropathy in uraemic patients caused by bovine arteriovenous shunt. J Neurol Neurosurg Psychiatry 42:810–814, 1979.

116. Bhasin HK, Dana CL. Spontaneous retroperitoneal hemorrhage in chronically hemodialyzed patients. Nephron 22:322–327, 1978.

117. Benz RL, Siegfried JW, Teehan BP. Carpal tunnel syndrome in dialysis patients: comparison between continuous ambulatory peritoneal dialysis and hemodialysis populations. Am J Kidney Dis 11:473–476, 1988.

118. Bicknell JM, Lim AC, Raroque HG Jr, Tzamaloukas AH. Carpal tunnel syndrome, subclinical median

mononeuropathy, and peripheral polyneuropathy: common early complications of chronic peritoneal dialysis and hemodialysis. Arch Phys Med Rehabil 72:378–381, 1991.

119. Chanard J, Lavaud S, Toupance O, Roujouleh H, Melin JP. Carpal tunnel syndrome and type of dialysis membrane used in patients undergoing long-term hemodialysis. Arthritis Rheum 29:1170–1171, 1986.

120. Charra B, Calemard E, Uzan M, Terrat JC, Vanel T, Laurent G. Carpal tunnel syndrome, shoulder pain and amyloid deposits in long-term hemodialysis patients [abstract]. Kidney Int 26:549, 1984.

121. McClure J, Bartley CJ, Ackrill P. Carpal tunnel syndrome caused by amyloid containing beta 2 microglobulin: a new amyloid and a complication of long term haemodialysis. Ann Rheum Dis 45: 1007–1011, 1986.

122. Gilbert MS, Robinson A, Baez A, Gupta S, Glabman S, Haimov M. Carpal tunnel syndrome in patients who are receiving long-term renal hemodialysis. J Bone Joint Surg Am 70:1145–1153, 1988.

123. Naito M, Ogata K, Goya T. Carpal tunnel syndrome in chronic renal dialysis patients: clinical evaluation of 62 hands and results of operative treatment. J Hand Surg [Br] 12:366–374, 1987.

124. Zamora JL, Rose JE, Rosario V, Noon GP. Hemodialysis-associated carpal tunnel syndrome: a clinical review. Nephron 41:70–74, 1985.

125. Wytrzes L, Markley HG, Fisher M, Alfred HJ. Brachial neuropathy after brachial artery–antecubital vein shunts for chronic hemodialysis. Neurology 37:1398–1400, 1987.

Chapter 10

NEUROLOGIC MANIFESTATIONS OF ACUTE HEPATIC FAILURE

For the most part, acute hepatic failure in critically ill patients occurs in the course of multiorgan failure. Acute hepatic failure as a primary presenting disorder is notably uncommon in medical intensive care units, and its cause may vary geographically. Acute hepatic failure is mostly encountered in patients with long-standing cirrhosis. These patients may be admitted with sudden onset of hepatic encephalopathy from acute gastrointestinal hemorrhage that causes rapid nitrogenous overload.

A particularly challenging management problem in the intensive care unit is sudden massive necrosis of the liver, a clinical entity known as fulminant hepatic failure.[1,2] The most important cause of fulminant hepatic failure is viral hepatitis, but it is also associated with acetaminophen overdose, halothane, carbon tetrachloride, hepatic vein occlusion (Budd-Chiari syndrome), Wilson's disease, and acute fatty liver of pregnancy. Reye's syndrome linked to aspirin use during a varicella or influenza-like illness has become virtually extinct, and treatable inborn errors of metabolism mimicking the disorder are now more likely.[3,4] The management of fulminant hepatic failure has evolved in surprising ways during recent years as a result of successful liver transplantation.

This chapter illustrates the clinical characteristics of acute hepatic encephalopathy but concentrates on the management of fulminant hepatic failure and treatment of cerebral edema.

GENERAL CONSIDERATIONS

Multiple organ involvement may occur in patients with acute liver failure requiring intensive care management, and if it does, mortality becomes extraordinarily high (up to 90%). Treatment options are very limited. In patients with fulminant hepatic failure, however, mortality can be reduced to 60% when liver transplantation is appropriately timed.[5–7] It appears that results of emergency liver transplantation depend on the degree of encephalopathy.

One series reported survival with good functional performance in 12 of 17 patients with fulminant hepatic failure in whom hepatic encephalopathy did not exceed stage I or II.[8] But in general, the likelihood of patients with stage IV encephalopathy surviving is low without urgent transplantation. (In the present classification of hepatic encephalopathy, stage IV indicates coma without further specification other than whether or not motor response to painful stimuli is present.)

Progression of the disorder to include

acute renal failure seriously complicates the clinical picture of liver failure. In patients with fulminant hepatic failure, oliguric renal failure coexists in approximately 75% of those who become comatose from liver failure, and deteriorating renal function may require hemodialysis.[9,10]

Another important consequence of acute hepatic failure is a coagulopathy that is often severe enough to warrant plasmapheresis or plasma infusions. Platelet infusions are usually indicated in patients with severe hemorrhage and in those about to undergo invasive procedures. Fresh-frozen plasma is used to replace coagulation factors, but its effect is short-lived.

Metabolic derangements can affect the level of consciousness. These include dilutional hyponatremia, hypoglycemia, and metabolic alkalosis. The effect of these acute metabolic changes on clinical staging of hepatic encephalopathy most likely is small because they are typically transient and rapidly corrected. Thus, progression into higher stages of hepatic encephalopathy in fulminant hepatic failure should not be readily attributed to multifactorial systemic factors, since it is often associated with the emergence of brain edema. Persistent hypotension may occur in patients who have hepatic failure that is associated with high cardiac output and low peripheral vascular resistance. Infusion of norepinephrine and vasopressin is required to overcome the systemic effects. Its effect on the brain is not known. Therefore, some factors other than the effects of hepatic failure alone could confound the clinical presentation and should be taken into account when the severity of hepatic encephalopathy is staged.

HEPATIC ENCEPHALOPATHY

Hepatic encephalopathy has been categorized in clinical stages of stepwise worsening. The description of each stage varies somewhat in the literature, but the differences between adjacent stages are clear enough to be helpful in clinical practice (Table 10–1). A formal interobserver and intraobserver variation study has not been performed, but there is no compelling reason to believe that this method of staging of hepatic encephalopathy is grossly invalid or poorly reproducible. It may be argued that additional use of the motor component of the Glasgow coma scale score may be useful and more exact.

Clinical Features

Psychiatric symptoms are prominent, and the earliest abnormality is apathy. Hypersomnia can be an early feature, with both prolongation of nocturnal sleep and extreme daytime sleepiness, but in others sleep inversion with agitated delirium at night may be obvious.[11,12] Personality changes, usually querulousness and impaired judgment, may be noted,[11] and even more surprising, eu-

Table 10–1. **Signs and Symptoms of Hepatic Encephalopathy**

Stage	Psychiatric	Neurologic
I	Apathy, anxiety, restlessness, short attention span, inverted sleep patterns, impaired calculations	Impaired handwriting, tremor, slowed coordination
II	Personality change, disorientation (time), poor recall, disobedience	Asterixis, ataxia, dysarthria, paratonia
III	Bizarre behavior, disorientation (place), delirium, paranoia, drowsy but arousable	Seizures, myoclonus, marked hyperreflexia, hyperpnea
IV	Coma	Coma (abnormal flexion or extensor responses, sluggish pupillary reactions to light), brisk oculocephalic responses

phoria with a transition to mania may be a presenting symptom.[13]

Progression into the next stages of hepatic encephalopathy is characterized by impairment of consciousness. Fluctuations in attention and slow responses to requests are typically present. Patients are incapable of registration, retention, and recall. The immediate memory span for digits is severely reduced. Overactivity and unrest, disorientation for place, delusions, and repetitive picking movements become evident in stage III hepatic encephalopathy. The paranoid content of delusions often results in panic reactions, which may be accompanied by tachycardia, facial flushing, and tremor. Outbursts of anger and hostility are fairly typical in this stage of encephalopathy,[14] causing marked difficulties in controlling the patient.

Patients with fulminant hepatic failure experience a very condensed process of clinical development of hepatic encephalopathy.[15] The disorder may begin with excitement and delirium. Traditionally, it has seldom been interrupted by focal or generalized tonic–clonic seizures. Endogenous benzodiazepines have been proposed as a possible explanation for the low incidence of clinically apparent seizures in hepatic encephalopathy. However, a recent study suggested subclinical electroencephalographic activity in 10 of 22 prospectively monitored patients with fulminant hepatic failure, and use of phenytoin muted the manifestations on electroencephalograms.[16] Indeed, epileptic activity may be more apparent than currently appreciated. A 10-year review of electroencephalography in patients with hepatic encephalopathy also documented epileptiform activity in 15% of patients without a structural cause evident by neuroimaging, which could potentially account for it.[17]

Multifocal myoclonus and startle responses can easily be produced by a clap of the hands. Asterixis (see Chapter 9) is infrequent in acute hepatic encephalopathy from fulminant hepatic necrosis. Fragmentary speech and paraphasic errors are noted in some patients, but localization of the abnormality has not been detected by conventional studies. Within 24 to 48 hr after the first manifestations, patients may lapse into coma with spontaneous extensor responses. They quickly become jaundiced, febrile, and dehydrated. Papilledema is absent but may appear early in patients with rapidly progressing brain edema.

The pupils of patients with early hepatic encephalopathy are normal, and light reflexes are preserved. In end-stage encephalopathy, the pupillary reaction becomes sluggish (admittedly an imprecise term) and, because of diffuse cerebral edema, eventually disappears as a consequence of progressive central brain herniation and brain stem displacement. Oculocephalic responses, although brisk, usually remain normal but may transiently disappear.[18] In occasional patients with higher stages of hepatic encephalopathy, these very brisk oculocephalic responses may give the impression that both globes are floating or rolling like ball bearings.

Transient ocular bobbing and dysconjugate gaze have been reported to occur and to disappear after treatment of hepatic encephalopathy and improvement of serum ammonia levels.[19] Plum and Posner[20] noted transient downward gaze in their series of patients with hepatic coma, a phenomenon also reported in postresuscitation encephalopathy (Chapter 8).[21] However, spontaneous eye movement abnormalities are rare and should point to other causes than fulminant hepatic failure.

Motor responses may fluctuate over time but are usually closely correlated with the depth of coma. The extensor posturing, albeit dramatic and characteristically seen in stage IV encephalopathy, may be completely reversible after correction of arterial ammonia and liver function.[22] The muscle tone in patients with hepatic encephalopathy is usually impressively increased, with gegenhalten, exaggerated tendon reflexes, and Babinski's signs. However, when extensor posturing occurs in the course of fulminant hepatic failure, brain death can be anticipated within a few hours. At this point, aggressive treatment of cerebral edema is indicated and may still completely reverse the clinical manifestations.

In general, the clinical presentation of hepatic encephalopathy may suggest a gloomy state, but the symptoms may resolve without any residual neurologic findings after liver transplantation or successful medical treatment.

Pathogenesis

The neuropathologic features of hepatic encephalopathy may vary between complete absence of any light microscopic features and presence of gross cerebral edema (Plate 10–1). Some glial changes, however, are distinctive in hepatic encephalopathy. Alzheimer type II astrocytes may occur in clusters and are identified by enlarged nuclei with inclusion bodies positive to periodic acid–Schiff testing. These changes are often found in the gray matter of the cerebrum and cerebellum and in the putamen and globus pallidus.

A unifying hypothesis of the biochemical changes and causes of hepatic encephalopathy has not yet emerged. A potential mechanism is depicted in Figure 10–1. Ammonia

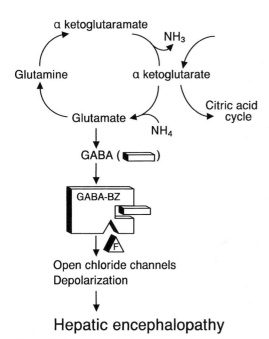

Figure 10–1. The γ-aminobutyric acid–benzodiazepine (GABA-BZ) receptor complex and its relation to hepatic encephalopathy. F, flumazenil. (Modified from Morris JC, Ferrendelli JA. Metabolic encephalopathy. In: Pearlman AL, Collins RC [eds]. Neurobiology of Disease. Oxford University Press, New York, 1990, pp 356–379. By permission of the publisher.)

is probably pivotal in the mechanism of hepatic encephalopathy and perhaps causes an imbalance of excitatory and inhibitory neurotransmitters. Ammonia is generated in the gastrointestinal tract from the degradation of amines, amino acids, and purines. Failure of liver clearance results in impaired conversion of ammonia to urea and glutamine and consequently a surfeit of glutamate. As a result of the linkage of ammonia with glutamate, γ-aminobutyric acid (GABA) is formed, which produces an inhibitory action after depolarization through the opening of chloride channels. It appears that the degree of hepatic encephalopathy is correlated with cerebrospinal fluid levels of GABA.[23]

The GABA–benzodiazepine receptor complex,[23] present in synaptic neural membranes, can be manipulated,[24] and this characteristic has created enthusiasm for a potential new rationale for treatment of hepatic encephalopathy. In the early studies, patients treated with drugs that antagonize the GABA–benzodiazepine receptor (for example, flumazenil) displayed both clinical and electroencephalographic improvement.[25–28] Further support for this hypothesis—the effect of benzodiazepines on GABA receptor neurotransmission—has been the discovery of an increase in endogenous benzodiazepines in animal models,[29] in body fluids in patients with hepatic encephalopathy,[30] and in uptake of benzodiazepine measured by positron emission tomography scanning.[31] Unfortunately, the evidence that flumazenil, a benzodiazepine receptor antagonist, may reverse hepatic encephalopathy is weak despite successful treatment with flumazenil in some uncontrolled series. Dramatic awakening from hepatic coma as soon as 30 sec after the injection of flumazenil and sustained remission after repeated injections have been reported.[32]

In a preliminary series of nine patients with fulminant hepatic failure, 6 of 11 episodes of hepatic encephalopathy were successfully reversed with flumazenil.[26] Unsuccessful treatment in stage IV encephalopathy has been tentatively explained by the existence of secondary factors, such as cerebral edema and effects of hypoglycemia. A placebo-controlled multicenter trial from Italy in 527 cirrhotic patients with grades III and IV hepatic encephalopathy found clinical and electroencephalographic improvement but only in a small proportion of patients (17.5% in grade III and 14.7% in grade IV, compared with 3.8% and 2.7%, respectively, in the placebo group).[33] Two smaller placebo-controlled studies from Germany and Holland showed marginal benefit in some patients only, with no apparent change on electroencephalographic variables.[34,35] Undoubtedly, flumazenil has an important role in patients with fulminant hepatic failure who have repeated injections of benzodiazepines, and administration may help in correctly assessing the stage of hepatic encephalopathy. This is particularly relevant when emergency transplantation is considered. Its efficacy in reversing hepatic encephalopathy seems minimal.

Other possible explanations of the mechanism of hepatic encephalopathy are controversial. Mercaptans (responsible for fetor hepaticus), short-chain fatty acids, and depletion of neurotransmitters, such as norepinephrine and dopamine, have been implicated.[36] The significance of these factors alone or in combination and whether they should represent avenues for potential pharmaceutical intervention remains uncertain.

An extensive survey of the possible toxins can be found in several excellent reviews on this subject[14,37] (Table 10–2).

Laboratory Tests

Both venous and arterial ammonia levels are somewhat correlated with degree of hepatic encephalopathy. The overlap is significant in venous samples, but ammonia in arterial samples tends to increase with worsening grades (Fig. 10–2).

Any of the four major acid–base abnormalities may be encountered in patients with hepatic encephalopathy, but respiratory or metabolic alkalosis is most frequent.[47] Most patients with fulminant hepatic failure hyperventilate, and the result is low Pa_{CO_2} with alkalemia. Respiratory alkalosis most likely results from increased respiratory drive triggered by accumulating toxins (such as ammonia). One study found that short-chain fatty acids, which are increased in hepatic encephalopathy, produced central hyperventilation in the rabbit.[48] The significance of alkalosis in hepatic encephalopathy was supported by Plum and Posner,[20] who cor-

---

Table 10–2. **Putative Factors in Hepatic Encephalopathy**

Substance	Evidence from Laboratory Studies
Ammonia (NH_3^+)	• Impairs postsynaptic inhibition in cortex, thalamus, and brain stem; interferes with chloride outward pumping[38,39]
	• Decreases (excitatory) glutaminergic synaptic function[40]
Glutamate	• Cultured astrocytes exposed to ammonia show diminished glutamate uptake[41]
	• Decreased high-affinity sites for glutamate in brain in portosystemic encephalopathy or experimental hyperammonia syndromes[42,43]
Serotonin	• Increased 5-hydroxytryptamine degradation by monoamine oxidase[44]
	• Grade of coma is correlated with cerebrospinal fluid level of indoleacetic acid (produced by tryptamine turnover)
Dopamine	• Loss of dopamine receptors in globus pallidus[45]
	• Increased dopamine metabolites, such as homovanillic acid and 3–methoxytyramine
Endogenous benzodiazepines	• Benzodiazepine ligands (e.g., flumazenil) reverse encephalopathy in some cases
	• Increased levels of diazepam-binding inhibitor in cerebrospinal fluid[46]

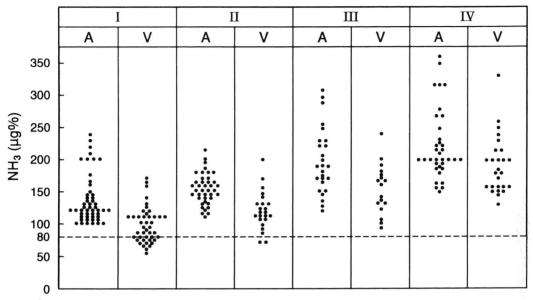

Figure 10–2. Arterial (A) and venous (V) ammonia levels in various stages of hepatic encephalopathy.

rectly implied that encephalopathy with respiratory or metabolic alkalosis most likely was hepatic in origin.

Somatosensory evoked potentials may be useful in fulminant hepatic failure. The bilateral absence of short latency cortical responses (see Chapter 8) appears to reflect poor outcome and development of brain edema. In these patients, liver transplantation may not reverse brain dysfunction.[49] The predictive value of somatosensory evoked potentials for outcome in hepatic encephalopathy is unresolved.[50] Experience in fulminant hepatic failure is limited, and we have not rejected donors for this reason.

Many investigators in this field claim that hepatic encephalopathy can be recognized early with abnormal visual evoked potentials, but in other studies of flash visual evoked responses, no sufficiently sensitive differences between patients with and those without encephalopathy could be demonstrated.[51–53]

Brain stem evoked potentials may be more promising for subclinical detection of hepatic encephalopathy. A study comparing auditory, somatosensory, and visual evoked potentials in 22 patients found that the brain stem evoked potentials were the most sensitive for detection of subclinical hepatic encephalopathy.[54]

Before the introduction of evoked responses in patients with hepatic encephalopathy, electroencephalography was the only objective method to measure the degree of hepatic encephalopathy. Spectral analysis of the electroencephalogram allows one to see small differences and shifts in patterns. A retrospective study noted a significant inverse correlation between the occurrence of delta waves and survival.[28] Triphasic wave patterns are defined as generalized, bilaterally synchronous, bifrontal periodic waves in patients with decreased level of consciousness, often associated with a background slowing[55,56] (Fig. 10–3). They can be used as prognostic indicators, because triphasic wave patterns have been associated with a 50% mortality in patients with metabolic encephalopathies, including hepatic encephalopathy.[55]

Magnetic resonance imaging (MRI) is helpful in assessing severity of liver disease. In approximately two-thirds of patients with advanced liver disease, hyperintensity in the globus pallidus is found on T1-weighted images and disappears after liver transplantation. An increase in extrapyramidal symp-

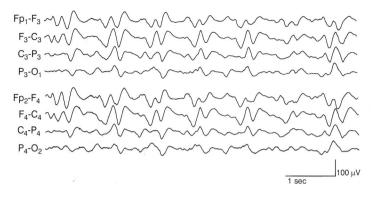

Figure 10–3. Typical triphasic waves (see text) common in hepatic encephalopathy but also described in Hashimoto's encephalopathy (Chapter 8) and postresuscitation encephalopathy (Chapter 8).

toms may occur but in many patients remains unnoticed. This change in paramagnetic properties in the globus pallidus, also seen in patients after prolonged parenteral feeding, most likely is due to abnormal manganese metabolism (Fig. 10–4). Higher blood concentrations of manganese were found in patients with these MRI abnormalities.[57] Iron deficiency may increase intestinal absorption of manganese and is an important factor.[57–60] Biochemical–pathologic correlation, which has not yet been performed, may provide an understanding of its clinical significance.[61]

Medical Management

Management of hepatic encephalopathy focuses on reduction of ammonia absorption from the intestinal lumen. Enemas with 20% lactose or 1% neomycin solutions adjusted to a pH of 4 usually thoroughly clean the gut. Dietary proteins are completely avoided to minimize the production of ammonia. Radical approaches in treatment-resistant patients with progressive hepatic encephalopathy include surgical exclusion of the colon and charcoal hemoperfusion, but success is only anecdotal.

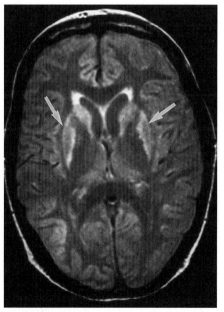
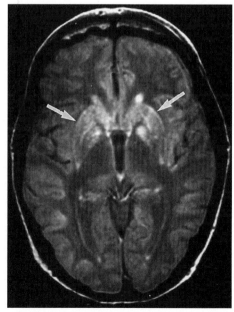

Figure 10–4. Hyperintensity in the globus pallidus in patient with hepatic encephalopathy on magnetic resonance imaging (arrows).

Table 10–3. **Basic Management of Hepatic Encephalopathy**

Correction of hypokalemia, metabolic alkalosis, hyponatremia, hypovolemia

Identification of possible bleeding site (e.g., varices, gastrointestinal tract)

Protein-free diet (1500–2000 cal/day)

Cathartics to clean protein from gut (oral magnesium citrate, 200 mL; sorbitol, 50 g/200 mL of water)

Vitamin supplementation: folate, 1 mg/day; vitamin K, 10 mg/day; thiamine and multivitamins

Decrease in absorption of gastrointestinal ammonia

    Neomycin, 1 g p.o. q.i.d.
    Lactulose, 10–30 mg p.o. t.i.d.
    Metronidazole, 250 mg t.i.d.

Data from Rothstein and McKhann.[12]

A meta-analysis of parenteral nutrition with branched-chain amino acids concluded that this regimen resulted in significant improvement in patients with hepatic coma, but further well-designed studies are needed to settle this matter.[62] The basic management of hepatic encephalopathy should therefore include measures to minimize production of ammonia (Table 10–3). Phenytoin prophylaxis requires confirmatory studies.[16]

Management of Brain Edema

The management of fulminant hepatic failure stands out because brain edema is a direct cause of mortality.[63,64] Predictors of brain edema may include a short interval between onset of jaundice and signs of encephalopathy and possibly early elevation of astroglial S-100 and neuron-specific enolase.[65–67]

PATHOPHYSIOLOGIC MECHANISMS

Brain edema is significant in most patients with stage III hepatic encephalopathy but only when caused by acute hepatic necrosis. Blei[68] summarized the potential mechanisms of brain edema in fulminant hepatic failure, which appear to involve both vasogenic and cytotoxic injuries. Animal stud-

ies have shown sodium accumulation within cells and swelling through inhibition of endothelial Na^+, K^+-ATPase after administration of sera from patients with stages III and IV encephalopathy.[69]

Before reviewing the factors proposed to be responsible for brain edema, it is essential to summarize the neuropathologic studies of brain edema in fulminant hepatic failure. Acute astrocyte swelling is observed early, suggesting that astrocytes are a primary target and the swelling mostly represents cytotoxic edema. In cytotoxic edema, impairment of cellular water and osmoregulation predominates, whereas in vasogenic edema, breakdown of the blood–brain barrier results in flooding of the extracellular space with serum protein and fluid. Kato and associates' landmark electron microscopic study[70] of brain edema in fulminant hepatic failure (most cases due to acetaminophen overdose) showed intracellular swelling of the astroglial foot processes with swollen mitochondria and dilated endoplasmic reticulum. Endothelial cells were swollen, and vesicles and vacuoles were present, suggesting macromolecule permeability, but these features of vasogenic edema were seen in terminal stages. Generally, no prominent disruption of the blood–brain barrier or extracellular edema was observed.[71]

What may cause this type of edema? Glutamine has been proposed as a major responsible substance. A fourfold to sixfold increase in glutamine in the brain preceding an increase in brain water has been documented in rat models.[72] This rapid rise due to increased removal of ammonia by ammonia detoxification and astrocyte localization of glutamine synthetase causes the introduction of a water-attracting osmolyte. When cellular increase in osmolality occurs, other osmolytes are removed. A recent study documented a decrease in the polyol/*myo*-inositol ratio, further strengthening the view that osmotic changes within the astrocyte are key.[73]

An alternative, much less convincing hypothesis suggests changes in regulation of cerebral circulation and development of brain ischemia. Toxic substances from the necrotic liver may impair vasoreactivity, and improvement after orthotopic liver transplantation has been documented by transcranial Doppler ultrasonography.[74] In addition, glutamate release by swollen astrocytes may further contribute to excitotoxicity.[75,76] Aquaporins, integral membrane proteins that are significantly expressed in astrocytes, may play a role. Deletion of aquaporin-4 in mice reduces cerebral edema, opening up pathways for possible inhibition.[77]

Diagnosis of brain edema is facilitated by measurements of intracranial pressure (ICP). Patients with increased ICP, decreased cerebral perfusion pressure, and fulminant hepatic failure may not have ominous signs such as sudden, transient dilated pupils and spontaneous extensor responses. Computed tomography (CT) scanning, however, may demonstrate effacement of cortical sulci and obliteration of basal cisterns. Two reports dismissed the value of CT scanning in detecting brain edema.[78,79] In a later study, however, systematic review of serial CT scanning and careful classification of the degree of edema showed a significant correla-

tion between the degree of cerebral edema and the degree of hepatic encephalopathy.[80] Patients whose condition worsened to stage III often had complete disappearance of the sylvian fissures and cortical sulci. In many patients with stage III hepatic encephalopathy, the clinical and radiologic signs of cerebral edema could be reversed with conventional treatment of increased ICP (Fig. 10–5). In others, cerebral edema progressed to brain death (Fig. 10–6).

Insertion of an ICP monitor in the epidural space is preferable. A miniaturized device composed of a small fiberoptic bundle has been developed to monitor ICP after insertion through a 2 mm bur hole, but the high risk of intracerebral hemorrhage at the site is an impediment (see Chapter 17). Attempts to overcome the coagulopathy by transfusion of fresh-frozen plasma or plasmapheresis result in only a very temporary correction of coagulopathy. Plasma exchange has the additional advantage of less volume loading when a hepatorenal syndrome exists. Blei and associates[81] surveyed all centers in the United States that performed liver transplantation and found that

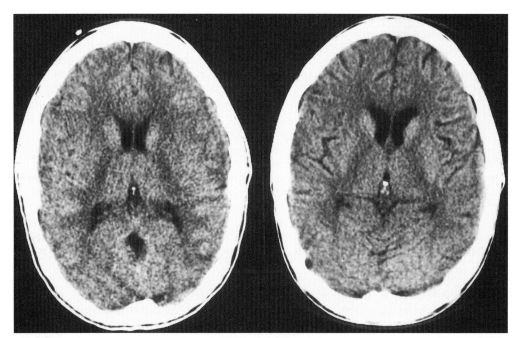

Figure 10–5. Computed tomography scans in a patient with fulminant hepatic failure. *Left*: Hepatic encephalopathy and evidence of cerebral edema (largely absent sulci and sylvian fissures). *Right*: After treatment of increased intracranial pressure and return to stage I encephalopathy. The sulci and sylvian fissures have reappeared.

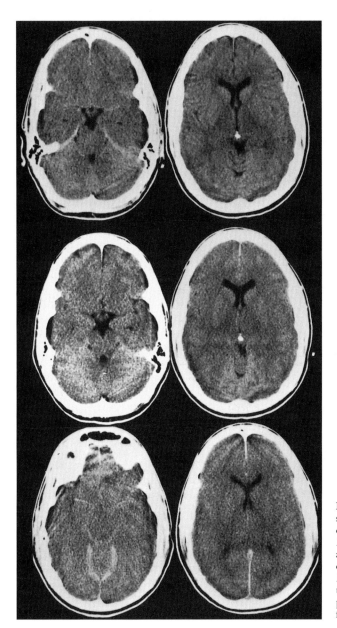

Figure 10–6. Serial computed tomography scans in a patient with rapid progression of cerebral edema. *Top row*: Normal findings. *Middle row*: Disappearance of cortical sulci and white matter discrimination of internal capsule; the third ventricle is barely visible. *Bottom row*: Complete effacement of basal cisterns, compression of lateral ventricles, and pseudosubarachnoid hemorrhage (patient fulfilled the clinical criteria for brain death).

1.3% of patients with epidurally placed ICP monitoring devices experienced fatal intracerebral hemorrhages; another 1.7% had nonfatal hemorrhages. Of patients with subdurally placed devices, on the other hand, 5% had fatal hemorrhages and 13%, nonfatal. When devices were placed directly in the brain parenchyma, 4% had fatal hemorrhages and 9%, nonfatal. These risks, although with considerable morbidity, remain small and are probably outweighed by the benefits of monitoring ICP and, equally important, cerebral perfusion pressure (difference between mean arterial pressure and ICP). Cerebral edema on CT scanning may further guide placement of the ICP monitor.

Sudden increases in ICP may hint at the development of cerebral edema, and, as expected, increases to >60 mm Hg are associated with poor outcome because of rapid downward movement of the brain stem or compression of the thalamus due to bilateral hemispheric edema.[82] The ICP values on insertion of the device were less predictive for outcome than the calculated cerebral perfusion pressures. Cerebral perfusion pressures of 40 mm Hg or less resulted in severe disability and death.

Monitoring ICP in patients with fulminant hepatic failure remains controversial, and many neurosurgeons are discouraged by the poor management results in some series and by the risk of intracerebral hematoma due to the coexisting coagulopathy. Moreover, aggressive treatment of ICP may not always lead to improvement in the degree of encephalopathy, because prolonged hypoglycemia and significant episodes of shock may have caused additional swelling from ischemic damage.

Several patterns of ICP may be observed during the clinical course of hepatic encephalopathy. A gradual increase in ICP is common and has been experimentally produced in pigs. Occasionally, brief increases and plateau waves may occur. These transient increases in ICP most likely indicate decreasing cerebral compliance but may also follow straining, coughing, or bucking of the ventilator. Surges of ICP occur in patients after reperfusion of the transplanted liver and extend during the first day after orthotopic liver transplantation.[83-85] This implies that ICP monitoring should continue at least until the second postoperative day.[86] Improvement in hepatic function usually coincides with resolution of increased intracranial pressure and, if present, with resolution of brain swelling on a CT scan. In our institution, an epidural catheter is placed when a CT scan indicates cerebral edema or when stage III hepatic encephalopathy is present.

When patients with fulminant hepatic failure are admitted to the liver transplantation unit, the decision to place an epidural catheter is typically based on the Glasgow coma sum score and CT scan findings. A Glasgow coma score of 8 or CT scan evidence of brain edema determines placement, but often the patient requires intubation for airway protection at the same time. As mentioned earlier, correction of a coagulopathy

with fresh–frozen plasma is preferable before placement (platelet counts <30,000, prothrombin ratio >1.3).

The first line of treatment of increased ICP is elevation of the head to 30°,[87,88] controlled hyperventilation, and osmotic therapy. Cerebral perfusion pressure should be maintained at 70 mm Hg or higher.

Short-term hyperventilation with an initial range for arterial P_{CO_2} between 28 and 35 mm Hg is preferable. As in many other circumstances, long-term hyperventilation is useless. In a clinical trial, prolonged hyperventilation in fulminant hepatic failure failed to decrease the number of episodes of increased ICP.[89] One group in Denmark used internal jugular bulb saturation monitoring to evaluate the efficacy of hyperventilation, but this cumbersome device is not universally used, nor is it of proven benefit.[90]

A difficult management problem in patients with fulminant hepatic failure is the potential for hepatorenal syndrome. Hyperosmolarity due to mannitol administration may exacerbate renal failure. Patients with severe renal failure thus may temporarily require ultrafiltration to remove mannitol and excess free water. In this situation, mannitol administration can be coupled with removal of about three times the given volume by ultrafiltration performed after 15 to 30 min.[91] Other difficulties with mannitol administration are hypokalemia and nonketotic hyperosmolar hyperglycemia. Nonetheless, the core therapy for ICP reduction remains restriction of free water intake and osmotic therapy. Mannitol in low doses (0.5 g/kg) may effectively reduce ICP and increase cerebral perfusion pressure within 10 to 20 min of infusion, and its effect may last 4 to 6 hr. The dose of mannitol should be titrated by plasma osmolality (ideal plasma osmolality: 310 to 320 mOsm/L). In patients with renal failure and in situations requiring prolonged treatment of ICP, use of tromethamine (THAM) should be strongly considered.

Sometimes, these measures result in lower ICP values and prevent sudden increases in ICP. Most patients, however, may need additional muscle relaxants, sedation, and barbiturates. A retrospective analysis of possible factors that preceded large increases in ICP found that fever, agitation, and arterial hypertension were significantly more common, but whether control of these factors halts progression to brain death is unclear.[92] Barbiturates can be of value in controlling ICP in fulminant hepatic failure due to reduction of cerebral blood flow, but several hours are required for them to take effect. A typical regimen of thiopental in a loading dose of 4 mg/kg and a maintenance dose of 1 mg/kg per hour can reduce blood flow by 50%[93] (Fig. 10–7). Forbes and associates[94] claimed a remarkable effect of thiopental infusion and complete recovery from stage IV encephalopathy in one-third of the patients, far better than the dismal figure of 5% reported earlier in patients with stage IV disease. The risk of systemic hypotension with thiopental administration can be overcome by a decrease in the rate of infusion or temporary use of vasopressors. Sudden surges in ICP should be treated with an intravenously delivered bolus of lidocaine or thiopental. Corticosteroids are of no use in the management of brain edema in patients with fulminant hepatic failure.

We now administer propofol first, a theoretically much better alternative than barbiturates. Administration of propofol can be discontinued quickly and the patient reassessed neurologically; accumulation is seldom seen, even after infusions. Our initial experience is that propofol in a dosage of 30 to 60 μg/kg per minute can control ICP.

However, 2 of our 12 patients treated with intravenous propofol progressed to brain death from cerebral edema despite moderate doses.[95] If tolerated, propofol can be pushed to its maximal dosage of 200 μg/kg per minute.

Moderate hypothermia should probably become standard in management of brain edema in fulminant hepatic failure after a randomized trial documents its efficacy. In one study, reduction of temperature by cooling blankets to 32°C or 33°C for at least 8 hr, with propofol or muscle relaxants used to reduce shivering, was followed by gradual rewarming in 1 to 2 hr. In this study, four patients were successfully shepherded to transplantation with good control of ICP.[96,97] A promising new treatment is intravenous administration of indomethacin.[98] Management of ICP is shown in Table 10–4.

Surgical Management and Bridging Devices

Liver transplantation remains the most definitive and the only viable therapeutic option in fulminant hepatic failure.[99–103] It should be considered in patients with otherwise low probability of survival (Table 10–5). Alternative therapies should be developed as bridges to liver transplantation, because despite urgent listing, 20% of patients deteriorate to brain death.

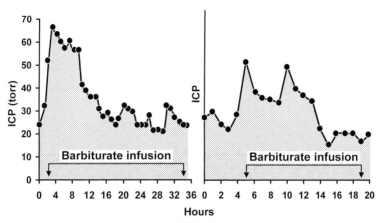

Figure 10–7. Barbiturate therapy in fulminant hepatic failure in two patients. Note delay in achieving control of intracranial pressure (ICP). (From Daas et al.[93] By permission of WB Saunders Company.)

Table 10–4. **Treatment Options of Brain Edema in Fulminant Hepatic Failure**

Propofol infusion (start with 30 mcg/kg per minute)

Moderate hypothermia (33°C–35°C) with cooling blankets, alcohol rubbings, and ice lavage

Pentobarbital bolus of 3–5 mg/kg intravenously followed by 1–3 mg/kg per hour up to normalizing of ICP, but avoid burst suppression or isoelectric electroencephalography

Mannitol, 0.5–1 g/kg every 6 hr if plasma osmolality is <310 mOsm/L

Tromethamine (1 mL/kg per hour)

Intravenously delivered indomethacin, 50 mg over 20 min

Two devices are currently being tested in phase 2 trials.[104] Pioneering work by Demetriou[105] has created a device that uses porcine hepatocytes attached to collagen microcarriers contained within the extracapillary space of a dialysis cartridge (bioartificial liver). The King's College group, led by Williams, utilize human hepatoblastoma cell lines (extracorporeal liver assist device).[106]

Patients undergo plasma separation and subsequent plasma perfusion through the artificial liver.

Other designs are modifications, and recently Dixit and Gitnick[107] suggested the use of microencapsulated porcine cells. Hepatocytes may improve surface area and membrane permeability characteristics and thus lead to better metabolic exchange of metabolytes with hepatocytes. Preliminary studies have shown successful bridging to transplantation (up to 7 hr with the bioartificial liver and 168 hr in one patient with the extracorporeal liver device), reduction in intracranial pressure, improvement in the grade of hepatic encephalopathy, and decrease in serum ammonia.[105,108,109] Prospective studies are under way.

Another bridging method that may gain acceptance is hepatocyte transplantation. Cryopreserved human hepatocytes are infused into the splenic artery from an advanced percutaneous femoral artery catheter. These isolated hepatocytes appear to survive and even proliferate in the spleen, resulting in a 40% to 60% reduction of ammonia levels.[110] The effect on survival of all the bridging methods is not yet known. Finally, adult-to-adult living donor transplantation through right lobectomy in a sibling has been reported.[111]

Table 10–5. **King's College Hospital Criteria for Expected Nonsurvival among Patients with Fulminant Hepatic Failure**

Patients Affected by Acetaminophen

PH <7.30 (irrespective of grade of encephalopathy)

or

Prothrombin time of >100 sec (INR, >6.5) and serum creatinine of >300 mmol/L (>3.4 mg/dL) in patients with stage III or IV encephalopathy

Patients Not Exposed to Acetaminophen

Prothrombin time of >100 sec (INR, >6.5) (irrespective of stage of encephalopathy)

or

Any three of the following variables (irrespective of stage of encephalopathy):

Age <10 or >40 years

Etiology: non-A, non-B hepatitis, halothane hepatitis, idiosyncratic drug reactions

Duration of jaundice before onset of encephalopathy of >7 days

Prothrombin time of >50 sec (INR, >3.5)

Serum bilirubin level of >300 mmol/L (>17.5 mg/dL)

INR, international normalized ratio.

CONCLUSIONS

Neurologists involved in the critical care of fulminant hepatic failure have had to rethink their laissez-faire attitude toward management of hepatic encephalopathy. Actually, hepatologists have been at the forefront, trying to convince neurologists (and neurosurgeons) that cerebral edema in fulminant hepatic failure is significant and not an epiphenomenon seen in only the fatal cases. Although CT scanning can demonstrate flattening of sulci, disappearance of white and gray matter differentiation, and obliteration of basal cisterns as evidence of cerebral edema, results can be normal in the early stages of encephalopathy. Aggressive treatment of increased ICP may prevent progression to brain death.

The timing of placement of an intracranial monitoring device is controversial. In clinical practice, a device is placed when a Glasgow coma sum score of 8 is reached, often at the same time that endotracheal intubation becomes necessary. Confounding factors (such as high doses of benzodiazepine, hypoglycemia, and hyponatremia) should be excluded first. An ICP monitor may be placed earlier in patients with CT scan features of edema, but normal findings on CT scan should not postpone the decision to place a monitoring device. The often rapid and clinically unexpected progression of signs of brain herniation in this situation justifies placement of a monitor. Every patient with fulminant hepatic failure has considerable coagulopathy, and intraparenchymal placement is not advised. Intracerebral hematomas, although surprisingly uncommon, have been reported with fatal outcome. These risks are low with an epidural ICP monitor.

After correction of ICP and maintenance of cerebral perfusion pressure at >60 mm Hg, monitoring should continue through the transplantation procedure, because marked surges in ICP during reperfusion and during the first 24 hr after return of the patient to the intensive care unit do occur. Treatment of ICP is at times complicated by coexisting renal failure, which precludes administration of mannitol. Propofol should be started not only to control agitation in many patients but also to control ICP. Aggressive management of cerebral edema in fulminant hepatic failure and emergency liver transplantation have improved survival and reduced morbidity. Regrettably, examples exist of patients with fulminant hepatic failure who were potential liver recipients but became brain dead donors of other vital organs and tissues.

REFERENCES

1. Rakela J, Lange SM, Ludwig J, Baldus WP. Fulminant hepatitis: Mayo Clinic experience with 34 cases. Mayo Clin Proc 60:289–292, 1985.
2. Hoofnagle JH, Carithers RL Jr, Shapiro C, Ascher N. Fulminant hepatic failure: summary of a workshop. Hepatology 21:240–252, 1995.
3. Meythaler JM, Varma RR. Reye's syndrome in adults. Diagnostic considerations. Arch Intern Med 147:61–64, 1987.
4. Belay ED, Bresee JS, Holman RC, Khan AS, Shahriari A, Schonberger LB. Reye's syndrome in the United States from 1981 through 1997. N Engl J Med 340:1377–1382, 1999.
5. Adams DH, Kirby RM, Clements D, Elias E, McMaster P. Fulminant hepatic failure treated by hepatic transplantation [letter]. Lancet 2:1037, 1986.
6. Brems JJ, Hiatt JR, Ramming KP, Quinones-Baldrich WJ, Busuttil RW. Fulminant hepatic failure: the role of liver transplantation as primary therapy. Am J Surg 154:137–141, 1987.
7. Emond JC, Aran PP, Whitington PF, Broelsch CE, Baker AL. Liver transplantation in the management of fulminant hepatic failure. Gastroenterology 96:1583–1588, 1989.
8. Bismuth H, Samuel D, Gugenheim J, et al. Emergency liver transplantation for fulminant hepatitis. Ann Intern Med 107:337–341, 1987.
9. Muñoz SJ, Ballas SK, Moritz MJ, et al. Perioperative management of fulminant and subfulminant hepatic failure with therapeutic plasmapheresis. Transplant Proc 21:3535–3536, 1989.
10. O'Grady JG, Gimson AE, O'Brien CJ, Pucknell A, Hughes RD, Williams R. Controlled trials of charcoal hemoperfusion and prognostic factors in fulminant hepatic failure. Gastroenterology 94:1186–1192, 1988.
11. Rothstein JD, Herlong HF. Neurologic manifestations of hepatic disease. Neurol Clin 7:563–578, 1989.
12. Rothstein JD, McKhann GM. Hepatic encephalopathy. Curr Ther Neurol Dis 3:352–356, 1990.
13. Zacharski LR, Litin EM, Mulder DW, Cain JC. Acute, fatal hepatic failure presenting with psychiatric symptoms. Am J Psychiatry 127:382–386, 1970.
14. Fraser CL, Arieff AI. Hepatic encephalopathy. N Engl J Med 313:865–873, 1985.
15. Ritt DJ, Whelan G, Werner DJ, Eigenbrodt EH, Schenker S, Combes B. Acute hepatic necrosis

with stupor or coma. An analysis of thirty-one patients. Medicine (Baltimore) 48:151–172, 1969.

16. Ellis AJ, Wendon JA, Williams R. Subclinical seizure activity and prophylactic phenytoin infusion in acute liver failure: a controlled clinical trial. Hepatology 32:536–541, 2000.

17. Ficker DM, Westmoreland BF, Sharbrough FW. Epileptiform abnormalities in hepatic encephalopathy. J Clin Neurophysiol 14:230–234, 1997.

18. Heubi JE, Daugherty CC, Partin JS, Partin JC, Schubert WK. Grade I Reye's syndrome—outcome and predictors of progression to deeper coma grades. N Engl J Med 311:1539–1542, 1984.

19. Caplan LR, Scheiner D. Dysconjugate gaze in hepatic coma. Ann Neurol 8:328–329, 1980.

20. Plum F, Posner JB. The Diagnosis of Stupor and Coma, 3rd ed. FA Davis, Philadelphia, 1980.

21. Keane JR, Rawlinson RG, Lu AT. Sustained downgaze deviation. Two cases without structural pretectal lesions. Neurology 26:594–595, 1976.

22. Conomy JP, Swash M. Reversible decerebrate and decorticate postures in hepatic coma. N Engl J Med 278:876–879, 1968.

23. Jones EA, Skolnick P, Gammal SH, Basile AS, Mullen KD. NIH conference. The gamma-aminobutyric acid A (GABA$_A$) receptor complex and hepatic encephalopathy. Some recent advances. Ann Intern Med 110:532–546, 1989.

24. Butterworth RF, Pomier Layrargues G. Benzodiazepine receptors and hepatic encephalopathy. Hepatology 11:499–501, 1990.

25. Bassett ML, Mullen KD, Skolnick P, Jones EA. Amelioration of hepatic encephalopathy by pharmacologic antagonism of the GABA$_A$-benzodiazepine receptor complex in a rabbit model of fulminant hepatic failure. Gastroenterology 93:1069–1077, 1987.

26. Grimm G, Ferenci P, Katzenschlager R, et al. Improvement of hepatic encephalopathy treated with flumazenil. Lancet 2:1392–1394, 1988.

27. Jones EA, Basile AS, Mullen KD, Gammal SH. Flumazenil: Potential implications for hepatic encephalopathy. Pharmacol Ther 45:331–343, 1990.

28. van der Rijt C, Schalm SW. Quantitative EEG analysis and survival in liver disease. Electroencephalogr Clin Neurophysiol 61:502–504, 1985.

29. Basile AS, Pannell L, Jaouni T, et al. Brain concentrations of benzodiazepines are elevated in an animal model of hepatic encephalopathy. Proc Natl Acad Sci U S A 87:5263–5267, 1990.

30. Mullen KD, Szauter KM, Kaminsky-Russ K. "Endogenous" benzodiazepine activity in body fluids of patients with hepatic encephalopathy. Lancet 336:81–83, 1990.

31. Samson Y, Bernuau J, Pappata S, Chavoix C, Baron JC, Maziere MA. Cerebral uptake of benzodiazepine measured by positron emission tomography in hepatic encephalopathy [letter]. N Engl J Med 316:414–415, 1987.

32. Scollo-Lavizzari G, Steinmann E, Bansky G, et al. Reversal of hepatic coma by benzodiazepine antagonist (Ro 15-1788) [letter]. Lancet 1:1324–1325, 1985.

33. Barbaro G, Di Lorenzo G, Soldini M, et al. Flumazenil for hepatic encephalopathy grade III

and IVa in patients with cirrhosis: an Italian multicenter double-blind, placebo-controlled, crossover study. Hepatology 28:374–378, 1998.

34. Gyr K, Meier R, Haussler J, et al. Evaluation of the efficacy and safety of flumazenil in the treatment of portal systemic encephalopathy: a double blind, randomised, placebo controlled multicentre study. Gut 39:319–324, 1996.

35. Groeneweg M, Gyr K, Amrein R, et al. Effect of flumazenil on the electroencephalogram of patients with portosystemic encephalopathy. Results of a double blind, randomised, placebo-controlled multicentre trial. Electroencephalogr Clin Neurophysiol 98:29–34, 1996.

36. Zieve L, Olsen RL. Can hepatic coma be caused by a reduction of brain noradrenaline or dopamine? Gut 18:688–691, 1977.

37. Jones EA, Gammal SH. Hepatic encephalopathy. In: Arias IM (ed). The Liver: Biology and Pathobiology, 2nd ed. Raven Press, New York, 1988, pp 985–1005.

38. Szerb JC, Butterworth RF. Effect of ammonium ions on synaptic transmission in the mammalian central nervous system. Prog Neurobiol 39:135–153, 1992.

39. Raabe W. Synaptic transmission in ammonia intoxication. Neurochem Pathol 6:145–166, 1987.

40. Fan P, Lavoie J, Le NL, Szerb JC, Butterworth RF. Neurochemical and electrophysiological studies on the inhibitory effect of ammonium ions on synaptic transmission in slices of rat hippocampus: evidence for a postsynaptic action. Neuroscience 37:327–334, 1990.

41. Norenberg MD, Mozes LW, Papendick RE, Norenberg L-OB. Effect of ammonia on glutamate, γ-aminobutyric acid, and rubidium uptake by astrocytes [abstract]. Ann Neurol 18:149, 1985.

42. Peterson C, Giguere JF, Cotman CW, Butterworth RF. Selective loss of N-methyl-D-aspartate-sensitive L-[^{3}H]glutamate binding sites in rat brain following portacaval anastomosis. J Neurochem 55:386–390, 1990.

43. Rao VL, Agrawal AK, Murthy CR. Ammonia-induced alterations in glutamate and muscimol binding to cerebellar synaptic membranes. Neurosci Lett 130:251–254, 1991.

44. Rao VL, Giguère JF, Layrargues GP, Butterworth RF. Increased activities of MAO$_A$ and MAO$_B$ in autopsied brain tissue from cirrhotic patients with hepatic encephalopathy. Brain Res 621:349–352, 1993.

45. Mousseau DD, Butterworth RF. Current theories on the pathogenesis of hepatic encephalopathy. Proc Soc Exp Biol Med 206:329–344, 1994.

46. Rothstein JD, McKhann G, Guarneri P, Barbaccia ML, Guidotti A, Costa E. Cerebrospinal fluid content of diazepam binding inhibitor in chronic hepatic encephalopathy. Ann Neurol 26:57–62, 1989.

47. Record CO, Iles RA, Cohen RD, Williams R. Acid-base and metabolic disturbances in fulminant hepatic failure. Gut 16:144–149, 1975.

48. Trauner DA, Huttenlocher PR. Short chain fatty acid-induced central hyperventilation in rabbits. Neurology 28:940–944, 1978.

49. Madl C, Grimm G, Ferenci P, et al. Serial recording of sensory evoked potentials: a noninvasive

prognostic indicator in fulminant liver failure. Hepatology 20:1487–1494, 1994.

50. Yang SS, Chu NS, Liaw YF. Somatosensory evoked potentials in hepatic encephalopathy. Gastroenterology 89:625–630, 1985.

51. Davies MG, Rowan MJ, Feely J. Flash visual evoked responses in the early encephalopathy of chronic liver disease. Scand J Gastroenterol 25:1205–1214, 1990.

52. Johansson U, Andersson T, Persson A, Eriksson LS. Visual evoked potential—a tool in the diagnosis of hepatic encephalopathy? J Hepatol 9:227–233, 1989.

53. Sandford NL, Saul RE. Assessment of hepatic encephalopathy with visual evoked potentials compared with conventional methods. Hepatology 8: 1094–1098, 1988.

54. Mehndiratta MM, Sood GK, Sarin SK, Gupta M. Comparative evaluation of visual, somatosensory, and auditory evoked potentials in the detection of subclinical hepatic encephalopathy in patients with nonalcoholic cirrhosis. Am J Gastroenterol 85:799–803, 1990.

55. Bahamon-Dussan JE, Celesia GG, Grigg-Damberger MM. Prognostic significance of EEG triphasic waves in patients with altered state of consciousness. J Clin Neurophysiol 6:313–319, 1989.

56. Fisch BJ, Klass DW. The diagnostic specificity of triphasic wave patterns. Electroencephalogr Clin Neurophysiol 70:1–8, 1988.

57. Hauser RA, Zesiewicz TA, Martinez C, Rosemurgy AS, Olanow CW. Blood manganese correlates with brain magnetic resonance imaging changes in patients with liver disease. Can J Neurol Sci 23:95–98, 1996.

58. Krieger D, Krieger S, Jansen O, Gass P, Theilmann L, Lichtnecker H. Manganese and chronic hepatic encephalopathy. Lancet 346:270–274, 1995.

59. Spahr L, Butterworth RF, Fontaine S, et al. Increased blood manganese in cirrhotic patients: relationship to pallidal magnetic resonance signal hyperintensity and neurological symptoms. Hepatology 24:1116–1120, 1996.

60. Malecki EA, Devenyi AG, Barron TF, et al. Iron and manganese homeostasis in chronic liver disease: relationship to pallidal T1-weighted magnetic resonance signal hyperintensity. Neurotoxicology 20:647–652, 1999.

61. Pujol A, Pujol J, Graus F, et al. Hyperintense globus pallidus on T1-weighted MRI in cirrhotic patients is associated with severity of liver failure. Neurology 43:65–69, 1993.

62. Naylor CD, O'Rourke K, Detsky AS, Baker JP. Parenteral nutrition with branched-chain amino acids in hepatic encephalopathy. A meta-analysis. Gastroenterology 97:1033–1042, 1989.

63. Ede RJ, Williams RW. Hepatic encephalopathy and cerebral edema. Semin Liver Dis 6:107–118, 1986.

64. Ware AJ, D'Agostino AN, Combes B. Cerebral edema: a major complication of massive hepatic necrosis. Gastroenterology 61:877–884, 1971.

65. O'Grady JG, Schalm SW, Williams R. Acute liver failure: redefining the syndromes. Lancet 342: 273–275, 1993.

66. Ytrebo LM, Ingebrigtsen T, Nedredal GI, et al. Protein S-100beta: a biochemical marker for increased intracranial pressure in pigs with acute hepatic failure. Scand J Gastroenterol 35:546–551, 2000.

67. Strauss GI, Knudsen GM, Christiansen M, Møller K, Hansen BA, Larsen FS. Neuronal and glial markers and their relation to cerebral herniation in fulminant hepatic failure [abstract]. Liver Transpl 6:C-37, 2000.

68. Blei AT. Cerebral edema and intracranial hypertension in acute liver failure: distinct aspects of the same problem. Hepatology 13:376–379, 1991.

69. Cordoba J, Blei AT. Brain edema and hepatic encephalopathy. Semin Liver Dis 16:271–280, 1996.

70. Kato M, Hughes RD, Keays RT, Williams R. Electron microscopic study of brain capillaries in cerebral edema from fulminant hepatic failure. Hepatology 15:1060–1066, 1992.

71. Livingstone AS, Potvin M, Goresky CA, Finlayson MH, Hinchey EJ. Changes in the blood–brain barrier in hepatic coma after hepatectomy in the rat. Gastroenterology 73.697–704, 1977.

72. Butterworth RF. Hepatic encephalopathy and brain edema in acute hepatic failure: does glutamate play a role? Hepatology 25:1032–1034, 1997.

73. Cordoba J, Gottstein J, Blei AT. Glutamine, myoinositol, and organic brain osmolytes after portocaval anastomosis in the rat: implications for ammonia-induced brain edema. Hepatology 24: 919–923, 1996.

74. Strauss G, Hansen BA, Kirkegaard P, Rasmussen A, Hjortrup A, Larsen FS. Liver function, cerebral blood flow autoregulation, and hepatic encephalopathy in fulminant hepatic failure. Hepatology 25:837–839, 1997.

75. Norenberg MD. Astrocytic-ammonia interactions in hepatic encephalopathy. Semin Liver Dis 16: 245–253, 1996.

76. Norenberg MD. Astroglial dysfunction in hepatic encephalopathy. Metab Brain Dis 13:319–335, 1998.

77. Manley GT, Fujimura M, Ma T, et al. Aquaporin-4 deletion in mice reduces brain edema after acute water intoxication and ischemic stroke. Nat Med 6:159–163, 2000.

78. Lidofsky SD, Bass NM, Prager MC, et al. Intracranial pressure monitoring and liver transplantation for fulminant hepatic failure. Hepatology 16:1–7, 1992.

79. Muñoz SJ, Robinson M, Northrup B, et al. Elevated intracranial pressure and computed tomography of the brain in fulminant hepatocellular failure. Hepatology 13:209–212, 1991.

80. Wijdicks EFM, Plevak DJ, Rakela J, Wiesner RH. Clinical and radiologic features of cerebral edema in fulminant hepatic failure. Mayo Clin Proc 70: 119–124, 1995.

81. Blei AT, Olafsson S, Webster S, Levy R. Complications of intracranial pressure monitoring in fulminant hepatic failure. Lancet 341:157–158, 1993.

82. Hanid MA, Davies M, Mellon PJ, et al. Clinical monitoring of intracranial pressure in fulminant hepatic failure. Gut 21:866–869, 1980.

83. Keays R, Potter D, O'Grady J, Peachey T, Alexander G, Williams R. Intracranial and cerebral perfusion

pressure changes before, during and immediately after orthotopic liver transplantation for fulminant hepatic failure. Q J Med 79:425–433, 1991.

84. LeRoux PD, Elliott JP, Perkins JD, Winn HR. Intracranial pressure monitoring in fulminant hepatic failure and liver transplantation [letter]. Lancet 335:1291, 1990.

85. Potter D, Peachey T, Eason J, Ginsberg R, O'Grady J. Intracranial pressure monitoring during orthotopic liver transplantation for acute liver failure. Transplant Proc 21:3528, 1989.

86. Detry O, Arkadopoulos N, Ting P, et al. Intracranial pressure during liver transplantation for fulminant hepatic failure. Transplantation 67:767–770, 1999.

87. Davenport A, Will EJ, Davison AM. Effect of posture on intracranial pressure and cerebral perfusion pressure in patients with fulminant hepatic and renal failure after acetaminophen self-poisoning. Crit Care Med 18:286–289, 1990.

88. Feldman Z, Kanter MJ, Robertson CS, et al. Effect of head elevation on intracranial pressure, cerebral perfusion pressure, and cerebral blood flow in head-injured patients. J Neurosurg 76:207–211, 1992.

89. Ede RJ, Gimson AE, Bihari D, Williams R. Controlled hyperventilation in the prevention of cerebral oedema in fulminant hepatic failure. J Hepatol 2:43–51, 1986.

90. Strauss GI, Moller K, Holm S, Sperling B, Knudsen GM, Larsen FS. Transcranial Doppler sonography and internal jugular bulb saturation during hyperventilation in patients with fulminant hepatic failure. Liver Transpl 7:352–358, 2001.

91. Williams R, Gimson AE. Intensive liver care and management of acute hepatic failure. Dig Dis Sci 36:820–826, 1991.

92. Muñoz SJ, Moritz MJ, Bell R, Northrup B, Martin P, Radomski J. Factors associated with severe intracranial hypertension in candidates for emergency liver transplantation. Transplantation 55:1071–1074, 1993.

93. Daas M, Plevak DJ, Wijdicks EFM, et al. Acute liver failure: results of a 5-year clinical protocol. Liver Transpl Surg 1:210–219, 1995.

94. Forbes A, Alexander GJ, O'Grady JG, et al. Thiopental infusion in the treatment of intracranial hypertension complicating fulminant hepatic failure. Hepatology 10:306–310, 1989.

95. Wijdicks EFM, Nyberg S. The role of propofol in management of intracranial pressure in fulminant hepatic failure (submitted for publication).

96. Cordoba J, Crespin J, Gottstein J, Blei AT. Mild hypothermia modifies ammonia-induced brain edema in rats after portacaval anastomosis. Gastroenterology 116:686–693, 1999.

97. Jalan R, Damink SWMO, Deutz NEP, Lee A, Hayes PC. Moderate hypothermia for uncontrolled intracranial hypertension in acute liver failure. Lancet 354:1164–1168, 1999.

98. Clemmesen JO, Hansen BA, Larsen FS. Indomethacin normalizes intracranial pressure in acute liver failure: a twenty-three-year-old woman treated with indomethacin. Hepatology 26:1423–1425, 1997.

99. Arkadopoulos N, Chen SC, Khalili TM, et al. Transplantation of hepatocytes for prevention of intracranial hypertension in pigs with ischemic liver failure. Cell Transplant 7:357–363, 1998.

100. Watanabe FD, Mullon CJ, Hewitt WR, et al. Clinical experience with a bioartificial liver in the treatment of severe liver failure. A phase I clinical trial. Ann Surg 225:484–491, 1997.

101. Eckhoff DE, Pirsch JD, D'Alessandro AM, et al. Pretransplant status and patient survival following liver transplantation. Transplantation 60:920–925, 1995.

102. Roger V, Balladur P, Honiger J, et al. Internal bioartificial liver with xenogeneic hepatocytes prevents death from acute liver failure: an experimental study. Ann Surg 228:1–7, 1998.

103. Kim SS, Utsunomiya H, Koski JA, et al. Survival and function of hepatocytes on a novel three-dimensional synthetic biodegradable polymer scaffold with an intrinsic network of channels. Ann Surg 228:8–13, 1998.

104. McLaughlin BE, Tosone CM, Custer LM, Mullon C. Overview of extracorporeal liver support systems and clinical results. Ann N Y Acad Sci 875:310–325, 1999.

105. Demetriou AA. Support of the acutely failing liver: state of the art. Ann Surg 228:14–15, 1998.

106. Riordan S, Williams R. Bioartificial liver support: developments in hepatocyte culture and bioreactor design. Br Med Bull 53:730–744, 1997.

107. Dixit V, Gitnick G. The bioartificial liver: state-of-the-art. Eur J Surg Suppl 582:71–76, 1998.

108. Ellis AJ, Hughes RD, Wendon JA, et al. Pilot-controlled trial of the extracorporeal liver assist device in acute liver failure. Hepatology 24:1446–1451, 1996.

109. Rozga J, Podesta L, LePage E, et al. A bioartificial liver to treat severe acute liver failure. Ann Surg 219:538–544, 1994.

110. Strom SC, Fisher RA, Thompson MT, et al. Hepatocyte transplantation as a bridge to orthotopic liver transplantation in terminal liver failure. Transplantation 63:559–569, 1997.

111. Marcos A, Ham JM, Fisher RA, et al. Emergency adult to adult living donor liver transplantation for fulminant hepatic failure. Transplantation 69:2202–2205, 2000.

Chapter 11

NEUROLOGIC COMPLICATIONS ASSOCIATED WITH DISORDERS OF THROMBOSIS AND HEMOSTASIS

Epidemiologic studies of coagulopathies targeted to neurologic complications in critically ill patients are notably few, and even in these studies they appear uncommon. In one comprehensive study, for instance, 2 of 118 patients with disseminated intravascular coagulation had neurologic complications.[1] Many unconfirmed clinical vignettes have been reported, and their significance in contributing to the spectrum of hematologic disorders in the intensive care unit (ICU) remains uncertain.

Thrombocytopenias or thrombocytopathies are likely to be the prime causes of bleeding disorders in the ICU. Thrombocytopenia (platelet count $<100,000/\mu L$) is common in critically ill patients and most of the time is due to decreased platelet production or increased platelet destruction. However, dilution (blood transfusion), altered distribution (splenomegaly), or even a spurious cause from insufficient anticoagulation of the blood sample, which causes platelet aggregation, should be considered.[2] Other triggers for thrombocytopenia are drugs (for example, heparin, antibiotics), massive blood transfusion, and intravascular coagulation with sepsis. In some instances, thrombocytopenia due to thrombotic thrombocytopenic purpura may coincide with neurologic manifestations. Thrombocytopathies, however, are often induced by uremia and cardiopulmonary bypass. Isolated factor deficiencies should be excluded in any event but are of limited relevance in this situation.

Multiorgan failure in critically ill patients is another important trigger of complex coagulopathies, and in some patients the point may be reached at which neurologic complications emerge. Conversely, catastrophic neurologic illness, predominantly traumatic brain injury and gunshots to the head, can initiate systemic activation of coagulation from entry of brain thromboplastin.[3]

Another major potential for bleeding in ICUs is the use of anticoagulation and thrombolytic therapy. Both have been used increasingly, and both may result in ominous neurologic complications.

This chapter attempts to draw all disparate observations into a coherent overview of the most commonly seen complications.

Table 11–1. **Causes of Disseminated Intravascular Coagulation in the Intensive Care Unit**

Sepsis or septic shock syndrome[4]

Massive blood transfusions

Burns

Aortic balloon pump or cardiopulmonary bypass

Infection after splenectomy

Toxic shock syndrome

Viremias (e.g., cytomegalovirus)[5]

Cancer (including acute leukemias)[6]

Massive tissue trauma

Aortic aneurysm*[7–9]

Head injury (often gunshot wounds)*[10–15]

Subarachnoid hemorrhage[16]

Neuroleptic malignant syndrome[17]

Cardiac arrest*[18]

*Many patients do not have clinical signs.

DISSEMINATED INTRAVASCULAR COAGULATION

Much morbidity in medical and surgical ICUs is related to acute disseminated intravascular coagulation (DIC). The conditions associated with DIC are summarized in Table 11–1. Failure to recognize these triggers results in self-perpetuation of the common pathways of clotting activation. The thrombotic coagulopathy is primarily responsible for significant end-organ damage.

Patients with DIC have clinical symptoms that pertain to both hemorrhage and thrombosis. Activation of the coagulation system is complex and partly unresolved, but systemic circulating thrombin and plasmin both have pivotal roles. Thrombin is a product of activation of the clotting cascade and, in turn, catalyzes the breakdown of fibrinogen into fibrin monomers. These monomers polymerize into fibrin, which leads to obstructive clots in the microvasculature. Furthermore, trapping of platelets into these fibrin clots results in considerable thrombocytopenia in this condition (often <50,000 platelets/μL). The laboratory diagnosis of DIC becomes likely when a decreased platelet count, decreased fibrinogen plasma level, and prolonged thrombin time are found. At the other end of the spectrum are the manifestations of proteolysis of fibrin by plasmin. Small fragments resulting from degradation of fibrinogen coat platelet membrane surfaces and contribute to defective platelet function in addition to the already existing thrombocytopenia. Demonstration of the fibrin degradation products by latex particle agglutination or hemagglutination test (often >40 μg/mL) is a strong indicator of DIC. The laboratory indicators of DIC are summarized in Table 11–2. More sophisticated laboratory tests can detect antithrombin III, increase in platelet 4, and increase in fibrinopeptide A. A recent analysis of 240 patients with DIC found that plasma levels of soluble fibrin monomer, D-dimer (D-dimers are formed after plasmin digestion of cross-linked fibrin), and thrombin–antithrombin complex were increased early during development of the disorder, and documentation of these components may be useful for screening.[21] Probably the most valuable test remains the D-dimer assay with monoclonal antibodies.[22]

The diagnosis of DIC is signaled by con-

Table 11–2. **Laboratory Support of Disseminated Intravascular Coagulation**

Indicator	Patients with This Finding (%)
Prolonged prothrombin time	65–75
Prolonged partial thromboplastin time	50–60
Thrombocytopenia (<60,000 platelets/μL)	80–90
Increase in fibrin degradation products	85–100
Red cell fragments	40–50

Data from Baker,[19] Bick,[20] and Siegal et al.[1]

tinued oozing of surgical wounds and arterial or venous puncture sites. In addition to these subtle clinical signs, petechiae, purpura, and large subcutaneous hematomas may develop. Intravascular fibrin and platelet deposition probably accounts for most of the clinical symptoms. Microthrombi compromise many organs and lodge particularly in the pulmonary and renal circulation. Thus, acute renal failure and acute respiratory distress syndrome are potential life-threatening complications that require urgent intervention. Signs of microvascular thrombosis may also involve the skin and result in superficial gangrene. Neurologic complications of DIC consist of intracerebral hemorrhage,[23] cerebral artery branch occlusions,[24–26] and, probably more common, cerebral sinus thrombosis.[27,28]

Cerebral Venous Thrombosis

Patients in a hypercoagulable state are also likely to have venous thrombi. Pathologic studies have thoroughly documented cerebral venous thrombosis in patients with rapid development of DIC. Little, however, is known of the risk in patients without terminal coagulopathy.

Clinical features of cerebral venous occlusion with involvement of large cerebral veins, such as the superior sagittal sinus and superficial middle cerebral vein, are characterized by a rapidly progressive decrease in consciousness without any warning localizing signs.[27] Initially, most patients (74%) present with severe headache, and approximately 50% display papilledema. If patients become drowsy or confused, it may signal development of areas of venous infarction. A considerable number have recurrent tonic–clonic seizures.

Cerebral venous sinus occlusion can be assessed by computed tomography (CT) scanning. A string-like hyperintensity may be seen but sometimes is too close to the occipital bone to be appreciated. This sign represents a clot in the transverse sinus. Other CT scan findings are unilateral or bilateral hypodensities or mixed densities suggesting hemorrhagic infarction and increased tentorial or gyral enhancement or an empty triangle-delta sign in contrast studies. Oc-

clusion of the internal cerebral veins may result in bilateral thalamic hypodensities or hemorrhages[29,30] (Fig. 11–1). Magnetic resonance imaging (MRI) with magnetic resonance venography is the preferred mode of imaging in assessment of cerebral venous thrombosis,[29,31,32] but transport of these critically ill patients may be very difficult.

Ischemic and Hemorrhagic Strokes

Ischemic strokes are less commonly seen, although microthrombi in small or medium-sized vessels are frequent histopathologic findings. Thrombi also may lodge in the choriocapillaris, causing visual loss and metamorphopsia, but fortunately, the condition is rare and transient.[33] Occlusion of major arterial branches, primarily the middle cerebral artery, may occur, but as dictated by small scattered thrombi, territorial involvement is small.[34]

Our recent review of 19 patients with critical medical illness and new-onset stroke showed that DIC was an associated finding in 60% of patients with ischemic stroke or hemorrhagic stroke.[35] Neurologic presentation in these patients with intravascular coagulation is commonly diffuse bihemispheric involvement resulting in various degrees of coma. Multiple cerebral infarcts initially caused hemiparesis, but coma intervened quickly. The CT scan was insufficient in documenting these infarcts, which were easily apparent on MRI (Fig. 11–2).

Anecdotal reports have mentioned subdural hematoma and subarachnoid hemorrhage. Subarachnoid hemorrhage is usually limited to the convexity.[23,26] Subcortical petechial hemorrhages have been reported on CT scans in patients with DIC and are identical to the pathologic descriptions[36] (Fig. 11–1B,C).

Treatment

The treatment of patients with neurologic manifestations of DIC, including an aggressive approach with subcutaneous administration of a low dose of heparin (80 U/kg every 4 to 6 hr), depends on the underlying

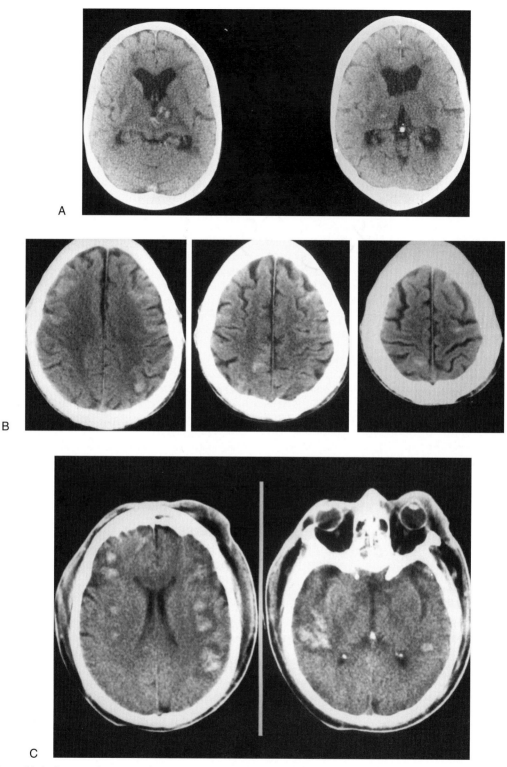

Figure 11–1. Computed tomography scan patterns in disseminated intravascular coagulation. *A*: Bilateral hemorrhagic thalamic infarction associated with deep cerebral vein thrombosis. *B*: Petechial hemorrhages in the white matter. *C*: Multiple small intracerebral hemorrhages. (Panels *B* and *C* from Wijdicks et al.[36] By permission of the American Society of Neuroradiology.)

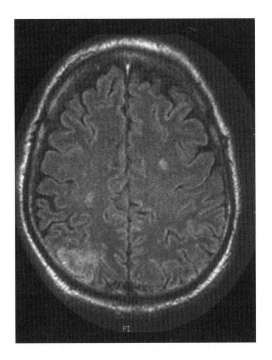

Figure 11–2. Multiple hyperintensities on fluid-attenuated inversion recovery (FLAIR) magnetic resonance image in a patient with florid disseminated intravascular coagulation.

cause.[19,20] Full intravenous heparin administration (activated partial thromboplastin time 2 × control value) is indicated in patients who have associated cerebral venous thrombosis.[37,38] A randomized trial (using 300 IU and 25,000 to 65,000 IU/day, with target partial thromboplastin time between 80 and 100 sec) demonstrated striking differences in morbidity and mortality and included patients who had already had hemorrhagic infarctions.[37] Most patients in the heparin group had complete clinical recovery, whereas in the control group, most patients remained severely disabled or died. Low-molecular-weight heparin is probably equally effective.[39]

Alternative treatment may be perfusion of the sinus with tissue-type plasminogen activator (tPA).[40,41] Preliminary series have documented successful recanalization, but this approach, mastered by interventional neuroradiologists, has not been performed in critically ill patients, predominantly because diagnosis of the disorder most likely signifies a critical terminal moment.

THROMBOLYSIS AND ANTICOAGULATION

Thrombolytic therapy and anticoagulation are widely used in medical and cardiac ICUs.[42–49] The efficacy of thrombolytic therapy has also been tested in patients with other critical illnesses, occlusion of vascular access shunts, thrombi from vascular grafts, and peripheral arterial thromboembolic disease, and promising results have been claimed. Its use in treatment of pulmonary emboli remains controversial, with no proven effect over intravenous heparin.[50–52] The current generation of thrombolytic agents has the potential to be more fibrin-specific and is less likely to cause a systemic response, but bleeding into the gastrointestinal tract, retroperitoneal space, and the brain occurs.

The evidence now available indicates that patients with acute myocardial infarction can substantially benefit from thrombolytic treatment (mostly tPA). The margin of benefit, however, may be smaller if coronary perfusion is not restored within 4 hr after occlusion. Thrombolytic therapy is usually combined with full doses of intravenously administered heparin for several days to prevent reocclusion, a combination that may in some cases account for the increased incidence of hemorrhagic complications.

Thrombolysis-Associated Cerebral Hemorrhage

Studies of thrombolysis-induced intracerebral hemorrhage have reported rates of 0.4% to 0.7%.[45,53–55] In most large clinical trials on thrombolysis, prevalence of intracerebral complications is biased by exclusion of patients with previous strokes and patients with moderate hypertension. Moreover, in most thrombolysis trials, one-third of the patients were not properly investigated and had strokes of undetermined origin.[56] Cerebral infarcts are equally frequent, and hemorrhagic transformation of a large cerebral infarct or hemorrhage in a previous infarct may also occur and cannot always be reliably differentiated from a spontaneous lobar hematoma. Subdural hematomas are rare (0.2% in the Thrombolysis in Myocardial Infarction, phase II [TIMI II] trial).

Intracerebral hemorrhage after administration of thrombolytic agents occurs within a few hours but has been reported up to 2 days after bolus injection, which weakens the association with these short-acting agents.[57–64] In the TIMI II trial, 65% of intracranial hematomas occurred within 12 hr and 83% within 24 hr after tPA infusion and continuous heparin treatment. In the National Registry of Myocardial Infarction 2, reliable data on intracerebral hematomas in 600 patients revealed that 74% occurred within 24 hr, 13% were between 24 and 48 hr, and 13% occurred 48 or more hr after treatment with tPA.[65]

Most hematomas are localized in the subcortical white matter. In some patients, additional lobar hematomas develop in previously infarcted areas of the brain. Less common sites are the putamen, vermis, cerebellar hemispheres,[66] and pons (Table 11–3), but this finding may reflect exclusion of patients with hypertension from treatment trials. The CT scan characteristics of thrombolysis-associated hemorrhage have been compared with those of other types of lobar hemorrhages (Fig. 11–3). More prevalent in thrombolysis-associated hemorrhages are fluid levels inside the hematoma (indicating continuing anticoagulation), multiple parenchymal hemorrhages, and hemorrhages in multiple intracranial compartments, including the intraventricular, subdural, and subarachnoid spaces. In one large study (Table 11–3), multiple sites of hemorrhage occurred in 45% of cases, but in our series 75% of the patients with thrombolysis-associated hemorrhages had hemorrhages in three or more compartments.[64] These characteristics are not unique to tPA or the combination with heparin, because the same pattern of multiple compartment involvement and fluid levels has been seen in warfarin-associated intracerebral hematomas.[67] Hemorrhage in only intraventricular or subarachnoid compartments without intraparenchymal hemorrhage is rare but has been described. In Uglietta and associates' series,[63] one patient had subdural hematoma in the posterior fossa and between hemispheres, both very uncommon locations.

The clinical course in many patients is devastating, and emergency neurosurgical intervention probably will be unsuccessful. In addition, early aggressive medical treatment may not prevent deterioration, because these hematomas rapidly enlarge[64] (Fig. 11–3B). Moreover, outcome is poor because many patients have large hematomas within hours after onset.[64]

Risk factors for intracerebral hematomas have been identified, and age of 70 years or more appears to be a major risk factor.[68,69] In a retrospective analysis, transient increased blood pressure (150/90 mm Hg or greater) tended to be more frequent in patients with intracerebral hemorrhage.[68] Only systolic blood pressure was statistically significant, a finding that suggested a systemic response rather than a direct cause of intracerebral hemorrhage.

Table 11–3. **Anatomical Distribution of Intracerebral Hematomas, after Thrombolysis for Acute Myocardial Infarction***

Location	No.	%
Lobe	229	77
Cerebellum	27	9
Putamen, internal capsule	24	8
Thalamus	9	3
Brain stem	9	3

*Total of 298 hemorrhages due to multiplicity in 54 (45%) patients.

From Gebel JM, Sila CA, Sloan MA, et al. Thrombolysis-related intracranial hemorrhage: a radiographic analysis of 244 cases from the GUSTO-1 trial with clinical correlation. Global Utilization of Streptokinase and Tissue Plasminogen Activator for Occluded Coronary Arteries. Stroke 29:563–569, 1998. By permission of Lippincott Williams & Wilkins.

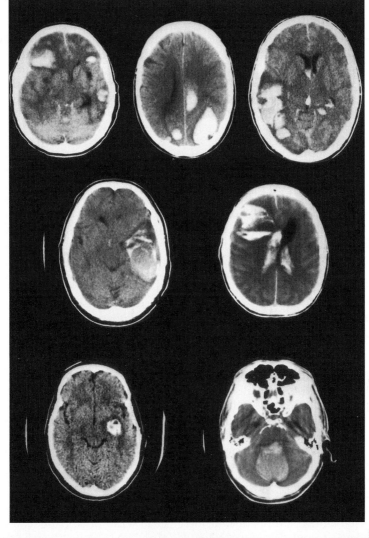

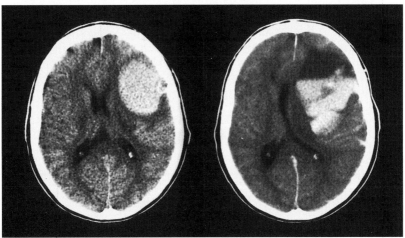

Figure 11–3. *A*: Patterns of intracerebral hematoma associated with tissue plasminogen activator. Multiple compartment hemorrhages are shown in the top row, lobar hemorrhages with prominent fluid levels in the middle row, and putamen and vermis hemorrhage in the bottom row. *B*: Sequential computed tomography scans (1 hr apart) in a patient with intracerebral hematoma associated with tissue plasminogen activator. Note extensive enlargement, fluid level, and shift. (From Wijdicks and Jack.[64] By permission of the American Heart Association.)

Also, the frequent lobar localization of the hemorrhages in thrombolysis-associated intracerebral hematomas argues against hypertension as a major contributing factor. Patients with hypertension usually have hematomas in the distribution of perforating vessels—sites such as the basal ganglia, posterior lateral thalamus, pons, and cerebellar hemispheres.

Kase and associates[59] found that activated partial thromboplastin time was excessively prolonged in two-thirds of their patient population with hemorrhages. In an analysis of 71,073 patients with myocardial infarction treated with tPA, Gurwitz and associates[65] found the following powerful risk factors for tPA-associated intracerebral hemorrhages: older patient (age over 75 years), low body weight, female sex, and black ethnicity. Appropriate weight-adjusted doses could reduce the risk.

The pathophysiologic mechanism of tPA-associated intracerebral hematoma is unresolved. However, we and others initially postulated that the increased incidence in the elderly and multiplicity and superficial lobar location of hematomas may support a role for severe cerebral amyloid angiopathy in this subset of patients. Amyloid angiopathy is much more prevalent in the octogenarian, but only a few patients have severe involvement with "leaky arteries" due to amyloid deposits. In a few patients with tPA-associated intracerebral hematoma, severe amyloid angiopathy has been found at autopsy when specifically looked for with Congo red stain under polarized light.[64] Severe amyloid angiopathy, pathologically characterized by fibroid necrosis and continuous blood leakage may cause only a lobar hemorrhage when the balance between clotting and hemorrhage is acutely disturbed by tPA and heparin. However, the role of advanced amyloid angiopathy in hemorrhages associated with thrombolytics or warfarin remains discordant, and study results are conflicting.[70,71]

Guidelines for management are summarized in Table 11–4. It is reasonable in the management of intracerebral hemorrhage to treat persistent hypertension (mean arterial pressure >120 mm Hg) in a patient with continuing bleeding. Hypertension is associated with catecholamine surges and can, therefore, probably be best managed with single doses of labetalol (20 to 80 mg intravenously) or esmolol (200 to 500 μg/kg). The principal agents for bleeding management are cryoprecipitate and fresh-frozen plasma, not antifibrinolytic drugs. Antifibrinolytic drugs carry the risk of coronary reocclusion and may cause extensive insoluble clots in the renal collecting system. Rapid progression of the hematoma may warrant neurosurgical evacuation, but this procedure seems only lifesaving.[72] Survivors are often markedly disabled. Recently, Sloan and associates[73] published an observational analysis of patients with intracerebral hematoma in which they predicted 30-day mortality in those with large-volume hematomas, low Glasgow coma scale sum scores, and early occurrence of hemorrhage after treatment (Table 11–5). A recently reported neurosurgical series of 46 patients with thrombolysis-associated hemorrhages suggested reduction in mortality and possible improved functional outcome after evacuation, but bias toward surgery in the least affected patients probably confounded the results. Nevertheless, neurosurgical consultation is war-

Table 11–4. **Guidelines for Treatment of Thrombolysis-Associated Intracerebral Hematomas**

Step 1	Cryoprecipitate	10 units
	Fresh frozen plasma	2 units
	Protamine	1 mg/100 U of heparin
Step 2	Bleeding time >9 min	Platelets, 10 units
Step 3	Repeat computed tomography scan 1 to 3 hr later; progression with shift	Consider neurosurgical evacuation or needle aspiration

Data from Eleff et al.[72]

ranted.[74] Good recovery after craniotomy has been reported, but only in patients with intracerebral hemorrhages of limited size without mass effect. Outcome was good in a report of successful needle aspiration of a tPA-associated hematoma with a fluid level.[75] We also were successful in draining a subdural hematoma in a patient with multiple compartmental hemorrhages (Fig. 11–4), and this patient reached functional independence.

The frequency of intracranial hemorrhage in the ICU after treatment of pulmonary emboli with thrombolysis has been reported. The incidence reached 2% in some studies, higher than that in myocardial infarction, but the overall figures of all reported studies combined were similar, averaging 1.2%.[76]

Anticoagulant Therapy

Anticoagulation with heparin or warfarin is used in critically ill patients who have evidence of systemic embolization. Heparin is also frequently used postoperatively in patients who had major cardiac or vascular procedures. Life-threatening bleeding complications from anticoagulation are relatively rare. The risk of bleeding complications has decreased by international normalized ratio measures and is 2.9% per year. The immediate risk of hemorrhage in the ICU is not known.[77]

Intracerebral hemorrhage may occur during initiation of anticoagulation. In a review of 24 patients with anticoagulation-associated intracerebral hemorrhage, Kase and co-workers,[78] found a predilection for

Table 11–5. Prediction of 30-Day Mortality after Thrombolysis-Associated Intracerebral Hemorrhage

AGE (YEARS)		GLASGOW COMA SCALE (GCS) SCORE		TIME FROM THROMBOLYSIS TO ONSET OF HEMORRHAGE (HR)		TOTAL HEMORRHAGIC VOLUME (MM³)*		Point Total†	Mortality Risk (%)
Age	Points	Score	Points	Time	Points	Volume	Points		
≤40	0	3	20	0	100	≤50	0	87	1
45	2	4	18	20	93	60	2	97	5
50	4	5	16	40	87	80	5	101	10
55	5	6	15	60	80	100	9	109	30
60	7	7	13	80	73	120	13	115	50
65	9	8	12	100	67	140	16	120	70
70	11	9	10	120	60	160	20	128	90
75	13	10	8	140	53	180	24	132	95
80	14	11	7	160	47	200	27	142	99
85	16	12	5	180	40	220	31		
90	18	13	3	200	33	240	35		
		14	2	220	27	260	38		
		15	0	240	20	280	42		
				260	13	300	46		
				280	7				
				≥300	0				

*The volume can be measured by the $ABC/2$ method. A is the maximum diameter, B is the diameter perpendicular to A, and C is the number of slices in which the hematoma is visible, assuming 10 mm slice thickness on computed tomography.

†Point total = Age + GCS score + Time to stroke + Volume.

From Sloan et al.[73] By permission of the American Heart Association.

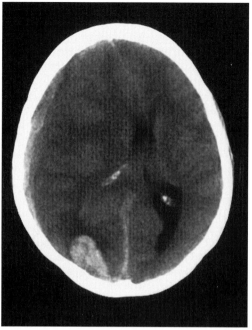
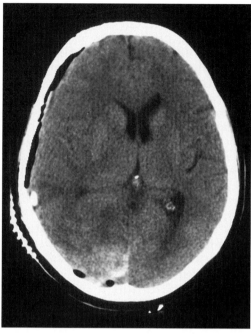

A   B

Figure 11–4. *A:* Serial computed tomography scans showing large subdural hematoma with significant shift and development of a contralateral hydrocephalus. The shift is determined by the subdural hematoma and not by the superficial occipital hematoma. *B:* After evacuation of the subdural hematoma, the parenchymal hematoma resolved and the ventricular system returned to normal size. The patient survived with a minimal deficit.

hemorrhage in the vermis of the cerebellum, but any location is possible. Patients with anticoagulant-associated intracerebral hemorrhage generally have higher incidences of mortality and morbidity. Advanced age (older than 75 years), intensity (international normalized ratio greater than 4.0), and concomitant antiplatelet agents or nonsteroidal anti-inflammatory drugs increase the risk of any hemorrhagic complication of warfarin therapy.[79]

Subdural hematomas, including those in the posterior fossa,[80,81] generally are more frequent in anticoagulated patients, often after trivial head trauma. Subarachnoid hemorrhage has frequently been mentioned in many review papers on neurologic complications of anticoagulation, but these isolated reports predate the routine use of CT scan. Most patients have subarachnoid blood in the sulci and not in the basal cisterns, and trauma is often implicated.

Intramedullary spinal cord hemorrhages have been described in several case reports.[82,83] Intraspinal hemorrhages may oc-

cur suddenly with maximal deficit at the onset, but a protracted course is possible. Neurosurgical evacuation may result in good ambulation and bladder control, but experience in nontraumatic intraspinal hemorrhages is small. The complexity of surgery may prompt neurosurgeons to wait with intervention if the deficit is small and stable.

Spinal epidural, subarachnoid, and subdural hematomas, often in association with lumbar puncture, have been described in many isolated reports.[83–97] Pain can be absent.[84] Spinal epidural hematomas may occur in patients who are anticoagulated and have an epidural catheter.[98] Most instances are associated with vascular surgery. It has been suggested that removal of the catheter may be traumatic and that heparin administration should be discontinued 1 to 2 hr before removal.[99] Urgent surgical decompression is warranted, but reversal of anticoagulation and conservative management have been successful in patients with extensive hematomas unsuitable for surgery. Conservative management in two patients who had extensive spinal intradural hematomas with clinically almost complete transverse myelopathy resulted in ambulation and normal bladder function.[100] It may be the only option in patients with additional critical morbidity.

Hematomas that cause compressive mononeuropathies or plexopathies are infrequent.[101] The relative infrequency may also suggest that these conditions are overlooked in the ICU and are overshadowed by systemic illness.

Femoral nerve compression in the psoas and iliac compartments has been well documented.[102–106] The anatomical relationship between the femoral nerve and the obturator nerve in the fascial compartments is outlined in Figure 11–5.

Clinically, femoral nerve paralysis is characterized by pain in the groin and thigh radiating into the patellar area. Weakness of the iliopsoas or quadriceps muscle, absent knee jerk, and sensory loss over the anteromedial region of the lower extremities are further hallmarks of this neuropathy. Many patients have an antalgic position of the hip (flexed, abducted, and externally rotated).

Computed tomography scanning[107,108] (Fig. 11–6) almost always demonstrates a retroperitoneal mass that may at times be bilateral.[104] Improvement after correction of the coagulopathy alone can be impressive. Surgical evacuation of a psoas hematoma may lead to immediate recurrence of the hematoma or bleeding into the retroperitoneal space when the tamponade is released. In addition, mobilization of the colon and difficult identification of a displaced ureter complicate the surgical procedure, so that it is not an attractive option.

Retroperitoneal hemorrhage is the most common anticoagulant-related hematoma, but hematoma in the gluteal muscles may cause severe hip pain and sudden weak foot from sciatic nerve compression. Outcome is excellent with conservative measures.[109–111]

Other compressive neuropathies are one of a kind. Two cases of acute carpal tunnel syndrome with anticoagulation have been reported.[112,113] Epineurolysis to release hematoma is often needed to relieve the excruciating pain. Generally, pain and diminished sensation in the wrist and fingers are experienced, and frank weakness of the opponens pollicis and abductor pollicis brevis is

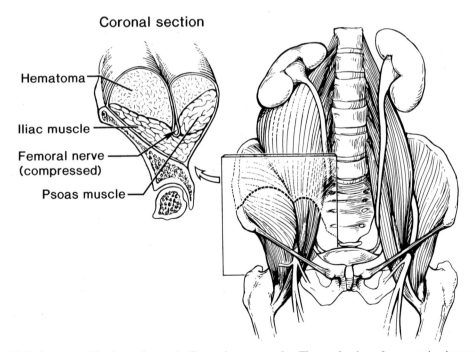

Figure 11–5. Anatomy of the femoral nerve in iliac and psoas muscles. The mechanism of compression in psoas hematoma is shown.

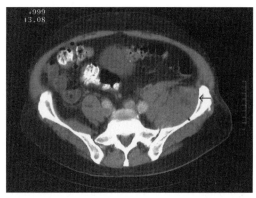

Figure 11–6. Psoas hematoma (arrow) demonstrated on abdominal computed tomography scan.

uncommon. Spontaneous occurrence but also association with axillary angiography have been reported in patients with brachial plexus neuropathy, all recognized by an ecchymosis overlying the shoulder and severe local and referred pain.[114] Recently, the first case of isolated ulnar neuropathy due to a diffuse muscular hematoma was reported.[115] Outcome of anticoagulation-associated neuropathies is good.[109–116]

THROMBOTIC THROMBOCYTOPENIC PURPURA

Moschcowitz's disease is viewed as unique because the systemic complications that accompany the disorder were fatal before the introduction of plasma exchange in the 1970s. Thrombotic thrombocytopenic purpura (TTP) is not rare (0.1 per 100,000 patients annually in the Rochester, Minnesota, area),[117] and the incidence may be increasing.[118] It occurs more often in females and has a peak incidence in the third and fourth decades. Treatment is complex, and mortality is substantial despite marked improvement after the introduction of plasma exchange. In this respect, many patients are cared for in medical ICUs, and neurologic manifestations are part of the manifestations of microangiopathic hemolytic anemia and thrombocytopenia. The disorder may be linked to infectious disease, vaccination, drugs (for example, ticlopidine or clopido-

grel[119]), rheumatologic disorders, malignant disease, and human immunodeficiency virus infection.[120]

PATHOPHYSIOLOGIC MECHANISMS

Microvascular thrombi are predominantly linked to the clinical manifestations, and they seem by histologic examination to be entirely composed of platelets. Any organ can be involved, although the kidney, brain, and retina appear to have a proclivity for these platelet aggregates. During acute episodes, lack of metalloproteinase activity exists. This protease cleaves von Willebrand's factor into circulating fragments, and failure to do so leaves large multimers, causing platelet agglutination. This sequence is important for our understanding, because removal of the antibody directed at this protinase or replacement of this inactive enzyme with fresh-frozen plasma may explain the rationale of plasma exchange. The development of a clinical assay for protease deficiency may allow a more specific and early diagnosis.

Clinical Features

The initial presentation of thrombotic thrombocytopenic purpura is abrupt, usually with bleeding and neurologic manifestations. Purpura is seldom the sole manifestation, and evidence of hemorrhage more often may include petechiae, ecchymoses, retinal hemorrhages, epistaxis, hemoptysis, and gastrointestinal hemorrhage. Of all the nonspecific symptoms, such as fatigue, arthralgia, and jaundice, fever is the most consistent, but it may be absent initially and at the time of neurologic manifestations.

Neurologic manifestations invariably punctuate the course of illness.[121–125] In a series of 102 patients, 64 had fluctuating neurologic signs at presentation, and neurologic abnormalities developed in 8 during the course of the illness.[126] Expressive aphasia of 2-day duration as a presenting symptom has been reported.[127]

Many patients have changes in level of consciousness associated with delirium and restlessness. Headache is common. The clinical presentations (Table 11–6) could represent ischemic strokes from occlusion of arterial branches. The waxing and waning of the neurologic deficits has been explained by brief ischemia caused by microthrombi composed of loose platelet aggregates occluding terminal arterioles and capillaries. Recently, two reports pointed out the possibility that confusion may actually indicate nonconvulsive status epilepticus. In these patients, however, seizures preceded nonconvulsive status epilepticus. Therefore, failure of patients to improve with plasma exchange should prompt electroencephalographic recording and video and electroencephalographic monitoring.[129,130] Despite claims of complete recovery, permanent neurologic deficits are not uncommon, even in the plasma exchange era.[131–134] Persistent multiple but small infarcts have been described. Occlusions of major arterial branches, including main stem middle cerebral artery thrombosis, are less common but do not exclude the link with TTP.[131]

Laboratory Findings and Neuroimaging

Initial laboratory tests should document moderately severe anemia, fragmented erythrocytes (Plate 11–1), increased blood levels of unconjugated bilirubin and lactic dehydrogenase, platelet counts around 20,000/μL, and increased reticulocyte counts (75%). Proteinuria, hematuria, increased creatinine and blood urea nitrogen, and abnormal liver function tests are also part of the laboratory profile.[132,133] The cerebrospinal fluid has only rarely been examined, because of the obvious dangers of inducing an epidural hematoma in a patient with hypocoagulable state.

Magnetic resonance imaging or CT scanning may demonstrate cerebral infarcts after neurologic signs have resolved, a suggestion of permanent damage rather than transient ischemic events.[123,135] Normal findings on CT scan seem to predict the potential for recovery in patients, including those with aphasia, hemiparesis, and visual field defects.[136] In addition, several MRI reports have documented signal changes in subcortical white matter that most likely represent edema due to hypoperfusion. These lesions disappear after plasma exchange.[137] Serial MRI (Fig. 11–7) may also show silent infarcts. Results of MRI, however, are most often normal in patients with waxing and waning level of consciousness alone.

The pathologic lesions of hyaline thrombi and occluded capillaries and arterioles may be demonstrated in 50% of gingiva biopsy specimens, but the finding is nonspecific. Kidney biopsy may be more diagnostic.[133]

Treatment

Treatment is plasmapheresis (1.5 plasma volume removal in 4 days).[126,133,134,138] The introduction of plasma exchange has not eliminated fatal outcome, and patients may succumb from multiorgan failure.[139] Additional use of aspirin and dipyridamole or additional high doses of corticosteroids (0.75 mg/kg twice a day)[140–142] are considered in the most severe cases. Cryosupernatant plasma, which depletes von Willebrand's factor multimers, does not further improve out-

Table 11–6. **Neurologic Manifestations of Thrombotic Thrombocytopenic Purpura**

Headache
Behavior changes, stupor
Hemiparesis, hemisensory findings, aphasia, hemianopia, cortical blindness
Focal and generalized seizures, nonconvulsive status epilepticus
Ischemic optic neuropathy, cotton-wool spots, retinal detachment
Cauda equina syndrome

Data from Ben-Yehuda et al.,[121] Petitt,[117] Rinkel et al.,[123] Silverstein,[124] Wijdicks,[125] and Melton and Spaide.[128]

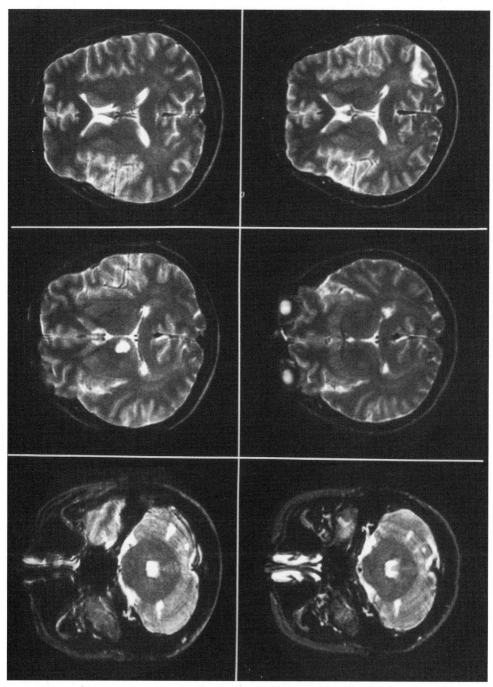

Figure 11–7. T2-weighted serial magnetic resonance images in a patient with thrombotic thrombocytopenic purpura. *Upper row:* Multiple cerebral infarcts in cerebellar hemispheres and thalamus. *Lower row:* "Silent" occipital infarct 6 months later and resolution of thalamic infarct. (From Wijdicks.[125] By permission of the American Heart Association.)

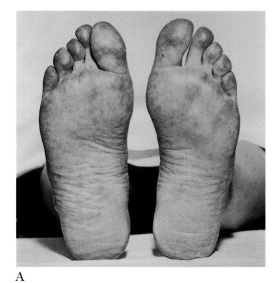

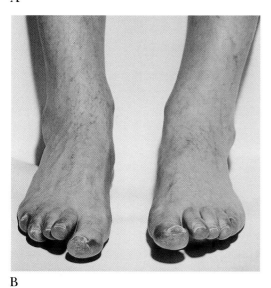

Plate 5–1. Blue toe syndrome (*A* and *B*) in cholesterol embolization.

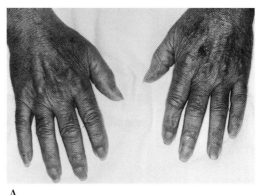

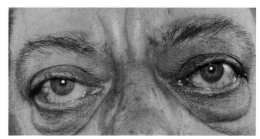

Plate 6–2. Hand muscle wasting (*A*) and prominence of the tibia due to atrophy (*B*) from critical illness polyneuropathy.

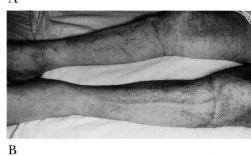

Plate 8–1. Proptosis and puffy eyelids in myxedema.

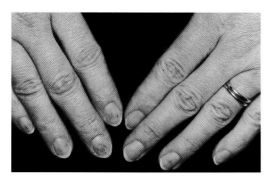

Plate 6–1. Splinter hemorrhages in nail bed from endocarditis.

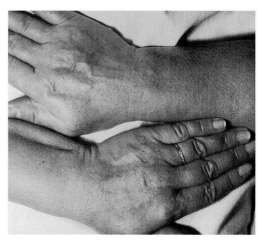

Plate 8–2. Pasty, puffy hands in myxedema.

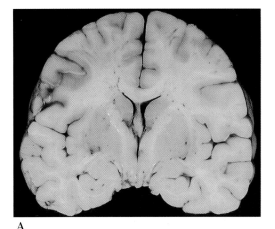

A

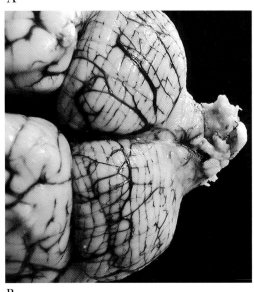

B

Plate 10–1. Brain edema in fulminant hepatic failure. Note slit-like ventricles and flattening of sulci (*A*) and tonsillar herniation (*B*). (Courtesy of Dr. E. A. Pfeifer.)

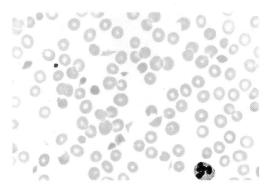

Plate 11–1. Peripheral blood smear showing scattered schistocytes and fragmented red blood cells in thrombotic thrombocytopenic purpura (Wright's Giemsa stain; ×1000).

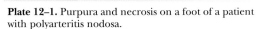

Plate 12–1. Purpura and necrosis on a foot of a patient with polyarteritis nodosa.

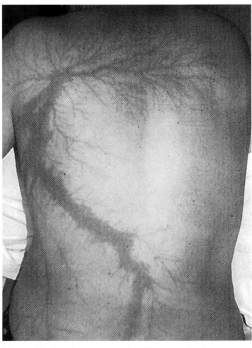

Plate 16–1. Cutaneous fernlike marks known as "Lichtenberg figures" in a patient struck by lightning. (From Domart Y, Garet E. Images in clinical medicine. N Engl J Med 343:1536, 2000. By permission of the Massachusetts Medical Society.)

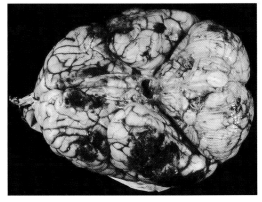

Plate 17–1. Multiple hemorrhagic contusions predominantly in frontal and temporal lobes.

come.[141] Relapse may occur within 30 days, and platelets need to be frequently monitored.

CONCLUSIONS

The addition of thrombolytic agents to the repertoire of the cardiologist has increased the incidence of hemorrhagic complications, particularly intracranial hemorrhages. The troublesome systemic side effects of thrombolytic agents, often easily overcome, contrast sharply with the considerable morbidity and mortality of intracranial hemorrhages. Hemorrhages in multiple compartments and fluid levels inside the hematomas suggest continuing anticoagulation. Neurosurgical intervention in multiple lesions is likely to be fruitless, but in a patient with a localized hematoma and sedimented blood from inability to form a firm clot, catheter placement or needle aspiration can be tried. Subdural hematomas should be evacuated if mass effect causes a decrease in the level of consciousness.

Another well-documented complication of anticoagulation is compression of the femoral nerve in the psoas and iliac compartments, which can be visualized on CT scan. The natural history is good, and thus a surgical approach to relieve compression is controversial.

REFERENCES

1. Siegal T, Seligsohn U, Aghai E, Modan M. Clinical and laboratory aspects of disseminated intravascular coagulation (DIC): a study of 118 cases. Thromb Haemost 39:122–134, 1978.
2. Drews RE, Weinberger SE. Thrombocytopenic disorders in critically ill patients. Am J Respir Crit Care Med 162:347–351, 2000.
3. Scherer RU, Spangenberg P. Procoagulant activity in patients with isolated severe head trauma. Crit Care Med 26:149–156, 1998.
4. Levi M, Ten Cate H. Disseminated intravascular coagulation. N Engl J Med 341:586–592, 1999.
5. Singh R, Singh MM, Hazra DK, et al. A study of disseminated intravascular coagulopathy in hepatic coma complicating acute viral hepatitis. Angiology 34:470–479, 1983.
6. Colman RW, Rubin RN. Disseminated intravascular coagulation due to malignancy. Semin Oncol 17:172–186, 1990.
7. Bieger R, Vreeken J, Stibbe J, Loeliger EA. Arterial aneurysm as a cause of consumption coagulopathy. N Engl J Med 285:152–154, 1971.
8. Fisher DF Jr, Yawn DH, Crawford ES. Preoperative disseminated intravascular coagulation associated with aortic aneurysms. A prospective study of 76 cases. Arch Surg 118:1252–1255, 1983.
9. Thompson RW, Adams DH, Cohen JR, Mannick JA, Whittemore AD. Disseminated intravascular coagulation caused by abdominal aortic aneurysm. J Vasc Surg 4:184–186, 1986.
10. Clark JA, Finelli RE, Netsky MG. Disseminated intravascular coagulation following cranial trauma. Case report. J Neurosurg 52:266–269, 1980.
11. Kaufman HH, Hui KS, Mattson JC, et al. Clinicopathological correlations of disseminated intravascular coagulation in patients with head injury. Neurosurgery 15:34–42, 1984.
12. Kaufman HH, Moake JL, Olson JD, et al. Delayed and recurrent intracranial hematomas related to disseminated intravascular clotting and fibrinolysis in head injury. Neurosurgery 7:445–449, 1980.
13. Olson JD, Kaufman HH, Moake J, et al. The incidence and significance of hemostatic abnormalities in patients with head injuries. Neurosurgery 24:825–832, 1989.
14. Pondaag W. Disseminated intravascular coagulation related to outcome in head injury. Acta Neurochir Suppl (Wien) 28:98–102, 1979.
15. Tikk A, Noormaa U. The significance of cerebral and systemic disseminated intravascular coagulation in early prognosis of brain injury. Acta Neurochir Suppl (Wien) 28:96–97, 1979.
16. Spallone A, Mariani G, Rosa G, Corrao D. Disseminated intravascular coagulation as a complication of ruptured intracranial aneurysms. Report of two cases. J Neurosurg 59:142–145, 1983.
17. Eles GR, Songer JE, DiPette DJ. Neuroleptic malignant syndrome complicated by disseminated intravascular coagulation. Arch Intern Med 144:1296–1297, 1984.
18. Mehta B, Briggs DK, Sommers SC, Karpatkin M. Disseminated intravascular coagulation following cardiac arrest: a study of 15 patients. Am J Med Sci 264:353–363, 1972.
19. Baker WF Jr. Clinical aspects of disseminated intravascular coagulation: a clinician's point of view. Semin Thromb Hemost 15:1–57, 1989.
20. Bick RL. Disseminated intravascular coagulation and related syndromes: a clinical review. Semin Thromb Hemost 14:299–338, 1988.
21. Wada H, Sakuragawa N, Mori Y, et al. Hemostatic molecular markers before the onset of disseminated intravascular coagulation. Am J Hematol 60:273–278, 1999.
22. Baglin T. Disseminated intravascular coagulation: diagnosis and treatment. BMJ 312:683–687, 1996.
23. Kawakami Y, Ueki K, Chikama M, Shimamura Y, Naito T. Intracranial hemorrhage associated with nontraumatic disseminated intravascular coagulation—report of four cases. Neurol Med Chir (Tokyo) 30:610–617, 1990.
24. Hill JB, Schwartzman RJ. Cerebral infarction and disseminated intravascular coagulation with pheochromocytoma. Arch Neurol 38:395, 1981.
25. Ryan FP, Timperley WR, Preston FE, Holdsworth CD. Cerebral involvement with disseminated in-

travascular coagulation in intestinal disease. J Clin Pathol 30:551–555, 1977.

26. Schwartzman RJ, Hill JB. Neurologic complications of disseminated intravascular coagulation. Neurology 32:791–797, 1982.

27. Buonanno FS, Cooper MR, Moody DM, Laster DW, Ball MR, Toole JF. Neuroradiologic aspects of cerebral disseminated intravascular coagulation. AJNR Am J Neuroradiol 1:245–250, 1980.

28. Grabowski EF, Zimmerman RD. Disseminated intravascular coagulation and the neuroradiologist. AJNR Am J Neuroradiol 12:344, 1991.

29. Gladstone DJ, Silver FL, Willinsky RA, Tyndel FJ, Wennberg R. Deep cerebral venous thrombosis: an illustrative case with reversible diencephalic dysfunction. Can J Neurol Sci 28:159–162, 2001.

30. Hagner G, Iglesias-Rozas JR, Kölmel HW, Gerhartz H. Hemorrhagic infarction of the basal ganglia. An unusual complication of acute leukemia. Oncology 40:387–391, 1983.

31. Nadel L, Braun IF, Kraft KA, Jensen ME, Laine FJ. MRI of intracranial sinovenous thrombosis: the role of phase imaging. Magn Reson Imaging 8:315–320, 1990.

32. Villringer A, Seiderer M, Bauer WM, Laub G, Haberl RL, Einhaupl KM. Diagnosis of superior sagittal sinus thrombosis by three-dimensional magnetic resonance flow imaging. Lancet 1:1086–1087, 1989.

33. Martin VA. Disseminated intravascular coagulopathy. Trans Ophthalmol Soc U K 98:506–507, 1978.

34. Weber MB. The neurological complications of consumption coagulopathies. Neurology 18:185–188, 1968.

35. Wijdicks EFM, Scott JP. Stroke in the medical intensive-care unit. Mayo Clin Proc 73:642–646, 1998.

36. Wijdicks EFM, Silbert PL, Jack CR, Parisi JE. Subcortical hemorrhage in disseminated intravascular coagulation associated with sepsis. AJNR Am J Neuroradiol 15:763–765, 1994.

37. Einhäupl KM, Villringer A, Meister W, et al. Heparin treatment in sinus venous thrombosis. Lancet 338:597–600, 1991.

38. Hanley DF, Feldman E, Borel CO, Rosenbaum AE, Goldberg AL. Treatment of sagittal sinus thrombosis associated with cerebral hemorrhage and intracranial hypertension. Stroke 19:903–909, 1988.

39. de Bruijn SF, Stam J. Randomized, placebo-controlled trial of anticoagulant treatment with low-molecular-weight heparin for cerebral sinus thrombosis. Stroke 30:484–488, 1999.

40. Barnwell SL, Higashida RT, Halbach VV, Dowd CF, Hieshima GB. Direct endovascular thrombolytic therapy for dural sinus thrombosis. Neurosurgery 28:135–142, 1991.

41. Frey JL, Muro GJ, McDougall CG, Dean BL, Jahnke HK. Cerebral venous thrombosis: combined intrathrombus rtPA and intravenous heparin. Stroke 30:489–494, 1999.

42. AIMS Trial Study Group. Long-term effects of intravenous anistreplase in acute myocardial infarction: final report of the AIMS study. Lancet 335:427–431, 1990.

43. Gruppo Italiano per lo Studio della Streptochinasi

44. Gruppo Italiano per lo Studio della Streptochinasi nell'Infarto Miocardico (GISSI). Effectiveness of intravenous thrombolytic treatment in acute myocardial infarction. Lancet 1:397–402, 1986.

44. Gruppo Italiano per lo Studio della Streptochinasi nell'Infarto Miocardico (GISSI). Long-term effects of intravenous thrombolysis in acute myocardial infarction: final report of the GISSI study. Lancet 2:871–874, 1987.

45. The International Study Group. In-hospital mortality and clinical course of 20,891 patients with suspected acute myocardial infarction randomised between alteplase and streptokinase with or without heparin. Lancet 336:71–75, 1990.

46. The I.S.A.M. Study Group. A prospective trial of intravenous streptokinase in acute myocardial infarction (I.S.A.M.). Mortality, morbidity, and infarct size at 21 days. N Engl J Med 314:1465–1471, 1986.

47. ISIS-3 (Third International Study of Infarct Survival) Collaborative Group. ISIS-3: a randomised comparison of streptokinase vs tissue plasminogen activator vs anistreplase and of aspirin plus heparin vs aspirin alone among 41,299 cases of suspected acute myocardial infarction. Lancet 339:753–770, 1992.

48. The TIMI Study Group. Comparison of invasive and conservative strategies after treatment with intravenous tissue plasminogen activator in acute myocardial infarction. Results of the thrombolysis in myocardial infarction (TIMI) phase II trial. N Engl J Med 320:618–627, 1989.

49. White HD, Norris RM, Brown MA, et al. Effect of intravenous streptokinase on left ventricular function and early survival after acute myocardial infarction. N Engl J Med 317:850–855, 1987.

50. Konstantinides S, Tiede N, Geibel A, Olschewski M, Just H, Kasper W. Comparison of alteplase versus heparin for resolution of major pulmonary embolism. Am J Cardiol 82:966–970, 1998.

51. Arcasoy SM, Kreit JW. Thrombolytic therapy of pulmonary embolism: a comprehensive review of current evidence. Chest 115:1695–1707, 1999.

52. Konstantinides S, Geibel A, Kasper W. Submassive and massive pulmonary embolism: a target for thrombolytic therapy? Thromb Haemost 82 (Suppl 1):104–108, 1999.

53. Anderson JL, Sorensen SG, Moreno FL, et al. Multicenter patency trial of intravenous anistreplase compared with streptokinase in acute myocardial infarction. The TEAM-2 Study Investigators. Circulation 83:126–140, 1991.

54. Gore JM, Sloan M, Price TR, et al. Intracerebral hemorrhage, cerebral infarction, and subdural hematoma after acute myocardial infarction and thrombolytic therapy in the Thrombolysis in Myocardial Infarction Study. Thrombolysis in Myocardial Infarction, Phase II, pilot and clinical trial. Circulation 83:448–459, 1991.

55. ISIS-2 (Second International Study of Infarct Survival) Collaborative Group. Randomised trial of intravenous streptokinase, oral aspirin, both, or neither among 17,187 cases of suspected acute myocardial infarction: ISIS-2. Lancet 2:349–360, 1988.

56. Sloan MA, Price TR. Intracranial hemorrhage fol-

lowing thrombolytic therapy for acute myocardial infarction. Semin Neurol 11:385–399, 1991.

57. De Jaegere PP, Arnold AA, Balk AH, Simoons ML. Intracranial hemorrhage in association with thrombolytic therapy: incidence and clinical predictive factors. J Am Coll Cardiol 19:289–294, 1992.

58. Kase CS, O'Neal AM, Fisher M, Girgis GN, Ordia JI. Intracranial hemorrhage after use of tissue plasminogen activator for coronary thrombolysis. Ann Intern Med 112:17–21, 1990.

59. Kase CS, Pessin MS, Zivin JA, et al. Intracranial hemorrhage after coronary thrombolysis with tissue plasminogen activator. Am J Med 92:384–390, 1992.

60. More RS, Vincent R. Intracerebral haemorrhage after thrombolytic therapy for acute myocardial infarction. Postgrad Med J 68:800–803, 1992.

61. Pendlebury WW, Iole ED, Tracy RP, Dill BA. Intracerebral hemorrhage related to cerebral amyloid angiopathy and t-PA treatment. Ann Neurol 29:210–213, 1991.

62. Ramsay DA, Penswick JL, Robertson DM. Fatal streptokinase-induced intracerebral haemorrhage in cerebral amyloid angiopathy. Can J Neurol Sci 17:336–341, 1990.

63. Uglietta JP, O'Connor CM, Boyko OB, Aldrich H, Massey EW, Heinz ER. CT patterns of intracranial hemorrhage complicating thrombolytic therapy for acute myocardial infarction. Radiology 181: 555–559, 1991.

64. Wijdicks EFM, Jack CR Jr. Intracerebral hemorrhage after fibrinolytic therapy for acute myocardial infarction. Stroke 24:554–557, 1993.

65. Gurwitz JH, Gore JM, Goldberg RJ, et al. Risk for intracranial hemorrhage after tissue plasminogen activator treatment for acute myocardial infarction. Participants in the National Registry of Myocardial Infarction 2. Ann Intern Med 129:597–604, 1998.

66. Partanen HJ, Nieminen MS. Intracerebellar fatal haemorrhage after thrombolytic therapy of suspected non-Q-wave myocardial infarction [letter]. Lancet 336:883, 1990.

67. Wijdicks EFM, Jack CR Jr. Intracerebral hemorrhage after fibrinolytic therapy for acute myocardial infarction: are fibrinolytic agents really the main instigators? [letter]. Stroke 25:713–714, 1994.

68. Anderson JL, Karagounis L, Allen A, Bradford MJ, Menlove RL, Pryor TA. Older age and elevated blood pressure are risk factors for intracerebral hemorrhage after thrombolysis. Am J Cardiol 68: 166–170, 1991.

69. Brass LM, Lichtman JH, Wang Y, Gurwitz JH, Radford MJ, Krumholz HM. Intracranial hemorrhage associated with thrombolytic therapy for elderly patients with acute myocardial infarction: results from the Cooperative Cardiovascular Project. Stroke 31:1802–1811, 2000.

70. Meschia JF, Chukwudelunzu FE, Dickson DW, et al. The relationship between cerebral amyloid angiopathy and lobar intracerebral hemorrhage in patients receiving anticoagulants and/or fibrinolytics. Neurology 52(Suppl 2):A502, 1999.

71. Rosand J, Hylek EM, O'Donnell HC, Greenberg SM. Warfarin-associated hemorrhage and cerebral amyloid angiopathy: a genetic and pathologic study. Neurology 55:947–951, 2000.

72. Eleff SM, Borel C, Bell WR, Long DM. Acute management of intracranial hemorrhage in patients receiving thrombolytic therapy: case reports. Neurosurgery 26:867–869, 1990.

73. Sloan MA, Sila CA, Mahaffey KW, et al. Prediction of 30-day mortality among patients with thrombolysis-related intracranial hemorrhage. Circulation 98:1376–1382, 1998.

74. Mahaffey KW, Granger CB, Sloan MA, et al. Neurosurgical evacuation of intracranial hemorrhage after thrombolytic therapy for acute myocardial infarction: Experience from the GUSTO-I trial. Global Utilization of Streptokinase and tissue-plasminogen activator (tPA) for Occluded Coronary Arteries. Am Heart J 138:493–499, 1999.

75. Longstreth WT Jr, Grady MS, Schmer G. Needle aspiration of an intracerebral hemorrhage complicating thrombolytic therapy for myocardial infarction. Stroke 25:712–714, 1994.

76. Kanter DS, Mikkola KM, Patel SR, Parker JA, Goldhaber SZ. Thrombolytic therapy for pulmonary embolism. Frequency of intracranial hemorrhage and associated risk factors. Chest 111:1241–1245, 1997.

77. Andrews TC, Peterson DW, Doeppenschmidt D, et al. Complications of warfarin therapy monitored by the International Normalized Ratio versus the prothrombin time ratio. Clin Cardiol 18:80–82, 1995.

78. Kase CS, Robinson RK, Stein RW, et al. Anticoagulant-related intracerebral hemorrhage. Neurology 35:943–948, 1985.

79. Sebastian JL, Tresch DD. Use of oral anticoagulants in older patients. Drugs Aging 16:409–435, 2000.

80. Capistrant T, Goldberg R, Shibasaki H, Castle D. Posterior fossa subdural haematoma associated with anticoagulant therapy. J Neurol Neurosurg Psychiatry 34:82–85, 1971.

81. Wintzen AR, Tijssen JG. Subdural hematoma and oral anticoagulant therapy. Arch Neurol 39:69–72, 1982.

82. Pullarkat VA, Kalapura T, Pincus M, Baskharoun R. Intraspinal hemorrhage complicating oral anticoagulant therapy: an unusual case of cervical hematomyelia and a review of the literature. Arch Intern Med 160:237–240, 2000.

83. Pisani R, Carta F, Guiducci G, Silvestro C, Davini MD. Hematomyelia during anticoagulant therapy. Surg Neurol 24:578–580, 1985.

84. Senelick RC, Norwood CW, Cohen GH. "Painless" spinal epidural hematoma during anticoagulant therapy. Neurology 26:213–225, 1976.

85. Bamford CR. Spinal epidural hematoma due to heparin. Arch Neurol 35:693–694, 1978.

86. Brandt M. Spontaneous intramedullary haematoma as a complication of anticoagulant therapy. Acta Neurochir (Wien) 52:73–77, 1980.

87. Dahlin PA, George J. Intraspinal hematoma as a complication of anticoagulant therapy. Clin Pharmacol 3:656–661, 1984.

88. Guthikonda M, Schmidek HH, Wallman LJ, Snyder TM. Spinal subdural hematoma: case report and review of the literature. Neurosurgery 5:614–616, 1979.

89. Harik SI, Raichle ME, Reis DJ. Spontaneously remitting spinal epidural hematoma in a patient on anticoagulants. N Engl J Med 284:1355–1357, 1971.

90. Hurst PG, Seeger J, Carter P, Marcus FI. Value of magnetic resonance imaging for diagnosis of cervical epidural hematoma associated with anticoagulation after cardiac valve replacement. Am J Cardiol 63:1016–1017, 1989.

91. Krolick MA, Cintron GB. Spinal epidural hematoma causing cord compression after tissue plasminogen activator and heparin therapy. South Med J 84:670–671, 1991.

92. Mayumi T, Dohi S. Spinal subarachnoid hematoma after lumbar puncture in a patient receiving antiplatelet therapy. Anesth Analg 62:777–779, 1983.

93. Metzger G, Singbartl G. Spinal epidural hematoma following epidural anesthesia versus spontaneous spinal subdural hematoma. Two case reports. Acta Anaesthesiol Scand 35:105–107, 1991.

94. Russell N, Maroun FB, Jacob JC. Spinal subdural hematoma in association with anticoagulant therapy. Can J Neurol Sci 8:87–89, 1981.

95. Toledo E, Shalit MN, Segal R. Spinal subdural hematoma associated with anticoagulant therapy in a patient with spinal meningioma. Neurosurgery 8:600–603, 1981.

96. Tomarken JL. Spinal subdural hematoma. Ann Emerg Med 14:261–263, 1985.

97. Tomarken JL. Spinal subdural hematoma: a case report and literature review. Am J Emerg Med 5:123–125, 1987.

98. Vandermeulen EP, Van Aken H, Vermylen J. Anticoagulants and spinal-epidural anesthesia. Anesth Analg 79:1165–1177, 1994.

99. Skilton RW, Justice W. Epidural haematoma following anticoagulant treatment in a patient with an indwelling epidural catheter. Anaesthesia 53:691–695, 1998.

100. Schwerdtfeger K, Caspar W, Alloussi S, Strowitzki M, Loew F. Acute spinal intradural extramedullary hematoma: a nonsurgical approach for spinal cord decompression. Neurosurgery 27:312–314, 1990.

101. Gilden DH, Eisner J. Lumbar plexopathy caused by disseminated intravascular coagulation. JAMA 237:2846–2847, 1977.

102. Jackson S. Femoral neuropathy secondary to heparin induced intrapelvic hematoma. A case report and review of the literature. Orthopedics 10:1049–1052, 1987.

103. Piazza I, Girardi A, Giunta G, Pappagallo G. Femoral nerve palsy secondary to anticoagulant induced iliacus hematoma. Int Angiol 9:125–126, 1990.

104. Stören EJ. Bilateral iliacus haematoma with femoral nerve palsy complicating anticoagulant therapy. Acta Chir Scand 144:181–183, 1978.

105. Zarranz JJ, Simon R, Salisachs P. Acute anticoagulant-induced compressive lumbar plexus neuropathy. A clinico-pathological study. Eur Neurol 20:469–472, 1981.

106. Ahuja R, Venkatesh P. Femoral neuropathy following anticoagulant therapy: a case report and discussion. Conn Med 63:69–71, 1999.

107. Hoyt TE, Tiwari R, Kusske JA. Compressive neuropathy as a complication of anticoagulant therapy. Neurosurgery 12:268–271, 1983.

108. Uncini A, Tonali P, Falappa P, Danza FM. Femoral neuropathy from iliac muscle hematoma induced by oral anticoagulation therapy. Report of three cases with CT demonstration. J Neurol 226:137–141, 1981.

109. Fleming RE Jr, Michelsen CB, Stinchfield FE. Sciatic paralysis. A complication of bleeding following hip surgery. J Bone Joint Surg Am 61:37–39, 1979.

110. Palliyath S, Buday J. Sciatic nerve compression: diagnostic value of electromyography and computerized tomography. Electromyogr Clin Neurophysiol 29:9–11, 1989.

111. Wallach HW, Oren ME. Sciatic nerve compression during anticoagulation therapy. Computerized tomography aids in diagnosis. Arch Neurol 36:448, 1979.

112. Copeland J, Wells HG Jr, Puckett CL: Acute carpal tunnel syndrome in a patient taking coumadin. J Trauma 29:131–132, 1989.

113. Nkele C. Acute carpal tunnel syndrome resulting from haemorrhage into the carpal tunnel in a patient on warfarin. J Hand Surg (Br) 11:455–456, 1986.

114. Frangides C, Kounis NG. Anticoagulant-induced shoulder hematoma producing brachial plexus neuropathy—case reports. Angiology 43:701–705, 1992.

115. Vijayakumar R, Nesathurai S, Abbott KM, Eustace S. Ulnar neuropathy resulting from diffuse intramuscular hemorrhage: a case report. Arch Phys Med Rehabil 81:1127–1130, 2000.

116. Blankenship JC. Median and ulnar neuropathy after streptokinase infusion. Heart Lung 20:221–223, 1991.

117. Petitt RM. Thrombotic thrombocytopenic purpura: a thirty year review. Semin Thromb Hemost 6:350–355, 1980.

118. Bukowski RM. Thrombotic thrombocytopenic purpura: a review. Prog Hemost Thromb 6:287–337, 1982.

119. Bennett CL, Connors JM, Carwile JM, et al. Thrombotic thrombocytopenic purpura associated with clopidogrel. N Engl J Med 342:1773–1777, 2000.

120. Leaf AN, Laubenstein LJ, Raphael B, Hochster H, Baez L, Karpatkin S. Thrombotic thrombocytopenic purpura associated with human immunodeficiency virus type 1 (HIV-1) infection. Ann Intern Med 109:194–197, 1988.

121. Ben-Yehuda D, Rose M, Michaeli Y, Eldor A. Permanent neurological complications in patients with thrombotic thrombocytopenic purpura. Am J Hematol 29:74–78, 1988.

122. de la Sayette V, Gallet E, Le Doze F, Charbonneau P, Morin P. Thrombotic thrombocytopenic purpura. A case diagnosed by MRI [in French]. Rev Neurol (Paris) 147:314–317, 1991.

123. Rinkel GJ, Wijdicks EFM, Hene RJ. Stroke in relapsing thrombotic thrombocytopenic purpura. Stroke 22:1087–1089, 1991.

124. Silverstein A. Thrombotic thrombocytopenic pur-

pura. The initial neurologic manifestations. Arch Neurol 18:358–362, 1968.

125. Wijdicks EFM. Silent brain infarct in thrombotic thrombocytopenic purpura. Stroke 25:1297–1298, 1994.

126. Rock GA, Shumak KH, Buskard NA, et al. Comparison of plasma exchange with plasma infusion in the treatment of thrombotic thrombocytopenic purpura. Canadian Apheresis Study Group. N Engl J Med 325:393–397, 1991.

127. D'Andrea CC, Chan L. Acute thrombotic thrombocytopenic purpura presenting as expressive aphasia. Am J Emerg Med 16:270–271, 1998.

128. Melton RC, Spaide RF. Visual problems as a presenting sign of thrombocytopenic purpura. Retina 16:78–80, 1996.

129. Garrett WT, Chang CW, Bleck TP. Altered mental status in thrombotic thrombocytopenic purpura is secondary to nonconvulsive status epilepticus. Ann Neurol 40:245–246, 1996.

130. Blum AS, Drislane FW. Nonconvulsive status epilepticus in thrombotic thrombocytopenic purpura. Neurology 47:1079–1081, 1996.

131. Kelly PJ, McDonald CT, Neill GO, Thomas C, Niles J, Rordorf G. Middle cerebral artery main stem thrombosis in two siblings with familial thrombotic thrombocytopenic purpura. Neurology 50:1157–1160, 1998.

132. Kwaan HC. Clinicopathologic features of thrombotic thrombocytopenic purpura. Semin Hematol 24:71–81, 1987.

133. Ruggenenti P, Remuzzi G. Thrombotic thrombocytopenic purpura and related disorders. Hematol Oncol Clin North Am 4:219–241, 1990.

134. Bosch T, Wendler T. Extracorporeal plasma treatment in thrombotic thrombocytopenic purpura and hemolytic uremic syndrome: a review. Ther Apher 5:182–185, 2001.

135. Gruber O, Wittig I, Wiggins CJ, von Cramon DY. Thrombotic thrombocytopenic purpura: MRI demonstration of persistent small cerebral infarcts after clinical recovery. Neuroradiology 42:616–618, 2000.

136. Kay AC, Solberg LA Jr, Nichols DA, Petitt RM. Prognostic significance of computed tomography of the brain in thrombotic thrombocytopenic purpura. Mayo Clin Proc 66:602–607, 1991.

137. Urushitani M, Seriu N, Udaka F, Kameyama M, Nishinaka K, Kodama M. MRI demonstration of a reversible lesion in cerebral deep white matter in thrombotic thrombocytopenic purpura. Neuroradiology 38:137–138, 1996.

138. Rock GA. Management of thrombotic thrombocytopenic purpura. Br J Haematol 109:496–507, 2000.

139. Druschky A, Erbguth F, Strauss R, Helm G, Heckmann J, Neundorfer B. Central nervous system involvement in thrombotic thrombocytopenic purpura. Eur Neurol 40:220–224, 1998.

140. Knobl P, Rintelen C, Kornek G, et al. Plasma exchange for treatment of thrombotic thrombocytopenic purpura in critically ill patients. Intensive Care Med 23:44–50, 1997.

141. Zeigler ZR, Shadduck RK, Gryn JF, et al. Cryoprecipitate poor plasma does not improve early response in primary adult thrombotic thrombocytopenic purpura (TTP). J Clin Apheresis 16:19–22, 2001.

142. George JN. How I treat patients with thrombotic thrombocytopenic purpura-hemolytic uremic syndrome. Blood 96:1223–1229, 2000.

Chapter 12

NEUROLOGIC COMPLICATIONS OF ACUTE VASCULITIC SYNDROMES

Innumerable occasions may arise for patients with a necrotizing vasculitis to be admitted to a medical or surgical intensive care unit (ICU). With every visceral and organ involvement comes a potentially life-threatening condition, and often they occur simultaneously. These conditions are ischemic ulceration of the gut, pulmonary hemorrhage due to small vessel vasculitis or capillaritis, necrotizing nephritis, and myocarditis. In some patients, the effects of immunosuppressive therapy to combat vasculitis may prompt intensive care. The disorders discussed in this chapter were chosen as typical of the problems that consulting neurologists may see in ICUs.

GENERAL CONSIDERATIONS

The pathologic lesion in vasculitis can be characterized as destructive inflammatory disease of any size of blood vessel, including arterioles and venules. Most clinicians prefer a clinicopathologic classification based on size and type of vessel involvement[1-3] (Fig. 12–1), and others classify vasculitis by whether an underlying disease is present. Lack of a cause in most patients with a vasculitic syndrome may indeed preclude classification, but in a review of 1337 patients with vasculitis, only 10% had a constellation of findings that could not be classified in one of the major histologic categories.[4] The vasculitic syndromes are very complex, consisting of a large group of heterogeneous disorders, and within the scope of this book cannot be dealt with in complete detail. Vasculitides with clinical courses that may become acutely lifethreatening are polyarteritis nodosa, Churg-Strauss syndrome, Wegener's granulomatosis, and drug-induced vasculitis.[5-7]

PATHOPHYSIOLOGIC MECHANISMS

Many mechanisms of endothelial cell injury have been proposed, each with solid experimental supportive data. Next to immunocomplex deposition in arterial walls in some patients, antiendothelial antibodies have been found, but they may be a consequence of vascular damage rather than pathogenic. Infectious agents, such as hepatitides B and C, human immunodeficiency virus, and parvovirus, may contribute, because they promote immunocomplex deposition, antigen presentation, and vascular inflammatory response. Antigens from chronic nasal carriage of *Staphylococcus aureus* may activate T cells and increase the risk of Wegener's granulomatosis.

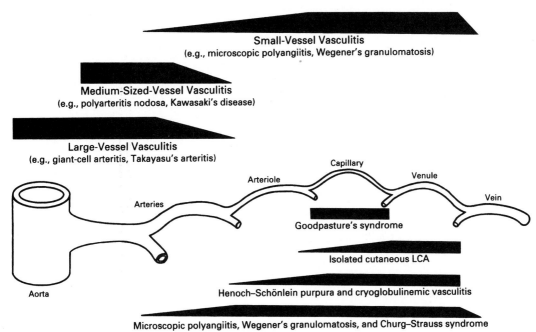

Figure 12–1. Preferred sites of vascular involvement by selected vasculitides. The widths of the trapezoids indicate the frequencies of involvement of various portions of the vasculature. LCA, leukocytoclastic angiitis. (From Jennette and Falk.[2] By permission of the Massachusetts Medical Society.)

Antineutrophil cytoplasmic autoantibodies are typical in active Wegener's granulomatosis, and the level appears to correlate with disease severity. They bind to proteinase 3, which is found in neutrophils, monocytes, and immature macrophages. This proteolytic serine protease may be responsible for vascular injury. These antibodies target neutrophil granules and monocyte lysosomes. Wegener's disease is associated with antiproteinase 3 antineutrophil cytoplasmic autoantibodies. Patients with microscopic polyangiitis or Churg-Strauss syndrome have antimyeloperoxidase antineutrophil cytoplasmic autoantibodies. Immunochemical assays can test for antimyeloperoxidase and antiproteinase 3.

The frequency of organ involvement is variable and wide-ranging. In some patients, only one organ is involved (Table 12–1).

POLYARTERITIS NODOSA

Polyarteritis is primarily a multisystem inflammatory disease of medium- and arteriolar-sized vessels. Pathologic examination characteristically shows infiltration of polymorphonuclear leukocytes, fibrinoid necrosis, and destruction of the media of the arterial wall. Aneurysm formation occurs at this stage and may lead to deadly rupture. However, after immunosuppression, unruptured aneurysms may vanish. Vasculitis in polyarteritis nodosa also results in circumferential proliferation of fibrous tissue and endothelial cells, eventually culminating in vascular occlusion and infarction. The most common reasons for ICU admission in patients with polyarteritis nodosa are perforation of the small or large bowel, gastro-intestinal hemorrhage from aneurysmal rupture, and congestive heart failure from coronary artery vasculitis and hypertension.

Clinical Features

Typical clinical findings in polyarteritis are palpable purpuric lesions, livedo reticularis, infarcted skin lesions (Plate 12–1), and necrotic digital tips.[8] Nodules along the course of arteries (from which the name "polyarteritis nodosa" is derived) represent

Table 12–1. **Neurologic and Organ Involvement in Vasculitides**

	APPROXIMATE FREQUENCY (%)			
Organ	Polyarteritis Nodosa	Churg-Strauss	Wegener's Granulomatosis	Drug-induced
CNS	15	<1	<1	5
PNS	60	30	15	<1
Lung	<1	95	95	10
Kidney	70	40	85	40
Heart	30	40	10	10
GI tract	40	40	<1	<1
Skin	40	70	45	100

CNS, central nervous system; GI, gastrointestinal; PNS, peripheral nervous system.
Data from Churg and Churg.[7]

local inflammatory exudates and are seen mostly, if ever, in fulminant cases.

Gastrointestinal involvement can be catastrophic. Abdominal pain and persistent vomiting and diarrhea may indicate pancreatitis or ischemic necrosis of the appendix, gallbladder, or bowel. Multiple aneurysms may lead to bleeding in the intra-abdominal cavity. Gastrointestinal bleeding or bowel infarction resulting in perforation often requires surgical intervention. Necrotizing glomerulonephritis is seldom fulminant but in occasional patients can produce malignant hypertension, and perhaps the early descriptions of "stupor and papilledema" in polyarteritis nodosa can be directly attributed to hypertensive encephalopathy. One-third of patients have overt cardiac disease caused by coronary artery vasculitis or pericarditis, but it seldom leads to myocardial infarction.

Polyarteritis nodosa can be diagnosed after sufficient clinical attributes of the disorder have been gathered. However, hepatitis B surface antigen, decreased concentration of C3 and C4 complement components, cryoglobulinemia, or antineutrophil cytoplasmic autoantibodies may suggest the diagnosis.[9] These laboratory tests may help in differentiating polyarteritis nodosa from other critical conditions that may strongly mimic polyarteritis, such as infective endocarditis, and left atrial myxoma.

Visceral angiography is the preferred procedure for confirming the diagnosis, but skin, rectum, kidney, skeletal muscle, and, possibly, nerve biopsies can determine the diagnosis with higher yield if these organs are clinically involved.[10,11] Only 30% of muscle biopsy specimens taken from muscles that are not particularly painful are positive.[12] The same holds true for any blind biopsy in other tissue (Table 12–2).

Kernohan and Woltman[13] noted in their seminal paper on periarteritis nodosa that neurologic involvement is one of the most

Table 12–2. **Biopsy in Necrotizing Vasculitis**

Site	Frequency of Positive Biopsy Results (%)
Symptomatic	
Skin	100
Sural nerve	70
Muscle	60
Kidney	100
Lung	100
Asymptomatic (or blind biopsy)	
Muscle	30
Sural nerve	15
Rectum	15
Liver	7

From Chakravarty K. Vasculitis by organ systems. Baillières Clin Rheumatol 11:357–393, 1997. By permission of WB Saunders Company.

consistent clinical features. A peripheral neuropathy usually evolves over weeks and may have an insidious course but becomes more prominent clinically when organ involvement reaches its zenith.

Peripheral Nervous System Involvement

Multiple mononeuropathies (mononeuritis multiplex) are traditionally associated with necrotizing angiitis.[14–21] Peripheral nerve involvement in polyarteritis nodosa is often heralded by transitory shooting pain and paresthesias in the toes and followed by sudden unilateral or bilateral footdrop.[8] Additional nerve involvement develops in many patients, predominantly in the radial or femoral nerve. Marked asymmetries during examination should point to multiple mononeuropathies rather than a polyneuropathy. Large hypesthetic patches in the distribution of cutaneous sensory nerves are often asymmetrically distributed over the body.

A distal sensory-motor polyneuropathy is more frequent than mononeuritis multiplex in polyarteritis nodosa. In Castaigne and associates' series of 27 patients,[16] 8 had mononeuropathy or multiple neuropathy, 17 had distal mixed motor-sensory polyneuropathy more pronounced in the legs than in the arms, and 2 had primarily sensory findings. Cranial nerves may be involved, most often the sixth, fifth, and third,[22] but involvement occurs mostly as part of an ischemic stroke of the brain stem. Internuclear ophthalmoplegia has been reported as an isolated finding with cerebellar signs almost certainly resulting from occlusive vertebrobasilar disease.[23] Several unusual unconfirmed manifestations have been reported in isolation, such as bilateral acoustic nerve involvement leading to sudden deafness[24] and visual loss due to posterior ischemic optic neuropathy.[25,26]

The extent of involvement of multiple mononeuropathies in polyarteritis nodosa varies greatly, but they may lead to a crippling and especially painful state. In a few patients, the cephalad progression of paresthesias and quadriplegia may suggest Guillain-Barré syndrome, but frequent alternating sequential involvement of isolated nerves clearly suggests mononeuritis multiplex. Muscle pain and red urine in association with quadriplegia may indicate rhabdomyolysis.[27]

PATHOPHYSIOLOGIC MECHANISMS

In the pathogenesis of vasculitis neuropathy, axonal degeneration remains a hallmark feature, but the mechanisms leading to small vessel injury remain to be elucidated. Endolethial cell adhesion molecules, such as intercellular adhesion molecule 1 and E-selectin, are expressed in microvessels surrounded by infiltrates, and they may become targets for therapy that is specific rather than just for neurologic manifestations. Cell-mediated cytotoxicity and genetic proclivity may play a role.[28,29] T cells and macrophages have been noted in cellular infiltrates in vascular walls. Satoi and associates[29] found expression of nitric oxide synthetase, cyclooxygenase-2, perforen, and matrix metalloproteinases in macrophages from nerve biopsy specimens in patients with vasculitis, suggesting that free radical nitric oxide, prostaglandins, and matrix metalloproteinases mediate inflammation and cytotoxicity.

The tendency of the disorder to unfold in exacerbation and remission is corroborated by the pathologic finding of different stages of vasculitis in biopsied tissue. Sural nerve biopsy has a high yield in patients with electrodiagnostic abnormalities and usually shows predominantly necrotizing vasculitis of the vasa vasorum with axonal degeneration[30] (Fig. 12–2).

The outcome of mononeuritis multiplex is difficult to predict, but recovery of the neuropathy often parallels control of the systemic vasculitis. Survival in patients with polyarteritis nodosa complicated by multiple mononeuropathies is not worse than that in patients whose nerves are spared.[18] Rapid remission of both mononeuritis multiplex and distal polyneuropathy occurs only in patients with limited involvement. Substantial recovery of nerve function, however, can be appreciated only after months and is less likely in patients with rapid onset and maximal

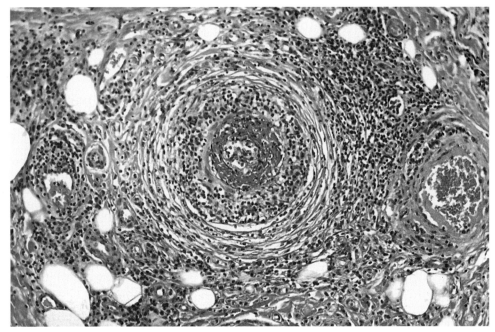

Figure 12–2. Photomicrograph of sural nerve. Large epineural artery with marked constriction, fibrinoid degeneration of intima, and cellular infiltration of media and aventitia, features typical of systemic necrotic vasculitis occurring in periarteritis nodosa, Churg-Strauss disease, Wegener's granulomatosis, and hypersensitivity angiitis. (Courtesy of Dr. P. Dyck, Peripheral Nerve Center, Mayo Clinic, Rochester, MN.)

deficits of the muscles innervated by the affected nerve. Unfortunately, many patients experience immense suffering from persisting pain and remain disabled from footdrop and wristdrop.

Cyclophosphamide (1 to 2 mg/kg orally) and prednisone (1 mg/kg per day) for 8 weeks followed by tapering treatment can be effective in patients with mononeuritis multiplex or distal polyneuropathy, but the individual response is hard to predict and determined by the degree of axonal loss.[31] In severe cases, additional treatment with plasma exchange, antiplatelet drugs, or azathioprine may seem reasonable, but its efficacy is uncertain. Plasma exchange may be a consideration as a last resort for patients in whom signs and symptoms progress despite adequate immunosuppression.

Neuropathic pain should be treated with gabapentin, 900 to 3600 mg/day.[32] Alternative agents include nortriptyline and amitriptyline, but they are less effective and have more adverse events. Carbamazepine and phenytoin are less effective in abolishing the severe pain with vasculitis. Finally, in refractory cases, intravenous administration of fentanyl can be considered.[33] Some recent evidence also suggests that pain can be relieved by a low dose of prednisone (10 mg/day) after initial high-dose therapy (60 mg/day).[34]

Central Nervous System Involvement

Patients may have a confusional state, visual impairment, and generalized tonic–clonic seizures that can be attributed to malignant hypertension. A reported instance of transient magnetic resonance imaging (MRI) abnormalities in the white matter can be fully explained by coexisting malignant hypertension.[35]

Virtually all arteries can be afflicted by necrosis, including large intracranial arteries, smaller meningeal arteries, and, occasionally, the temporal artery. Autopsy studies have reported well-documented cases of cerebral or brain stem infarction associated with occlusive vasculitic disease, in many already evident intra vitam on cerebral angiograms or MRI (Fig. 12–3). In Ford and Siekert's series,[36] 13% of the 114 patients with polyarteritis nodosa had cerebral infarction or hemorrhage. Stroke occurred more often in patients with multiple organ involvement and rarely as a presenting feature. Cerebral infarcts have been located in the distribution of both the anterior and the posterior circulation. Infarction of the basal ganglia has led to an acute Parkinson's syndrome.[37] These earlier studies may be biased toward the worst cases because of lack of aggressive therapy. A recent review of the literature of polyarteritis nodosa claimed a frequent occurrence of lacunar syndromes (capsule, striatum, centrum semiovale) attributed to hypertension, a thrombotic microangiopathy, or associated antiphospholipid antibodies.[38,39] Next to specific treatment of the disorder itself, antiplatelet agents might be the drugs of choice to prevent recurrent attacks, but long-term treatment with warfarin is indicated if anticardiolipin antibodies are demonstrated.

Intracerebral hemorrhage due to hypertension from renal failure is commonly localized in the putamen. Subarachnoid hemorrhage may be caused by dissection through necrotic and destroyed media.[40] However, intracranial aneurysms, in contrast to visceral arteries, are less common.[41,42] On the other hand, Munn and associates[43] found that at 3 months to 10 years after the presenting diagnosis of subarachnoid hemorrhage, four of six patients had evidence of vasculitis in other vascular beds.

Patients with sudden spinal cord syndrome should undergo emergency MRI because an extradural hematoma compressing the spinal cord has been reported in polyarteritis.[44] In other anecdotal cases, necrotizing arteritis of spinal cord arteries resulted in spinal cord infarction.[45]

CHURG-STRAUSS SYNDROME

Churg and Strauss[46] pathologically established a distinctive clinical syndrome with

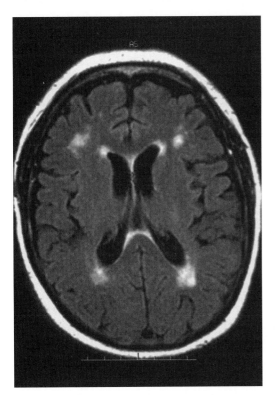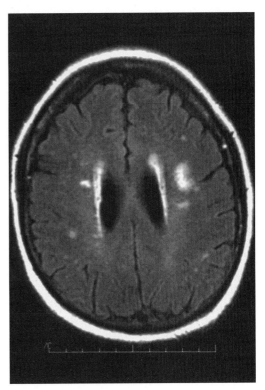

Figure 12–3. Magnetic resonance images of the brain (fluid-attenuated inversion recovery) in a patient with transient focal signs and proven periarteritis nodosa. Note scattered small hyperintensities indicating infarcts.

systemic vasculitis, similar to polyarteritis nodosa, but with tissue infiltration by eosinophils, a vasculitic process extending into venules and capillaries, and predominant pulmonary involvement.[47–49]

Clinical Features

Late-onset asthma (third decade) is a defining feature in this disorder. Systemic vasculitis may occur years after recurrent rhinorrhea, pansinusitis, and repeated nasal polypectomies.

Patients with Churg-Strauss disease may be admitted to the medical ICU because of an initially puzzling pulmonary disorder, or patients with congestive heart failure are seen in a coronary care unit. Respiratory failure from acute lung injury results in urgent need for mechanical ventilation in many patients and causes death in 10%. Chest radiographs may demonstrate bilateral confluent or nodular infiltrates with pleural effusions that contain massive numbers of eosinophils, but the clinical and radiographic presentation may resemble that of many of the community-acquired pneumonias.[50] Diffuse interstitial or miliary lesions have been reported, but without cavitary lesions. Alveolar hemorrhage may suddenly worsen gas exchange, but its occurrence is not specific for this disorder.[51]

Congestive heart failure is a major cause of death in Churg-Strauss disease from involvement of the epicardium and may be clinically detected by a loud friction rub. Other cardiac manifestations that have certainly been known to occur are eosinophilic myocarditis with restrictive cardiomyopathy and coronary arteritis with myocardial infarction. For some unknown reason, renal disease and acute hypertension are less common in Churg-Strauss syndrome. The diagnosis of Churg-Strauss syndrome can be made after renal, skin, and muscle biopsies. Typical granulomas surrounded by eosinophils are seen. Open lung biopsy specimens are often nonspecific but may show granulomas surrounded by eosinophils. Most of the laboratory evaluation is similar to that in polyarteritis nodosa. Clinical remission can be expected in more than 90% of patients after immunosuppression.[52]

Peripheral Nervous System Involvement

Mononeuritis multiplex may seem less frequent in Churg-Strauss syndrome than in polyarteritis but nevertheless affects a third of patients. The common peroneal nerve is often involved, followed by the ulnar and radial nerves.[52] Asthma and other atopic signs typically antedate the onset of neuropathy, but the interval varies (average, 7 years).[53] The clinical manifestations are similar to those in polyarteritis nodosa, but involvement is more extensive, as reflected by a potential for recovery of only 50%. Sehgal and colleagues[53] reported the Mayo Clinic experience of 47 patients with Churg-Strauss syndrome. Of 25 patients with a polyneuropathy, 17 had evidence of multiple mononeuropathy, 7 had a distal symmetrical polyneuropathy, and 1 had generalized polyneuropathy with asymmetrical findings. Cramping in calf muscles, caused by myositis, may be an overwhelming complaint in some patients. Muscle biopsy examination is rarely diagnostic, because typical granulomas are difficult to sample. Isolated cranial nerve involvement (II, III, VII, VIII) has been noted. In the Mayo Clinic series, a symmetrical trigeminal neuropathy was noted, but there were no other instances of multicranial nerve involvement.[53] Transient monocular blindness or permanent retinal infarcts[54] may be manifestations of vasculitis or artery-to-artery embolism. Bilateral optic neuropathy resulting in profound visual loss in rapid succession in both eyes with peripapillary hemorrhage has been reported.[55] Recovery in visual acuity is not expected despite aggressive treatment.

Treatment of Churg-Strauss syndrome is similar to that of polyarteritis nodosa. The response can be brisk, and remission is expected within weeks of corticosteroid therapy.[56] As noted previously, outcome in mononeuritis multiplex or distal polyneuropathy is less favorable. Long-term high-dose corticosteroid therapy (3 to 6 months, 1 mg/kg per day) is preferred in patients with mononeuritis multiplex, and tapering of the dosage even when the systemic manifestations subside should be postponed for some months to allow for aggressive control of the inflammatory neuropathy.

Central Nervous System Involvement

Central nervous system involvement seems rare in Churg-Strauss syndrome, and other mechanisms should be sought in patients with a manifestation such as confusion, seizures, or coma. Intracerebral hemorrhage has been reported but without further clinical or computed tomography (CT) details. In Lanham and associates' series of 50 patients,[49] 16% had intracranial hemorrhage. Cerebral infarcts have been reported but without pathologic confirmation of vasculitis. Because cardiomyopathy develops in a sizable proportion of patients with Churg-Strauss disease, a cardiac embolic source should be considered in these patients.[53] Among the 96 patients with Churg-Strauss syndrome reported by Guillevin and associates[52] of the French Vasculitis Study Group, ischemic stroke developed in 6%. Whether a vasculitis triggered an ischemic stroke in these cases remained unknown, because cerebral angiography was performed in only one patient, who had no abnormalities.

WEGENER'S GRANULOMATOSIS

Wegener's triad (simultaneous involvement of upper and lower respiratory tract and kidneys) often points to the diagnosis, but the lesions of Wegener's granulomatosis may involve nearly any organ.[57–59]

Clinical Features

Pulmonary infiltrates and sinusitis initially characterize the disease. Involvement of the respiratory tract can rapidly become life threatening. Multiple nodular and cavitary infiltrates are radiologic features of Wegener's granulomatosis, but in some patients

fulminant pulmonary hemorrhage prompts intensive care admission. Other emergency conditions are spontaneous pneumothorax, severe subglottic stenosis from pseudotumors, and massive epistaxis.

Although necrotizing glomerulonephritis is commonly seen in classic Wegener's granulomatosis, it is seldom reported as a cause of acute progressive renal failure. The diagnosis of Wegener's granulomatosis is greatly facilitated by the finding of cytoplasm-staining antineutrophil cytoplasmic autoantibodies, which have a reported sensitivity of 66% and specificity of more than 90%. Open lung biopsy is preferred for pathologic diagnosis, but granulomatous foci may be found in virtually any tissue. Unfortunately, despite the easy accessibility of nasal mucosa, the diagnostic yield of nasal tissue biopsies is low.

In approximately one-third of patients with Wegener's granulomatosis, a neurologic manifestation develops during the course of the illness. Wegener's granulomatosis may be particularly considered in a patient with a new neurologic finding. In a review series of 324 cases from the Mayo Clinic, cranial neuropathy (usually ophthalmoplegia), temporal arteritis (without giant cells), and ischemic stroke were common conditions at presentation.[60,61]

Peripheral Nervous System Involvement

Mononeuritis multiplex or asymmetrical sensory-motor polyneuropathy occurred in 16% of patients in the Mayo Clinic series, a remarkably lower incidence than that in other systemic vasculitides.[61] The interval between onset of Wegener's granulomatosis and diagnosis of neuropathy is short, approximately 1 year. The peroneal or tibial nerve is most commonly affected, followed in order by the ulnar, median, radial, and femoral nerves. The second, sixth, and seventh cranial nerves are often involved separately, but multiple cranial neuropathy may occur and can be unilateral when caused by local invasion by destructive granulomatous tumors.

Central Nervous System Involvement

Granulomatous masses arising in the paranasal sinuses may cause destruction of the cavernous sinus manifested by ophthalmoplegia. A large localized mass may also compress the carotid artery and result in ischemic stroke. Some plausible anecdotal cases suggest that vasculitis of cerebral arteries may cause ischemic or hemorrhagic stroke in Wegener's granulomatosis.[62,63] Extensive involvement of the anterior cerebral artery due to contiguous invasion from the nasal cavity may lead to bilateral frontal infarcts and be recognized by abulia and personality changes.[64] However, multiple cerebral infarcts from vasculitic involvement of small arteries may occur. Cerebral angiography in patients with cerebral infarcts in Wegener's disease may be nondiagnostic for this reason, and brain biopsy may be needed for confirmation. On MRI, central nervous system vasculitis in Wegener's granulomatosis may be demonstrated by multiple T2-weighted signal abnormalities in frontal, parietal, and occipital lobes in the cortex and at the gray–white matter junction[65] and also by dural thickening and meningeal enhancement, including the spinal cord.[66] Meningeal enhancement may disappear with appropriate treatment.[67] Wegener's granulomatosis can be accompanied by multiple granulomatous lesions that markedly diminish in size after treatment with cyclophosphamide, prednisone, trimethoprim, and sulfamethoxazole.[68–70] When the entire vessel is inflamed, it may rupture and produce a subarachnoid hemorrhage or intracerebral hemorrhage.[71,72]

DRUG-INDUCED VASCULITIS

Drug-induced vasculitis is categorized together with other hypersensitivity vasculitides (postinfectious Henoch-Schönlein syndrome in children and mixed cryoglobulinemia). Drug-induced vasculitis often is based on circumstantial evidence. Commonly implicated drugs are antibiotics, nonsteroidal antiinflammatory agents, sulfonamides, and anti-epileptic drugs. A fulminant vasculitis may develop 7 to 10 days after drug injection. It remains a rare occurrence in the ICU.

Examination of tissue with a fully developed lesion shows leukoclastic (polymorphonuclear necrotizing and fragmentary nuclei) small veins, particularly the postcapillary venules in the dermis. The skin is most commonly involved, and virtually all types of lesions can occur. None is specific for one drug category. Frequently, palpable patches of purpura that can be nodular, urticarial, ulcerative, and vesicular are found on the legs, but in other patients, maculopapular or erythema multiforme rashes are more characteristic.[73] Nasal and oral mucosae may not be spared. Renal failure is common. Gastrointestinal abnormalities and lung and cardiac involvement are uncommon, although in some patients, multiorgan involvement may be a direct cause of death. Fortunately, the disorder is frequently self-limiting. Treatment is supportive, but patients probably should receive a course of prednisone.

With the almost complete disappearance of acute serum sickness, which has traditionally been associated with encephalopathy, polyneuropathy, plexopathy, seizures, and coma,[74] neurologic manifestations of drug-induced vasculitis are rare, but they could be underreported. Numbness and painful paresthesias are common, but pruritus and burning sensations may be caused by the skin lesion itself rather than from a sensory-motor polyneuropathy or a developing mononeuritis multiplex. In a review of case reports by Mullick and associates,[75] sensory-motor polyneuropathy was reported anecdotally in 4 of 70 patients with drug-related vasculitis. Well-documented cases with histologic or electrodiagnostic confirmation are not available.

Focal or generalized seizures have been reported, usually without a known cause. In one patient with an allopurinol-associated vasculitis, seizures could be linked to central nervous system vasculitis and infarction documented on CT scan and highly suggestive cerebral angiograms.[76] There is little systematic study of neurologic complications in this type of vasculitis, and whether associations exist is difficult to gauge because of its rarity.

CONCLUSIONS

The peripheral nervous system becomes involved in severe forms of acute vasculitis syndromes with acute respiratory or renal failure. The principal goal in treatment is to achieve rapid remission of the neuropathy that may cause severe disability. In general, the efficacy of immunosuppressive medication (cyclophosphamide, 1 to 2 mg/kg, and prednisone, 1 mg/kg per day) is best demonstrated in improvement of distal polyneuropathy and mononeuritis multiplex. Central nervous system involvement in Wegener's granulomatosis may be due to invasion of nasal granulomas, remote granulomas compressing cranial nerves, or vasculitis of the intracranial tree.

In Wegener's granulomatosis, cranial neuropathy, temporal arteritis, and ischemic stroke may be presenting features. Vasculitis of cerebral vessels may produce intracranial hemorrhages or multiple territory cerebral infarcts. Ischemic stroke, lacunar infarcts, and deep hemorrhages (from associated hypertension) are predominantly found in polyarteritis nodosa and Churg-Strauss syndrome.

REFERENCES

1. Jennette JC, Falk RJ. Do vasculitis categorization systems really matter? Curr Rheumatol Rep 2:430–438, 2000.
2. Jennette JC, Falk RJ. Small-vessel vasculitis. N Engl J Med 337:1512–1523, 1997.
3. Hunder G. Vasculitis: diagnosis and therapy. Am J Med 100:37S-45S, 1996.
4. Lie JT. Diagnostic histopathology of major systemic and pulmonary vasculitic syndromes. Rheum Dis Clin North Am 16:269–292, 1990.
5. Specks U, DeRemee RA. Granulomatous vasculitis. Wegener's granulomatosis and Churg-Strauss syndrome. Rheum Dis Clin North Am 16:377–397, 1990.
6. Walker GL. Neurological features of polyarteritis nodosa. Clin Exp Neurol 15:237–247, 1978.
7. Churg A, Churg J (eds). Systemic Vasculitides. Igaku-Shoin, New York, 1991.
8. Cohen RD, Conn DL, Ilstrup DM. Clinical features, prognosis, and response to treatment in polyarteritis. Mayo Clin Proc 55:146–155, 1980.
9. Falk RJ, Jennette JC. Anti-neutrophil cytoplasmic autoantibodies with specificity for myeloperoxidase in patients with systemic vasculitis and idiopathic necrotizing and crescentic glomerulonephritis. N Engl J Med 318:1651–1657, 1988.
10. Panegyres PK, Blumbergs PC, Leong AS, Bourne AJ. Vasculitis of peripheral nerve and skeletal muscle: clinicopathological correlation and immunopathic mechanisms. J Neurol Sci 100:193–202, 1990.
11. Wees SJ, Sunwoo IN, Oh SJ. Sural nerve biopsy in systemic necrotizing vasculitis. Am J Med 71:525–532, 1981.
12. Fort JG, Griffin R, Tahmoush A, Abruzzo JL. Muscle involvement in polyarteritis nodosa: report of a patient presenting clinically as polymyositis and review of the literature. J Rheumatol 21:945–948, 1994.
13. Kernohan JW, Woltman HW. Periarteritis nodosa: a clinicopathologic study with special reference to the nervous system. Arch Neurol Psychiatry 39:655–686, 1938.
14. Belsole RJ, Lister GD, Kleinert HE. Polyarteritis: a cause of nerve palsy in the extremity. J Hand Surg (Am) 3:320–325, 1978.
15. Bouche P, Leger JM, Travers MA, Cathala HP, Castaigne P. Peripheral neuropathy in systemic vasculitis: clinical and electrophysiologic study of 22 patients. Neurology 36:1598–1602, 1986.
16. Castaigne P, Burnet P, Hauw JJ, Leger JM, Gherardi R, Guillevin L. Peripheral nervous system and panarteritis nodosa. Review of 27 cases [in French]. Rev Neurol (Paris) 140:343–352, 1984.
17. Chang RW, Bell CL, Hallett M. Clinical characteristics and prognosis of vasculitic mononeuropathy multiplex. Arch Neurol 41:618–621, 1984.
18. Frohnert PP, Sheps SG. Long-term follow-up study of periarteritis nodosa. Am J Med 43:8–14, 1967.
19. Harati Y, Niakan E. The clinical spectrum of inflammatory-angiopathic neuropathy. J Neurol Neurosurg Psychiatry 49:1313–1316, 1986.
20. Kissel JT, Slivka AP, Warmolts JR, Mendell JR. The clinical spectrum of necrotizing angiopathy of the peripheral nervous system. Ann Neurol 18:251–257, 1985.
21. Moore PM, Cupps TR. Neurological complications of vasculitis. Ann Neurol 14:155–167, 1983.
22. Hagen NA, Stevens JC, Michet CJ Jr. Trigeminal sensory neuropathy associated with connective tissue diseases. Neurology 40:891–896, 1990.
23. Kirkali P, Topaloglu R, Kansu T, Bakkaloglu A. Third nerve palsy and internuclear ophthalmoplegia in periarteritis nodosa. J Pediatr Ophthalmol Strabismus 28:45–46, 1991.
24. Lake-Bakaar G. Polyarteritis nodosa presenting with bilateral nerve deafness. J R Soc Med 71:144–147, 1978.
25. Hutchinson CH. Polyarteritis nodosa presenting as posterior ischaemic optic neuropathy. J R Soc Med 77:1043–1046, 1984.
26. Long SM, Dolin P. Polyarteritis nodosa presenting as acute blindness. Ann Emerg Med 24:523–525, 1994.
27. Smith DL, Kim JA, Wang B. Polyarteritis nodosa-induced quadriplegia [letter]. Ann Intern Med 122:731–732, 1995.
28. Coll-Vinent B, Cebrian M, Cid MC, et al. Dynamic pattern of endothelial cell adhesion molecule expression in muscle and perineural vessels from patients with classic polyarteritis nodosa. Arthritis Rheum 41:435–444, 1998.

29. Satoi H, Oka N, Kawasaki T, Miyamoto K, Akiguchi I, Kimura J. Mechanisms of tissue injury in vasculitic neuropathies. Neurology 50:492–496, 1998.

30. Hawke SH, Davies L, Pamphlett R, Guo YP, Pollard JD, McLeod JG. Vasculitic neuropathy. A clinical and pathological study. Brain 114:2175–2190, 1991.

31. Fauci AS, Katz P, Haynes BF, Wolff SM. Cyclophosphamide therapy of severe systemic necrotizing vasculitis. N Engl J Med 301:235–238, 1979.

32. Laird MA, Gidal BE. Use of gabapentin in the treatment of neuropathic pain. Ann Pharmacother 34:802–807, 2000.

33. Dellemijn PL, Vanneste JA. Randomised double-blind active-placebo-controlled crossover trial of intravenous fentanyl in neuropathic pain. Lancet 349:753–758, 1997.

34. Bradley WG, Verma A. Painful vasculitic neuropathy in HIV-1 infection: relief of pain with prednisone therapy. Neurology 47:1446–1451, 1996.

35. Koppensteiner R, Base W, Bognar H, Kiss A, al Mubarak M, Tscholakoff D. Course of cerebral lesions in a patient with periarteritis nodosa studied by magnetic resonance imaging. Klin Wochenschr 67:398–401, 1989.

36. Ford RG, Siekert RG. Central nervous system manifestations of periarteritis nodosa. Neurology 15:114–122, 1965.

37. Mayo J, Arias M, Leno C, Berciano J. Vascular parkinsonism and periarteritis nodosa [letter]. Neurology 36:874–875, 1986.

38. Morelli S, Perrone C, Paroli M. Recurrent cerebral infarctions in polyarteritis nodosa with circulating antiphospholipid antibodies and mitral valve disease. Lupus 7:51–52, 1998.

39. Reichhart MD, Bogousslavsky J, Janzer RC. Early lacunar strokes complicating polyarteritis nodosa: thrombotic microangiopathy. Neurology 54:883–889, 2000.

40. Gherardi GJ, Lee HY. Localized dissecting hemorrhage and arteritis. Renal and cerebral manifestations. JAMA 199:219–220, 1967.

41. Iaconetta G, Benvenuti D, Lamaida E, Gallicchio B, Signorelli F, Maiuri F. Cerebral hemorrhagic complication in polyarteritis nodosa. Case report and review of the literature. Acta Neurol (Napoli) 16:64–69, 1994.

42. Oran I, Memis A, Parildar M, Yunten N. Multiple intracranial aneurysms in polyarteritis nodosa: MRI and angiography. Neuroradiology 41:436–439, 1999.

43. Munn EJ, Alloway JA, Diffin DC, Arroyo RA. Polyarteritis with symptomatic intracerebral aneurysms at initial presentation. J Rheumatol 25:2022–2025, 1998.

44. Haft H, Finneson BE, Cramer H, Fiol R. Periarteritis nodosa as a source of subarachnoid hemorrhage and spinal cord compression: report of a case and review of the literature. J Neurosurg 14:608–616, 1957.

45. Ojeda VJ. Polyarteritis nodosa affecting the spinal cord arteries. Aust N Z J Med 13:287–289, 1983.

46. Churg J, Strauss L. Allergic granulomatosis, allergic angiitis, and periarteritis nodosa. Am J Pathol 27:277–301, 1951.

47. Chumbley LC, Harrison EG Jr, DeRemee RA. Allergic granulomatosis and angiitis (Churg-Strauss syndrome). Report and analysis of 30 cases. Mayo Clin Proc 52:477–484, 1977.

48. Lanham JG, Churg J. Churg-Strauss syndrome. In: Churg A, Churg J (eds). Systemic Vasculitides. Igaku-Shoin Medical Publishers, New York, 1991, pp 101–120.

49. Lanham JG, Elkon KB, Pusey CD, Hughes GR. Systemic vasculitis with asthma and eosinophilia: a clinical approach to the Churg-Strauss syndrome. Medicine (Baltimore) 63:65–81, 1984.

50. Degesys GE, Mintzer RA, Vrla RF. Allergic granulomatosis: Churg-Strauss syndrome. AJR Am J Roentgenol 135:1281–1282, 1980.

51. Clutterbuck EJ, Pusey CD. Severe alveolar haemorrhage in Churg-Strauss syndrome. Eur J Respir Dis 71:158–163, 1987.

52. Guillevin L, Cohen P, Gayraud M, Lhote F, Jarrousse B, Casassus P. Churg-Strauss syndrome: clinical study and long-term follow-up of 96 patients. Medicine 78:26–37, 1999.

53. Sehgal M, Swanson JW, DeRemee RA, Colby TV. Neurologic manifestations of Churg-Strauss syndrome. Mayo Clin Proc 70:337–341, 1995.

54. Dagi LR, Currie J. Branch retinal artery occlusion in the Churg-Strauss syndrome. J Clin Neuroophthalmol 5:229–237, 1985.

55. Acheson JF, Cockerell OC, Bentley CR, Sanders MD. Churg-Strauss vasculitis presenting with severe visual loss due to bilateral sequential optic neuropathy. Br J Ophthalmol 77:118–119, 1993.

56. MacFadyen R, Tron V, Keshmiri M, Road JD. Allergic angiitis of Churg and Strauss syndrome. Response to pulse methylprednisolone. Chest 91:629–631, 1987.

57. Fahey JL, Leonard E, Churg J, Godman GC. Wegener's granulomatosis. Am J Med 17:168–179, 1954.

58. Fauci AS, Haynes BF, Katz P, Wolff SM. Wegener's granulomatosis: prospective clinical and therapeutic experience with 85 patients for 21 years. Ann Intern Med 98:76–85, 1983.

59. Godman GC, Churg J. Wegener's granulomatosis: pathology and review of the literature. Arch Pathol 58:533–553, 1954.

60. Nishino H, DeRemee RA, Rubino FA, Parisi JE. Wegener's granulomatosis associated with vasculitis of the temporal artery: report of five cases. Mayo Clin Proc 68:115–121, 1993.

61. Nishino H, Rubino FA, DeRemee RA, Swanson JW, Parisi JE. Neurological involvement in Wegener's granulomatosis: an analysis of 324 consecutive patients at the Mayo Clinic. Ann Neurol 33:4–9, 1993.

62. Lucas FV, Benjamin SP, Steinberg MC. Cerebral vasculitis in Wegener's granulomatosis. Cleve Clin Q 43:275–281, 1976.

63. Yamashita Y, Takahashi M, Bussaka H, Miyawaki M, Tosaka K. Cerebral vasculitis secondary to Wegener's granulomatosis: computed tomography and angiographic findings. J Comput Tomogr 10:115–120, 1986.

64. Satoh J, Miyasaka N, Yamada T, et al. Extensive cerebral infarction due to involvement of both anterior cerebral arteries by Wegener's granulomatosis. Ann Rheum Dis 47:606–611, 1988.

65. von Scheven E, Lee C, Berg BO. Pediatric Wegener's granulomatosis complicated by central nervous system vasculitis. Pediatr Neurol 19:317–319, 1998.

66. Murphy JM, Gomez-Anson B, Gillard JH, et al. Wegener granulomatosis: MR imaging findings in brain and meninges. Radiology 213:794–799, 1999.

67. Spranger M, Schwab S, Meinck H-M, et al. Meningeal involvement in Wegener's granulomatosis confirmed and monitored by positive circulating antineutrophil cytoplasm in cerebrospinal fluid. Neurology 48:263–265, 1997.

68. Miller KS, Miller JM. Wegener's granulomatosis presenting as a primary seizure disorder with brain lesions demonstrated by magnetic resonance imaging. Chest 103:316–318, 1993.

69. Oimomi M, Suehiro I, Mizuno N, Baba S, Okada S, Kanazawa Y. Wegener's granulomatosis with intracerebral granuloma and mammary manifestation. Report of a case. Arch Intern Med 140:853–854, 1980.

70. Payton CD, Jones JM. Cortical blindness complicating Wegener's granulomatosis. Br Med J 290:676, 1985.

71. Drachman DA. Neurological complications of Wegener's granulomatosis. Arch Neurol 8:145–155, 1963.

72. Hearne CB, Zawada ET Jr. Survival after intracerebral hemorrhage in Wegener's granulomatosis. West J Med 137:431–434, 1982.

73. Aboobaker J, Greaves MW. Urticarial vasculitis. Clin Exp Dermatol 11:436–444, 1986.

74. Park AM, Richardson JC. Cerebral complications of serum sickness. Neurology 3:277–283, 1953.

75. Mullick FG, McAllister HA Jr, Wagner BM, Fenoglio JJ Jr. Drug related vasculitis. Clinicopathologic correlations in 30 patients. Hum Pathol 10:313–325, 1979.

76. Weiss EB, Forman P, Rosenthal IM. Allopurinol-induced arteritis in partial HGPRTase deficiency: atypical seizure manifestation. Arch Intern Med 138:1743–1744, 1978.

Chapter 13

NEUROLOGIC COMPLICATIONS IN THE CRITICALLY ILL PREGNANT PATIENT

A pregnant woman slipping into a life-threatening condition remains one of the most trying of all presentations. Obstetric admissions to the intensive care unit are the most common peripartum emergencies and often include obstetric hemorrhage and uncontrolled hypertension.[1]

Pregnancy-specific disorders such as (pre) eclampsia, HELLP syndrome (**h**emolysis, **el**evated **l**iver enzymes, and **l**ow **p**latelet count), amniotic fluid embolism, and neurologic manifestations of tocolytic agents are the most common causes of admission to the intensive care unit. These are the main focus of this chapter. Other typical manifestations of critical illness in pregnancy, such as sepsis, are discussed in Chapter 6. Neurologists should work in concert with gynecologists

and should have a working knowledge of these illnesses of pregnancy. The objective of delivery of a viable fetus remains highly probable, yet there is a serious impact on maternal mortality.[2,3]

ECLAMPSIA

Eclampsia is more common in patients with preexisting hypertension or renal disease, prior episodes of eclampsia, nulliparity or multiple gestation, triploidy, molar pregnancy, and hydrops fetalis.[4] Curiously, a paternal component exists. Both men and women are predisposed to have children born of a pregnancy complicated by preeclampsia if they were born of a preeclamptic pregnancy themselves.[5]

Hypertension is prevalent in pregnancies (approximately 10%), but eclampsia is broadly defined as seizures or coma in a hypertensive patient. A working group on high blood pressure in pregnancy defined preeclampsia as occurrence of hypertension, proteinuria, or pitting edema after 20 weeks of gestation. *Hypertension* is defined as blood pressure above 140/90 mm Hg on two occasions 4 hr apart and *proteinuria* as urinary excretion of protein exceeding 300 mg in 24 hr.[6] More than 75% of patients with eclampsia present before partus, or intrapartum and postpartum eclampsia may occur up to 7 days after delivery.

PATHOPHYSIOLOGIC MECHANISMS

The crucial component in the pathology of eclampsia is endothelial cell damage. In response to this vascular injury, a cascade of vasoconstriction and intravascular coagulation occurs involving renal, hepatic, and hematopoietic systems. The prostaglandins thromboxane (from trophoblastic tissue) and prostacyclin (from endothelial cells) work in opposite ways. Thromboxane causes vasoconstriction and clumping of platelets; prostacyclin causes vasodilation and inhibits platelet aggregation. A reversal of the normal balanced ratio has been considered one of the possible mechanisms.

Circulating human chorionic gonadotropin (hCG) and thrombomodulin may reflect the severity of endothelial injury. The changes in placental tissue are postulated to alter the syncytiotrophoblast and cytotrophoblast and thus alter hCG secretion. In addition, thrombomodulin, a soluble endothelial surface glycoprotein, is released after damage to the endothelium and is a cofactor for thrombin-catalyzed activation of protein C.

Clinical Features

Antepartum preeclampsia or eclampsia may be manifested not only by hypertension or proteinuria but also by edema, which may become generalized, including pitting edema in the hands and facial edema. Headaches become gradually severe and pounding, and eventually they may be associated with sudden obscurations if papilledema emerges. The clinical presentation is indistinguishable from hypertensive encephalopathy and also supported by similar radiologic hallmarks (see Chapter 9 for details).

Generalized tonic–clonic seizures are defining but also dreaded moments in the evolution of eclampsia. Flurries of seizures (for example, three or four in one day) may occur but rarely turn into status epilepticus.[7] Other causes, albeit rare, should be considered if seizures continue (Table 13–1).

Visual disturbances may be the primary clinical presentation and evolve into cortical

Table 13–1. Seizures and Status Epilepticus in Pregnancy

Eclampsia
Arteriovenous malformation
Aneurysmal rupture
Encephalitis
Meningitis (*Listeria*)
Cerebral infarct
Puerperal cerebral venous thrombosis
Illicit drug use or withdrawal
Water intoxication

blindness.[8,9] Cortical blindness with denial (Anton's syndrome) is less common,[7,9,10] but blindness, when present, is frequently associated with excruciating headache and persistently increased blood pressures. If untreated, it may be a prelude to seizures, and patients may lapse into any degree of altered state of consciousness. Profound coma may be a manifestation in eclampsia, but most patients are obtuse and inattentive. Generalized brain edema with transtentorial herniation was noted in one patient from a large study of patients with eclampsia, but this is uncommon.[11] Localizing neurologic findings are not expected from eclampsia alone and may suggest it has been complicated by a stroke.

Pregnancies terminating with eclampsia are more commonly complicated by ischemic and hemorrhagic strokes.[12–14] In a study in the Ile de France region, eclampsia accounted for a surprising 44% of intraparenchymal hemorrhages and 47% of ischemic strokes in a cohort with more than 300,000 deliveries.[15] Intraparenchymal hemorrhage, as expected, occurred in typical locations associated with hypertension, including the putamen, brain stem, and cerebellum.

Postpartum eclampsia, however, may be more subtle. Raps and associates[16] convincingly documented white matter abnormalities on magnetic resonance imaging (MRI) in four postpartum women with hypertension but no proteinuria or edema, suggesting that at least for neurologic manifestations, the criteria may be too stringent.

Neuroimaging

Computed tomography (CT) scanning results were normal in 42% of the patients, but this finding may represent differences in technique and quality of CT scans.[7] The MRI findings are abnormal in patients who present with blindness. Characteristic findings are hyperintense signal abnormalities in occipital lobes,[17,18] but these brightly outlined lesions may also be noted in the basal ganglia and periventricular white matter and without clinical accompaniment. Frontal and temporal lobe lesions and petechial hemorrhages without the typical symmetrical distribution of the occipital lesions in eclampsia have been described (Fig. 13–1). Intracerebral hematomas may appear on MRI but were much less common (6%) in cases reviewed by Thomas.[7] Small lobar hemorrhages, cortical petechiae, and subarachnoid hemorrhage were found at autopsy in patients who had been gravely ill. Lesions in the subcortical white matter that follow the gyri may be found.[19,20]

Complete resolution of the abnormalities is characteristic after treatment, supporting the notion that the lesions mentioned above are either from edema due to increased intracellular fluid secondary to transient cellular ischemia or from edema due to a disruption of the blood–brain barrier. The increased apparent diffusion coefficient value on diffusion-weighted MR images in a 23-year-old primigravida indicated that vasogenic edema was the predominant mechanism.[18]

Management

Management of seizures and hypertension is a key component to management of eclampsia. Obstetricians emphasize induction of delivery, and when feasible, this should be the most appropriate approach.

The choice of magnesium sulfate over phenytoin has been questioned,[21–23] but judged by any standard, magnesium sulfate has been found superior to phenytoin and diazepam.[22] The therapeutic level needed to prevent seizures is 4 to 6 mEq/L. It can be achieved after a loading dose of 4 g of magnesium sulfate followed by a maintenance infusion of 1 g/hr (Fig. 13–2). Rapid infusion of magnesium sulfate results in sweating, sensations of warmth, and flushing due to peripheral vasodilatation. Recurrent seizures are treated with an individual bolus of 2 to 4 g of magnesium sulfate given over 5 min. The toxicity of magnesium sulfate can be substantial, but because tendon reflexes disappear before symptoms of toxicity appear, frequent testing of the tendon reflexes is an important monitoring procedure. However, severe muscular and respiratory weakness occurs when serum levels are allowed to increase more than 12 mg/dL, and cardiac arrest has been noted with severe toxicity. In these circumstances, calcium gluconate (10%; 10 mL) counters magnesium toxicity. For antepartum eclampsia, administration of magnesium sulfate is continued until 24 hr after delivery, and for postpartum eclampsia, it is discontinued 24 hr after the last seizure, preferably when electroencephalography shows no epileptogenic focus.

PATHOPHYSIOLOGIC MECHANISMS

The mechanism by which magnesium sulfate has its effect has been partly elucidated; several beneficial actions to the brain could be operative. Magnesium antagonizes and suppresses seizures mediated by N-methyl-D-aspartate (NMDA).[24] Neuronal burst firing and electroencephalographic spike generation are markedly suppressed. Magnesium sulfate also acts on the neuromuscular junction by decreasing the amount of acetylcholine liberated from the presynaptic junction, decreasing the sensitivity of the motor end plate to acetylcholine, and reducing the muscle membrane excitability. Magnesium sulfate dilates vessels, including the cerebral arteries. Magnesium sulfate opposes calcium-dependent arterial constriction and relieves vasospasm associated with this disorder. Other effects are increased production of the endothelial vasodilator prostacyclin and inhibition of platelet activation.[25,26]

Treatment with magnesium sulfate resulted in better seizure control, lower mortality, and

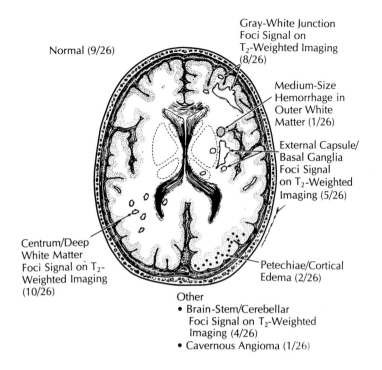

Normal (9/26)

Gray-White Junction
Foci Signal on
T$_2$-Weighted Imaging
(8/26)

Medium-Size
Hemorrhage in
Outer White
Matter (1/26)

External Capsule/
Basal Ganglia
Foci Signal
on T$_2$-Weighted
Imaging (5/26)

Centrum/Deep
White Matter
Foci Signal on T$_2$-
Weighted Imaging
(10/26)

Petechiae/Cortical
Edema (2/26)

Other
• Brain-Stem/Cerebellar
  Foci Signal on T$_2$-Weighted
  Imaging (4/26)
• Cavernous Angioma (1/26)

A

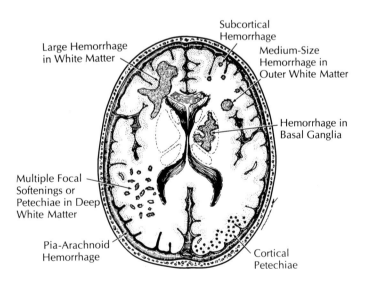

Subcortical
Hemorrhage

Large Hemorrhage
in White Matter

Medium-Size
Hemorrhage in
Outer White Matter

Hemorrhage in
Basal Ganglia

Multiple Focal
Softenings or
Petechiae in Deep
White Matter

Pia-Arachnoid
Hemorrhage

Cortical
Petechiae

B

Figure 13–1. Magnetic resonance imaging (*A*) and autopsy (*B*) findings in eclampsia based on 16 women with severe preeclampsia and 10 women with eclampsia. (From Digre et al.[17] By permission of the American Medical Association.)

241

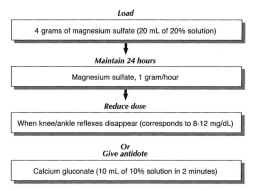

Figure 13–2. Management of eclampsia with magnesium sulfate.

reduced need for mechanical ventilation and, therefore, less risk of ventilator-associated pneumonia. There is no documented detriment to the child. In fact, Apgar scores are higher in magnesium sulfate-treated patients than those in phenytoin-treated patients.[27] Seizures may also be terminated with small intravenous doses of thiopental (50 mg) or diazepam (5 mg) in the period before the therapeutic level of magnesium is attained. Long-term administration of antiepileptic agents is not needed, because late seizures should be very rare.

Increased intracranial pressure, including herniation, may occur from cerebral edema or an intracerebral hemorrhage with mass effect. As mentioned earlier, diffuse cerebral edema remains an uncommon explanation for most clinical presentations (6% in 175 women), but patients have been described who have had a flurry of seizures preceding coma and abnormal motor responses due to cerebral edema.[11] There is only experience with traditional management of cerebral edema, which involves elevation of the head of the bed, hyperventilation, and administration of mannitol or loop diuretics.

HELLP SYNDROME

The acronym "HELLP" was introduced by Weinstein[28] to delineate a syndrome within the population of patients with eclampsia who in addition had hemolytic anemia, liver dysfunction, and thrombocytopenia (he-molysis, **e**levated **l**iver enzymes, and **l**ow **p**latelet count).[29] With an incidence of 3% to 25%, the syndrome remains one of the most common causes of maternal mortality.[30] The laboratory criteria are summarized in Table 13–2. The syndrome can be subclassified on the basis of platelet count, and studies have suggested that the actual platelet count may predict rapidity of postpartum recovery,[31,32] recurrent risk of HELLP syndrome, perinatal outcome, and need for plasma exchange (class I: platelet count, $<50,000/\mu L$; class II: 50,000 to $100,000/\mu L$; class III: 100,000 to $150,000/\mu L$ with hemolysis and elevated liver enzymes).

Clinical Features

Neurologic manifestations are more profound and severe in HELLP syndrome. The disorder may begin with nonspecific malaise, epigastric or right upper quadrant pain, and nausea and vomiting but without hypertension, which comes several days later. Early presentation with gum bleeding, gastrointestinal bleeding, hematuria, and jaundice

Table 13–2. **Essential and Associated Features of HELLP Syndrome**

Essential

Thrombocytopenia (platelets, $<100 \times 10^9/L$)

Increased aspartate transaminase, alanine transaminase

Hemolysis on blood smear

Associated

Abdominal pain (right upper quadrant)

Nausea, vomiting

Headaches

Renal failure

Intrauterine growth retardation or death

Placental abruption

Disseminated intravascular coagulation

Premature delivery

Postpartum hemorrhage

HELLP, **h**emolysis, **e**levated **l**iver enzymes, and **l**ow **p**latelet count.

may occur, but it is more likely that the diagnosis has been delayed and not recognized because of its nonspecific presentation mimicking a flulike illness.

Seizures, cortical blindness, and reduced level of consciousness are the most common manifestations. There is an increased risk for intracerebral hemorrhage due to hypertension and thrombocytopenia.

Neuroimaging

Neuroimaging in HELLP syndrome has rarely been reported, but a combination of subarachnoid hemorrhage and white matter lesions seems apparent. CT and MRI correlations in one example are shown in Figure 13–3. Subarachnoid hemorrhage is located in sulci and rarely in the basal cisterns, a finding expected in a coagulation-associated subarachnoid hemorrhage.[33] Serial CT scanning may show resolving features of white matter hypodensities and resorption of subarachnoid hemorrhage. If a subarachnoid hemorrhage is diagnosed by CT, it is not likely that aneurysmal rupture plays a role, and transfer for a cerebral angiogram may unnecessarily jeopardize patient safety and monitoring in the intensive care unit.

Management

Delivery remains key to resolution of the syndrome. Expectant management in selected cases may be considered to enhance fetal lung maturity, but a preliminary result from the International HELLP-Multicenter-Study showed significantly higher maternal complications.[34] Management of seizures is similar to that in eclampsia. The complex management of HELLP syndrome, which includes additional potent antihypertensive agents (labetalol or nicardipine), dexamethasone,[35] and aggressive fluid management, is not further discussed here. The use of epidural anesthesia to support delivery may be problematic because of thrombocytopenia, but after platelet infusion most anesthesiologists consider a platelet count of 100,000/μL to be safe.[36]

AMNIOTIC FLUID EMBOLISM

One of the most catastrophic disorders of pregnancy is amniotic fluid embolism, which may occur in 1 in 8000 to 1 in 80,000 deliveries. Mortality approaches 80%. The diagnosis is typically made at autopsy by demonstration of squamous cells or debris in the pulmonary artery vasculature.[37–41] The neurologic manifestations are severe, with therapy-resistant seizures and a severe anoxic–ischemic impact to the brain.

Clinical Features

At any time during pregnancy, amniotic fluid embolization may occur, varying from the first trimester to 48 hr postpartum. The critical condition immediately becomes apparent because of hypotension, depressed ventricular function, and profound hypoxemia. Hypoxemia is from initial pulmonary vasospasm and may result in death in 50% of the patients. If patients survive, a marked acute respiratory distress syndrome develops with major hemodynamic alterations. Disseminated intravascular coagulation often accompanies cardiorespiratory collapse.[42] Seizures occurred in half the patients in a large series analyzed from a national registry[39] in which most patients were resuscitated for cardiopulmonary arrest.

Approximately 50% of patients who survive incur anoxic–ischemic brain injury. Coma after cardiopulmonary resuscitation due to amniotic fluid embolization has a very poor outcome despite urgent cesarean section. The fetus in all likelihood may have had an anoxic injury too, and neonatal outcome is similarly poor.

Management

In some patients, successful therapy includes mechanical ventilation, blood pressure support, and replacement, by use of cryoprecipitate or fresh-frozen plasma, of essential factors depleted by disseminated intravascular coagulation. After correction of hypotension, fluid therapy should be restricted to maintain a normal fluid balance to minimize

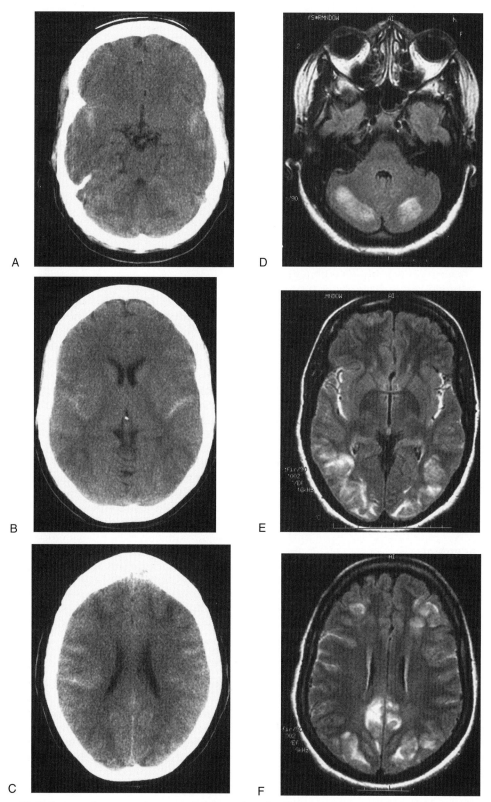

Figure 13–3. Computed tomography scans of diffuse subarachnoid hemorrhage and white matter abnormalities (*A–C*) with corresponding but more evident magnetic resonance changes (*D–F*) in patients with HELLP (**h**emolysis, **e**levated **l**iver enzymes, **l**ow **p**latelet count) syndrome.

244

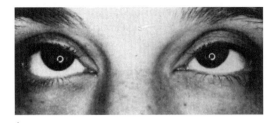 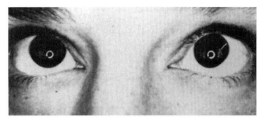

A   B

Figure 13–4. Ptosis (*A*) with complete resolution (*B*) in a woman receiving magnesium sulfate intravenously for tocolysis. (From Digre et al.[44] By permission of Mosby.)

further pulmonary edema. Seizures may recur, and therapy is with conventional antiepileptic drugs (see Chapter 3).

NEUROLOGIC COMPLICATIONS OF TOCOLYTIC AGENTS

Premature labor may be inhibited by tocolytic agents, although the therapeutic impact on the incidence of premature delivery is controversial. A variety of drugs are known, each with a plausible effect on presumed mediators, such as oxytocin, prostaglandins, and other smooth muscle contractants.[43] The most commonly used tocolytic agents are beta agonists (stimulate beta receptors in myometrium, decrease intracellular calcium), prostaglandin synthetase inhibitors (assuming a pivotal role for prostaglandin), calcium channel blockers (inhibit smooth muscle contractility and relax uterine muscle), and, most favored, magnesium sulfate (calcium antagonist, thus inhibiting myometrial contractility mediated by calcium).[43] Magnesium sulfate may produce bilateral symmetrical ptosis (Fig. 13–4) with no involvement of the levator function, an implication that the mechanism is supranuclear. Often an accommodation and convergence disturbance is found as well. Blurred vision, diplopia, and photophobia are common. End-gaze nystagmus and hypometric saccades were also noted in most of 13 patients studied.[44]

Myasthenia gravis should be suspected when weakness is out of proportion to the dose administered and also when weakness does not subside with calcium gluconate. At least two convincing cases with quadriplegia and bifacial weakness (but no ptosis) have

been reported,[45,46] but the condition should be extremely uncommon.

Approximately 25% of patients treated with tocolytic agents complain of nonspecific malaise, weakness, lethargy, and visual blurring, with no objective substrate, quick resolution, and insufficient severity to warrant cessation of therapy.[47]

The side effects of beta agonists (ritodrine, terbutaline, hexoprenaline) are mostly systemic, and pulmonary edema is well established and unique to beta agonist use for this indication. Severe hypoxia may occur, but no neurologic complications have been reported.

A history of migraine may precipitate a migraine attack, most likely from rebound vasospasm, and focal neurologic symptoms may result. In two reported cases of minor stroke associated with terbutaline, migraine headaches were known in the family or began in childhood. It remains unclear whether terbutaline is contraindicated in patients with migraine, and no other reports have appeared since this case report in 1982.[48]

CONCLUSIONS

Management of seizures predominates in the care of the critically ill pregnant patient with eclampsia. Magnesium sulfate (and not phenytoin) has been established as the therapeutic agent of choice. Preeclampsia and HELLP syndrome are best ended by delivery, and when this is done within 48 hr of diagnosis, maternal mortality is decreased. Fortunately, these admissions represent a fraction of all deliveries, but in so many ways confrontation with this rapidly developing emergency in young women defies description.

REFERENCES

1. Mahutte NG, Murphy-Kaulbeck L, Le Q, Solomon J, Benjamin A, Boyd ME. Obstetric admissions to the intensive care unit. Obstet Gynecol 94:263–266, 1999.
2. Panchal S, Arria AM, Labhsetwar SA. Maternal mortality during hospital admission for delivery: a retrospective analysis using a state-maintained database. Anesth Analg 93:134–141, 2001.
3. Sawhney H, Aggarwal N, Biswas R, Vasishta K, Gopalan S. Maternal mortality associated with eclampsia and severe preeclampsia of pregnancy. J Obstet Gynaecol Res 26:351–356, 2000.
4. Sibai BM. Eclampsia. VI. Maternal–perinatal outcome in 254 consecutive cases. Am J Obstet Gynecol 163:1049–1054, 1990.
5. Esplin MS, Fausett MB, Fraser A, et al. Paternal and maternal components of the predisposition to preeclampsia. N Engl J Med 344:867–872, 2001.
6. National High Blood Pressure Education Program Working Group Report on High Blood Pressure in Pregnancy. Am J Obstet Gynecol 163:1691–1712, 1990.
7. Thomas SV. Neurological aspects of eclampsia. J Neurol Sci 155:37–43, 1998.
8. Cunningham FG, Fernandez CO, Hernandez C. Blindness associated with preeclampsia and eclampsia. Am J Obstet Gynecol 172:1291–1298, 1995.
9. Torres PJ, Antolin E, Gratacos E, Chamorro A, Cararach V. Cortical blindness in preeclampsia: diagnostic evaluation by transcranial Doppler and magnetic resonance imaging techniques. Acta Obstet Gynecol Scand 74:642–644, 1995.
10. Borromeo CJ, Blike GT, Wiley CW, Hirsch JA. Cortical blindness in a preeclamptic patient after a cesarean delivery complicated by hypotension. Anesth Analg 91:609–611, 2000.
11. Cunningham FG, Twickler D. Cerebral edema complicating eclampsia. Am J Obstet Gynecol 182:94–100, 2000.
12. Simolke GA, Cox SM, Cunningham FG. Cerebrovascular accidents complicating pregnancy and the puerperium. Obstet Gynecol 78:37–42, 1991.
13. Witlin AG, Friedman SA, Egerman RS, Frangieh AY, Sibai BM. Cerebrovascular disorders complicating pregnancy—beyond eclampsia. Am J Obstet Gynecol 176:1139–1145, 1997.
14. Maymon R, Fejgin M. Intracranial hemorrhage during pregnancy and puerperium. Obstet Gynecol Surv 45:157–159, 1990.
15. Sharshar T, Lamy C, Mas JL. Incidence and causes of strokes associated with pregnancy and puerperium. A study in public hospitals in Ile de France. Stroke in Pregnancy Study Group. Stroke 26:930–936, 1995.
16. Raps EC, Galetta SL, Broderick M, Atlas SW. Delayed peripartum vasculopathy: cerebral eclampsia revisited. Ann Neurol 33:222–225, 1993.
17. Digre KB, Varner MW, Osborn AG, Crawford S. Cranial magnetic resonance imaging in severe preeclampsia vs eclampsia. Arch Neurol 50:399–406, 1993.
18. Kanki T, Tsukimori K, Mihara F, Nakano H. Diffusion-weighted images and vasogenic edema in eclampsia. Obstet Gynecol 93:821–823, 1999.
19. Rooholamini SA, Au AH, Hansen GC, et al. Imaging of pregnancy-related complications. Radiographics 13:753–770, 1993.
20. Sanders TG, Clayman DA, Sanchez-Ramos L, Vines FS, Russo L. Brain in eclampsia: MR imaging with clinical correlation. Radiology 180:475–478, 1991.
21. Appleton MP, Kuehl TJ, Raebel MA, Adams HR, Knight AB, Gold WR. Magnesium sulfate versus phenytoin for seizure prophylaxis in pregnancy-induced hypertension. Am J Obstet Gynecol 165:907–913, 1991.
22. Eclampsia Trial Collaborative Group. Which anticonvulsant for women with eclampsia? Evidence from the Collaborative Eclampsia Trial. Lancet 345:1455–1463, 1995.
23. Robson SC. Magnesium sulphate: the time of reckoning. Br J Obstet Gynecol 103:99–102, 1996.
24. Cotton DB, Hallak M, Janusz C, Irtenkauf SM, Berman RF. Central anticonvulsant effects of magnesium sulfate on N-methyl-D-aspartate-induced seizures. Am J Obstet Gynecol 168:974–978, 1993.
25. McGiff JC, Carroll MA. Eicosanoids in preeclampsia-eclampsia: the effects of magnesium. Hypertens Pregnancy 13:217–226, 1994.
26. Sipes SL, Weiner CP, Gellhaus TM, Goodspeed JD. Effects of magnesium sulfate infusion upon plasma prostaglandins in preeclampsia and preterm labor. Hypertens Pregnancy 13:293–302, 1994.
27. Crowther C. Magnesium sulphate versus diazepam in the management of eclampsia: a randomized controlled trial. Br J Obstet Gynaecol 97:110–117, 1990.
28. Weinstein L. Syndrome of hemolysis, elevated liver enzymes, and low platelet count: a severe consequence of hypertension in pregnancy. Am J Obstet Gynecol 142:159–167, 1982.
29. Stone JH. HELLP syndrome: hemolysis, elevated liver enzymes, and low platelets. JAMA 280:559–562, 1998.
30. Geary M. The HELLP syndrome. Br J Obstet Gynaecol 104:887–891, 1997.
31. Martin JN Jr, Blake PG, Lowry SL, Perry KG Jr, Files JC, Morrison JC. Pregnancy complicated by preeclampsia–eclampsia with the syndrome of hemolysis, elevated liver enzymes, and low platelet count: how rapid is postpartum recovery? Obstet Gynecol 76:737–741, 1990.
32. Martin JN Jr, Blake PG, Perry KG Jr, McCaul JF, Hess LW, Martin RW. The natural history of HELLP syndrome: patterns of disease progression and regression. Am J Obstet Gynecol 164:1500–1509, 1991.
33. Imaizumi H, Nara S, Kaneko M, Chiba S, Tamakawa M. Magnetic resonance evaluation of brainstem dysfunction in eclampsia and the HELLP syndrome. J Emerg Med 13:191–194, 1995.
34. Faridi A, Heyl W, Rath W. Preliminary results of the International HELLP-Multicenter-study. Int J Gynecol Obstet 69:279–280, 2000.
35. Isler CM, Barrilleaux PS, Magann EF, Bass JD, Martin JN Jr. A prospecitve, randomized trial comparing the efficacy of dexamethasone and betametha-

sone for the treatment of antepartum HELLP (hemolysis, elevated liver enzymes, and low platelet count) syndrome. Am J Obstet Gynecol 184:1332–1337, 2001.

36. Crosby ET, Preston R. Obstetrical anaesthesia for a parturient with preeclampsia, HELLP syndrome and acute cortical blindness. Can J Anaesth 45:452–459, 1998.

37. Clark SL. Arachidonic acid metabolites and the pathophysiology of amniotic fluid embolism. Semin Reprod Endocrinol 3:253–257, 1985.

38. Clark SL. New concepts of amniotic fluid embolism: a review. Obstet Gynecol Surv 45:360–368, 1990.

39. Clark SL, Hankins GD, Dudley DA, Dildy GA, Porter TF. Amniotic fluid embolism: analysis of the national registry. Am J Obstet Gynecol 172:1158–1167, 1995.

40. Liban E, Raz S. A clinicopathologic study of fourteen cases of amniotic fluid embolism. Am J Clin Pathol 51:477–486, 1969.

41. Plauche WC. Amniotic fluid embolism [letter]. Am J Obstet Gynecol 147:982–983, 1983.

42. Clark SL, Montz FJ, Phelan JP. Hemodynamic alterations associated with amniotic fluid embolism: a reappraisal. Am J Obstet Gynecol 151:617–621, 1985.

43. McCombs J. Update on tocolytic therapy. Ann Pharmacother 29:515–522, 1995.

44. Digre KB, Varner MW, Schiffman JS. Neuroophthalmologic effects of intravenous magnesium sulfate. Am J Obstet Gynecol 163:1848–1852, 1990.

45. Bashuk RG, Krendel DA. Myasthenia gravis presenting as weakness after magnesium administration. Muscle Nerve 13:708–712, 1990.

46. Cohen BA, London RS, Goldstein PJ. Myasthenia gravis and preeclampsia. Obstet Gynecol 48 (Suppl): 35S-37S, 1976.

47. Dudley D, Gagnon D, Varner M. Long-term tocolysis with intravenous magnesium sulfate. Obstet Gynecol 73:373–378, 1989.

48. Rosene KA, Featherstone HJ, Benedetti TJ. Cerebral ischemia associated with parenteral terbutaline use in pregnant migraine patients. Am J Obstet Gynecol 143:405–407, 1982.

NEUROLOGIC COMPLICATIONS OF AORTIC SURGERY

Centers of excellence have specific intensive care provisions to systematically accommodate patients operated on for thoracoabdominal aneurysm. After aortic surgery, triage out of the intensive care unit (ICU) may be accomplished rather quickly, but ischemic colitis and renal failure may intervene and extend the stay in the surgical intensive care unit. Extensive surgical reconstructive repairs of the aorta increase the risk of ischemic injury to the viscera and spinal cord. Spinal cord infarction,[1–6] in one of the largest series reported, occurred in 16% of 1509 patients who had elective surgery of the descending aorta,[7] but some recent series have suggested a reduction in rate to less than 10% (Table 14–1). Paraplegia after

emergency repair for traumatic or acute spontaneous rupture is much more prevalent, is difficult to avert because of sudden shock, and ranges from 20% to 30%.[15,16]

Spinal cord injury from aortic surgery is crushing for the patient and surgical team. Once the damage is done, therapeutic intervention seems futile and the handicap from paraplegia is expected to be permanent. Thus prevention of spinal cord injury, if possible at all, during repair of thoracoabdominal aneurysm remains a challenge to the skills of vascular surgeons and monitoring anesthesiologists. Novel methods of spinal cord protection, such as selective intercostal arterial perfusion using motor evoked potentials, epidural cooling of the cord, and noninvasive detection of the critical artery of Adamkiewicz by magnetic resonance angiography, have appeared and may potentially affect the incidence of spinal cord infarction. Clinical trials of any real significance have not been performed. The diagnostic approach, validity of intraoperative monitoring, and therapeutic options are discussed in this chapter.

VASCULAR ANATOMY OF THE SPINAL CORD

The blood supply to the spinal cord is provided by intercostal or lumbar arterial branches that give rise to anterior and posterior radicular arteries. These arteries branch to three longitudinal arterial trunks, the anterior spinal artery and both posterior spinal arteries, which regulate the blood sup-

Table 14–1. Incidence of Paraplegia in Large Series of Patients (>100) with Elective Repair of Thoracoabdominal Aortic Aneurysms

Series	Paraplegia (%)
Carlson et al., 1983[8]	5
Svensson et al., 1993[7]	16
Gilling-Smith et al., 1995[9]	8
Coselli et al., 1996[10]	5
Safi and Miller, 1999[11]	7
Galla et al., 1999[12]	13
Cambria et al., 2000[13]	7
Von Segesser et al., 2001[14]	8

ies pass through the central sulcus to the middle part of the cord. Each so-called sulcal artery supplies one side of the cord and provides flow to the gray matter, which harbors the cells of the origin of the ventral root fibers, preganglionic cells for the autonomic nervous system, and incoming posterior horn fibers. Zülch and Kurth-Schumacher[21] postulated that the posterior horns are situated in a watershed area between the sulcal arteries and branches of the posterior spinal artery, but posterior horn infarcts are rare, and neurons in the central region are much more vulnerable to episodes of hypoperfusion. The sulcal artery also supplies most of the lateral corticospinal tract, including the hand and arm areas. More peripherally located tracts, however, may also receive blood of tributaries from the coronal arteries, which arise from the anterior spinal artery or branches of the posterior spinal artery.

The paired posterior spinal arteries sup-

ply to the entire spinal cord[17–20] (Fig. 14–1). The anterior spinal artery supplies approximately 75% of the blood to the cord. From this major contributing artery, sets of arter-

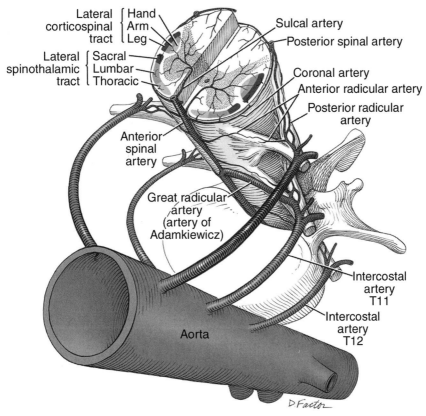

Figure 14–1. Vascularization of the spinal cord (see text for explanation).

ply major parts of the posterior columns of the white matter. The lateral spinothalamic tracts, which convey pain and temperature sensation, receive their vascular supply through the coronal arteries and are therefore not spared in a typical anterior spinal artery syndrome.

In the longitudinal plane (Fig. 14–2), a fairly consistent pattern of vascularization has been recognized. Three major segments of arterial organization of the spinal cord have been defined, but anatomical variations at various levels are the rule. The cervicothoracic territory includes the cervical cord

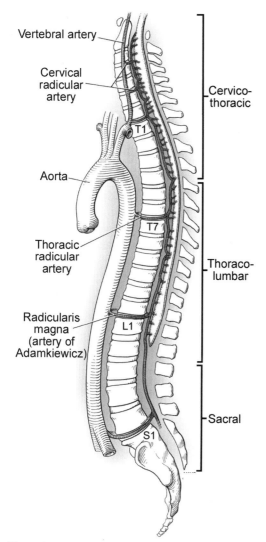

Figure 14–2. Segmental vascularization of the spinal cord (see text for explanation).

and first two or three thoracic segments. The anterior spinal artery and posterior spinal arteries are branches of the vertebral arteries and costocervical trunk. Below the T3 level, the intercostal arteries from the aorta supply the thoracic segments and are highly variable in number. One human cadaver study found a range of 2 to 17 (mean, 8) intercostal arteries. At T7, a large thoracic radicular artery frequently contributes to the anterior spinal artery. The thoracolumbar territory derives its supply from the artery of Adamkiewicz,[22] which typically originates between T5 and L2 but varies in its origin and in 75% of cases is identified between T9 and T12, in 15% between T5 and T8, and in 10% between L1 and L2. The terminal portions of the spinal cord and cauda equina depend on branches from the internal iliac or middle sacral artery.

Although the lengthwise division of the vascularization of the spinal cord may imply that a vulnerable watershed area is present in the midthoracic region (T4 to T8), any level in the thoracic region may become affected.[23] Spinal cord perfusion depends on the number of radicular arteries and not so much on the number of intercostal arteries that arise from the aorta. The vulnerability of the thoracic region is plausible when one considers the scarce supply derived from one to three anterior radicular arteries more widely spaced in the thoracic area than in other regions. In addition, sulcal arteries, although abundant in the cervical and lumbar regions, are poorly represented in the thoracic region.[18] Pathologic studies found that in some areas in the thoracic region, one segment was supplied by one sulcal artery and another segment was supplied by small ascending and descending branches from adjacent segments. Thus perfusion of the thoracic spinal cord is largely guaranteed by the great radicular artery of Adamkiewicz.

SCOPE OF THE PROBLEM

Complications of thoracoabdominal aneurysmectomy have been reported through use of the Crawford classification system.[24,25] The estimated risks of paraplegia have been 12%, 6%, 3%, and 3% in types I, II, III, and IV, respectively (Fig. 14–3). Familiarity with

I   II   III   IV

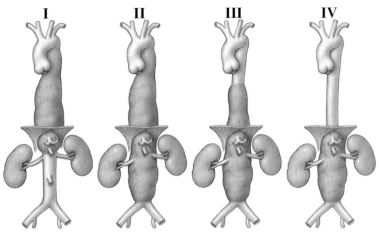

Figure 14–3. In the Crawford classification of thoracoabdominal aneurysms,[24] *type I* is a thoracic aneurysm that extends inferiorly to the extent that it involves the visceral vessels, *type II* is a diffuse thoracoabdominal aneurysm with extensive involvement of the aorta both above and below the visceral arteries, *type III* has aneurysmal changes starting below the middle of the thoracic aorta, and *type IV* consists of aneurysmal changes that start at the level of the diaphragm and involve the visceral vessels and infrarenal aorta.

anesthetic techniques during repair of the thoracoabdominal aorta is necessary to understand the risks of spinal cord injury.

Swan-Ganz catheter measurements have shown that immediately after aortic cross-clamping, arterial blood pressure increases, stroke volume and cardiac output decrease, and pulmonary artery wedge pressure increases. Also during cross-clamping, cerebrospinal fluid pressure increases markedly,[26] probably from increased intraspinal venous blood volume that is a result of venous back pressure. Indeed, Svensson and associates[27] evaluated cerebrospinal fluid (CSF) alterations in patients who underwent thoracic and thoracoabdominal aortic surgery and found that in addition to significant increases during induction of general anesthesia and intubation, CSF pressures correlated linearly with central venous pressures. This marked increase in CSF pressure may result in a decrease of the perfusion pressure of the spinal cord (perfusion pressure = spinal cord arterial pressure − CSF pressure). Furthermore, a decrease in spinal cord arterial pressure resulting from exclusion of the aorta or use of vasodilators to overcome hypertension may contribute to spinal cord ischemia and merits notice.[27,28]

The spinal cord is particularly at risk for ischemic damage after aortic declamping.

Release of the abdominal aortic cross-clamp may cause hypotension. Reperfusion of the ischemic, vasodilated, and vasomotor-paralyzed lower extremity and pelvic arteries may be the operative mechanism of decrease in blood pressure.[29] Intravascular volume amplification before this procedure generally prevents hypotension, but if it occurs, it rapidly responds to phenylephrine. Additionally, anesthesiologists reduce the concentration of inhalation agents before clamp release.

The risk factors for spinal cord injury in thoracoabdominal repair have been rather consistently identified. Repair of extensive abdominal aneurysms implies a long duration of aortic cross-clamping. There is no doubt that prolonged clamping increases the risk of postoperative spinal cord injury, suggesting that surgical skill and speed may be factors (Table 14-2). Multiple logistic regression analyses revealed that age (64 years and older), aortic clamp time (over 45 min), and postoperative hypotension (<100 mm Hg systolic) were independent significant risk factors for postoperative paraplegia.[24]

Many cardiothoracic surgeons routinely implant the intercostal arteries, but others question whether the incidence of paraplegia with such a time-consuming procedure can be reduced. The cardiothoracic surgeon

Table 14–2. **Incidence of Paraplegia in Relation to Cross-Clamp Time**

Time (min)	Patients (no.)	Paraplegia (%)
0–15	8	0
16–30	142	3
31–45	90	10
46–60	16	13
>60	4	25

Modified from Livesay et al.[30] By permission of the Society of Thoracic Surgeons.

therefore is faced with the dilemma of reimplanting as many intercostal arteries as possible (an estimated 10 min for end-to-end anastomosis) with the assumption that one or more critical intercostal arteries are included or proceeding directly with replacing the aneurysm within a short clamping time.

The merit of preoperative localization of so-called critical intercostal arteries, including the great radicular artery of Adamkiewicz, is controversial.[31] Early claims to have visualized the artery of Adamkiewicz in most patients were offset by a later study of selective spinal arteriography in which the origin was found in a much lower percentage (55%).[31] Furthermore, patients without paraplegia have been reported who have had the artery of Adamkiewicz sacrificed. A group at Baylor perfected a new technique of intraoperative localization of segmental arteries important in spinal cord supply.[32] The method involves intrathecal placement of a platinum electrode that senses hydrogen. Saline saturated with hydrogen is injected into several segmental artery ostia, and "positive arteries" are reanastomosed. In a pilot study of eight patients, five did well despite long total clamp time. One patient died, and delayed paraplegia associated with hypotension developed in two patients.[32] A promising technique is the use of magnetic resonance angiography and gadolinium bolus injection to visualize the artery of Adamkiewicz. Yamada and associates[33] claimed to have identified the Adamkiewicz arteries in 69% of 26 patients, none of whom became paraplegic. This study, however, demonstrated limited spatial resolution, and its validity requires confirmation.

Revascularization resulted in a much lower incidence of paraplegia than that in historical controls. Williams and co-workers[31] hypothesized that patients with extensive aneurysm of the descending and abdominal aorta and a large patent great radicular artery arising from a large intercostal branch at the center of the aneurysm are at risk for spinal cord injury. Again, whether reimplantation results in better neurologic outcome and whether laboratory tests to identify intercostal arteries may increase the total duration of ischemia are unsettled issues.

Most patients with spinal cord injuries awaken with paraplegia, but several large surgical series reported a fair number of patients in whom onset of a spinal cord lesion was delayed.[34] In Crawford and associates' experience,[24] this rather unusual presentation is transient, occurs up to 3 weeks after the operation, and is related to hypovolemia (for example, due to hemorrhage from the gastrointestinal tract), low cardiac output during arrhythmias, or respiratory acidosis. Loss of spinal cord perfusion due to arterial spasm, progressive aortic dissection, or thrombosis in a graft limb has also been suggested as an alternative mechanism of delayed spinal cord injury. However, a study in rabbits documented that the incidence of delayed-onset paraplegia was related to ischemia time and most likely not to thrombosis or embolization in spinal arteries.[34] This variant of delayed onset of paraplegia has important implications for postoperative monitoring of patients, particularly those with long aortic clamp times who awaken neurologically intact. Monitoring CSF pressure in the postoperative period therefore makes logical sense, but its value has not been demonstrated in randomized trials.

PATHOPHYSIOLOGIC MECHANISMS

To a large extent, the pathophysiology of spinal cord ischemia can be explained by altered blood flow mechanics. During aortic cross-clamping, the spinal cord is extremely sensitive to ischemia from reduced blood flow distal to the clamp. Two distinct ischemic insults exist to the spinal cord. Ischemic injury occurs from aortic cross-clamping and is due to devascularization associated with loss of critical blood supply. The hyperemic phase of cord reperfusion may be operative as well and has led to trials of hypothermic protection or amelioration with epidural cooling techniques.

Opioid receptors and N-methyl-D-aspartate receptors may be involved and have led to trials of neuroprotection with naloxone. There is considerable evidence of increased glutamate and aspartate in the CSF, particularly during reperfusion and cross-clamping. Glycene, known to enhance the excitotoxic effects of increased glutamate, appeared elevated in one study.[35]

It has been well acknowledged that the incidence of paraplegia is very low in reconstruction of the aortic arch, of the high thoracic aorta, and particularly in the aortoiliac region. At the Mayo Clinic, the incidence of paraplegia after aortoiliac reconstruction was 0.1% (2 of 1901 patients) after elective repair and 1.4% (3 of 210 patients) after emergency repair.[36] However, the incidence of spinal cord infarction steeply increases in thoracoabdominal aneurysmal repair.[37]

NEUROLOGIC FEATURES OF SPINAL CORD INFARCTION

The typical clinical presentation of spinal cord injury is postoperative flaccid paralysis, loss of tendon reflexes, and analgesia caudal to the lesion. Total spinal cord infarction (Fig. 14–4A) is common, but other spinal cord syndromes with distinctive clinical features after aortic surgery have been described. Very few patients recover, and in most patients this complication evolves to spastic paraplegia with eventually some improvement of lower extremity sensation.

Anterior Spinal Artery Syndrome

If paired posterior spinal arteries with extensive collateral blood supply are functional, clamping of the thoracic aorta may result in spinal cord infarction of only the anterior two-thirds of the spinal cord (Fig. 14–4B). Involvement of the corticospinal, pyramidal, and spinothalamic tracts and anterior horns results in loss of any muscle ac-

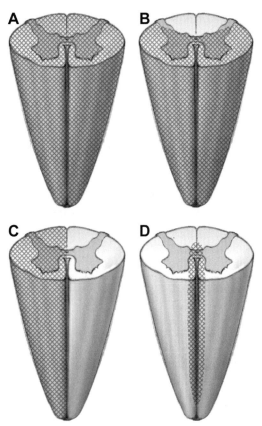

Figure 14–4. Patterns of spinal cord infarction after aortic repair. *A*: Complete infarction. *B*: Anterior spinal artery syndrome. *C*: Brown-Séquard syndrome. *D*: Central cord syndrome.

tivity in the legs. Many patients have fine fasciculations in the lower limbs that usually resolve within 1 or 2 days. Decreased reactions to pin prick and to hot and cold sensation are present, but light touch and position sense are preserved. Vibration sense may be decreased at the toes and ankles merely because the prevalence of diabetes is relatively high in patients undergoing thoracoabdominal repair (13% in a large series).[7] Lesions of the spinal cord after aortic surgery are very often located at the T4 level—an area of reduced sensation to the nipples—but sensory levels may range from T10 to L2. The tendon reflexes are absent. Abdominal reflexes, often useful in localizing the level of damage in the longitudinal axis, are usually difficult to interpret in these patients with large abdominal incisions and may not be helpful. The rectal sphincters are usually paralyzed, and the genital reflexes are lost.

Because the descending thermoregulatory fibers supplying the sweat glands are closely localized to the corticospinal tracts, anhydrosis may be present. This may cause a marked increase in temperature and falsely suggest a postoperative infection.

Brown-Séquard Syndrome

A few instances of a Brown-Séquard-like syndrome (Fig. 14–4C) are on record.[38] The classic presentation of this unilateral transverse lesion is ipsilateral limb weakness, loss of position and vibration sensation, and contralateral loss of pain and temperature sensation. At the level of the lesion, some patients have a small ipsilateral area of anesthesia. Occlusion of a single sulcal artery may explain this phenomenon. A Brown-Séquard-like syndrome may also develop during resolution of complete paraplegia.[39] In general, unilateral leg weakness is unusual after aortic surgery and when present may more frequently point to a possible plexopathy from postoperative lumbosacral bleeding and psoas hematoma (see Chapter 11).

Central Cord Syndrome

A central cord–like syndrome (Fig. 14–4D) has been clinically described and pathologically confirmed. These infarcts are located in the thoracolumbar spinal cord and produce a pencil-like softening.[21] The only way to explain this odd anatomical lesion is embolization to both central sulcus arteries with collateral compensation through the coronal arteries. These proximal branches of the anterior spinal artery have their major supply zones in the periphery of the spinal cord and distribute blood to the spinothalamic tracts that represent the sacral dermatomes.

The clinical picture is similar to that of the anterior spinal artery syndrome, but the sacral dermatomes (S3 to S5) are spared.[40] The anal reflex is often preserved, and a reflex bladder contractility predominates. Outcome in these patients, albeit incidentally reported, is poor.

DIAGNOSTIC EVALUATION OF SPINAL CORD INFARCTION

Spinal cord infarction remains a clinical diagnosis, and before magnetic resonance imaging (MRI) there were no methods of confirming spinal cord ischemia other than postmortem examination. Monitoring of somatosensory evoked potentials has become routine during surgery in many institutions, and early detection of abnormal amplitude and latency may help to identify segmental arteries that need reattachment and to manage distal aortic perfusion techniques.

Magnetic Resonance Imaging

Magnetic resonance imaging of the spinal cord can be diagnostic of infarction. A typical MRI with intensity changes throughout the cord is depicted in Figure 14–5. Certain MRI patterns have been described, and these patterns possibly may be used to predict the chance of recovery.[5]

In 17 of 24 imaged patients, magnetic resonance studies showed four types of signal abnormalities (Fig. 14–6). Twelve patients had a clinically completed spinal cord infarction, and T2-weighted images showed diffuse signal abnormality of the entire cross section of the spinal cord (Fig. 14–6D). Patients with focal abnormalities involving the anterior horns of the gray matter ("owl's eyes") (Fig. 14–6A) became ambulant.

These types of spinal cord involvement represent the range of severity of impact. Focal abnormalities (example A) have been linked to "spinal transient ischemic attack" and "spinal reversible ischemic neurologic deficit" and in an early postoperative episode may indicate a potential for recovery. Any other pattern seems to be associated with a permanent deficit.

Monitoring Techniques

Somatosensory evoked potentials (SSEPs) may monitor development of cord ischemia in patients undergoing thoracoabdominal surgery. Enthusiasm has slightly diminished because a prospective study from Baylor College of Medicine showed that the incidences

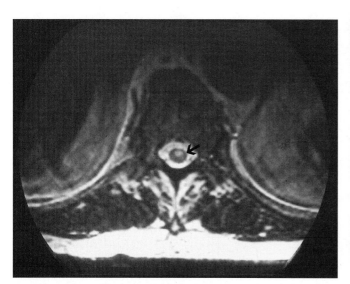 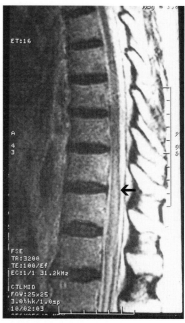

Figure 14–5. Magnetic resonance images of spinal cord infarction (arrows).

of false-negative and false-positive responses were considerable (Table 14–3). In addition, some unconvinced investigators argue that the vulnerable lateral and ventral columns of the central gray matter are not primarily monitored by SSEPs, which are generated in the dorsal columns.

Many studies have explored the value of SSEP recording in establishing potential ischemic damage.[12,41–43] The most detailed studies are those of Laschinger and colleagues[44] and Cunningham and associates.[45] Four SSEP responses were recognized.

TYPE I SSEP RESPONSE

This response, noted in some patients, is characterized by a gradual diminution of SSEP amplitude and increased latency 7 to 30 min after aortic cross-clamping. Usually, distal aortic perfusion pressure is <30 mm Hg. The incidence of paraplegia is considered to be high, occurring in more than one-third of the patients. Unclamping may restore conduction velocity and amplitude, but they commonly fail to reappear.

TYPE II SSEP RESPONSE

Essentially, a normal SSEP associated with adequate distal aortic perfusion pressure is maintained throughout the clamping procedure. In the study by Cunningham and colleagues,[45] spinal cord infarction did not develop in these patients, but in Crawford and associates' study[41] of a larger group of patients, 5% had immediate postoperative paraplegia.

TYPE III SSEP RESPONSE

Disappearance or significant decrease of the SSEP amplitude after placement of the distal aortic clamp has been linked to inclusion of critical intercostal vessels. Reimplantation of intercostal arteries may result in return of the SSEP response, even in patients in whom the SSEP response has been lost for more than 30 min. None of the patients with return of SSEP responses had neurologic deficits, but it is difficult to determine what would have happened if reconstruction had not been done.

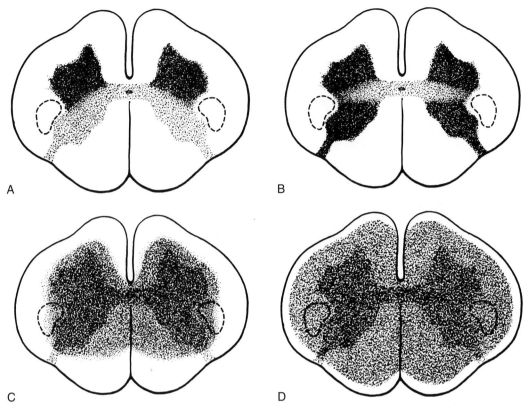

Figure 14–6. Schematic patterns of magnetic resonance images of spinal cord infarction. *A*: Anterior horn involvement (owl's eyes). *B*: Anterior and posterior horn involvement. *C*: Involvement of entire gray matter and adjacent central white matter. *D*: Diffuse signal abnormality of entire cross section of spinal cord. (From Mawad et al.[5] By permission of the American Society of Neuroradiology.)

TYPE IV SSEP RESPONSE

This response is characterized by gradual fade-out of SSEP tracings, sometimes associated with overzealous use of nitroprusside, and is associated with inadequate distal aortic perfusion pressure. Fade-out occurs in patients with long clamping times and often takes 1/2 hr to become clearly evident. Restoration of distal perfusion after un-

Table 14–3. Relation of Spinal Cord Infarction to Intraoperative Somatosensory Evoked Potential (SSEP) Recording in 99 Patients

SSEP Response*	No. of Patients	PATIENTS WITH PARAPARESIS AND PARAPLEGIA	
		No.	%
No change	53	7	13
Change with return	11	3	27
Change with fluctuating return of response	10	2	20
Change with no return	25	8	32

*Change in SSEP response is defined as latency increase of not more than 10% and amplitude decrease of not more than 25% for 10 min. All patients had temporary bypass and distal perfusion pressure of 60 mm Hg or greater.
Modified from Crawford et al.[41] By permission of Mosby.

clamping results in a prompt return of SSEP but may falsely suggest normal cord function, because paraplegia may occur.

The current experience with SSEP recording may guide the vascular surgeon, but it has not been clearly demonstrated that measures taken to improve spinal cord perfusion will decrease the incidence of postoperative paraplegia. Whether catheter-type electrodes should be placed in the subarachnoid space for SSEP stimulation in unstable patients to monitor possible postoperative deterioration is unresolved.[46]

Monitoring with motor evoked potentials, an exciting but cumbersome technique, deserves further study of its validity in predicting spinal cord ischemia. Levy[47] noted that in a preliminary study of 45 spinal cord operations, motor evoked potentials correctly predicted spinal cord injury in all cases. Preliminary animal data suggest that in prediction of spinal cord injury, loss of motor evoked potentials has a high sensitivity (90%).[48]

de Haan and associates[49] studied the use of motor evoked potentials in the selection of critical segmental arteries. These preliminary results were confirmed in a study of 38 patients.[50] Progressive decrease of motor evoked potentials (<25% change in amplitude) guided intercostal or lumbar artery reattachment or, when these vessels were not apparent, endarterectomy of the aortic wall with selective grafts to segmental arteries. Restoration of flow resulted in reappearance of the motor evoked potential. Paraplegia did not develop in any patient. Simultaneously recorded SSEP responses were falsely positive (fade-out pattern) in 39% of patients. This very promising study needs confirmation. Similarly, Sueda and colleagues[51] used motor evoked potentials to reconstruct intercostal arteries. In a study of five cases, motor evoked potential amplitude dampened after clamping but recovered after selective perfusion of the intercostal arteries, which were subsequently attached.

THERAPEUTIC OPTIONS

Numerous studies have claimed the potential usefulness of reimplantation of intercostal arteries, use of bypass or shunts, or, more recently, fractionated double-clamp-

ing to counteract steal from the spinal cord circulation. None of these studies has convincingly shown a decrease in the incidence of spinal cord infarction.[30,52–55] There is accumulating evidence that moderate hypothermia (30°C) decreases spinal cord injury. However, epidural cooling is not generally used as a preventive measure.[56–58] Cambria and co-workers[13] noted a possible reduction in spinal cord ischemic complications when iced (4°C) normal saline was administered by epidural catheter, but this finding was not confirmed in a recent sutdy from Switzerland.[14] Attention has focused on CSF drainage to prevent spinal cord injury, assuming that drainage may improve spinal perfusion pressure by decreasing the counteracting CSF pressure.[59] A prospective study, however, did not demonstrate a reduction in the incidence of paraplegia with continuous drainage of lumbar spinal fluid and maintenance of normal to nearly normal CSF pressures.[60]

The addition of intrathecally delivered papaverine to dilate the anterior spinal artery and increase spinal cord blood flow had no marked effect on spinal cord ischemia in a preliminary study.[61,62] Intravenous administration of naloxone has shown promising results in reversal of neurologic deficits,[63] but prospective studies are not available. A single high dose of methylprednisolone (30 mg/kg) in patients with anticipated extensive repairs and long clamping times may be another therapeutic consideration. Animal studies support a protective effect despite lack of effect on spinal blood flow.[64] However, there is no clinical evidence of benefit from methylprednisolone in aortic surgery.

To summarize, the postoperative management of patients with thoracoabdominal repairs may include monitoring of CSF pressure for at least 24 hr, provision of both adequate oxygenation and systemic pulse pressure, and immediate action when these variables change. Generally, 20 to 50 mL of CSF is withdrawn with a closed draining system. The manometric system can be kept at a level that allows increases in CSF pressure above 10 mm Hg to result in drainage, which may amount to 200 to 300 mL/day. Drainage of CSF has also been claimed to reverse delayed paraplegia.[65] Cooling with ice may be promising, but further feasibility studies are needed. The possible neuroprotective effect of tacrolimus is currently being investigated.[66]

PLEXOPATHIES

Unlike direct compression of the lumbosacral plexus by large aneurysms of the common iliac artery,[67] rupture of abdominal aneurysms may result in extensive retroperitoneal hematomas with damage to the femoral and obturator nerves.[68–71] Other potential mechanisms for nerve damage may be hemorrhagic extension into the nerve sheath or compression of the distal femoral nerve segment against the inguinal ligament through enlarged anterior fascial pockets.

Fasciotomy may be indicated in the first 24 hr. The approach in patients with coagulopathies is different and, because of recurrent bleeding, more likely to be conservative (see Chapter 11).

The clinical entity of unilateral or bilateral ischemic plexopathy after aortic repairs is poorly defined. It would appear virtually impossible to compromise perfusion of the lumbosacral plexus, because its vascular anatomy is characterized by a rich network of collaterals. Nevertheless, patients may have unilateral leg weakness with electromyographic abnormalities that are very suggestive of a lumbosacral plexopathy. In general, these patients tend to have a more favorable outcome and a high probability of becoming ambulant within 1 year.[36]

AORTIC DISSECTION

Acute aortic dissection is one of the major vascular emergencies[72,73] and is also due to involvement of other arterial systems.[74] A tear in the aortic intima allows blood to track into the aortic media and force itself through the entire length of the aorta, including arteries branching off the arch. Predisposing factors are hypertension, cannulation during cardiac surgery, angiographic catheterization, trauma, and cardiac valve replacement. Aortic dissections can be categorized according to DeBakey's classification (Fig. 14–7).[75] Severe migrating chest pain is one of the salient features and may be asso-

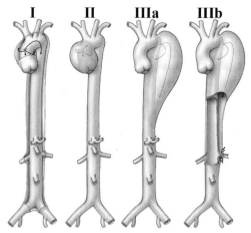

Figure 14–7. Classification of dissection (DeBakey) and incidence of neurologic complications. The arrows indicate the direction of propagation of the dissection. In the DeBakey classification system, *type I* dissection involves the ascending aorta, arch, and any length of the descending aorta; *type II* dissection is confined to the ascending aorta; *type IIIa* dissection involves the descending thoracic aorta; and *type IIIb* dissection involves the descending aorta but progresses into the abdominal aorta and may occlude the renal artery (small arrows).

ciated with loss of a femoral pulse. Signs of aortic insufficiency or cardiac tamponade may be present.

Neurologic Manifestations

Neurologic complications are uncommon in acute aortic dissections[74–78] (Table 14–4). The reported incidences of stroke and spinal cord ischemia according to DeBakey's types are 7% and 4% in types I and III, respectively, and occurrence is understandably much less common in type II when the dissection is confined to the ascending aorta. Preoperative hypotension triples the risk of stroke.[80] The surprisingly high incidence of decreased consciousness or coma is unexplained but perhaps is due to global hypoperfusion or multiple hemispheric infarcts.

When the dissection extends into the common carotid artery, the inequality of the carotid pulses and unilateral tenderness over the left carotid may be helpful signs. Nissim[81] noted a unilateral reduplication in pul-

Table 14–4. Neurologic Manifestations of Aortic Dissection*

Findings	PATIENTS	
	No.	%
Decreased level of consciousness or coma	26	5
Hemiplegia	10	2
Paraplegia	27	5
Transient blindness	4	0.8
Horner's syndrome	3	0.6

*Based on 505 cases from the literature compiled by Hirst and associates.[79]

sations of the carotid artery (that is, two beats in quick succession on the right for every single beat on the left). This effect has been attributed to a difference in the velocity of the pulse wave through the lumen and through the dissecting aneurysm. Carotid dissection may lead to Horner's syndrome and tongue deviation from, respectively, sympathetic nerve and hypoglossal nerve involvement. Innominate occlusion may result in right hemispheric infarction and may be followed by paraparesis after extension of the dissection to the thoracic and abdominal portions of the aorta.

Very uncommon manifestations in aortic dissection include putaminal hemorrhage, probably related to marked surges in blood pressure.[78] Transient blindness reported in older series may be a result of ophthalmic artery involvement by artery-to-artery embolism from occlusion of the common carotid.[82]

Spinal cord damage has been well recognized in many series, but it is generally not related to the extent of intercostal artery involvement in the dissection. The most common mechanism may be hypoperfusion of the spinal cord associated with shock. Concomitant infarction of the vertebral bodies that can be recognized on plain radiographs may accompany paraplegia.[83] Outcome of paraplegia in dissection of the aorta is similarly poor. In their collection of 11 cases, Weisman and Adams[82] drew attention to ischemic necrosis of the peripheral nerves caused by obstruction of the iliac arteries.

Most patients had a pulseless, cold extremity with weakness, anesthesia, and areflexia.

Diagnosis and Management

Transesophageal echocardiography may diagnose aortic dissection with high accuracy.[84–86] However, angiography remains the mainstay for confirming the diagnosis.

Acute aortic dissections are treated medically with a regulated infusion of nitroprusside to control hypertension. A short-acting drug such as labetalol is often also considered. Inability to control hypertension is an indication for emergency surgery, including proximal dissections.

Patients who present with acute ischemic stroke, often right-sided, and acute type A aortic dissection at the same time are particularly difficult to manage. In one reported case, treatment with tissue plasminogen activator was successful.[87] Emergency replacement of the ascending aorta may produce reperfusion damage or hemorrhagic transformation, and, indeed, this was reported in two of seven patients who had emergency surgery.[88]

CONCLUSIONS

Surgical repairs of thoracoabdominal aneurysm may result in paraplegia in 10% to 20% of patients after elective surgery; in acute spontaneous or traumatic rupture, the incidence doubles. Aortoiliac repair, however, is uncommonly complicated by spinal cord or plexus injury (<1%).

Several pathologic types of spinal cord infarction have been reported, but anterior spinal artery syndrome or complete spinal cord infarction at the midthoracic to low-thoracic level is most frequent. Magnetic resonance imaging can demonstrate signal changes in the spinal cord that not only confirm the ischemic damage but in some instances may predict recovery when only anterior horn abnormalities (owl's eyes) are present.

No study in humans has shown that measures such as hypothermia, CSF drainage, intrathecally delivered papaverine, or combinations of treatments have actually decreased the incidence of paraplegia. All reported series have used historical controls. A reasonable approach in patients with major risk factors (aged 64 years or older, aortic clamp time over 45 min) and abnormal SSEP or motor evoked potential responses during surgery is CSF drainage, moderate cooling to 30°C, and very careful maintenance of adequate systemic blood pressure and normal acid–base balance. All risks cannot be eliminated, but every effort should be made to reduce the dangers of spinal cord ischemia. Some surgeons advocate aggressive reattachment of intercostal arteries until SSEP signals reappear.

Prevention of spinal cord injury begins in the operating theater, but some patients awaken neurologically intact only to deteriorate days later. Hypovolemia, hypotension, and respiratory acidosis have accompanied this delayed-onset paraplegia. In addition, drainage of CSF (the increase in CSF pressure may result in a decrease of spinal cord perfusion pressure) should logically be the first action when leg function begins to deteriorate.

Another major vascular catastrophe in the surgical ICU is aortic dissection. The risk of neurologic complications is related to extension of the dissection. Ischemic stroke, occurring in approximately 6% of patients, may be traced to extension into the carotid artery.

REFERENCES

1. Adams HD, van Geertruyden HH. Neurologic complications of aortic surgery. Ann Surg 144:574–609, 1956.
2. Hogan EL, Romanul FC. Spinal cord infarction occurring during insertion of aortic graft. Neurology 16:67–74, 1966.
3. Lynch C, Weingarden SI. Paraplegia following aortic surgery. Paraplegia 20:196–200, 1982.
4. Lynch DR, Dawson TM, Raps EC, Galetta SL. Risk factors for the neurologic complications associated with aortic aneurysms. Arch Neurol 49:284–288, 1992.
5. Mawad ME, Rivera V, Crawford S, Ramirez A, Breitbach W. Spinal cord ischemia after resection of thoracoabdominal aortic aneurysms: MR findings in 24 patients. AJNR Am J Neuroradiol 11:987–991, 1990.
6. Szilagyi DE, Hageman JH, Smith RF, Elliott JP. Spinal cord damage in surgery of the abdominal aorta. Surgery 83:38–56, 1978.
7. Svensson LG, Crawford ES, Hess KR, Coselli JS, Safi HJ. Experience with 1509 patients undergoing thoracoabdominal aortic operations. J Vasc Surg 17:357–368, 1993.
8. Carlson DE, Karp RB, Kouchoukos NT. Surgical treatment of aneurysms of the descending thoracic aorta: an analysis of 85 patients. Ann Thorac Surg 35:58–69, 1983.
9. Gilling-Smith GL, Worswick L, Knight PF, Wolfe JH, Mansfield AO. Surgical repair of thoracoabdominal aortic aneurysm: 10 years' experience. Br J Surg 82:624–629, 1995.
10. Coselli JS, Plestis KA, La Francesca S, Cohen S. Results of contemporary surgical treatment of descending thoracic aortic aneurysms: experience in 198 patients. Ann Vasc Surg 10:131–137, 1996.
11. Safi HJ, Miller CC III. Spinal cord protection in descending thoracic and thoracoabdominal aortic repair. Ann Thorac Surg 67:1937–1939, 1999.
12. Galla JD, Ergin MA, Lansman SL, et al. Use of somatosensory evoked potentials for thoracic and thoracoabdominal aortic resections. Ann Thorac Surg 67:1947–1952, 1999.
13. Cambria RP, Davison JK, Carter C, et al. Epidural cooling for spinal cord protection during thoracoabdominal aneurysm repair: a five-year experience. J Vasc Surg 31:1093–1102, 2000.
14. von Segesser LK, Marty B, Mueller X, et al. Active cooling during open repair of thoraco-abdominal aortic aneurysms improves outcome. Eur J Cardiothorac Surg 19:411–415, 2001.
15. Katz NM, Blackstone EH, Kirklin JW, Karp RB. Incremental risk factors for spinal cord injury following operation for acute traumatic aortic transection. J Thorac Cardiovasc Surg 81:669–674, 1981.
16. Sturm JT, Billiar TR, Dorsey JS, Luxenberg MG, Perry JF Jr. Risk factors for survival following surgical treatment of traumatic aortic rupture. Ann Thorac Surg 39:418–421, 1985.
17. Hassler O. Blood supply to human spinal cord. A microangiographic study. Arch Neurol 15:302–307, 1966.
18. Herren RY, Alexander L. Sulcal and intrinsic blood vessels of human spinal cord. Arch Neurol Psychiatry 41:678–687, 1939.
19. Lazorthes G, Gouaze A, Zadeh JO, Santini JJ, Lazorthes Y, Burdin P. Arterial vascularization of the spinal cord: recent studies of the anastomotic substitution pathways. J Neurosurg 35:253–262, 1971.
20. Turnbull IM. Blood supply of the spinal cord: normal and pathological considerations. Clin Neurosurg 20:56–84, 1973.
21. Zülch KJ, Kurth-Schumacher R. The pathogenesis of "intermittent spinovascular insufficiency" (spinal claudication of Dejerine) and other vascular syndromes of the spinal cord. Vasc Surg 4:116–136, 1970.
22. Wadouh F, Lindemann EM, Arndt CF, Hetzer R, Borst HG. The arteria radicularis magna anterior as a decisive factor influencing spinal cord damage during aortic occlusion. J Thorac Cardiovasc Surg 88:1–10, 1984.
23. Dommisse GF. The blood supply of the spinal cord. A critical vascular zone in spinal surgery. J Bone Joint Surg (Br) 56:225–235, 1974.
24. Crawford ES, Crawford JL, Safi HJ, et al. Thoracoabdominal aortic aneurysms: preoperative and intraoperative factors determining immediate and

long-term results of operations in 605 patients. J Vasc Surg 3:389–404, 1986.

25. Crawford ES, Hess KR, Cohen ES, Coselli JS, Safi HJ. Ruptured aneurysm of the descending thoracic and thoracoabdominal aorta. Analysis according to size and treatment. Ann Surg 213:417–425, 1991.

26. Hantler CB, Knight PR. Intracranial hypertension following cross-clamping of the thoracic aorta. Anesthesiology 56:146–147, 1982.

27. Svensson LG, Rickards E, Coull A, Rogers G, Fimmel CJ, Hinder RA. Relationship of spinal cord blood flow to vascular anatomy during thoracic aorta cross-clamping and shunting. J Thorac Cardiovasc Surg 91:71–78, 1986.

28. Svensson LG, Von Ritter CM, Growneveld HT, et al. Cross-clamping of the thoracic aorta. Influence of aortic shunts, laminectomy, papaverine, calcium channel blocker, allopurinol, and superoxide dismutase on spinal cord blood flow and paraplegia in baboons. Ann Surg 204:38–47, 1986.

29. Marini CP, Grubbs PE, Toporoff B, et al. Effect of sodium nitroprusside on spinal cord perfusion and paraplegia during aortic cross-clamping. Ann Thorac Surg 47:379–383, 1989.

30. Livesay JJ, Cooley DA, Ventemiglia RA, et al. Surgical experience in descending thoracic aneurysmectomy with and without adjuncts to avoid ischemia. Ann Thorac Surg 39:37–46, 1985.

31. Williams GM, Perler BA, Burdick JF, et al. Angiographic localization of spinal cord blood supply and its relationship to postoperative paraplegia. J Vasc Surg 13:23–33, 1991.

32. Svensson LG, Patel V, Robinson MF, Ueda T, Roehm JO Jr, Crawford ES. Influence of preservation or perfusion of intraoperatively identified spinal cord blood supply on spinal motor evoked potentials and paraplegia after aortic surgery. J Vasc Surg 13:355–365, 1991.

33. Yamada N, Okita Y, Minatoya K, et al. Preoperative demonstration of the Adamkiewicz artery by magnetic resonance angiography in patients with descending or thoracoabdominal aortic aneurysms. Eur J Cardiothorac Surg 18:104–111, 2000.

34. Moore WM Jr, Hollier LH. The influence of severity of spinal cord ischemia in the etiology of delayed-onset paraplegia. Ann Surg 213:427–431, 1991.

35. Brock MV, Redmond JM, Ishiwa S, et al. Clinical markers in CSF for determining neurologic deficits after thoracoabdominal aortic aneurysm repairs. Ann Thorac Surg 64:999–1003, 1997.

36. Gloviczki P, Cross SA, Stanson AW, et al. Ischemic injury to the spinal cord or lumbosacral plexus after aortoiliac reconstruction. Am J Surg 162:131–136, 1991.

37. Lintott P, Hafez HM, Stansby G. Spinal cord complications of thoracoabdominal aneurysm surgery. Br J Surg 85:5–15, 1998.

38. Decroix JP, Ciaudo-Lacroix C, Lapresle J. Brown-Séquard syndrome caused by a spinal cord infarction [in French]. Rev Neurol 140:585–586, 1984.

39. Ferguson LR, Bergan JJ, Conn J Jr, Yao JS. Spinal ischemia following abdominal aortic surgery. Ann Surg 181:267–272, 1975.

40. Byrne TN, Waxman SG. Spinal Cord Compression: Diagnosis and Principles of Management. FA Davis, Philadelphia, 1990, pp 21–65.

41. Crawford ES, Mizrahi EM, Hess KR, Coselli JS, Safi HJ, Patel VM. The impact of distal aortic perfusion and somatosensory evoked potential monitoring on prevention of paraplegia after aortic aneurysm operation. J Thorac Cardiovasc Surg 95:357–367, 1988.

42. Drenger B, Parker SD, McPherson RW, et al. Spinal cord stimulation evoked potentials during thoracoabdominal aortic aneurysm surgery. Anesthesiology 76:689–695, 1992.

43. Kaplan BJ, Friedman WA, Alexander JA, Hampson SR. Somatosensory evoked potential monitoring of spinal cord ischemia during aortic operations. Neurosurgery 19:82–90, 1986.

44. Laschinger JC, Izumoto H, Kouchoukos NT. Evolving concepts in prevention of spinal cord injury during operations on the descending thoracic and thoracoabdominal aorta. Ann Thorac Surg 44:667–674, 1987.

45. Cunningham JN Jr, Laschinger JC, Spencer FC. Monitoring of somatosensory evoked potentials during surgical procedures on the thoracoabdominal aorta. IV. Clinical observations and results. J Thorac Cardiovasc Surg 94:275–285, 1987.

46. Okamoto Y, Murakami M, Nakagawa T, Murata A, Moriya H. Intraoperative spinal cord monitoring during surgery for aortic aneurysm: application of spinal cord evoked potential. Electroencephalogr Clin Neurophysiol 84:315–320, 1992.

47. Levy WJ Jr. Clinical experience with motor and cerebellar evoked potential monitoring. Neurosurgery 20:169–182, 1987.

48. Tanaka S, Fujimoto Y, Sasaki M, Oka S, Ikuta Y, Sueda T. Effect of spinal cord ischemia on spinal cord evoked potentials. J Electrodiagn Spinal Cord 19:21–24, 1997.

49. de Haan P, Kalkman CJ, de Mol BA, Ubags LH, Veldman DJ, Jacobs MJ. Efficacy of transcranial motor-evoked myogenic potentials to detect spinal cord ischemia during operations for thoracoabdominal aneurysms. J Thorac Cardiovasc Surg 113:87–100, 1997.

50. Meylaerts SA, Jacobs MJ, van Iterson V, De Haan P, Kalkman CJ. Comparison of transcranial motor evoked potentials and somatosensory evoked potentials during thoracoabdominal aortic aneurysm repair. Ann Surg 230:742–749, 1999.

51. Sueda T, Morita S, Okada K, Orihashi K, Shikata H, Matsuura Y. Selective intercostal arterial perfusion during thoracoabdominal aortic aneurysm surgery. Ann Thorac Surg 70:44–47, 2000.

52. Colon R, Frazier OH, Cooley DA, McAllister HA. Hypothermic regional perfusion for protection of the spinal cord during periods of ischemia. Ann Thorac Surg 43:639–643, 1987.

53. Murray MJ, Werner E, Oliver WC Jr, Bower TC, Gloviczki P. Anesthetic management of thoracoabdominal aortic aneurysm repair: effects of CSF drainage and mild hypothermia [abstract]. Anesthesiology 71:62A, 1989.

54. Wadouh F, Wadouh R, Hartmann M, Crisp-Lindgren N. Prevention of paraplegia during aortic operations. Ann Thorac Surg 50:543–552, 1990.

55. Wakabayashi A, Connolly JE. Prevention of paraplegia associated with resection of extensive thoracic aneurysms. Arch Surg 111:1186–1189, 1976.

56. Berguer R, Porto J, Fedoronko B, Dragovic L. Selective deep hypothermia of the spinal cord prevents paraplegia after aortic cross-clamping in the dog model. J Vasc Surg 15:62–71, 1992.

57. Svensson LG, Crawford ES, Patel V, McLean TR, Jones JW, DeBakey ME. Spinal oxygenation, blood supply localization, cooling, and function with aortic clamping. Ann Thorac Surg 54:74–79, 1992.

58. Davison JK, Cambria RP, Vierra DJ, Columbia MA, Koustas G. Epidural cooling for regional spinal cord hypothermia during thoracoabdominal aneurysm repair. J Vasc Surg 20:304–310, 1994.

59. Woloszyn TT, Marini CP, Coons MS, et al. Cerebrospinal fluid drainage and steroids provide better spinal cord protection during aortic cross-clamping than does either treatment alone. Ann Thorac Surg 49:78–82, 1990.

60. Crawford ES, Svensson LG, Hess KR, et al. A prospective randomized study of cerebrospinal fluid drainage to prevent paraplegia after high-risk surgery on the thoracoabdominal aorta. J Vasc Surg 13:36–45, 1991.

61. Svensson LG, Grum DF, Bednarski M, Cosgrove DM III, Loop FD. Appraisal of cerebrospinal fluid alterations during aortic surgery with intrathecal papaverine administration and cerebrospinal fluid drainage. J Vasc Surg 11:423–429, 1990.

62. Svensson LG, Stewart RW, Cosgrove DM III, et al. Intrathecal papaverine for the prevention of paraplegia after operation on the thoracic or thoracoabdominal aorta. J Thorac Cardiovasc Surg 96:823–829, 1988.

63. Acher CW, Wynn MM, Archibald J. Naloxone and spinal fluid drainage as adjuncts in the surgical treatment of thoracoabdominal and thoracic aneurysms. Surgery 108:755–761, 1990.

64. Laschinger JC, Cunningham JN Jr, Cooper MM, Krieger K, Nathan IM, Spencer FC. Prevention of ischemic spinal cord injury following aortic cross-clamping: use of corticosteroids. Ann Thorac Surg 38:500–507, 1984.

65. Widman MD, DeLucia A, Sharp J, Richenbacher WE. Reversal of renal failure and paraplegia after thoracoabdominal aneurysm repair. Ann Thorac Surg 65:1153–1155, 1998.

66. Lang-Lazdunski L, Heurteaux C, Dupont H, Rouelle D, Widmann C, Mantz J. The effects of FK506 on neurologic and histopathologic outcome after transient spinal cord ischemia induced by aortic cross-clamping in rats. Anesth Analg 92:1237–1244, 2001.

67. Wilberger JE Jr. Lumbosacral radiculopathy secondary to abdominal aortic aneurysms. Report of three cases. J Neurosurg 58:965–967, 1983.

68. Boontje AH, Haaxma R. Femoral neuropathy as a complication of aortic surgery. J Cardiovasc Surg (Torino) 28:286–289, 1987.

69. Merchant RF Jr, Cafferata HT, DePalma RG. Ruptured aortic aneurysm seen initially as acute femoral neuropathy. Arch Surg 117:811–813, 1982.

70. Owens ML. Psoas weakness and femoral neuropathy: neglected signs of retroperitoneal hemorrhage from ruptured aneurysm. Surgery 91:363–366, 1982.

71. Razzuk MA, Linton RR, Darling RC. Femoral neuropathy secondary to ruptured abdominal aortic aneurysms with false aneurysms. JAMA 201:817–820, 1967.

72. Kawahito K, Adachi H, Yamaguchi A, Ino T. Preoperative risk factors for hospital mortality in acute type A aortic dissection. Ann Thorac Surg 71:1239–1243, 2001.

73. Hagan PG, Nienaber CA, Isselbacher EM, et al. The International Registry of Acute Aortic Dissection (IRAD): new insights into an old disease. JAMA 283:897–903, 2000.

74. Chase TN, Rosman NP, Price DL. The cerebral syndromes associated with dissecting aneurysm of the aorta. A clinicopathological study. Brain 91:173–190, 1968.

75. DeBakey ME, McCollum CH, Crawford ES, et al. Dissection and dissecting aneurysms of the aorta: twenty-year follow-up of five hundred twenty-seven patients treated surgically. Surgery 92:1118–1134, 1982.

76. DeSanctis RW, Doroghazi RM, Austen WG, Buckley MJ. Aortic dissection. N Engl J Med 317:1060–1067, 1987.

77. Gerber O, Heyer EJ, Vieux U. Painless dissections of the aorta presenting as acute neurologic syndromes. Stroke 17:644–647, 1986.

78. Moersch FP, Sayre GP. Neurologic manifestations associated with dissecting aneurysm of the aorta. JAMA 144:1141–1148, 1950.

79. Hirst AE Jr, Johns VJ Jr, Kime SW Jr. Dissecting aneurysm of the aorta: a review of 505 cases. Medicine (Baltimore) 37:217–279, 1958.

80. Safi HJ, Miller CC III, Reardon MJ, et al. Operation for acute and chronic aortic dissection: recent outcome with regard to neurologic deficit and early death. Ann Thorac Surg 66:402–411, 1998.

81. Nissim JA. Dissecting aneurysm of the aorta: a new sign. Br Heart J 8:203–206, 1946.

82. Weisman AD, Adams RD. The neurological complications of dissecting aortic aneurysm. Brain 67:69–92, 1944.

83. Hill CS Jr, Vasquez JM. Massive infarction of spinal cord and vertebral bodies as a complication of dissecting aneurysm of the aorta. Circulation 25:997–1000, 1962.

84. Erbel R, Engberding R, Daniel W, Roelandt J, Visser C, Rennollet H. Echocardiography in diagnosis of aortic dissection. Lancet 1:457–461, 1989.

85. Farah MG, Suneja R. Diagnosis of circumferential dissection of the ascending aorta by transesophageal echocardiography. Chest 103:291–292, 1993.

86. Petasnick JP. Radiologic evaluation of aortic dissection. Radiology 180:297–305, 1991.

87. Fesler AJ, Alberts MJ. Stroke treatment with tissue plasminogen activator in the setting of aortic dissection. Neurology 54:1010, 2000.

88. Fann JI, Sarris GE, Miller DC, et al. Surgical management of acute aortic dissection complicated by stroke. Circulation 80:I-257–I-263, 1989.

Chapter 15

NEUROLOGIC COMPLICATIONS
OF CARDIAC SURGERY

GENERAL CONSIDERATIONS
ISCHEMIC STROKE
Predictive Factors
Clinical Features
Neuroimaging
Management
NEUROPSYCHOLOGIC IMPAIRMENT
RETINAL DAMAGE
PERIPHERAL NERVE DAMAGE
CONCLUSIONS

Advances in cardiac surgery have improved long-term outcome in patients with coronary and valvular disease, but some of the gains have been counterbalanced by damage to the brain. Use of cardiopulmonary bypass in either coronary artery bypass grafting (CABG) or open heart surgery greatly increases the risk for neurologic complications.[1-4]

Even more broadly, the clinical profile of patients undergoing coronary bypass surgery is changing. Mortality may have declined from increased use of left internal mammary artery grafts, multiple arterial conduits, and warm blood cardioplegia,[5] but there is a clear shift toward a greater prevalence of patients who are older than 70 years and have diabetes mellitus. Consequently, neurologic morbidity may increase along with other systemic perioperative complications.[6] These neurologic complications considerably delay hospital dismissal and return to work or in severe cases necessitate daily living assistance, all with personal and social costs.

Particular risks for neurologic complications that have been identified include duration of cardiopulmonary bypass and prior stroke. Occlusive disease of the carotid arteries and the ascending aorta is an additional risk factor for postoperative stroke. However, no evidence exists that unambiguously supports carotid endarterectomy in an asymptomatic patient and, by the same token, it has not been convincingly established whether modification of techniques in patients with severe atheromatous aortic arch disease reduces the risk of postoperative ischemic stroke.

This chapter reviews the most important neurologic complications of cardiac surgery, highlights the possible pathophysiologic mechanisms, and discusses the relevance to clinical practice and management. Any future therapy needs to affect the degree of microembolization during cardiac surgery or improve ischemic tolerance of the brain.

GENERAL CONSIDERATIONS

As a starting point for the consulting neurologist, some knowledge about the condition of the patient on cardiopulmonary bypass is required.

The extracorporeal perfusion system is depicted in Figure 15–1. Essentially, venous return from two connecting catheters placed in the superior and inferior venae cavae passes through an oxygenator, and a nonocclusive roller pump returns blood to the ascending aorta. Additional left ventricular

263

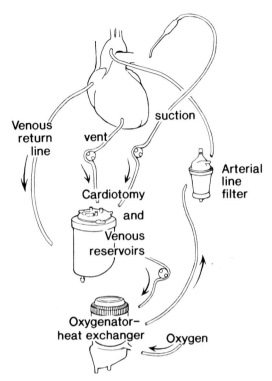

Figure 15–1. Extracorporeal circulation.

may also be associated with the stress response of the procedure itself, use of pressor agents, and infusion of large volumes of dextrose solutions. In a brain challenged by decreased blood flow and possible widespread ischemia, hyperglycemia may lead to exaggerated neuronal damage and failure to fuel recovery as a result of enhanced extracellular glutamate accumulation.[8] Other serious problems with a potential for central nervous system injury are bubble expansion and subsequent air embolism during the cooling phase of bypass, hypotension during the procedure, increased intracranial pressure resulting from obstruction of the vena cava cannula, and decrease in hematocrit. Increase in blood viscosity may also occur from the effect of hypothermia or from infusion of hyperosmolar solutions.

These concerns have led to a rekindling of the use of warm blood cardioplegia. Warm heart surgical techniques have been evaluated by randomized clinical trials.[9,10] The advantages of warm blood cardioplegia are related to myocardial protection due to reduction of reperfusion injuries, particularly in complex cardiac procedures. However, the results of these trials conflict with at least one other study claiming a similar effect or better protection with mild hypothermia.[11]

The pathophysiology of global cerebral injury in patients undergoing cardiopulmonary bypass is complicated and has been only partly elucidated. Factors associated with increased incidence of cognitive deficits are intracardiac procedures, duration of bypass, use of bubble oxygenation,[12] and absence of arterial filters.[13]

Hemodynamic threats and danger of microemboli remain major problems during cardiac surgery. During cardiopulmonary bypass, cerebral blood flow is altered by shifts in temperature, hemodynamic changes induced by anesthetic pharmacologic agents, and changes in P_{CO_2}.[14–17] Cerebral autoregulation, however, remains intact. A scholarly account of cerebrovascular physiology during bypass can be found in a review by Schell and associates.[18]

A history of stroke or transient ischemic attacks indicates a predisposition for stroke after cardiac surgery. Whether a possible hemodynamic compromise exists in patients with unilateral or bilateral carotid stenosis

stenting is used in some cardiac centers. Two types of oxygenators are commonly used: bubble oxygenators with very efficient oxygenation at low cost, and membrane oxygenators with the additional advantages of prolonged use and virtual absence of blood cell disruption that is otherwise created by gas bubbling. Filters may be placed on both sides of the system to ensure a low risk of infusing debris and air bubbles into the circulation. The extracorporeal system is primed with a heparinized and buffered physiologic salt solution, which is followed by administration of a cardioplegia solution through one of the roller heads on the pump oxygenator. Usually, a large dose of potassium cardioplegia solution is used.

Cold crystalloid cardioplegia and cold reperfusion may permit adequate central nervous system protection.[7] Nevertheless, other physiologic changes occur that can result in significant risks to the brain. One of the most important changes—a decreased response of insulin to hypothermia—potentially causes hyperglycemia. Hyperglycemia has not been systematically studied. A transcranial Doppler study done at the time of bypass found that blood flow velocity may decrease just after the onset of cardiopulmonary bypass ipsilateral to a carotid stenosis, but reduced cerebral perfusion was not observed despite a marked drop in arterial blood pressure to <50 mm Hg during the first minutes of bypass.[19] Intuitively, hemodynamic hazards during the various stages of cardiopulmonary bypass may contribute to cerebral injury, but recent evidence suggests that microemboli may be more relevant in the genesis of global brain injury.

Interposition of a filter in the arterial line of the extracorporeal circuit may diminish but not eliminate neurologic complications.[20] Clinical studies have been conflicting. Pugsley and associates,[21] in a small group of patients with grafts who randomly received filtered (40 μm self-venting blood filter) or nonfiltered cardiopulmonary bypass, assessed the effects with a battery of neuropsychologic tests and transcranial Doppler (TCD) ultrasonography. Significantly fewer microembolic events were detected by TCD examination in the patients in the filtered group, who also had significantly better neuropsychologic performance. In contrast, a randomized study from Spain in which 20 μm filters were used in the arterial line could not demonstrate any change in postoperative cerebral impairment.[22]

Microemboli may come from several sources: ventricular air,[23] atheromatous debris dislodged during insertion of the cannula, fat globules, platelet aggregates,[24] and perhaps also particulate emboli from glove powder, foam products, and the lining of tubes.

The TCD examination of the middle cerebral artery during bypass has greatly improved the recognition of these particles, but TCD ultrasonography cannot differentiate between particulate and gaseous emboli.[12] The TCD monitoring of the middle cerebral artery blood velocities during bypass may identify high-amplitude flow disturbance signals that produce a chirping sound superimposed on a nearly silent band created by nonpulsatile flow of the bypass. Repeated emboli are commonly heard during continuous TCD monitoring.

The end of bypass has been identified as the most critical period for embolization.[25] The number of embolic events significantly increases during filling of the beating heart rather than immediately after declamping of the aorta (Fig. 15–2). The clinical value of this finding may remain uncertain, but meticulous draining before filling of the empty heart may reduce this complication. Prospective studies that correlate the prevalence of embolic showers with postoperative stroke or neuropsychologic deficit are needed.

The neuropathologic counterpart of microemboli has been described. Neuropathologic investigation of patients who died after the procedure revealed many focal small capillary and arteriolar dilatations (so-called SCADs) in the cortical and deep nuclear gray matter.[26] These abnormalities have not been found in patients without bypass procedures and represent microgaseous or, perhaps more likely, lipid microemboli. In a study of cardiopulmonary bypass in dogs, clear microspheres and black microspheres were injected to possibly link SCADS to cardiopulmonary bypass, and indeed, these pathologic phenomena could be reproduced (Fig. 15–3). Serial magnetic resonance images (MRIs) have not detected abnormalities linked to neuropsychologic deficits,[27] but correlative studies with TCD ultrasonography have not been performed.

Monitoring during bypass graft surgery offers the possibility of recognizing damage to the cerebral cortex. Except for numerous studies that have tried to correlate EEG abnormalities with postoperative neuropsychologic or neurologic complications, convincing data are not available to support routine use of monitoring. Part of the question is whether aggressive intervention after detection of abnormalities during cardiac surgery can be successful. Indeed, Arom and associates[28] carefully correlated computed EEG recordings with postoperative deficits and found that intervention (consisting of increase in cerebral perfusion pressure, increase in bypass pump flow, and use of pressors) resulted in improvement of EEG variables and, more important, decreased the incidence of postoperative neuropsychologic deficits. Alternatively, somatosensory evoked potentials may have no application in cold

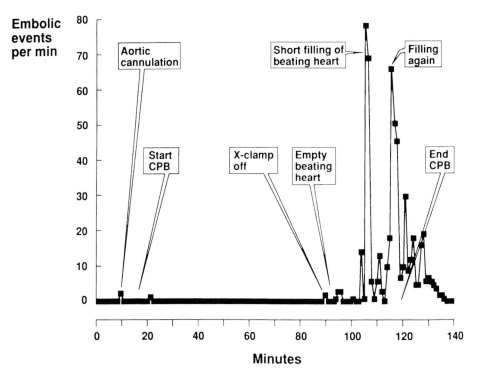

Figure 15–2. Transcranial Doppler recording of emboli during open heart surgery, indicating maximal embolic events during redistribution of blood when the heart is beginning to eject. CPB, cardiopulmonary bypass. (From van der Linden and Casimir-Ahn.[25] By permission of the Society of Thoracic Surgeons.)

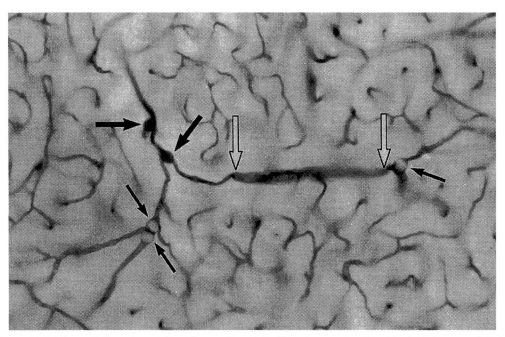

Figure 15–3. Microemboli causing small capillary and arteriolar dilatations are "bracketed in time" by sequentially injected microspheres of different colors. Clear microspheres (small black arrows), a long fat embolus (between white arrows), and black microspheres (large black arrows) can be seen in distal to proximal order in a single arteriolar complex. In this experiment, clear spheres were injected into the carotid artery of a dog, followed in succession by injection of corn oil and then black spheres. Direction of blood flow in the arteriole is from top to bottom. (Alkaline phosphatase-stained 100-μm-thick celloidin section; microspheres = 15 μm.) (From Moody DM, Brown WR, Challa VR, Stump DA, Reboussin DM, Legault C. Brain microemboli associated with cardiopulmonary bypass: a histologic and magnetic resonance imaging study. Ann Thorac Surg 59:1304–1307, 1995. By permission of the Society of Thoracic Surgeons.)

266

cardioplegia, because marked hypothermia attenuates or may even abolish the cortical response.[29,30]

Few clinical trials have assessed the neurologic outcome with agents that may protect the brain during cardiopulmonary bypass surgery. Much of the gathered data are from animal studies. Reports of large trials, two with thiopental loading, have been published (Table 15–1). Nussmeier and associates' study[31] found a significantly lower incidence of stroke and neuropsychologic deficits in patients treated with thiopental loading, but a later study[32] reached the opposite conclusion. Important differences in patient selection (open heart or CABG) and cardiopulmonary bypass conditions (normothermic or hypothermic, arterial filters or no arterial filter, glucose priming or plasma solution primer) may have accounted for some of the differences but are not likely to explain the major differences in results. A recent study evaluated propofol in a sufficiently high dose to create a burst–suppression pattern on EEG during cardiac valve replacement.[33] (Burst suppression has been assumed to indicate neuroprotection through reduction of the cerebral metabolic rate.) However, no improvement in neurologic outcome was found, and, worse, there was a tendency toward a greater incidence of early neurologic deficit, possibly associated with propofol-induced hypotension.[33]

PATHOPHYSIOLOGIC MECHANISMS

Much mystification remains about the mechanisms leading to the decline in processing of cognitive information in patients undergoing cardiopulmonary bypass. The least likely cause, although simple in concept, is a reduction of cerebral blood flow. Normal cerebral blood flow is estimated at 40 to 60 mL $\cdot$ 100 g$^{-1} \cdot$ mL $\cdot$ min^{-1}, with a bypass-induced reduction of 20 to 60 mL $\cdot$ 100 g$^{-1} \cdot$ min^{-1} when the standard setting is used on bypass machines.[34] In itself, therefore, the reduction of cerebral blood flow is still significantly higher than the ischemia threshold set by Astrup and associates[34] ($\leq$10 mL $\cdot$ 100 g$^{-1} \cdot$ min^{-1}).

Embolic load may seem responsible for neuropsychologic changes. More likely, microbubbles of air produce these effects, because their small size (25 mm) may allow them to pass through the 40 mm filters.

Management of pH during cardiopulmonary bypass may contribute, changing cerebral blood flow and, possibly indirectly, increasing delivery of microemboli. Acid–base management may be divided into "pH-stat" (plasma pH at 7.4 regardless of temperature) and "alpha-stat" (permitting relative alkalosis when the patient is cooled). The pH-stat technique artificially increases the carbon dioxide content, causing higher cerebral blood flow, hyper-

Table 15–1. Barbiturate Cerebral Protection Studies

Characteristics	Nussmeier et al. Study[31]	Zaidan et al. Study[32]
Patients (no.)	182	300
Procedure	Open chamber	CABG
History of stroke	No	No
Oxygenation	Bubble	Membrane
Arterial filter	No	Yes
Temperature (°C)	>34	28
Duration of CPB (min)	50	90
Pump flow rate (L/min)	3.0–4.4	2.5
Thiopental dose (mg/kg)	39 ± 8	33 ± 11
EEG burst suppression	Yes	Yes
Mean arterial pressure (mm Hg)	40–90	50–100
Priming	5% dextrose	Plasmalyte
Stroke, thiopental/placebo	0/6	5/2

CABG, coronary artery bypass grafting; CPB, cardiopulmonary bypass; EEG, electroencephalographic.

emia, and possibly cerebral edema. With the pH-stat technique, cerebral blood flow is pressure-passive and moves with perfusion pressure. The tight coupling between cerebral blood flow and cerebral metabolic rate may become mismatched, and cerebral autoregulation may be lost.

With alpha-stat management, cerebral autoregulation is preserved, and lesser cerebral blood flow than that with pH-stat probably reduces cerebral emboli. A randomized study on pH- and alpha-stat management settled the issue. Cognitive dysfunction was significantly greater at 2 months in the pH-stat group but only when bypass times were longer than 90 min.[35]

ISCHEMIC STROKE

The incidence of ischemic stroke after CABG may approach 5%,[36–43] but it has been as low as 1.5% in more recent studies. After open heart surgery involving valve replacement, the risk of stroke is markedly higher (increasing to 10%).[1] Fortunately, permanent disabling deficit from ischemic stroke occurs in fewer than 2% of the patients, and only a minority of the patients actually die from brain swelling.

Predictive Factors

Many risk factors have been identified. First, perioperative stroke seems more prevalent in warm blood cardioplegia. In a published trial,[39] perioperative stroke was 3% in "warm blood cardioplegia" as opposed to 1% in "cold blood cardioplegia," but no significant difference was found in delayed-onset stroke. This trial can be criticized for poor definition of neurologic events.

Second, four large studies (Table 15–2) found that previous history of stroke, carotid artery disease, prolonged bypass time (often over 2 hr), and postoperative atrial fibrillation were significantly more common in patients who had an ischemic stroke after CABG.[40–43] Gardner and associates[40] emphasized that atherosclerosis of the ascending aorta may predispose patients to stroke. Although the diagnosis of a "shaggy aorta" ideally should be made by transesophageal echocardiography, this examination is not routinely done, and more often the condi-

Table 15–2. Risk Factors for Stroke after Coronary Artery Bypass Grafting

Factors	Gardner et al.[40]	Reed et al.[41]	D'Agostino et al.[42]	Stamou et al.[43]
Age >60 years	+	+		+
History				
Myocardial infarction	−	+	−	+
Cardiac failure	NA	−	NA	+
Diabetes mellitus	−	−	+	+
Stroke or transient ischemic attack	+	+	+	+
Atherosclerosis of ascending aorta and arch	+	NA	+	+
Carotid bruits or stenosis	NA	+	+	+
Aorta clamp time	NA	−	NA	+
Protracted bypass time	+	+	+	+
Perioperative hypotension	+	−	NA	NA
Perioperative flow rates	−	NA	NA	NA
Postoperative				
Atrial fibrillation	NA	+	+	+
Hematocrit	NA	−	NA	NA
Platelet count	NA	−	NA	NA

NA, not assessed; +, significant increased risk; −, no increased risk.

tion is revealed at the time of insertion of bypass cannulae. Intraoperative epiaortic scanning visualizing the distal ascending aorta, often poorly seen by transesophageal echocardiography, could be more sensitive.

A link between the severity of atheromatous disease of the thoracic aorta and a particular vulnerability for postoperative stroke in patients with atheroma with mobile components has been documented[45] (Fig. 15–4). Although carotid artery disease was not evaluated in this study, a recent study did not find a correlation between severity of carotid stenosis and degree of aortic atheromatous disease in a subgroup of 435 patients with carotid disease.[46] If this correlation is confirmed, atheromatous disease of the ascending aorta may be an independent factor.

A study from Massachusetts General Hospital again stressed the risk of stroke in patients with carotid bruit, implying carotid artery disease and stenosis, a major controversy for years.[41]

When carotid artery disease is routinely screened for in prospective patients for CABG, the true proportion of those with significant carotid artery disease is between 2% and 16%, but this figure obviously is determined by referral patterns (Table 15–3). Furthermore, many other studies usually based their incidences of severe carotid disease on noninvasive angiographic studies in patients selected only because they had carotid bruits or a history of transient ischemic attack or stroke.[53,54] A carotid bruit is poorly related to the severity of carotid stenosis whether evaluated by duplex ultrasonography[55,56] or more definitively by cerebral angiography. Approximately two-thirds of patients who have severe carotid stenosis (defined as >50% reduction in diameter) probably do not have carotid bruits. In patients with transient ischemic attacks, carotid bruits are absent in more than one-third of those with 70% to 99% carotid artery stenosis.[57] Thus, carotid auscultation lacks some utility in prediction of carotid stenosis.

With the current available data, it is difficult to give strong recommendations for management of *asymptomatic* carotid stenosis in patients with CABG. Previous studies have not identified patients whose risk is sufficiently high to justify a trial of prophylactic endarterectomy.[58] Several prospective studies of CABG could not substantiate an increased risk of stroke in patients with asymptomatic stenosis.[59] Nonetheless, asymptomatic carotid disease significantly increases the risk of perioperative deaths, including those caused by myocardial infarction. A retrospective study found that older patients (aged 60 years or older) with severe carotid stenosis are at risk.[41] It is not known whether prophylactic carotid endarterectomy, staged or combined, decreases the overall risk of stroke. Ideally, one should conduct a clinical trial in which all patients undergo noninvasive testing before cardiac surgery and randomly receive prophylactic carotid endarterectomy when severe unilateral or bilateral disease has been identified. The logistic problems of such a trial with an estimated initial patient pool of 20,000 to 30,000 are enormous (these large numbers are needed to recruit enough patients with severe stenosis and to demonstrate a reduction with sufficient statistical power in postoperative stroke). Currently, no evidence supports prophylactic carotid repair of any

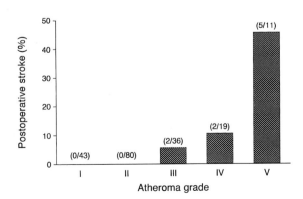

Figure 15–4. One-week stroke rate as a function of atheroma grade in 189 patients with coronary artery bypass grafting. Atheroma grade I, normal or mild intimal thickening; grade II, severe intimal thickening without protruding atheroma; grade III, atheroma protruding less than 5 mm; grade IV, atheroma protruding more than 5 mm; grade V, atheroma of any size but with mobile components. (From Hartman et al.[45] By permission of the International Anesthesia Research Society.)

Table 15–3. Severe Asymptomatic Stenosis in Unselected Series of Coronary Artery Bypass Grafting

Series	No. of Patients	Method of Assessment	PATIENTS WITH SEVERE CAROTID STENOSIS		Degree of Carotid Stenosis (%)
			No.	%	
Barnes et al., 1981[47]	324	Doppler	40	12	>50
Breslau et al., 1981[48]	78	Doppler	5	6	>50
Balderman et al., 1983[49]	500	OPG, angiography	9	2	≥80
Brener et al., 1987[50]	4047	OPG, Doppler	153	4	>50
Faggioli et al., 1990[51]	539	Doppler	47	9	>75
D'Agostino et al., 1996[42]	1212	Doppler	195	16	>50
Hill et al., 1999[52]	200	Doppler	16	8	≥80

OPG, oculoplethysmography.

degree of carotid artery stenosis in asymptomatic patients scheduled for cardiac surgery. Evidence is also lacking in elective stenting of the carotid artery. In a recent study in 50 patients, stenting reduced carotid stenosis from a mean of 78% to 13% but at the expense of three transient ischemic attacks and two strokes.[60] There is insufficient evidence to recommend repair of asymptomatic carotid artery disease before or during cardiac surgery. In these patients, it seems more appropriate to view both conditions separately and not in conjunction with each other.

The management of *symptomatic* carotid stenosis before planning of CABG is another major controversy. Previous studies have indicated that the risk of postoperative stroke in symptomatic carotid stenosis is significantly higher than that in the entire population. In a study of 126 patients with a history of stroke who underwent CABG, 13% had a new stroke or worsening of previous deficits.[61] Worsening of hemiparesis usually occurred in patients with recent strokes (within 3 months before open heart surgery). Symptoms persisted for 2 weeks in some patients but cleared within a few days in many others. However, in this particular clinical setting of cardiac surgery, it is unknown whether prophylactic carotid endarterectomy, proven to be effective in prevention of stroke in selected patients with severe symptomatic stenosis (70% to 99% in diameter on carotid angiograms),[62,63] decreases the incidence of postoperative stroke. Nor is it clearly known what management is appropriate in patients with previous transient ischemic attacks, in patients with bilateral carotid artery disease of more than 50% with or without contralateral occlusion, or in patients with a high-grade carotid stenosis and prior stroke.[64]

It seems reasonable to consider carotid endarterectomy in symptomatic patients with severe carotid stenosis who are eligible for cardiac surgery. However, aside from increased risk of postoperative stroke, there is a considerable risk for postoperative cardiac failure and life-threatening myocardial infarction after carotid surgery in patients with still uncorrected triple coronary artery disease. Fatal myocardial infarction or cardiac death after carotid endarterectomy was about 1% in large series of carotid endarterectomy, even after patients with severe cardiac disease were excluded.[62,63,65] Thus, it seems more logical to proceed with carotid endarterectomy during coronary reconstruction (combined approach)[66–69] because the risks may be blended in one operation, but only in institutions with an acceptable record of complications that are known after a comprehensive internal audit.

Given what is now known, one should also consider other important supplemental observations and place them in a broad context. Postoperative strokes or transient ischemic attacks are often not evident on the first postoperative day. In a large series from Massachusetts General Hospital, ischemic stroke developed in less than half the patients on the first postoperative day. The remaining patients had first signs of ischemic stroke up to 12 days after cardiac surgery. At the Mayo Clinic, 21 of 25 patients with CABG had a stroke at least 2 days after surgery.[70] In a more recent study, 61% of patients had a stroke by day 2 and 39% between days 3 and 9.[71] Why ischemic strokes occur several days after the procedure remains unknown. Possibly, focal signs are detected when the infarct matures or when sedation is discontinued, but these published series continue to claim an asymptomatic interval.[70,72] Postoperative atrial fibrillation after CABG has been significantly associated with ischemic stroke. Ischemic stroke occurred days after acute onset of atrial fibrillation, suggesting a therapeutic possibility. Unfortunately, however, a prospective study in 418 consecutive patients admitted for elective CABG failed to identify predictive factors for atrial fibrillation after CABG.[73] Therefore, anticoagulation cannot be tailored to individual patients but should be considered in patients with acutely manifested atrial fibrillation.

The second potential source of cardiac embolus is left ventricular thrombi in patients undergoing open heart surgery. A retrospective study from the Cleveland Clinic found that the incidence of stroke was approximately 10% in patients with intraluminal defects on left ventriculography but only 2% in patients without left ventricular thrombi.[74] Maslow and associates[75] recently published an account of four patients in whom intraoperative transesophageal echocardiography detected ventricular thrombi. Detection should prompt removal of protruding or mobile thrombi before discontinuation of the bypass. Evaluation for thrombi should be strongly considered in patients with a history of myocardial infarction. Otherwise, because of meticulous operative care, the chance of ventricular thrombi is comparatively small, and it is certainly an insult to the cardiac surgeon if it is tangentially suggested by the consulting neurologist.

As alluded to previously, atherosclerosis of the ascending aorta[45] may be an equally important source for CABG-associated stroke. The incidence of moderate-to-severe atherosclerosis of the aorta (defined as circumferential involvement of most of the ascending aorta and protruding atheroma) was 20% in an unselected series of cardiac surgical patients.[76] This finding prompted at least one group to replace this aortic segment, and there were no postoperative ischemic complications in a preliminary series of 27 patients.[76] Another, more recent study from New York University School of Medicine of 43 patients with aortic arch endarterectomy reported a disquieting 35% incidence of postoperative stroke.[77]

Although hemodynamic changes are frequently encountered during the operation or in the immediate postoperative course, cerebral infarctions associated with hypotension are rare after cardiac surgery. Border zone infarcts between major vascular territories occur in a minority of the patients only but can be a major cause of failure to awaken (Chapter 1). Cerebral infarction in single territories is far more frequent.

In summary, several mechanisms may be involved in early postoperative stroke, the most likely of which is manipulation during surgery. In delayed ischemic stroke, the type of stroke suggests embolization of retained emboli in the heart or fractured thrombi in the ascending aorta from clamping or catheter placement associated with cardiopulmonary bypass surgery. Intraoperative echocardiography may detect severe aortic atherosclerotic disease in segments not visualized on preoperative transesophageal echocardiography. Alternative surgical techniques may be used to avoid plaque disruptions.[46]

Clinical Features

Cardiogenic embolus may be predicted from its clinical presentation. On the basis of a synthesis of the literature, the Cerebral Embolism Task Force provided guidelines for diagnosing cardiogenic embolus,[78–80] although they should be interpreted with caution. Three possibly discriminating features for cardiac embolic stroke were suggested: (1) recent systemic embolism, (2) abrupt onset, defined as a neurologic deficit occurring during the first 10 min and no subsequent deterioration for the first 24 hr, and (*3*) decreased level of consciousness.[81]

Typically, the clinical course in a patient with a cardiogenic brain embolus is marked by a maximal sudden and unheralded neurologic deficit. These emboli tend to lodge in medium-sized branches and involve considerable territories. Aphasia (not infrequently initially misinterpreted as postoperative confusion) and hemiparesis are common presenting signs. The level of consciousness is often diminished at onset. Impaired consciousness is generally not related to horizontal displacement by edematous infarcted tissue but more likely is related to bilateral hemispheric dysfunction associated with either cardiac arrhythmia-induced hypotension or multiple emboli. Visual field defects are usually the only neurologic abnormalities in patients with emboli in the posterior cerebral artery and are detected by the intensive care unit (ICU) nursing staff. Partial or complete occipital infarction is often recognized, but quadrantanopia that reflects infarction in more distal parts of the optic radiation may go unnoticed by the patient and physician.[82] Occasionally, patients awaken with blindness after cardiac surgery.[83] Partial seizures resulting in hallucinations of flashing red lights or vivid, detailed images of persons have been noted before loss of vision due to cortical blindness.[84] Macular sparing is common in patients with large infarcts involving the upper and lower calcarine cortex or optic radiations. A gradually progressive or stuttering clinical course over hours or days may occur in patients with ischemic strokes in the posterior cerebral artery territory. For example, Aldrich and associates[83] found gradual visual deterioration in 6 of 25 patients with cortical blindness after cardiac surgery.

Neuroimaging

The limited data available do not identify computed tomography (CT) patterns that are highly specific for cardiogenic embolization,[85,86] although infarction in the posterior cerebral artery territory has commonly been associated with emboli from cardiac sources, particularly cardiac surgery. Indeed, a study in 1960 that used antifoam emboli showed that most end up in the posterior cerebral circulation.[87]

In addition, infarcts in the superior cerebellar artery territory have been specifically linked to a cardiogenic source.[88] A recent study of 24 patients over a 4-year period found a predilection for the posterior cerebral circulation and a high incidence of multiple infarcts linked to mobile aortic plaque early after surgery. Single territory infarcts were present in patients with a delayed stroke[89] (Table 15–4). Similar findings were present in our review of 25 ischemic strokes occurring after coronary bypass surgery, with most ischemic infarcts located in the middle cerebral artery territory.[70] Not awakening was most often associated with multiple territory strokes, which traditionally have been linked to a cardiogenic source[86] (Fig. 15–5). Late strokes (more than 2 days), however, occurred mostly in single territories.[70]

Watershed cerebral infarcts may also be embolic. These infarcts occur in the border zones between two large cerebral artery territories and have traditionally been linked to a hemodynamic compromise during cardiac surgery. However, some investigators have taken an opposing view in explaining bilateral border zone infarction by showers of microemboli.[90]

Magnetic resonance imaging may be more sensitive and may also show multiple ischemic changes in the white matter (Fig. 15–6). However, several serial magnetic resonance studies found no new abnormalities or minor lesions imperceptible after clinical examination.[91–93] Diffusion-weighted MRI may be more sensitive as shown in a series of 14 patients in whom multiple small infarcts were found, including patients with encephalopathy alone.[94] Cerebral swelling has been observed after normothermic cardiopulmonary bypass but without any clinical correlate and with return to normal within days. Neither its mechanism nor its relation to acid–base management (see "Pathophysiologic Mechanisms") is known.[95]

Management

The effect of ischemic stroke on outcome is significant, leading to a prolonged stay in the ICU. Mortality at 6 months is also substan-

Table 15–4. **Frequency of Territorial and Border Zone Infarcts in Patients with Cardiac Surgery**

Time	Vascular Territory Affected*	No.	%
Within first operative day (group 1, $n = 19$)	Cerebellum	15	79
	PCA	14	74
	PCA-MCA	10	53
	MCA branch	11	58
	Posterior	7	37
	Anterior	6	32
	Deep	3	16
	Multiple	5	26
	Parasagittal watershed	5	26
	MCA–ACA	2	11
	ACA	0	0
Beyond first operative day (group 2, $n = 5$)	Cerebellum	2	40
	PCA	1	20
	MCA branch	1	20
	Parasagittal	1	20

ACA, anterior cerebral artery; MCA, middle cerebral artery; MCA–ACA, anterior watershed territory; PCA, posterior cerebral artery; PCA–MCA, posterior watershed territory.
*In group 1, 16 infarcts were multiple and 3 were single-territory. In group 2, infarcts were single-territory only.
Modified from Barbut et al.[89] By permission of the Society of Thoracic Surgeons.

tially higher.[96] Single territory ischemic strokes are fixed in time and resolve spontaneously. It is prudent to fully anticoagulate patients for 2 to 4 weeks to allow for restoration of the damaged ascending aorta. Long-term anticoagulation is indicated if transesophageal echocardiography shows a retained intramural clot. Thrombolysis can be considered when ischemic stroke occurs weeks after surgery, but neither its benefit nor its risk of major hemorrhage in the postoperative period is known.

Brain swelling may occur in large territorial infarcts, and medical management is unsuccessful, including that with osmotic diuretics, barbiturates, hyperventilation, and combination therapy. Promising but unproven new avenues are moderate hypothermia (33°C) and decompressive craniectomy with duraplasty, but only as a last resort and in younger patients without comorbidity who can sustain a long rehabilitation.

Finally, there is a widely held dictum that cardiac surgery after a recent stroke may significantly exacerbate the neurologic deficit. The problem of management in this subset of patients has been addressed in only a few studies. One review found no deterioration in patients with remote or recent strokes (defined as 3 months before the day of open heart surgery).[61] Zisbrod and associates[97] operated on 15 patients with recent strokes (within 2 to 28 days), and again, none of the patients had worsening of the deficit after the procedure. In another study, new focal signs from ischemic stroke developed in only 1 of 41 patients with coronary artery bypass and previous stroke.[98] These results suggest that heparinization during bypass is not harmful in this subset of patients and that surgery should proceed in neurologically stable patients despite a recent stroke. However, uniform management guidelines are difficult to give in patients with a recent ischemic stroke, and most cardiovascular surgeons think it more prudent to defer cardiac surgery, if feasible, for 6 to 8 weeks.

NEUROPSYCHOLOGIC IMPAIRMENT

A heavier burden of cardiac surgery is cognitive decline, and neuropsychologic impairment may be found in 30% of patients.[99–102] Intellectual deterioration may vary from overt memory deficits to difficulties in attention

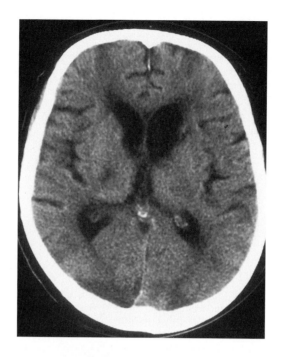

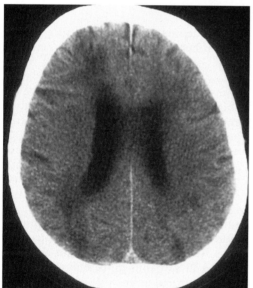
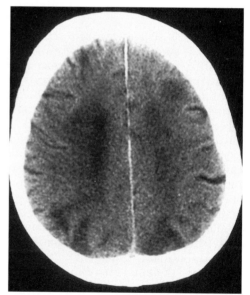

Figure 15–5. Multiple ischemic strokes, some of which are in watershed areas.

and concentration in more demanding tasks. Decreased attention span, decreased motor speed, and problems with immediate retrieval of memory develop. Savageau and associates[103,104] found no definite risk factors for neuropsychologic involvement, but patients older than 60 years with enlarged heart, long aortic cross-clamp time, or extensive postoperative blood loss appeared to be significantly more at risk.[102] A follow-up study 6 months later found that in more than 80% of the patients with abnormal performance, these abnormalities subsided.[102] Marked improvement is noted in the first year and gradual

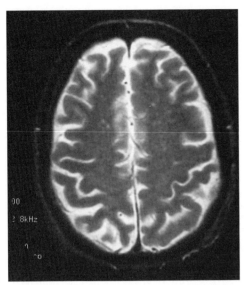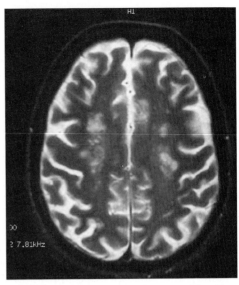

A   B

Figure 15–6. Magnetic resonance images before (A) and immediately after (B) coronary artery bypass grafting. Note emergence of white matter changes on postoperative image.

further improvement up to 5 years in all neuropsychologic dimensions. Other studies were less optimistic, and a 3-year follow-up assessment of 97 patients showed an overall incidence of any neurologic or cognitive dysfunction of 35%.[105]

The Johns Hopkins University study, under the direction of McKhann,[106] found evidence of further cognitive decline at 5 years, predominantly in the domain of visuoconstruction. Cognitive impairment remains uncertain in nature and may be confounded by fatigue and depression, which possibly influence test results. However, psychologic abnormalities were consistently absent in a control group of patients undergoing major vascular surgical procedures without the concomitant use of cardiopulmonary bypass. The selection of tests may be important, and comparisons between studies may be difficult.[107] Also, the older population may be at risk for development of Alzheimer's disease.

A recently completed longitudinal assessment of 261 patients at Duke University Medical Center found that a surprisingly high proportion of patients (53%) had abnormal scores on tests of neurocognitive function at dismissal but that the incidence declined to 24% at 6 months. At 5 years, however, 42% of these patients had scores below the baseline, indicating not only that the course is biphasic but also that cognitive decline immediately after CABG seems to predispose to later decline. Possible explanations are increased vulnerability of the brain after initial injury, effects of aging on the brain, cerebrovascular disease,[108] and genetic predisposition. A correlative study of outcome from Duke Medical Center found that patients with apolipoprotein E-epsilon 4 had a higher risk of cognitive dysfunction.[109] These results, with numbers almost too high to be accurate, need confirmation.

Whether warm blood cardioplegia increases the risk of neuropsychologic abnormalities is not known. A subgroup analysis of 150 patients in a study at Emory University found no differences between warm and cold blood cardioplegia.[39] Two recent randomized trials confirmed the absence of any significant increase in cognitive dysfunction with temperature modulation.[110,111]

RETINAL DAMAGE

The proportion of patients with neuro-ophthalmologic sequelae after cardiopulmonary bypass may be as high as 25%[112–117] (Table 15–5). In a prospective study in which

Table 15–5. Neuro-ophthalmologic Findings after Cardiopulmonary Bypass

Retinal cotton-wool spots
Ischemic optic neuropathy
Transient macular edema
Cortical blindness
Homonymous hemianopia
Altitudinal hemianopia
Isolated quadrantanopia

bedside neurologic assessment was done in patients who underwent CABG, areas of retinal infarction were most frequently found.[113] Cotton-wool spots, produced by occlusion of small vessels supplying the inner nerve layer of the retina, occurred in 54 of 312 patients (17%). Only half the patients, including those with multiple lesions, were aware of visual symptoms, most likely because of the spottiness of these tiny foci. Usually, retinal infarcts are manifested by blurred vision, haziness in the peripheral parts of the visual field, or difficulty reading. A lodged embolus may be seen by direct ophthalmoscopy. Both platelet-fibrin microaggregates and gaseous microbubbles could produce this retinal damage, but theoretically this phenomenon—so characteristic in patients undergoing cardiopulmonary bypass—may also be the result of a regional maldistribution of perfusion. An elegant study in patients undergoing elective CABG with use of bubble oxygenators found retinal abnormalities in all patients serially studied with retinal fluorescein angiography.[114] New cotton-wool spots, however, were noted in only 10% of the patients. The clinical significance is uncertain. In this study, most patients did not experience profound visual loss, and neuropsychologic and neurologic complications were similar in patients with more severe retinal artery occlusions. This condition is considered to be benign, with few, if any, persistent residual deficits. Return to normal vision takes at least a few weeks.

Unilateral altitudinal field defect (sharp border along the horizontal meridian) is an uncommon visual field deficit. In the Cleve-land Clinic experience,[116] 7 of 7685 patients were found to have bilateral involvement. In each patient, a swollen and pale optic nerve disc could be demonstrated. This ischemic optic neuropathy was caused by infarction in the laminar anterior portion of the optic nerve. Most of the patients had considerable blood loss from hemorrhage and shock.[117] Ischemic optic neuropathy may occur from decreased blood flow of the distal optic nerve due to decreased velocity and sludging associated with hypothermia.[118] Outcome is very guarded, and patients who become blind remain so permanently.

PERIPHERAL NERVE DAMAGE

Cardiovascular surgeons are primarily concerned with the potential deleterious effects on the central nervous system, but damage to peripheral nerves, particularly the brachial plexus, is equally important.[54,119–121]

The incidence of brachial plexus injury is less than 10% in major series (Table 15–6). Approximately half of patients with cardiac postsurgical plexopathy have disabling dysesthesias and pain or marked weakness at onset.[122] Usually, the lower trunk or medial cord fibers are involved. Burning pain and numbness can be specifically present in the C8 and T1 to T2 dermal segments, and many patients have profound weakness of the intrinsic hand muscles and long finger flexors. Reflexes are usually normal, but finger flexion and triceps reflex may be reduced. Horner's syndrome may accompany a lower trunk injury. Outcome is generally good, and the neurologic deficits resolve within 3 months; major improvement is already apparent within the first 6 weeks, in some patients even within a week. In those patients with persisting complaints, transaxillary resection of the first rib may result in resolution of the nerve injury, but this treatment is not common practice.

The mechanism of brachial plexus injury is thought to be related to the position of the sternal retractors and the extent to which the halves are opened. An autopsy study postulated that when the retractor is opened to its fullest extent (which may occur in patients with grafting of an internal mammary artery), the lower trunk of the bra-

Table 15–6. **Incidence of Unilateral Brachial Plexus Injury after Cardiac Surgery**

Series	No. of Patients	BRACHIAL PLEXUS INJURY	
		No.	%
Vander Salm et al., 1980[123]	188	35	19
Morin et al., 1982[121]	958	10	1
Hanson et al., 1983[124]	531	25	5
Shaw et al., 1985[3]	312	21	7
Tomlinson et al., 1987[125]	335	16	5
Vahl et al., 1991[122]	1000	27	3

chial plexus is pinched between the first rib and the clavicle[126] (Fig. 15–7). Vander Salm and associates[123] suggested that fractures of the first rib related to placement of the cephalad blade of the retractor at the level of the second intercostal space may contribute to nerve damage. Rib fractures may not be evident on conventional chest roentgenograms but may be visualized by bone scans.[127] Fractures were avoided after a more caudal placement of the retractor. Traction on the brachial plexus is preventable and may be related to the type of retractor. In a prospective study using Favaloro retractors for harvesting of the internal mammary artery as a graft for CABG, the incidence of brachial plexopathy increased to 10%.[122] With somatosensory evoked potential monitoring, it was found recently that the Delacroix-Chevalux retractor reduced damage to the plexus.[128] Less abnormality in somatosensory evoked potential amplitude than that with other retractors was attributed to the unique asymmetrical opening mechanism that reduced lateral force to the plexus. Other possible preventive measures,

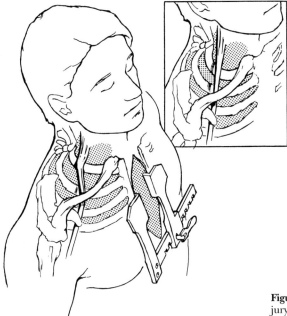

Figure 15–7. Possible mechanism of brachial plexus injury after use of retractors during cardiac surgery (*inset* shows normal anatomy).

such as hands-up positioning, did not reduce plexus injury.[129] Somatosensory evoked potentials could possibly predict intraoperative injury to the brachial plexus.[130] The validity of somatosensory evoked potential monitoring during surgery has not been established, and in later studies, changes in somatosensory evoked potential were not correlated with postoperative injury.[131]

Mononeuropathy may be more frequent than previously appreciated. In a prospective study, mononeuropathies were found in 17 of 312 patients (5%) who underwent elective coronary artery bypass.[132] Ulnar and lateral femoral cutaneous nerves were most frequently affected, and all instances might have been preventable. Ulnar nerve palsy is common after cardiac surgery. However, compression at the cubital tunnel during surgery can be remarkably diminished, as shown in nerve conduction studies, by placing the patient's arms above the head with the elbows flexed, but, as mentioned, this does not prevent plexus injury.[110] One report suggested that meralgia paresthetica associated with lateral femoral cutaneous nerve involvement was caused by placing the thighs in the frog-leg position during this procedure.[133] A preventable wrist-drop from radial nerve damage was reported in two obese patients.[134,135] The supporting post of the retractor presumably compressed the upper arm in both patients. Full recovery was noted.

A report from the Mayo Clinic found that 6 of more than 23,000 patients who underwent cardiac surgery had sciatic neuropathy.[136] Because four of the six patients required intra-aortic balloon pump insertion, blood flow to the nerves may have been compromised. The patients had pain and sensory loss below the knee and posterior thigh, with involvement of temperature sense more than touch or pain in most of the foot, weakness of the toes, and reduced dorsiflexion, extension, and supination of the foot. A watershed arterial zone exists in the midthigh, and the absence of hamstring muscle involvement in these patients supports this explanation.[136]

Another important hazard of hypothermia during open heart surgery is bilateral diaphragmatic paralysis. In a prospective study that used phrenic nerve conduction, ultrasonography of the diaphragm, and chest radiographs, 24 of 92 patients (26%) had phrenic neuropathy, but none required prolonged mechanical ventilation and most had resolution within 1 year.[137] In other studies, the incidence of this complication was only 2%.[137-140] Electrophysiologic evaluation of the function of the phrenic nerve and diaphragm showed that no marked changes in nerve conduction occurred during surgery. The lowest myocardial temperature recorded in patients with phrenic nerve palsy was similar to that in the other patients, but the duration of cardiopulmonary bypass was significantly longer. These findings suggested that prolonged pericardial stretch of the phrenic nerve during the operation may be the main cause.

Local hypothermia may also be a contributing factor, because filling of the pericardial sac with ice and saline to protect the myocardium during periods of ischemic arrest was strongly linked to bilateral diaphragmatic paralysis and compromised recovery in many patients. Ice slush used for topical cooling of the myocardium is a major risk factor, increasing the risk of phrenic nerve damage eightfold.[141] Warm blood cardioplegia has eliminated phrenic nerve injury.[142,143]

CONCLUSIONS

Initially it appears that for most patients, CABG is a surgical procedure without neurologic complications. However, for many (estimated in prospective series to be up to 50%), cognitive function is worse after the operation than before. Rather than substantial intellectual loss, problems with executive functions, such as decision making, are common and may pass unnoticed in the postoperative days. Fortunately, despite contradictory reports, these abnormalities subside in 6 months in most patients. The origin is still uncertain but has been linked to microemboli during cardiopulmonary bypass.

On average severe coexisting carotid disease is present in 10% of patients scheduled for CABG surgery. The lack of a prospective, randomized study of prophylactic carotid endarterectomy hampers our ability to give sound scientific advice. The incidence of stroke after CABG surgery is very low (probably <2%), and when it occurs, it does so days after surgery—timing that questions the role of carotid artery disease in postoperative stroke. Thrombi from damage to an atherosclerotic aorta associated with clamping or postoperative atrial fibrillation are the main causes in delayed-onset stroke.

In patients with proven symptomatic carotid disease and the need for repair of both carotid and coronary arteries, it seems reasonable to proceed with carotid endarterectomy or stenting in one surgical session or after coronary reconstruction.

Brachial plexopathy from use of sternal retractors is occasionally observed in the ICU. Recovery to full function can be expected after conservative management.

REFERENCES

1. Furlan AJ, Breuer AC. Central nervous system complications of open heart surgery. Stroke 15: 912–915, 1984.
2. Gilman S. Cerebral disorders after open-heart operations. N Engl J Med 272:489–498, 1965.
3. Shaw PJ, Bates D, Cartlidge NE, Heaviside D, Julian DG, Shaw DA. Early neurological complications of coronary artery bypass surgery. Br Med J 291:1384–1387, 1985.
4. Shaw PJ, Bates D, Cartlidge NE, et al. Neurologic and neuropsychological morbidity following major surgery: comparison of coronary artery bypass and peripheral vascular surgery. Stroke 18:700–707, 1987.
5. Abramov D, Tamariz MG, Fremes SE, et al. Trends in coronary artery bypass surgery results: a recent, 9-year study. Ann Thorac Surg 70:84–90, 2000.
6. Jones EL, Weintraub WS, Craver JM, Guyton RA, Cohen CL. Coronary bypass surgery: is the operation different today? J Thorac Cardiovasc Surg 101:108–115, 1991.
7. Ehrlich MP, McCullough J, Wolfe D, et al. Cerebral effects of cold reperfusion after hypothermic circulatory arrest. J Thorac Cardiovasc Surg 121: 923–931, 2001.
8. Li PA, Shuaib A, Miyashita H, He QP, Siesjo BK, Warner DS. Hyperglycemia enhances extracellular glutamate accumulation in rats subjected to forebrain ischemia. Stroke 31:183–192, 2000.
9. Christakis GT, Koch JP, Deemar KA, et al. A randomized study of the systemic effects of warm heart surgery. Ann Thorac Surg 54:449–457, 1992.
10. Jacquet LM, Noirhomme PH, Van Dyck MJ, et al. Randomized trial of intermittent antegrade warm blood versus cold crystalloid cardioplegia. Ann Thorac Surg 67:471–477, 1999.
11. Kaukoranta P, Lepojarvi M, Nissinen J, Raatikainen P, Peuhkurinen KJ. Normothermic versus mild hypothermic retrograde blood cardioplegia: a prospective, randomized study. Ann Thorac Surg 60:1087–1093, 1995.
12. Padayachee TS, Parsons S, Theobold R, Linley J, Gosling RG, Deverall PB. The detection of microemboli in the middle cerebral artery during cardiopulmonary bypass: a transcranial Doppler ultrasound investigation using membrane and bubble oxygenators. Ann Thorac Surg 44:298–302, 1987.
13. Padayachee TS, Parsons S, Theobold R, Gosling RG, Deverall PB. The effect of arterial filtration on reduction of gaseous microemboli in the middle cerebral artery during cardiopulmonary bypass. Ann Thorac Surg 45:647–649, 1988.
14. Lundar T, Froysaker T, Lindegaard KF, et al. Some observations on cerebral perfusion during cardiopulmonary bypass. Ann Thorac Surg 39:318–323, 1985.
15. Lundar T, Lindegaard KF, Froysaker T, Aaslid R, Wiberg J, Nornes H. Cerebral perfusion during nonpulsatile cardiopulmonary bypass. Ann Thorac Surg 40:144–150, 1985.
16. Lundar T, Lindegaard KF, Froysaker T, et al. Cerebral carbon dioxide reactivity during nonpulsatile cardiopulmonary bypass. Ann Thorac Surg 41: 525–530, 1986.
17. Prough DS, Rogers AT, Stump DA, Mills SA, Gravlee GP, Taylor C. Hypercarbia depresses cerebral oxygen consumption during cardiopulmonary bypass. Stroke 21:1162–1166, 1990.
18. Schell RM, Kern FH, Greeley WJ, et al. Cerebral blood flow and metabolism during cardiopulmonary bypass. Anesth Analg 76:849–865, 1993.
19. von Reutern GM, Hetzel A, Birnbaum D, Schlosser V. Transcranial Doppler ultrasonography during cardiopulmonary bypass in patients with severe carotid stenosis or occlusion. Stroke 19:674–680, 1988.
20. Henriksen L, Hjelms E. Cerebral blood flow during cardiopulmonary bypass in man: effect of arterial filtration. Thorax 41:386–395, 1986.
21. Pugsley W, Kliner L, Paschalis C, et al. Microemboli and cerebral impairment during cardiac surgery. Vasc Surg 24:34–43, 1990.
22. Aris A, Solanes H, Camara ML, Junque C, Escartin A, Caralps JM. Arterial line filtration during cardiopulmonary bypass. Neurologic, neuropsychologic, and hematologic studies. J Thorac Cardiovasc Surg 91:526–533, 1986.
23. Mills NL, Ochsner JL. Massive air embolism during cardiopulmonary bypass. Causes, prevention, and management. J Thorac Cardiovasc Surg 80: 708–717, 1980.
24. Parker FB Jr, Marvasti MA, Bove EL. Neurologic complication following coronary artery bypass. The role of atherosclerotic emboli. Thorac Cardiovasc Surg 33:207–209, 1985.
25. van der Linden J, Casimir-Ahn H. When do cerebral emboli appear during open heart operations? A transcranial Doppler study. Ann Thorac Surg 51:237–241, 1991.
26. Moody DM, Bell MA, Challa VR, Johnston WE, Prough DS. Brain microemboli during cardiac surgery or aortography. Ann Neurol 28:477–486, 1990.
27. Schmidt R, Fazekas F, Offenbacher H, et al. Brain magnetic resonance imaging in coronary artery bypass grafts: a pre- and postoperative assessment. Neurology 43:775–778, 1993.

28. Arom KV, Cohen DE, Strobl FT. Effect of intraoperative intervention on neurological outcome based on electroencephalographic monitoring during cardiopulmonary bypass. Ann Thorac Surg 48:476–483, 1989.

29. Aren C, Badr G, Feddersen K, Radegran K. Somatosensory evoked potentials and cerebral metabolism during cardiopulmonary bypass with special reference to hypotension induced by prostacyclin infusion. J Thorac Cardiovasc Surg 90:73–79, 1985.

30. Coles JG, Taylor MJ, Pearce JM, et al. Cerebral monitoring of somatosensory evoked potentials during profoundly hypothermic circulatory arrest. Circulation 70:I-96–I-102, 1984.

31. Nussmeier NA, Arlund C, Slogoff S. Neuropsychiatric complications after cardiopulmonary bypass: cerebral protection by a barbiturate. Anesthesiology 64:165–170, 1986.

32. Zaidan JR, Klochany A, Martin WM, Ziegler JS, Harless DM, Andrews RB. Effect of thiopental on neurologic outcome following coronary artery bypass grafting. Anesthesiology 74:406–411, 1991.

33. Roach GW, Newman MF, Murkin JM, et al. Ineffectiveness of burst suppression therapy in mitigating perioperative cerebrovascular dysfunction. Multicenter Study of Perioperative Ischemia (McSPI) Research Group. Anesthesiology 90:1255–1264, 1999.

34. Astrup J, Symon L, Branston NM, Lassen NA. Cortical evoked potential and extracellular K^+ and H^+ at critical levels of brain ischemia. Stroke 8:51–57, 1977.

35. Murkin JM, Martzke JS, Buchan AM, Bentley C, Wong CJ. A randomized study of the influence of perfusion technique and pH management strategy in 316 patients undergoing coronary artery bypass surgery. II. Neurologic and cognitive outcomes. J Thorac Cardiovasc Surg 110:349–362, 1995.

36. Breuer AC, Furlan AJ, Hanson MR, et al. Central nervous system complications of coronary artery bypass graft surgery: prospective analysis of 421 patients. Stroke 14:682–687, 1983.

37. Borger MA, Ivanov J, Weisel RD, Rao V, Peniston CM. Stroke during coronary bypass surgery: principal role of cerebral macroemboli. Eur J Cardiothorac Surg 19:627–632, 2001.

38. Gonzalez-Scarano F, Hurtig HI. Neurologic complications of coronary artery bypass grafting: case–control study. Neurology 31:1032–1035, 1981.

39. Martin TD, Craver JM, Gott JP, et al. Prospective, randomized trial of retrograde warm blood cardioplegia: myocardial benefit and neurologic threat. Ann Thorac Surg 57:298–302, 1994.

40. Gardner TJ, Horneffer PJ, Manolio TA, et al. Stroke following coronary artery bypass grafting: a ten-year study. Ann Thorac Surg 40:574–581, 1985.

41. Reed GL III, Singer DE, Picard EH, DeSanctis RW. Stroke following coronary-artery bypass surgery. A case–control estimate of the risk from carotid bruits. N Engl J Med 319:1246–1250, 1988.

42. D'Agostino RS, Svensson LG, Newmann DJ, Balkhy HH, Williamson WA, Shahian DM. Screening carotid ultrasonography and risk factors for stroke in coronary artery surgery patients. Ann Thorac Surg 62:1714–1723, 1996.

43. Stamou SC, Hill PC, Dangas G, et al. Stroke after coronary artery bypass: incidence, predictors, and clinical outcome. Stroke 32:1508–1513, 2001.

44. Taylor GJ, Malik SA, Colliver JA, et al. Usefulness of atrial fibrillation as a predictor of stroke after isolated coronary artery bypass grafting. Am J Cardiol 60:905–907, 1987.

45. Hartman GS, Yao FS, Bruefach M III, et al. Severity of aortic atheromatous disease diagnosed by transesophageal echocardiography predicts stroke and other outcomes associated with coronary artery surgery: a prospective study. Anesth Analg 83:701–708, 1996.

46. Trehan N, Mishra M, Kasliwal RR, Mishra A. Surgical strategies in patients at high risk for stroke undergoing coronary artery bypass grafting. Ann Thorac Surg 70:1037–1045, 2000.

47. Barnes RW, Liebman PR, Marszalek PB, Kirk CL, Goldman MH. The natural history of asymptomatic carotid disease in patients undergoing cardiovascular surgery. Surgery 90:1075–1083, 1981.

48. Breslau PJ, Fell G, Ivey TD, Bailey WW, Miller DW, Strandness DE Jr. Carotid arterial disease in patients undergoing coronary artery bypass operations. J Thorac Cardiovasc Surg 82:765–767, 1981.

49. Balderman SC, Gutierrez IZ, Makula P, Bhayana JN, Gage AA. Noninvasive screening for asymptomatic carotid artery disease prior to cardiac operation. Experience with 500 patients. J Thorac Cardiovasc Surg 85:427–433, 1983.

50. Brener BJ, Brief DK, Alpert J, Goldenkranz RJ, Parsonnet V. The risk of stroke in patients with asymptomatic carotid stenosis undergoing cardiac surgery: a follow-up study. J Vasc Surg 5:269–279, 1987.

51. Faggioli GL, Curl GR, Ricotta JJ. The role of carotid screening before coronary artery bypass. J Vasc Surg 12:724–729, 1990.

52. Hill AB, Obrand D, Steinmetz OK. The utility of selective screening for carotid stenosis in cardiac surgery patients. J Cardiovasc Surg (Torino) 40:829–836, 1999.

53. Ivey TD, Strandness E, Williams DB, Langlois Y, Misbach GA, Kruse AP. Management of patients with carotid bruit undergoing cardiopulmonary bypass. J Thorac Cardiovasc Surg 87:183–189, 1984.

54. Keates JR, Innocenti DM, Ross DN. Mononeuritis multiplex: a complication of open-heart surgery. J Thorac Cardiovasc Surg 69:816–819, 1975.

55. Chambers BR, Norris JW. Outcome in patients with asymptomatic neck bruits. N Engl J Med 315:860–865, 1986.

56. Hennerici M, Hulsbomer HB, Hefter H, Lammerts D, Rautenberg W. Natural history of asymptomatic extracranial arterial disease. Results of a long-term prospective study. Brain 110:777–791, 1987.

57. Sauve JS, Thorpe KE, Sackett DL, et al. Can bruits distinguish high-grade from moderate symptomatic carotid stenosis? The North American Symptomatic Carotid Endarterectomy Trial. Ann Intern Med 120:633–637, 1994.

58. Barnes RW, Marszalek PB. Asymptomatic carotid disease in the cardiovascular surgical patient: is prophylactic endarterectomy necessary? Stroke 12:497–500, 1981.

59. Furlan AJ, Craciun AR. Risk of stroke during coronary artery bypass graft surgery in patients with internal carotid artery disease documented by angiography. Stroke 16:797–799, 1985.

60. Waigand J, Gross CM, Uhlich F, et al. Elective stenting of carotid artery stenosis in patients with severe coronary artery disease. Eur Heart J 19:1365–1370, 1998.

61. Rorick MB, Furlan AJ. Risk of cardiac surgery in patients with prior stroke. Neurology 40:835–837, 1990.

62. European Carotid Surgery Trialists' Collaborative Group. MRC European Carotid Surgery Trial: interim results for symptomatic patients with severe (70–99%) or with mild (0–29%) carotid stenosis. Lancet 337:1235–1243, 1991.

63. North American Symptomatic Carotid Endarterectomy Trial Collaborators. Beneficial effect of carotid endarterectomy in symptomatic patients with high-grade carotid stenosis. N Engl J Med 325:445–453, 1991.

64. Lazar HL, Menzoian JO. Coronary artery bypass grafting in patients with cerebrovascular disease. Ann Thorac Surg 66:968–974, 1998.

65. Hobson RW II, Weiss DG, Fields WS, et al. Efficacy of carotid endarterectomy for asymptomatic carotid stenosis. The Veterans Affairs Cooperative Study Group. N Engl J Med 328:221–227, 1993.

66. Cambria RP, Ivarsson BL, Akins CW, Moncure AC, Brewster DC, Abbott WM. Simultaneous carotid and coronary disease: safety of the combined approach. J Vasc Surg 9:56–64, 1989.

67. Cosgrove DM, Hertzer NR, Loop FD. Surgical management of synchronous carotid and coronary artery disease. J Vasc Surg 3:690–692, 1986.

68. Crawford ES, Palamara AE, Kasparian AS. Carotid and noncoronary operations: simultaneous, staged, and delayed. Surgery 87:1–8, 1980.

69. Hertzer NR, Loop FD, Taylor PC, Beven EG. Combined myocardial revascularization and carotid endarterectomy. Operative and late results in 331 patients. J Thorac Cardiovasc Surg 85:577–589, 1983.

70. Wijdicks EFM, Jack CR. Coronary artery bypass grafting-associated ischemic stroke: a clinical and neuroradiological study. J Neuroimaging 6:20–22, 1996.

71. Libman RB, Wirkowski E, Neystat M, Barr W, Gelb S, Graver M. Stroke associated with cardiac surgery. Determinants, timing, and stroke subtypes. Arch Neurol 54:83–87, 1997.

72. Hogue CW Jr, Murphy SF, Schechtman KB, Dávila-Román VG. Risk factors for early or delayed stroke after cardiac surgery. Circulation 100:642–647, 1999.

73. Crosby LH, Pifalo WB, Woll KR, Burkholder JA. Risk factors for atrial fibrillation after coronary artery bypass grafting. Am J Cardiol 66:1520–1522, 1990.

74. Breuer AC, Franco I, Marzewski D, Soto-Velasco J. Left ventricular thrombi seen by ventriculography are a significant risk factor for stroke in open-heart surgery [abstract]. Ann Neurol 10:103–104, 1981.

75. Maslow A, Lowenstein E, Steriti J, Leckie R, Cohn W, Haering M. Left ventricular thrombi: intraoperative detection by transesophageal echocardiography and recognition of a source of post CABG embolic stroke: a case series. Anesthesiology 89:1257–1262, 1998.

76. Wareing TH, Davila-Roman VG, Daily BB, et al. Strategy for the reduction of stroke incidence in cardiac surgical patients. Ann Thorac Surg 55:1400–1407, 1993.

77. Stern A, Tunick PA, Culliford AT, et al. Protruding aortic arch atheromas: risk of stroke during heart surgery with and without aortic arch endarterectomy. Am Heart J 138:746–752, 1999.

78. Cerebral Embolism Study Group. Cardioembolic stroke, early anticoagulation, and brain hemorrhage. Arch Intern Med 147:636–640, 1987.

79. Cerebral Embolism Task Force. Cardiogenic brain embolism. Arch Neurol 43:71–84, 1986.

80. Cerebral Embolism Task Force. Cardiogenic brain embolism. The second report of the Cerebral Embolism Task Force. Arch Neurol 46:727–743, 1989.

81. Kittner SJ, Sharkness CM, Price TR, et al. Infarcts with a cardiac source of embolism in the NINCDS Stroke Data Bank: historical features. Neurology 40:281–284, 1990.

82. Taugher PJ. Visual loss after cardiopulmonary bypass. Am J Ophthalmol 81:280–288, 1976.

83. Aldrich MS, Alessi AG, Beck RW, Gilman S. Cortical blindness: etiology, diagnosis, and prognosis. Ann Neurol 21:149–158, 1987.

84. Pessin MS, Lathi ES, Cohen MB, Kwan ES, Hedges TR III, Caplan LR. Clinical features and mechanism of occipital infarction. Ann Neurol 21:290–299, 1987.

85. Hise JH, Nipper ML, Schnitker JC. Stroke associated with coronary artery bypass surgery. AJNR Am J Neuroradiol 12:811–814, 1991.

86. Ringelstein EB, Koschorke S, Holling A, Thron A, Lambertz H, Minale C. Computed tomographic patterns of proven embolic brain infarctions. Ann Neurol 26:759–765, 1989.

87. Cassie AB, Riddell AG, Yates PO. Hazard of antifoam emboli from a bubble oxygenator. Thorax 15:22–29, 1960.

88. Amarenco P, Roullet E, Goujon C, Cheron F, Hauw JJ, Bousser MG. Infarction in the anterior rostral cerebellum (the territory of the lateral branch of the superior cerebellar artery). Neurology 41:253–258, 1991.

89. Barbut D, Grassineau D, Lis E, Heier L, Hartman GS, Isom OW. Posterior distribution of infarcts in strokes related to cardiac operations. Ann Thorac Surg 65:1656–1659, 1998.

90. Torvik A, Skullerud K. Watershed infarcts in the brain caused by microemboli. Clin Neuropathol 1:99–105, 1982.

91. Sellman M, Hindmarsh T, Ivert T, Semb BK. Magnetic resonance imaging of the brain before and after open heart operations. Ann Thorac Surg 53:807–812, 1992.

92. Simonson TM, Yuh WT, Hindman BJ, Embrey RP, Holloran JI, Behrendt DM. Contrast MR of the

brain after high-perfusion cardiopulmonary bypass. AJNR Am J Neuroradiol 15:3–7, 1994.

93. Vik A, Brubakk AO, Rinck PA, Sande E, Levang OW, Sellevold O. MRI: a method to detect minor brain damage following coronary bypass surgery? Neuroradiology 33:396–398, 1991.

94. Wityk RJ, Goldsborough MA, Hillis A, et al. Diffusion- and perfusion-weighted brain magnetic resonance imaging in patients with neurologic complications after cardiac surgery. Arch Neurol 58:571–576, 2001.

95. Harris DN, Oatridge A, Dob D, Smith PL, Taylor KM, Bydder GM. Cerebral swelling after normothermic cardiopulmonary bypass. Anesthesiology 88:340–345, 1998.

96. Almassi GH, Sommers T, Moritz TE, et al. Stroke in cardiac surgical patients: determinants and outcome. Ann Thorac Surg 68:391–397, 1999.

97. Zisbrod Z, Rose DM, Jacobowitz IJ, Kramer M, Acinapura AJ, Cunningham JN Jr. Results of open heart surgery in patients with recent cardiogenic embolic stroke and central nervous system dysfunction. Circulation 76:V109–V112, 1987.

98. Beall AC Jr, Jones JW, Guinn GA, Svensson LG, Nahas C. Cardiopulmonary bypass in patients with previously completed stroke. Ann Thorac Surg 55:1383–1384, 1993.

99. Aberg T, Ronquist G, Tyden H, et al. Adverse effects on the brain in cardiac operations as assessed by biochemical, psychometric, and radiologic methods. J Thorac Cardiovasc Surg 87:99–105, 1984.

100. Smith PL, Treasure T, Newman SP, et al. Cerebral consequences of cardiopulmonary bypass. Lancet 1:823–825, 1986.

101. Sotaniemi KA. Brain damage and neurological outcome after open-heart surgery. J Neurol Neurosurg Psychiatry 43:127–135, 1980.

102. Sotaniemi KA, Mononen H, Hokkanen TE. Long-term cerebral outcome after open-heart surgery. A five-year neuropsychological follow-up study. Stroke 17:410–416, 1986.

103. Savageau JA, Stanton BA, Jenkins CD, Frater RW. Neuropsychological dysfunction following elective cardiac operation. Part II. A six-month reassessment. J Thorac Cardiovasc Surg 84:595–600, 1982.

104. Savageau JA, Stanton BA, Jenkins CD, Klein MD. Neuropsychological dysfunction following elective cardiac operation. Part I. Early assessment. J Thorac Cardiovasc Surg 84:585–594, 1982.

105. Murkin JM, Baird DL, Martzke JS, Adams SJ, Lok P. Long-term neurological and neuropsychological outcome 3 years after coronary artery bypass surgery [abstract]. Anesth Analg 82:S328, 1996.

106. Selnes OA, Royall RM, Grega MA, Borowicz LM Jr, Quaskey S, McKhann GM. Cognitive changes 5 years after coronary artery bypass grafting: is there evidence of late decline? Arch Neurol 58:598–604, 2001.

107. Selnes OA, Goldsborough MA, Borowicz LM, McKhann GM. Neurobehavioural sequelae of cardiopulmonary bypass. Lancet 353:1601–1606, 1999.

108. Newman MF, Kirchner JL, Phillips-Bute B, et al. Longitudinal assessment of neurocognitive function after coronary-artery bypass surgery. N Engl J Med 344:395–402, 2001.

109. Tardiff BE, Newman MF, Saunders AM, et al. Preliminary report of a genetic basis for cognitive decline after cardiac operations. The Neurologic Outcome Research Group of the Duke Heart Center. Ann Thorac Surg 64:715–720, 1997.

110. Plourde G, Leduc AS, Morin JE, et al. Temperature during cardiopulmonary bypass for coronary artery operations does not influence postoperative cognitive function: a prospective, randomized trial. J Thorac Cardiovasc Surg 114:123–128, 1997.

111. Regragui I, Birdi I, Izzat MB, et al. The effects of cardiopulmonary bypass temperature on neuropsychologic outcome after coronary artery operations: a prospective randomized trial. J Thorac Cardiovasc Surg 112:1036–1045, 1996.

112. Shahian DM, Speert PK. Symptomatic visual deficits after open heart operations. Ann Thorac Surg 48:275–279, 1989.

113. Shaw PJ, Bates D, Cartlidge NE, et al. Neuro-ophthalmological complications of coronary artery bypass graft surgery. Acta Neurol Scand 76:1–7, 1987.

114. Blauth CI, Arnold JV, Schulenberg WE, McCartney AC, Taylor KM. Cerebral microembolism during cardiopulmonary bypass. Retinal microvascular studies in vivo with fluorescein angiography. J Thorac Cardiovasc Surg 95:668–676, 1988.

115. Moster ML. Visual loss after coronary artery bypass surgery. Surv Ophthalmol 42:453–457, 1998.

116. Sweeney PJ, Breuer AC, Selhorst JB, et al. Ischemic optic neuropathy: a complication of cardiopulmonary bypass surgery. Neurology 32:560–562, 1982.

117. Tice DA. Ischemic optic neuropathy and cardiac surgery [letter]. Ann Thorac Surg 44:677, 1987.

118. Lund PE, Madsen K. Bilateral blindness after cardiopulmonary bypass. J Cardiothorac Vasc Anesth 8:448–450, 1994.

119. Honet JC, Raikes JA, Kantrowitz A, Pursel SE, Rubenfire M. Neuropathy in the upper extremity after open-heart surgery. Arch Phys Med Rehabil 57:264–267, 1976.

120. Lederman RJ, Breuer AC, Hanson MR, et al. Peripheral nervous system complications of coronary artery bypass graft surgery. Ann Neurol 12:297–301, 1982.

121. Morin JE, Long R, Elleker MG, Eisen AA, Wynands E, Ralphs-Thibodeau S. Upper extremity neuropathies following median sternotomy. Ann Thorac Surg 34:181–185, 1982.

122. Vahl CF, Carl I, Muller-Vahl H, Struck E. Brachial plexus injury after cardiac surgery. The role of internal mammary artery preparation: a prospective study on 1000 consecutive patients. J Thorac Cardiovasc Surg 102:724–729, 1991.

123. Vander Salm TJ, Cereda JM, Cutler BS. Brachial plexus injury following median sternotomy. J Thorac Cardiovasc Surg 80:447–452, 1980.

124. Hanson MR, Breuer AC, Furlan AJ, et al. Mechanism and frequency of brachial plexus injury in open-heart surgery: a prospective analysis. Ann Thorac Surg 36:675–679, 1983.

125. Tomlinson DL, Hirsch IA, Kodali SV, Slogoff S. Protecting the brachial plexus during median sternotomy. J Thorac Cardiovasc Surg 94:297–301, 1987.

126. Kirsh MM, Magee KR, Gago O, Kahn DR, Sloan H. Brachial plexus injury following median ster-

notomy incision. Ann Thorac Surg 11:315–319, 1971.

127. Baisden CE, Greenwald LV, Symbas PN. Occult rib fractures and brachial plexus injury following median sternotomy for open-heart operations. Ann Thorac Surg 38:192–194, 1984.

128. Jellish WS, Blakeman B, Warf P, Slogoff S. Somatosensory evoked potential monitoring used to compare the effect of three asymmetric sternal retractors on brachial plexus function. Anesth Analg 88:292–297, 1999.

129. Jellish WS, Blakeman B, Warf P, Slogoff S. Hands-up positioning during asymmetric sternal retraction for internal mammary artery harvest: a possible method to reduce brachial plexus injury. Anesth Analg 84:260–265, 1997.

130. Hickey C, Gugino LD, Aglio LS, Mark JB, Son SL, Maddi R. Intraoperative somatosensory evoked potential monitoring predicts peripheral nerve injury during cardiac surgery. Anesthesiology 78: 29–35, 1993.

131. Seal D, Balaton J, Coupland SG, et al. Somatosensory evoked potential monitoring during cardiac surgery: an examination of brachial plexus dysfunction. J Cardiothorac Vasc Anesth 11:187–191, 1997.

132. Wey JM, Guinn GA. Ulnar nerve injury with open-heart surgery. Ann Thorac Surg 39:358–360, 1985.

133. Parsonnet V, Karasakalides A, Gielchinsky I, Hochberg M, Hussain SM. Meralgia paresthetica after coronary bypass surgery. J Thorac Cardiovasc Surg 101:219–221, 1991.

134. Guzman F, Naik S, Weldon OG, Hilton CJ. Transient radial nerve injury related to the use of a self retaining retractor for internal mammary artery dissection. J Cardiovasc Surg (Torino) 30:1015–1016, 1989.

135. Rao S, Chu B, Shevde K. Isolated peripheral radial nerve injury with the use of the Favaloro retractor. J Cardiothorac Anesth 1:325–327, 1987.

136. McManis PG. Sciatic nerve lesions during cardiac surgery. Neurology 44:684–687, 1994.

137. DeVita MA, Robinson LR, Rehder J, Hattler B, Cohen C. Incidence and natural history of phrenic neuropathy occurring during open heart surgery. Chest 103:850–856, 1993.

138. Chandler KW, Rozas CJ, Kory RC, Goldman AL. Bilateral diaphragmatic paralysis complicating local cardiac hypothermia during open heart surgery. Am J Med 77:243–249, 1984.

139. Markand ON, Moorthy SS, Mahomed Y, King RD, Brown JW. Postoperative phrenic nerve palsy in patients with open-heart surgery. Ann Thorac Surg 39:68–73, 1985.

140. Mickell JJ, Oh KS, Siewers RD, Galvis AG, Fricker FJ, Mathews RA. Clinical implications of postoperative unilateral phrenic nerve paralysis. J Thorac Cardiovasc Surg 76:297–304, 1978.

141. Dimopoulou I, Daganou M, Dafni U, et al. Phrenic nerve dysfunction after cardiac operations: electrophysiologic evaluation of risk factors. Chest 113:8–14, 1998.

142. Tolis GA, Astras G, Sfyras N, Georgiou G. Experience with warm blood cardioplegia in 480 patients. Cardiovasc Surg 3:175–180, 1995.

143. Maccherini M, Davoli G, Sani G, et al. Warm heart surgery eliminates diaphragmatic paralysis. J Card Surg 10:257–261, 1995.

Chapter 16

NEUROLOGIC COMPLICATIONS OF ACUTE ENVIRONMENTAL INJURIES

The forces of nature or hostile outdoor enrivonments may create treacherous conditions. Any of these geographical hazards may seriously endanger lives. Environmental injuries may occur in several persons at the same time, and reconstruction of the event may be difficult because of panic-stricken bystanders. Such an event often triggers a disaster plan. Other situations are more foreseeable, subtle, and closer to home. In children and young adults, accidental in-

juries are one of the leading causes of death and disability. These injuries have a propensity for pulmonary, cardiovascular, and renal involvement. Morbidity is commonly determined by an additional insult to the brain or spinal cord. However, certain types of environmental injuries can produce specific neurologic manifestations. An exhaustive overview of environmental injury to the nervous system has been offered in several well-respected texts.[1,2] This chapter presents an overview of the most common neurologic presentations in environmental injuries severe enough to have resulted in intensive care admission. Our understanding of management strategies has not developed for some of the injuries.

THERMAL BURNS

The medical complexity of patients with major burns and the need for multidisciplinary care fit well into the definition of critical illness.[3] Patients with extensive burns should be managed in specialized burn centers, but major referral centers are occasionally challenged with the intensive care management of thermal or electrical burns. One may expect neurologic complications of major thermal burns in a number of patients, but their recognition may be overshadowed by metabolic derangements and developing infections. Neurologic complications are frequently appreciated only after the patient's critical condition has abated.

Morbidity and mortality in patients with major burns depend on the extent of third-

or second-degree burn surface and possibly are increased in women aged 30 to 59 years.[4] The extent of the burn can be assessed by the so-called rule of nine in adults. It may exaggerate the size of the burn, and less clinical experience with estimating the size of burns may reduce the reliability of this rating system.[5] Nonetheless, when the extent of injury determined by this simple guide approximates 50% of the total skin surface area, significant sequelae in survivors or early mortality can be expected (Fig. 16–1).

In patients with third-degree burns over a large surface area, a hypermetabolic response exists that may triple energy needs. This hypermetabolic phase is characterized by fever, massive weight loss, and protein catabolism similar to sepsis syndrome (see Chapter 6). Nutrition, therefore, should meet the demands and include adequate vitamin supplements.

Perhaps one of the most important pathophysiologic changes in patients with major burns is the alteration of pharmacokinetics.[6,7] Predisposing factors are protein loss from the burn wound, hepatic failure from hypovolemic shock, sepsis, toxic inhalation, and renal failure from myoglobinuria.

Martyn[8] pioneered the pharmacokinetic studies in burn patients at a Shriners hospital. Important drug-binding proteins such as albumin may be reduced to 50% of baseline, although another, equally important, drug-binding protein, α_1-globulin, may decrease considerably in the first weeks after burn injury. An acute decrease in the protein-binding capacity of drugs results in an increase in free drug concentration. As referred to in Chapter 2, in patients with signs of toxic drug levels, one should measure free drug concentrations rather than the more commonly measured total drug concentration, which includes the bound fraction. An overview of drugs that may interfere with neurologic assessment in the intensive care unit (ICU) in patients with hypoalbuminemia is shown in Table 16–1. It is apparent that many antiepileptic drugs may easily increase to toxic levels, but the serum levels of opioids remain the same or even decrease. That a significant percentage of patients with major burns may have epilepsy is of particular concern, because concentrations of bound

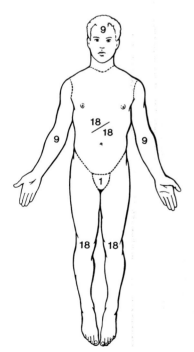

Data Obtained from Specialized Burn Facilities for Mean Survival Rate (%) Comparing Age and Burn Size

Burn size (%)	Age (yr)				
	5-34	35-49	50-59	60-74	>75
0-10	>95	>95	>95	95	90
10-20	>95	>90	>85	80	50
20-30	95	90	75	50	25
30-40	90	80	60	30	<10
40-50	80	60	40	10	<5
50-60	60	45	30	<10	<5
60-70	40	20	15	<5	0
70-80	25	10	5	0	0
80-90	10	<10	<5	0	0
90-100	<5	<5	0	0	0

Figure 16–1. Extent of second- or third-degree burns assessed by the rule of nine and correlation with survival rate. The drawing shows the rule of nine and distribution over the body surface. The table can be used to assess survival rate when the percentage of burned skin surface has been calculated.

Table 16–1. **Change in Serum Drug Concentrations after Burns**

Drug	Expected Change
Diazepam	Increase
Chlordiazepoxide	Increase
Lorazepam	Same
Phenytoin	Increase
Phenobarbital	Increase
Valproate	Increase
Morphine	Same
Meperidine	Decrease
Imipramine	Decrease
Pancuronium	Decrease
Suxamethonium	Increase

Data from Martyn;[8] Brown and Bell;[9] Martyn et al.;[10,11] Pugh;[12] and Stanford and Pine.[13]

antiepileptic drugs may change in persons suddenly exposed to skin loss.

Central nervous system complications in severely burned patients are largely derived from autopsy studies. In autopsy studies by Winkelman and Galloway,[14] central nervous system infections and hypoxic–ischemic encephalopathy were most common and may have been preventable.

Another life-threatening condition is wound infection resulting in sepsis, multiorgan failure, or endocarditis. *Staphylococcus aureus*, *Klebsiella pneumoniae*, *Pseudomonas aeruginosa*, and *Candida* infections may develop in burn patients and may result in endocarditis and septic emboli to the brain.

Burn Encephalopathy

The neurologic presentation of patients with extensive burns is often muddled by systemic factors, none of which is specific for burns. Severe burns result in hypovolemic shock from fluid loss in the burn surface, and direct myocardial depression from increased sympathetic tone may result in decreased cardiac output. Both factors may cause a robust reduction in cerebral tissue perfusion and readily predispose burn victims to ischemic encephalopathy.

Severely burned patients tend to have fluctuating levels of consciousness.[15–18] In ap-

proximately 30% of the patients, agitation, visual hallucinations, and coarse tremor develop in association with burn delirium.[16–19] Systemic factors may initiate a delirious state, but in most patients, fever is already an important trigger in itself. Massive facial swelling and eye bandages to treat corneal damage may contribute to deprivation, and the long-term use of lorazepam given intravenously may well give rise to delirium when withdrawn.[13]

Burn encephalopathy is an imperfectly delineated clinical syndrome and may occur more frequently in children.[16,20] It may be a mixture of structural brain lesions manifested as a more or less diffuse and global encephalopathy and likely is not a separate entity. Many other more common and certainly better defined disorders should be excluded (Table 16–2). Central pontine myelinolysis has been reported in patients with burns after correction of hyponatremia[14,21] (see Chapter 8). Reduced level of consciousness was a common first sign; in some patients, narcotic overdose was deemed likely until magnetic resonance imaging (MRI) abnormalities with punched-out ventral pons lesions appeared.

The neurologic manifestation of burn encephalopathy usually involves generalized tonic–clonic seizures, drowsiness, or stupor with unpredictable onset. Onset may be weeks after the burn injury, even, at times, when fever and metabolic derangements have subsided. Seizures are often associated with hyponatremia, usually as a result of iatrogenic fluid loading overshooting the fluid demands in patients in a hypovolemic state.[22] A fortunately rare complication of extensive burns is acute blindness.[23–26]

Table 16–2. **Differential Diagnosis in Burn Encephalopathy**

Central nervous system infections
Cerebral venous thrombosis
Ischemic encephalopathy
Central pontine myelinolysis or osmotic demyelination syndrome
Severe hyponatremia
Nonketotic hyperosmolar hyperglycemia
Wernicke's encephalopathy

Blindness in children and young adults commonly occurs in the second or third week after the ravaging burns. Blindness may be due to either bilateral occipital infarcts associated with shock or anterior ischemic neuropathy. Outcome for patients with either of these conditions is not necessarily poor, and recovery has been reported, sometimes in only one eye.

Autopsy has not been particularly revealing. Neuropathologic findings consisting of small areas of demyelination, degeneration of axons, and scattered hemorrhages have been found at autopsy in severely burned patients, but it is not certain whether these represent one of the pathologic correlates of burn encephalopathy. In some patients with documented sepsis, bacterial colonies have been found in small vessels, but they may not necessarily explain the clinical manifestations. In others, massive cerebral edema is prominent. As this suggests, burn encephalopathy remains a captivating but poorly elucidated manifestation of extensive burns.

Central Nervous System Infections

Wound infection is common in patients with burns that cover more than 30% of total body surface area. However, the frequency of central nervous system infections in patients with systemic infection is not known, and most data are derived only from autopsy studies. Winkelman and Galloway's comprehensive autopsy series[14] noted that all patients with intracranial infections had systemic signs of sepsis syndrome, many with positive blood cultures (Table 16–3). The most common organisms causing both significant multiorgan failure and cerebral microabscesses, septic infarcts, and meningitis were *S. aureus*, *P. aeruginosa*, and *Candida* species. All patients with *S. aureus* cerebritis also had *S. aureus* endocarditis. *S. aureus* may hematogenously spread to the vertebral venous plexus from infected femoral and pelvic veins in burned legs and eventually contribute to development of epidural abscesses.[27] Epidural localization of an abscess should be strongly considered in a burned patient whose condition is complicated by staphylococcal bacteremia and sudden paraparesis (Chapter 6).

In Winkelman and Galloway's autopsy series, bacterial meningitis was most frequently associated with nosocomially acquired *P. aeruginosa*, a generally unusual pathogen for meningitis.[14] No significant relation was found with face or scalp burns. Cerebral infarcts that may potentially have been caused by local invasion of the organism in penetrating blood vessels were found in half the patients with *P. aeruginosa* meningitis. Cerebrospinal fluid confirmation of *Pseudomonas* involvement is important, but a lumbar puncture could be hard to justify in patients with extensive burns, and then treatment should probably be guided by physical findings and confirmation from blood cultures. Treatment of *Pseudomonas* meningitis is complex and involves ceftazidime and parenterally administered anti-*Pseudomonas* penicillins or intrathecally administered aminoglycosides (see Chapter 6 for dose schedules).

Table 16–3. **Central Nervous System Complications of Fatal Burns in 143 Patients**

	PATIENTS	
Complication	No.	%
Central nervous system infection	22	15
Ischemic stroke	15	10
Hypoxic–ischemic encephalopathy	18	13
Central pontine myelinolysis	11	8
Cerebral hemorrhage	5	3

Data from Winkelman and Galloway.[14]

Candida infection may be widespread throughout the nervous system, and the infection is very difficult to diagnose or establish through cultures. *Candida* infections of the brain may result in microabscesses (often too small to detect with current imaging methods), meningitis, or spinal osteomyelitis.[28]

Peripheral Neuropathies

The incidence of peripheral neuropathy is derived from retrospective analysis. Common themes are close relation with severity of burn and frequent presence of mononeuritis multiplex. Prolonged use of vancomycin has been implicated,[29,30] but it is very unlikely that this agent is a crucial factor in a patient population that will at some point, whatever the critical illness, be treated with antibiotics. Other contributing factors have been suggested, including chromium, thiamine, vitamin B$_6$, and phosphate deficiencies.[31–33]

In a series of 800 patients, a mononeuritis multiplex was found in 11 of 19 patients with a neuropathy, probably explained by protein denaturation and clumping within nerve arterioles in extensive skin burns.[30] Multiple compression neuropathies were considered unlikely, although conditions such as faulty position, incorrect splinting, and tight dressing were favorable. Surprisingly, in that study, a critical illness neu-

ropathy was seldom seen despite a high incidence of sepsis, but it may have escaped detection. A recent study from the Harborview Medical Center Burn Unit including patients with a mean total body surface burn of 24% found no correlation of peripheral neuropathy with medication, nutritional status, or infection.[34] However, a statistically significant relationship was found between C-reactive protein and electrophysiologic testing, suggesting a direct relationship with thermal burns rather than with a complication or treatment of severe burns.

SMOKE INHALATION

Severe burns may be associated with inhalation of toxic products of combustion, mostly carbon monoxide and cyanide. Facial burns should point to the possibility of smoke inhalation. Oxygenation may become compromised by lung damage from direct inhalation, and smoke inhalation may also bring the development of an acute respiratory distress syndrome.

Carbon Monoxide

Smoke from fires may contain up to 10% carbon monoxide.[35] Signs of carbon monoxide poisoning may not be immediately obvious in patients who have large burns and who are in hypovolemic shock. Concentrations of

Table 16–4. Carboxyhemoglobin Concentrations in Relation to Symptoms

Carboxyhemoglobin Concentration (%)	Clinical Effect
0–10	None
10–20	Mild headache, fatigue
20–30	Throbbing headache, blurred vision, irritability, impaired motor dexterity
30–40	Weakness, dizziness, confusion, excitement, blurred vision
40–50	Weakness, ataxia, hallucinations
50–70	Seizures, coma
>70	Respiratory failure, death

Modified from Bryson PD. Comprehensive Review in Toxicology for Emergency Clinicians, 3rd ed. Taylor & Francis, Washington, DC, 1996, p 340. By permission of the publisher.

carboxyhemoglobin that are >40% result in coma (Table 16–4). In the lower range, these concentrations are poorly correlated with the level of consciousness, and in many patients small traces are related to cigarette smoking. The effects of carbon monoxide poisoning can be profound when the gas is inhaled for a considerable period and when minute ventilation is increased, such as during physical exercise. The cardiac effects are potentially serious, and electrocardiograms may show patterns indicative of myocardial ischemia. Patients with underlying coronary artery disease may be particularly vulnerable to small amounts of carbon monoxide.

Manifestations of carbon monoxide intoxication are variable.[36] Earliest signs of carbon monoxide poisoning are personality changes with loss of orderliness, snapping at people, and outbursts of anxiety but also profound headache and diminished responsiveness when carboxyhemoglobin concentration increases. The classic cherry red coloring sign is very infrequently seen,[36,37] and because of tissue hypoxia, many patients are more likely to be cyanotic and tachypneic at presentation. Severe papilledema with splinter hemorrhages may occur,[38] sometimes as a direct result of asphyxia.

brain, such as Sommer's sector of Ammon's horn of the hippocampus, anterior portion of the globus pallidus, and centrum semiovale. The delayed response may be due to production of free radicals, an increase in brain lipid peroxidation, or a decrease in cytochrome oxidase activity.[1]

Computed tomography (CT) scanning or MRI may demonstrate the characteristic symmetrical lucencies in the globus pallidus (Fig. 16–2), centrum semiovale, and hippocampus but also in the cerebellum.[39–42] White matter hypodensities, often seen in comatose patients and patients with exposure of long duration, predict poor outcome and may be associated with development of later parkinsonism.[43] Globus pallidus lesions are generally less prognostic.[39,40]

Treatment of acute carbon monoxide poisoning[44] is 100% oxygen and, if that is unsuccessful, hyperbaric oxygen. High oxygen concentrations are achieved because of increased atmospheric pressure, but no evidence exists of improvement in neurologic function.[45] Criteria for hyperbaric oxygen therapy (limited in availability and requiring air transport) are carboxyhemoglobin concentration >30%, coma, acute signs of myo-

PATHOPHYSIOLOGIC MECHANISMS

The half-life of carbon monoxide in blood is 20 min in contrast to 80 to 100 min with 100% oxygen. Carbon monoxide binds to hemoglobin with a great affinity, resulting in the compound carboxyhemoglobin and effectively reducing the capacity of hemoglobin to carry oxygen to tissue. The bond of carbon monoxide to the heme group, however, remains reversible and is released by high concentrations of oxygen. Additional significant effects are a leftward shift in the oxyhemoglobin dissociation curve, particularly at concentrations of >50%, reducing oxygen release from remaining oxyhemoglobin. Less affinity exists to other heme proteins, such as myoglobin (reducing oxygen availability to the heart) and cytochromes (impairing the electron transport chain and cellular respiration). Tissue hypoxia and hypotension produce abnormalities in vulnerable areas of the

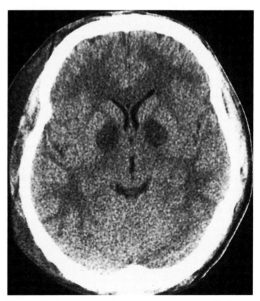

Figure 16–2. Computed tomography image of pallidal lesions in comatose patient with carbon monoxide poisoning.

Cyanide

Smoke inhalation victims may have significant blood levels of cyanide as a result of combustion of organic nitrogen-containing materials common in plastics and wood.[46–49] Both cyanide poisoning and carbon monoxide inhalation frequently occur in residential fires,[46] and cyanide has been detected in the sera of firefighters.[50]

Cyanide inhibits reoxidation of cytochrome oxidase and blocks oxidative phosphorylation and adenosine triphosphate formation, essentially blocking aerobic metabolism. Cyanosis does not occur, and patients die with pink skin.

Cyanide inhalation (blood concentration >1 μg/mL) results in rapid development of dilated pupils, ataxia, generalized "violent" tonic–clonic seizures, coma with absent motor responses, and, very often, death at the scene. Poor oxygenation may result in bright red retinal veins, obscuring the difference from retinal arteries. Delayed striatal degeneration with parkinsonism and dystonia and an anatomical substrate very similar to that in carbon monoxide has been reported.[51]

Laboratory diagnosis of cyanide inhalation is difficult. The detection of cyanide in blood is technically cumbersome and may take hours. High serum concentrations of lactate causing anion gap metabolic acidosis are suggestive of cyanide poisoning in patients without burns.

Treatment of cyanide exposure due to smoke inhalation is immediate administration of high-flow oxygen.[52] The administration of sodium thiosulfate produces a conversion in thiocyanate that is much less toxic and is excreted in urine. It is supplemented by amyl nitrite, which acts by converting hemoglobin to methemoglobin and has a high affinity for cyanide. A dose of 12.5 g of sodium thiosulfate (Lilly cyanide antidote kit) is followed by amyl nitrite when life-threatening cardiac arrhythmias and seizures persist. Hydroxocobalamin is less toxic and less expensive for the treatment of cyanide poisoning, and strong arguments have been made for out-of-hospital use as well.[49]

ELECTRICAL BURNS

Direct neurologic complications of deep conductive electrical injury are well documented, but a fall caused by sudden collapse may result in very significant head trauma or spine injury.[53] Sustained tetanic contraction may also contribute to vertebral fractures with a mechanism similar to that in patients with status epilepticus[54] (see Chapter 3). The most common presentations of electrical burns are related to peripheral nerve damage (Table 16–5), but the severity of the effects most likely depends on the voltage of the electric shock.

Spinal Cord Damage

It has long been recognized that spinal cord damage can occur in patients with electrical burns,[53,56–60] and electrical heating probably causes necrosis of the cord, predominantly

Table 16–5. **Neurologic Complications of Electrical Burns in 90 Patients**

	PATIENTS	
Findings	**No.**	**%**
Acute peripheral neuropathy	21	23
Delayed peripheral neuropathy	11	12
Seizures	3	3
Transient hemiparesis	1	1

Data from Grube et al.[55]

Table 16–6. Incidence of Spinal Cord Injury after Electrical Burns in Large Series of Patients

	PATIENTS		
Series	Total	No.	%
DiVincenti et al., 1969[62]	65	2	3
Butler and Gant, 1977[63]	182	3	2
Varghese et al., 1986[64]	85	5	6
Grube et al., 1990[55]	90	0	0

in the thoracic region. Demyelination of corticospinal tracts, lateral columns, and both fasciculi is usually found at autopsy, but in patients with delayed onset of spinal cord injury, thrombosis of the supplying arteries to the spinal cord has been postulated as the mechanism.[61] The clinical picture may vary from short-lived paresthesias or sensory deficit, mild proximal leg weakness, and extensor plantar responses that resolve within 24 hr to severe permanent quadriplegia. The electrical injury may have a more striking course, characterized by ascending paralysis.

After electrical shocks with high voltage, clinical features similar to those of amyotrophic lateral sclerosis have been reported, with severe upper extremity muscle wasting, fasciculations, and spastic paraplegia without sensory involvement. Spinal cord injury varies in incidence, remains uncommon, and in one large series was surprisingly absent[55] (Table 16–6). Delayed onset of spinal cord injury—within days, months, or years after the injury—typically results in permanent damage. In addition, significant recovery is not expected in patients with a complete spinal cord lesion after a symptom-free episode. When spinal cord injury is limited and the patient can continue walking, there is a chance of recovery.[64]

Peripheral Neuropathy

Polyneuropathy, mononeuropathy, and plexopathies have been described in association with major and minor electrical burns.[62,63,65] In series from Engrav and associates[66] and Grube and associates,[55] acute peripheral nerve injury developed in a third of the patients, most frequently in the median and ulnar nerves. The mechanism of injury after electrical contact may be indirect due to prominent muscle swelling causing nerve entrapment.[67,68] Many surgeons are inclined to immediately decompress the carpal tunnel and Guyon's canal, but the effectiveness of preventing permanent damage has not been demonstrated, and spontaneous resolution has been reported.

Central Nervous System Manifestations

Typically, electrical shocks produce sudden loss of consciousness followed by a confusional state.[69] Neurologic sequelae are rare, but homonymous hemianopia and hemiparesis from associated ischemic stroke have been described.[70] Delayed onset of coma was linked to thrombotic occlusion of the basilar artery in one case report.[71]

High-voltage exposure produces cardiac arrest and often diffuse anoxic–ischemic brain injury.[72] The victims are immediately unresponsive and remain in a persistent vegetative state if they survive the initial impact at all.

LIGHTNING INJURY

If not electrocuted, victims of a lightning strike (estimated 1000 deaths worldwide annually) may suffer serious neurologic morbidity.[73–77] The surge of current may traverse the brain, causing direct parenchymal damage, or the current may flow through the heart and lungs, resulting in cardiac arrest leading to anoxic–ischemic brain injury, not different from any other type of cardiac standstill.

PATHOPHYSIOLOGIC MECHANISMS

Five mechanisms cause lightning injury. (1) In a direct hit or strike, lightning passes through a person's body, possibly facilitated by a carried metal object, such as an umbrella. Exit and entry sites can be found, but occurrence is rare. (2) Splash is much more frequent. The current jumps to the person from, for example, a tree or building used by the victim for shelter, but it also can jump from another person. (3) Contact occurs when an object held by the person is hit by lightning. The person may be thrown for a considerable distance. (4) In step voltage, a ground wave hits the person's feet and may ascend. (5) Blunt trauma is an indirect consequence; the explosive force may cause traumatic brain injury, such as epidural, subdural, or contrecoup hematoma, often with a demonstrable skull fracture.[78]

A demographic profile seems to have emerged: male, younger than 35 years, struck during recreation in mountains and forested areas, often near mountain tops or in the open, near vehicles, or close to the water, apparently during the afternoon.[79] Lightning strike, therefore, should be initially considered in patients with coma of undetermined cause found under these circumstances.

Clinical Features

The clinical manifestations of lightning injury are protean and may be confounded by brain injury from the associated fall or cardiac arrest. The degree of impact can be extrapolated from entry and exit points (if present) and lightning ("Lichtenberg") figures,[80] dendritic ferning forms ("evergreen tree pattern") that are caused by electron showers and are not true burns to the skin (Plate 16–1). These patterns may disappear

in a few hours but usually last 1 to 2 days. Other lightning-associated skin burns are superficial, consisting of linear burns at places where sweat or water accumulates and punctate burns in a rosette-like fashion.

The neurologic manifestations have been divided by Cherington[81] into immediate or delayed. Moreover, these features may be a consequence of trauma due to being propelled into the air and thrown down. Typically, the immediate manifestations are transient and not prolonged and permanent. The delayed manifestations could be progressive.[81]

The immediate neurologic manifestations in survivors of lightning strike include dysesthesias in the affected limbs, muscular pain from rhabdomyolysis, diminished hearing (one or both tympanic membranes may be ruptured), blindness, and abnormalities of mood, memory, and affect.[82] Absent red reflex, most likely from intravitreal hemorrhage, has been incidentally noted.[83]

Loss of consciousness can be brief, and patients may be dazed, stunned, and disoriented, with no recall of the strike. Seizures may occur, but when confusion persists or waxes and wanes, nonconvulsive status epilepticus should be one of the first considerations.[82]

Many patients have keraunoparalysis (a term coined by Charcot).[84] This condition, fairly characteristic for lightning strikes, consists of transient limb weakness (hemiparesis, paraparesis, or quadriparesis) and a blue, mottled, cold, pulseless appearance from vasospasm and sympathetic overdrive. Although limb gangrene seems imminent, recovery is often prompt, and these vasomotor manifestations disappear in 1 to 2 hr after the patient is hit.

The clinical manifestations of direct injury to the neuraxis are often related to a post-resuscitation encephalopathy. If the brain is in the pathway of current, not only the brain tissue but also the blood vessels may be damaged, leading to subarachnoid hemorrhage. Intraparenchymal hematoma (often in the basal ganglia) or simply a few minute hemorrhages may be seen on neuroimaging studies.[81,85–88] However, the blunt injury associated with lightning strike frequently results in typical CT findings of traumatic brain injury.[75] Isolated spinal cord damage has been reported in a few instances.[89,90]

Peripheral nervous system injury is mostly presented in the literature as a plexopathy and mononeuropathy, but clinical documentation of these disorders is scarce or nonconvincing. Later neurologic consequences of lightning have been reported, but the interval of many years and the overall frequent occurrence of these disorders (Parkinson's disease, amyotrophic lateral sclerosis, demyelinating disorders) make the association putative at best.

Management

Management of a victim of lightning injury follows the guidelines for management of coma described in Chapter 1. Several specific problems, however, can be encountered. Seizures and status epilepticus may continue to emerge in the first days, and a seizure disorder may evolve from the strike. Immediate intravenous loading with phenytoin should suffice.

Diffuse cerebral edema may have its origin in anoxic–ischemic damage, and thus monitoring of intracranial pressure or aggressive management may be of no use in patients with immediate coma (Chapter 7). However, in patients with associated hemorrhagic contusions, it is important to place a monitor early to follow the progression of intracranial pressure. Preliminary reports suggested that delayed brain edema develops, resulting in increased intracranial pressure, and conventional therapies, such as hyperventilation and administration of osmotic agents, are effective.[91–93] A recent study of two patients struck by lightning who had profound visual loss to light perception only showed that treatment with methylprednisolone led to complete improvement.[94]

ACCIDENTAL HYPOTHERMIA

Accidental hypothermia most frequently follows cold water immersion, winter outdoor exposure, and poisoning.[55] Primary hypothalamic disorders may result in spontaneous episodic hypothermia but remain extremely rare causes for hypothermia.

Most patients admitted to the ICU have hypothermia after cold water or environmental exposure.[95] One of the largest series of neurologic manifestations of hypothermia has been reported from San Francisco, where it can become deceptively cold (30°F) in the summer at night. Hypothermia may affect the relatively high proportion of homeless people in this city.

Clinical Features

The neurologic findings in patients with accidental hypothermia may simulate severe damage to the central nervous system and may include absence of brain stem reflexes. In all instances, however, core temperature should be corrected before brain damage is assessed.[95–98] The dictum "no one is dead until warm and dead" should be applied to every patient with accidental hypothermia.

The clinical changes produced by hypothermia are fairly typical. The level of consciousness is for the most part substantially decreased with core temperatures of less than 32°C. During rapid cooling, confusion and combative behavior may prevail. Neurologic abnormalities are only subtle above 32°C, and muscle tone may be slightly increased. Thus, additional causes, particularly suicidal ingestion of drugs, intracranial structural lesions, and severe hypothyroidism, should be actively sought when at temperatures above 32°C, patients can be aroused only with vigorous stimuli. For example, the frequent association of accidental hypothermia with alcohol abuse in a confused and disoriented patient could point to Wernicke's encephalopathy, particularly if nystagmus or oculomotor abnormalities and cerebellar dysfunction are present. Rapid volume expansion with glucose may also exacerbate signs of Wernicke's encephalopathy in patients with marginal thiamine stores. Coma, however, is very infrequent in Wernicke-Korsakoff syndrome. In Victor and associates' series of 229 patients, only 2 patients were in coma at presentation.[99]

Neurologic signs may begin to develop in patients with moderate hypothermia (34°C to 36°C) (Fig. 16–3), but the clinical presentation may still be limited to drowsiness and diminished judgment at these levels of hypothermia. Depressed or absent brain

Hypothermia

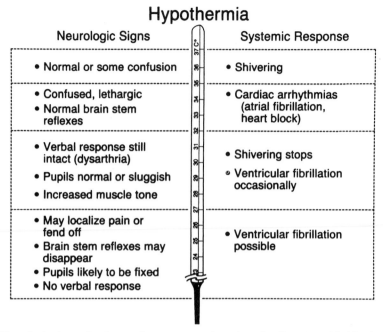

Neurologic Signs		Systemic Response
• Normal or some confusion		• Shivering
• Confused, lethargic • Normal brain stem reflexes		• Cardiac arrhythmias (atrial fibrillation, heart block)
• Verbal response still intact (dysarthria) • Pupils normal or sluggish • Increased muscle tone		• Shivering stops • Ventricular fibrillation occasionally
• May localize pain or fend off • Brain stem reflexes may disappear • Pupils likely to be fixed • No verbal response		• Ventricular fibrillation possible

Figure 16–3. Neurologic signs of and systemic responses to hypothermia. (Data from Fischbeck and Simon.[95])

stem reflexes appear in patients with severe hypothermia (<27°C), but this cutoff point is not absolute. Some patients may have absent brain stem reflexes and apnea, closely mimicking brain death. Muscle tone, however, is markedly increased rather than flaccid and may be misinterpreted as rigor mortis by novices. Cold, stiff, and blue patients may not be dead.

Neurologic diagnostic tests may not be very helpful. Electroencephalographic recordings in severe hypothermia may show many patterns, such as increased delta activity, triphasic waves, and, occasionally, isoelectricity.[100,101] However, MRI may show changes associated with prior trauma and cerebellar shrinkage involving both hemispheres and vermis, often from long-standing alcohol or drug abuse.

Cardiac arrhythmias are more common and may show characteristic electrocardiographic features, such as an Osborne wave ("camel's hump") in the QRS complex, that can easily be recognized.[102] These abnormal waves may occur with core temperatures of 32°C or less and often with sinus bradycardia (Fig. 16–4).

Treatment and Outcome

Most hypothermic patients are rewarmed by simple insulation with blankets. This method results in a 7°C core temperature increase per hour. High doses of thiamine (100 mg parenterally daily) should be administered to any alcoholic patient with hypothermia, and if thiamine deficiency is contributing, improvement can be expected within hours. Another major pitfall is myxedema coma, which should be considered in patients who fail to rewarm (see

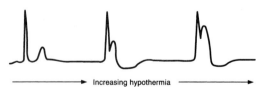

Increasing hypothermia

Figure 16–4. First tracing shows normal QRS complex. With increasing hypothermia, the QRS complex widens and an ST elevation is seen, with features of a "camel's hump" (Osborne wave). The hump increases with increasing hypothermia. Often a muscle artifact from shivering is observed.

Table 16–7. Factors Suggesting Poor Prognosis in Hypothermia

Increased potassium levels (>10 mmol/L)
Prehospital cardiac arrest
Low or absent blood pressure
Increased blood urea nitrogen
Severe underlying disease

Data from Schaller et al.[107]

Chapter 8). A large bolus of levothyroxine (500 μg) along with corticosteroid coverage is the first step in treatment.

Peritoneal lavage or cardiopulmonary bypass may be indicated.[103] Long-term outcome in a recently published series of 15 survivors managed with extracorporeal blood warming was good despite prolonged coma, amnesia, aphasia, ataxia, and spasticity in the early recovery period in these patients; mean interval of more than 2 1/2 hr from discovery of the patient to rewarming; and apnea and lack of a pulse in half the patients.[104]

Poor prognostic factors that have been described are impractical at the time of deciding whether to continue resuscitation in the emergency department[105–107] (Table 16–7). Neurologic outcome can be remarkably good even after prolonged cardiac resuscitation,[108] core temperature of 20°C or lower,[109] and absent brain stem reflexes. Any decision to discontinue resuscitation in a patient without brain stem reflexes who has severe hypothermia should be deferred until core temperature is at least above 32°C and preferably normal.

HEAT STROKE

Heat stroke should be considered a medical emergency,[110] and early treatment is crucial to prevent neurologic complications. A clear history and consistent recording of a rectal temperature above 40°C guide the diagnosis of heat stroke.[111–113] Well-known predisposing conditions are exertion in a hot environment and sudden heat waves in urban areas. Drugs that impair heat loss are often implicated, the most common of which are anticholinergic agents, phenothiazine deriva-

tives, tricyclic antidepressants, amphetamines, and monoamine oxidase inhibitors.[114] Cocaine, which increases heat production, may contribute as well.[115] The incidence of heat stroke is unknown, mainly because many patients die early from cardiovascular compromise caused by high ambient temperatures.

Severe hyperthermia leads to multiorgan failure. Many patients are profoundly hypotensive from dehydration, and the direct effect of hyperthermia results in progressive hepatic failure, usually within a few days after the temperature has surged. Bone marrow suppression leads to marked thrombocytopenia, but disseminated intravascular coagulation more likely produces the hypocoagulable state. Other typical findings are rhabdomyolysis with renal failure and severe electrolyte abnormalities (hypocalcemia, hyponatremia, hypophosphatemia), all of which could confound the neurologic assessment.

Clinical Features

Prodromes of heat stroke are acute confusional state, and a fair proportion of the patients may be psychotic, with vivid and often terrifying hallucinations. Headache and severely painful cramps in the truncal muscles may be present, often in association with hyponatremia from sweating. Patients should have hot and dry skin, but many already have had wet towels for cooling during transportation, obscuring this key clinical sign.

In heat stroke, progression into deep stages of coma is rapid. Most patients have small pupils, profound rigidity, and spontaneous extensor responses.[116]

In most patients with heat stroke and a fatal course, generalized tonic–clonic seizures occur at presentation. Any focal neurologic sign should point to a primary central nervous system disorder that may have directly contributed to hyperthermia, usually because the patient has been unable to prevent further deterioration by taking cover or rehydrating. For example, traumatic brain injury or pontine hemorrhage may cause hyperthermia and may falsely suggest heat stroke when patients are found under implicative circumstances.

Neuroimaging studies are usually nonrevealing except for some cortical effacement due to diffuse cerebral edema. In the only instance on record, central pontine myelinolysis detected by MRI was attributed to rapid shifts in serum osmolality.[117] Cerebrospinal fluid may show mild pleocytosis but is more often normal.

Treatment and Outcome

Treatment is supportive. Surface cooling (water and fan) should begin immediately after the airway is secured.[118,119] Other therapeutic options are gastric lavage with cool saline, cold intravenous fluids, groin and axillary ice packs, alcohol rubs, and a variety of antipyretic agents.[120] Rehydration is crucial in the first hours. Although effective in many other causes of hyperthermia, dantrolene is not useful.[121]

Neurologic outcome is often poor, and patients who remain comatose after cooling die or have severe cognitive deficits. However, coma on presentation is not necessarily a sign of poor prognosis (Table 16–8). In 54 patients with heat stroke, only a minority, including 40% of the patients with a Glasgow coma scale score of 3, had neurologic sequelae.[123] Death or neurologic morbidity is more likely in patients with extreme hyperthermia (>42°C), although survivors have been reported.[124] Coagulopathy, hypovolemic shock, increased serum lactate levels, metabolic acidosis, association with predisposing medication, and electrolyte abnormalities may indicate a poor prognosis.

Cerebellar signs are frequent neurologic findings in survivors of heat stroke,[47] probably because hyperthermia may directly result in damage to Purkinje's cells, but as communicated in Chapter 7, the cerebellar cortex is also exquisitely sensitive to anoxic–ischemic episodes. The neuropathologic correlates are petechiae in the walls of the third and fourth ventricles and degenerative changes, most strikingly in the cerebellum, cerebral cortex, and basal ganglia.[125,126] These findings may be a consequence of severe liver failure and coagulopathy. Many patients have slowed and scanning speech. Sitting in a chair while being weaned from the ventilator may unmask truncal instability and a tendency to fall to one side. The prospects of recovery are minimal. Functional impairment at dismissal not only persists but also leads to increased mortality within the first 10 years.[115]

NEAR-DROWNING

Patients entering the emergency department or ICU after nearly drowning are unusually difficult to manage. Excellent survival can be expected in some aggressively resuscitated patients, but other patients remain in a persistent vegetative state. After resuscitation, general measures should focus on prevention of secondary brain damage from hypoxia and hypoglycemia, both common accompanying conditions in near-drowning victims.

Clinical Features

Neurologic examination of the rescued drowned patient may not produce reliable

Table 16–8. **Series of Patients with Heat Stroke**

| | | NO. OF PATIENTS | | | | |
| | | PRESENTING FEATURES | | OUTCOME | | |
Series	Total	Stupor or Coma	Seizures	Died	Disabled	Recovered
Tucker et al., 1985[113]	34	26	2	6	3	25
Yaqub et al., 1986[122]	30	15	2	3	2	25
Bouchama et al., 1991[121]	52	20	6	1	4	47
Dematte et al., 1998[115]	58	33	9	12	15	31

findings. Many patients display hypothermia from submersion in ice water, and some have drug or alcohol intoxication. The patient may have a severe hyponatremia from having swallowed large amounts of water, and this condition may potentially trigger seizures. Comatose patients with flaccid limbs unresponsive to pain may be the most unfortunate, particularly if recovery halts in the first 48 hr. Quadriplegia may also be caused by burst fractures of the cervical spine during submersion.

CT scan is often initially normal, but diffuse cerebral edema may occur. Effacement of sulci and tailoring of ventricles are noted in the most severe cases. However, differentiation of subtle cerebral edema on CT from normal findings in young patients can be extremely difficult because of the presence of a few sulci and generally small ventricles in this age group.

Management and Outcome

Critical care management is focused on respiratory care.[127–130] In many patients, respiratory failure develops from acute respiratory distress syndrome or pulmonary infection that is caused by aspiration of contaminated water. These conditions may lead to sustained hypoxia in the first hours after resuscitation, but it is not clear whether neurologic outcome is less favorable when this happens.

Monitoring of intracranial pressure has been used, usually as part of an aggressive management approach, but successful control of intracranial pressure, if elevated at all, has not led to increased survival or recovery.[131]

Intracranial pressure monitoring in patients has demonstrated only occasional decreases in cerebral perfusion pressure in the first 3 days after near-drowning. Initially increased intracranial pressure may predict poor outcome, but consistently normal intracranial pressure values have been found in patients who remained comatose.[132]

The general opinion is that use of intracranial pressure monitoring in victims of near-drowning is of no value. This conclusion implies that aggressive measures with agents that can lower intracranial pressure, such as osmotic diuretics, steroids, and bar-

Table 16–9. Poor Prognostic Indicators in Near-Drowning*

Apnea on admission to the emergency department
Pupils fixed to light
Glasgow coma scale sum score of <5
Submersion for more than 5 min
Metabolic acidosis of pH <7.1

*Largely pediatric series.[133]

biturates, are also probably of no therapeutic use.

Outcome of near-drowning is difficult to predict, but the same rules of prognostication as those in coma after cardiac resuscitation may apply (see Chapters 7 and 19) (Table 16–9). However, in this category of patients, a major confounding factor can be hypothermia. In fact, outcome in hypothermic survivors is significantly better only when patients are immersed in ice water. Normal findings on pulmonary examination and a Glasgow coma scale score of 13 or 14 have been associated with the best outcome in childhood drowning.[134] Attempts to prolong the protective effect of hypothermia with high doses of barbiturates have been unsuccessful and in addition may aggravate neutropenia and sepsis.[135]

CONCLUSIONS

Three important points can be made in patients with neurologic involvement of environmental injury. First, the reliability of neurologic evaluation should be questioned in any patient with hypothermia, whether from outdoor exposure or from near-drowning. Every circumstance is different, and compounding factors, such as acute drug intoxication or an unexpected acute structural central nervous system lesion that has led to the injury, should be excluded. Core body temperatures should be around 32°C before a reliable neurologic assessment is attempted.

Second, care should be taken to prevent compression neuropathy in immobilized patients. Especially in burn patients, the incidence of peripheral neuropathy may be increased when appropriate measures are taken (for example, splinting, dressing changes).

Third, prognostication in these victims can be assessed and may determine the level of care—aggressive or minimal. For most injured patients, prognostic factors have been identified that can ascertain the level of functioning in those who survive resuscitation.

REFERENCES

1. Spencer PS, Schaumburg HH, Ludolph AC. Experimental and Clinical Neurotoxicology, 2nd ed. Oxford University Press, New York, 2000.
2. Feldman RG. Occupational and Environmental Neurotoxicology. Lippincott-Raven, Philadelphia, 1999.
3. Demling RH. Burns. N Engl J Med 313:1389–1398, 1985.
4. O'Keefe GE, Hunt JL, Purdue GF. An evaluation of risk factors for mortality after burn trauma and the identification of gender-dependent differences in outcomes. J Am Coll Surg 192:153–160, 2001.
5. Wachtel TL, Berry CC, Wachtel EE, Frank HA. The inter-rater reliability of estimating the size of burns from various burn area chart drawings. Burns 26:156–170, 2000.
6. Bloedow DC, Hansbrough JF, Hardin T, Simons M. Postburn serum drug binding and serum protein concentrations. J Clin Pharmacol 26:147–151, 1986.
7. Bowdle TA, Neal GD, Levy RH, Heimbach DM. Phenytoin pharmacokinetics in burned rats and plasma protein binding of phenytoin in burned patients. J Pharmacol Exp Ther 213:97–99, 1980.
8. Martyn JAJ. Acute Management of the Burned Patient. WB Saunders, Philadelphia, 1990.
9. Brown TC, Bell B. Electromyographic responses to small doses of suxamethonium in children after burns. Br J Anaesth 59:1017–1021, 1987.
10. Martyn JA, Abernethy DR, Greenblatt DJ. Plasma protein binding of drugs after severe burn injury. Clin Pharmacol Ther 35:535–539, 1984.
11. Martyn J, Goldhill DR, Goudsouzian NG. Clinical pharmacology of muscle relaxants in patients with burns. J Clin Pharmacol 26:680–685, 1986.
12. Pugh CB. Phenytoin and phenobarbital protein binding alterations in a uremic burn patient. Drug Intell Clin Pharm 21:264–267, 1987.
13. Stanford GK, Pine RH. Postburn delirium associated with use of intravenous lorazepam. J Burn Care Rehabil 9:160–161, 1988.
14. Winkelman MD, Galloway PG. Central nervous system complications of thermal burns. A postmortem study of 139 patients. Medicine (Baltimore) 71:271–283, 1992.
15. Haynes BW Jr, Bright R. Burn coma: a syndrome associated with severe burn wound infection. J Trauma 7:464–475, 1967.
16. Mohnot D, Snead OC III, Benton JW Jr. Burn encephalopathy in children. Ann Neurol 12:42–47, 1982.
17. Rosenbloom C, Kravath R. Neurological disturbances following minor burns. Lancet 2:1423, 1969.
18. Sanders R. Neurological disturbances and minor burns. Lancet 2:1133, 1969.
19. Andreasen NJ, Hartford CE, Knott JR, Canter A. EEG changes associated with burn delirium. Dis Nerv Syst 38:27–31, 1977.
20. Antoon AY, Volpe JJ, Crawford JD. Burn encephalopathy in children. Pediatrics 50:609–616, 1972.
21. Cohen BJ, Jordon MH, Chapin SD, Cape B, Laureno R. Pontine myelinolysis after correction of hyponatremia during burn resuscitation. J Burn Care Rehabil 12:153–156, 1991.
22. Hughes JR, Cayaffa JJ, Boswick JA Jr. Seizures following burns of the skin. III. Electroencephalographic recordings. Dis Nerv Syst 36:443–447, 1975.
23. Resch CS, Sullivan WG. Unexplained blindness after a major burn. Burns Incl Therm Inj 14:225–227, 1988.
24. Salz JJ, Donin JF. Blindness after burns. Can J Ophthalmol 7:243–246, 1972.
25. Williams IM. Neuro-ophthalmic deterioration after burns. Proc Aust Assoc Neurol 11:49–56, 1974.
26. Xiao J, Xu H, Kong FY. Bilateral visual loss after severe burns in a child. Burns 17:423–424, 1991.
27. Still JM, Abramson R, Law EJ. Development of an epidural abscess following staphylococcal septicemia in an acutely burned patient: case report. J Trauma 38:958–959, 1995.
28. Mullins RF, Still JM Jr, Savage J, Davis JB, Law EJ. Osteomyelitis of the spine in a burn patient due to *Candida albicans*. Burns 19:174–176, 1993.
29. Leibowitz G, Golan D, Jeshurun D, Brezis M. Mononeuritis multiplex associated with prolonged vancomycin treatment. BMJ 300:1344, 1990.
30. Marquez S, Turley JJ, Peters WJ. Neuropathy in burn patients. Brain 116:471–483, 1993.
31. Henderson B, Koepke GH, Feller I. Peripheral polyneuropathy among patients with burns. Arch Phys Med Rehabil 52:149–151, 1971.
32. Helm PA, Johnson ER, Carlton AM. Peripheral neurological problems in acute burn patient. Burns 3:123–125, 1977.
33. Brown RO, Forloines-Lynn S, Cross RE, Heizer WD. Chromium deficiency after long-term total parenteral nutrition. Dig Dis Sci 31:661–664, 1986.
34. Margherita AJ, Robinson LR, Heimbach DM, Fishfader VL, Schneider VA, Jones D. Burn-associated peripheral polyneuropathy. A search for causative factors. Am J Phys Med Rehabil 74:28–32, 1995.
35. Dolan MC. Carbon monoxide poisoning. CMAJ: Canadian Medical Association Journal 133:392–399, 1985.
36. Bour H, Tutin M, Pasquier P. The central nervous system and carbon monoxide poisoning. I. Clinical data with reference to 20 fatal cases. Prog Brain Res 24:1–30, 1967.
37. Simini B. Cherry-red discolouration in carbon monoxide poisoning [letter]. Lancet 352:1154, 1998.
38. Pye IF, Blandford RL. Papilloedema associated with respiratory failure. Postgrad Med J 53:704–709, 1977.
39. Miura T, Mitomo M, Kawai R, Harada K. CT of the brain in acute carbon monoxide intoxication: characteristic features and prognosis. AJNR Am J Neuroradiol 6:739–742, 1985.

40. Nardizzi LR. Computerized tomographic correlate of carbon monoxide poisoning. Arch Neurol 36:38–39, 1979.

41. Taylor R, Holgate RC. Carbon monoxide poisoning: asymmetric and unilateral changes on CT. AJNR Am J Neuroradiol 9:975–977, 1988.

42. O'Donnell P, Buxton PJ, Pitkin A, Jarvis LJ. The magnetic resonance imaging appearances of the brain in acute carbon monoxide poisoning. Clin Radiol 55:273–280, 2000.

43. Sohn YH, Jeong Y, Kim HS, Im JH, Kim JS. The brain lesion responsible for parkinsonism after carbon monoxide poisoning. Arch Neurol 57:1214–1218, 2000.

44. Norkool DM, Kirkpatrick JN. Treatment of acute carbon monoxide poisoning with hyperbaric oxygen: a review of 115 cases. Ann Emerg Med 14:1168–1171, 1985.

45. Juurlink DN, Stanbrook MB, McGuigan MA. Hyperbaric oxygen for carbon monoxide poisoning (Cochrane Review). In: The Cochrane Library, Issue 3, 2001. Oxford: Update Software.

46. Baud FJ, Barriot P, Toffis V, et al. Elevated blood cyanide concentrations in victims of smoke inhalation. N Engl J Med 325:1761–1766, 1991.

47. Hall AH, Rumack BH. Clinical toxicology of cyanide. Ann Emerg Med 15:1067–1074, 1986.

48. Jones J, McMullen MJ, Dougherty J. Toxic smoke inhalation: cyanide poisoning in fire victims. Am J Emerg Med 5:317–321, 1987.

49. Sauer SW, Keim ME. Hydroxocobalamin: improved public health readiness for cyanide disasters. Ann Emerg Med 37:635–641, 2001.

50. Symington IS, Anderson RA, Thomson I, Oliver JS, Harland WA, Kerr JW. Cyanide exposure in fires. Lancet 2:91–92, 1978.

51. Rosenberg NL, Myers JA, Martin WR. Cyanide-induced parkinsonism: Clinical, MRI, and 6-fluorodopa PET studies. Neurology 39:142–144, 1989.

52. Hart GB, Strauss MB, Lennon PA, Whitcraft DD III. Treatment of smoke inhalation by hyperbaric oxygen. J Emerg Med 3:211–215, 1985.

53. Panse F. Electrical lesions of the nervous system. In: Vinken PJ, Bruyn GW (eds). Handbook of Clinical Neurology, Vol. 7: Diseases of Nerves. North-Holland Publishing, Amsterdam, 1970, pp 344–387.

54. Layton TR, McMurtry JM, McClain EJ, et al. Multiple spine fractures from electric injury. J Burn Care Rehabil 5:373–375, 1984.

55. Grube BJ, Heimbach DM, Engrav LH, Copass MK. Neurologic consequences of electrical burns. J Trauma 30:254–258, 1990.

56. Kanitkar S, Roberts AH. Paraplegia in an electrical burn: a case report. Burns Incl Therm Inj 14:49–50, 1988.

57. Langworthy OR. Neurological abnormalities produced by electricity. J Nerv Ment Dis 84:13–26, 1936.

58. Levine NS, Atkins A, McKeel DW Jr, Peck SD, Pruitt BA Jr. Spinal cord injury following electrical accidents: case reports. J Trauma 15:459–463, 1975.

59. Naville F, de Morsier G. Symptômes neurologiques consécutifs aux électrocutions industrielles. Rev Neurol (Paris) 1:337–355, 1932.

60. Silversides J. The neurological sequelae of electrical injury. Can Med Assoc J 91:195–204, 1964.

61. Holbrook LA, Beach FX, Silver JR. Delayed myelopathy: a rare complication of severe electrical burns. Br Med J 4:659–660, 1970.

62. DiVincenti FC, Moncrief JA, Pruitt BA Jr. Electrical injuries: a review of 65 cases. J Trauma 9:497–507, 1969.

63. Butler ED, Gant TD. Electrical injuries, with special reference to the upper extremities. A review of 182 cases. Am J Surg 134:95–101, 1977.

64. Varghese G, Mani MM, Redford JB. Spinal cord injuries following electrical accidents. Paraplegia 24:159–166, 1986.

65. Hanumadass ML, Voora SB, Kagan RJ, Matsuda T. Acute electrical burns: a 10-year clinical experience. Burns Incl Therm Inj 12:427–431, 1986.

66. Engrav LH, Gottlieb JR, Walkinshaw MD, Heimbach DM, Trumble TE, Grube BJ. Outcome and treatment of electrical injury with immediate median and ulnar nerve palsy at the wrist: a retrospective review and a survey of members of the American Burn Association. Ann Plast Surg 25:166–168, 1990.

67. Justis DL, Law EJ, MacMillan BG. Tibial compartment syndromes in burn patients. A report of four cases. Arch Surg 111:1004–1008, 1976.

68. Rosenberg DB. Neurologic sequelae of minor electric burns. Arch Phys Med Rehabil 70:914–915, 1989.

69. Christensen JA, Sherman RT, Balis GA, Wuamett JD. Delayed neurologic injury secondary to high-voltage current, with recovery. J Trauma 20:166–168, 1980.

70. Gans M, Glaser JS. Homonymous hemianopia following electrical injury. J Clin Neuroophthalmol 6:218–223, 1986.

71. Haase E, Luhan JA. Protracted coma from delayed thrombosis of basilar artery following electrical injury. Arch Neurol 1:195–202, 1959.

72. Critchley M. Neurological effects of lightning and of electricity. Lancet 1:68–72, 1934.

73. Cherington M, Yarnell P, Lammereste D. Lightning strikes: nature of neurological damage in patients evaluated in hospital emergency departments. Ann Emerg Med 21:575–578, 1992.

74. Cherington M, Yarnell PR, London SF. Neurologic complications of lightning injuries. West J Med 162:413–417, 1995.

75. Graber J, Ummenhofer W, Herion H. Lightning accident with eight victims: case report and brief review of the literature. J Trauma 40:288–290, 1996.

76. Frayne JH, Gilligan RS. Neurological sequelae of lightning strike. Clin Exp Neurol 24:195–200, 1987.

77. Lynch MJG, Shorthouse PH. Injuries and death from lightning. Lancet 1:473–478, 1949.

78. Steinbaum S, Harviel JD, Jaffin JH, Jordan MH. Lightning strike to the head: case report. J Trauma 36:113–115, 1994.

79. Lopez RE, Holle RL. Demographics of lightning casualties. Semin Neurol 15:286–295, 1995.

80. Resnik BI, Wetli CV. Lichtenberg figures. Am J Forensic Med Pathol 17:99–102, 1996.

81. Cherington M. Central nervous system complications of lightning and electrical injuries. Semin Neurol 15:233–240, 1995.

82. Kotagal S, Rawlings CA, Chen SC, Burris G, Npuriouri S. Neurologic, psychiatric, and cardiovascular complications in children struck by lightning. Pediatrics 70:190–192, 1982.

83. Castrén JA, Kytilä J. Eye symptoms caused by lightning. Acta Ophthalmol (Kobenhavn) 42:139–143, 1964.

84. ten Duis HJ, Klasen HJ. Keraunoparalysis, a 'specific' lightning injury. Burns Incl Therm Inj 12:54–57, 1986.

85. Kleinschmidt-DeMasters BK. Neuropathology of lightning-strike injuries. Semin Neurol 15:323–328, 1995.

86. Stanley LD, Suss RA. Intracerebral hematoma secondary to lightning strike: case report and review of the literature. Neurosurgery 16:686–688, 1985.

87. Mann H, Kozic Z, Boulos MI. CT of lightning injury. AJNR Am J Neuroradiol 4:976–977, 1983.

88. Cherington M, Yarnell P, Hallmark D. MRI in lightning encephalopathy. Neurology 43:1437–1438, 1993.

89. Sharma M, Smith A. Paraplegia as a result of lightning injury. Br Med J 2:1464–1465, 1978.

90. Davidson GS, Deck JH. Delayed myelopathy following lightning strike: a demyelinating process. Acta Neuropathol 77:104–108, 1988.

91. Lehman LB. Successful management of an adult lightning victim using intracranial pressure monitoring. Neurosurgery 28:907–910, 1991.

92. Ghezzi KT. Lightning injuries. A unique treatment challenge. Postgrad Med 85:197–198; 201–203; 207–208, 1989.

93. Kandt RS, Rossitch JC, Trippett TM, Turlington KW, Rossitch E Jr, Oakes WJ. Intracranial pressure (ICP) monitoring as a guide to prognosis in a lightning-injured, comatose child. Childs Nerv Syst 4:370–372, 1988.

94. Norman ME, Younge BR. Association of high-dose intravenous methylprednisolone with reversal of blindness from lightning in two patients. Ophthalmology 106:743–745, 1999.

95. Fischbeck KH, Simon RP. Neurological manifestations of accidental hypothermia. Ann Neurol 10:384–387, 1981.

96. Niazi SA, Lewis FJ. Profound hypothermia in man: report of a case. Ann Surg 147:264–266, 1958.

97. Nozaki R, Ishibashi K, Adachi N, Nishihara S, Adachi S. Accidental profound hypothermia [letter]. N Engl J Med 315:1680, 1986.

98. Reuler JB. Hypothermia: pathophysiology, clinical settings, and management. Ann Intern Med 89:519–527, 1978.

99. Victor M, Adams RD, Collins GH. The Wernicke-Korsakoff Syndrome and Related Neurologic Disorders Due to Alcoholism and Malnutrition, 2nd ed. FA Davis, Philadelphia, 1989.

100. Reutens DC, Dunne JW, Gubbay SS. Triphasic waves in accidental hypothermia. Electroencephalogr Clin Neurophysiol 76:370–372, 1990.

101. Scott JW, McQueen D, Callahagn JC. The effect of lowered body temperature on the EEG [abstract]. Electroencephalogr Clin Neurophysiol 5:465, 1953.

102. Patel A, Getsos J. Images in clinical medicine. Osborn waves of hypothermia. N Engl J Med 330:680, 1994.

103. Farstad M, Andersen KS, Koller M, Grong K, Segadal L, Husby P. Rewarming from accidental hypothermia by extracorporeal circulation. A retrospective study. Eur J Cardiothorac Surg 20:58–64, 2001.

104. Walpoth BH, Walpoth-Aslan BN, Mattle HP, et al. Outcome of survivors of accidental deep hypothermia and circulatory arrest treated with extracorporeal blood warming. N Engl J Med 337:1500–1505, 1997.

105. Danzl DF, Hedges JR, Pozos RS. Hypothermia outcome score: development and implications. Crit Care Med 17:227–231, 1989.

106. Danzl DF, Pozos RS, Auerbach PS, et al. Multicenter hypothermia survey. Ann Emerg Med 16:1042–1055, 1987.

107. Schaller MD, Fischer AP, Perret CH. Hyperkalemia. A prognostic factor during acute severe hypothermia. JAMA 264:1842–1845, 1990.

108. Southwick FS, Dalglish PH Jr. Recovery after prolonged asystolic cardiac arrest in profound hypothermia. A case report and literature review. JAMA 243:1250–1253, 1980.

109. Gilbert M, Busund R, Skagseth A, Nilsen PA, Solbo JP. Resuscitation from accidental hypothermia of 13.7 degrees C with circulatory arrest [letter]. Lancet 355:375–376, 2000.

110. Salem SN. Neurological complications of heatstroke in Kuwait. Ann Trop Med Parasitol 60:393–400, 1966.

111. Austin MG, Berry JW. Observations on 100 cases of heatstroke. JAMA 161:1525–1529, 1956.

112. Gauss H, Meyer KA. Heat stroke: report of one hundred and fifty eight cases from Cook County Hospital, Chicago. Am J Med Sci 154:554–564, 1917.

113. Tucker LE, Stanford J, Graves B, Swetnam J, Hamburger S, Anwar A. Classical heatstroke: clinical and laboratory assessment. South Med J 78:20–25, 1985.

114. Sarnquist F, Larson CP Jr. Drug-induced heat stroke. Anesthesiology 39:348–350, 1973.

115. Dematte JE, O'Mara K, Buescher J, et al. Near-fatal heat stroke during the 1995 heat wave in Chicago. Ann Intern Med 129:173–181, 1998.

116. Freeman W, Dumoff SE. Cerebral syndrome following heat stroke. Arch Neurol Psychiatry 51:67–71, 1944.

117. McNamee T, Forsythe S, Wollmann R, Ndukwu IM. Central pontine myelinolysis in a patient with classic heat stroke [letter]. Arch Neurol 54:935–936, 1997.

118. Graham BS, Lichtenstein MJ, Hinson JM, Theil GB. Nonexertional heatstroke. Physiologic management and cooling in 14 patients. Arch Intern Med 146:87–90, 1986.

119. Vicario SJ, Okabajue R, Haltom T. Rapid cooling in classic heatstroke: effect on mortality rates. Am J Emerg Med 4:394–398, 1986.

120. Gaffin SL, Gardner JW, Flinn SD. Cooling methods for heatstroke victims [letter]. Ann Intern Med 132:678, 2000.

121. Bouchama A, Cafege A, Devol EB, Labdi O, el-Assil K, Seraj M. Ineffectiveness of dantrolene sodium in the treatment of heatstroke. Crit Care Med 19:176–180, 1991.

122. Yaqub BA, Al-Harthi SS, Al-Orainey IO, Laajam

MA, Obeid MT. Heat stroke at the Mekkah pilgrimage: clinical characteristics and course of 30 patients. Q J Med 59:523–530, 1986.

123. Mehta AC, Baker RN. Persistent neurological deficits in heat stroke. Neurology 20:336–340, 1970.

124. Slovis CM, Anderson GF, Casolaro A. Survival in a heat stroke victim with a core temperature in excess of 46.5 C. Ann Emerg Med 11:269–271, 1982.

125. Malamud N, Haymaker W, Custer RP. Heat stroke: a clinico-pathologic study of 125 fatal cases. Mil Surg 99:397–449, 1946.

126. Snider RS, Thomas W, Snider SR. Focal brain hyperthermia. I. The cerebellar cortex. Experientia. 34:479–481, 1978.

127. Fields AI. Near-drowning in the pediatric population. Crit Care Clin 8:113–129, 1992.

128. Modell JH. Drowning. N Engl J Med 328:253–256, 1993.

129. Modell JH, Graves SA, Ketover A. Clinical course of 91 consecutive near-drowning victims. Chest 70:231–238, 1976.

130. Orlowski JP. Drowning, near-drowning, and ice-water submersions. Pediatr Clin North Am 34:75–92, 1987.

131. Sarnaik AP, Preston G, Lieh-Lai M, Eisenbrey AB. Intracranial pressure and cerebral perfusion pressure in near-drowning. Crit Care Med 13:224–227, 1985.

132. Dean JM, McComb JG. Intracranial pressure monitoring in severe pediatric near-drowning. Neurosurgery 9:627–630, 1981.

133. Quan L, Wentz KR, Gore EJ, Copass MK. Outcome and predictors of outcome in pediatric submersion victims receiving prehospital care in King County, Washington. Pediatrics 86:586–593, 1990.

134. Causey AL, Tilelli JA, Swanson ME. Predicting discharge in uncomplicated near-drowning. Am J Emerg Med 18:9–11, 2000.

135. Bohn DJ, Biggar WD, Smith CR, Conn AW, Barker GA. Influence of hypothermia, barbiturate therapy, and intracranial pressure monitoring on morbidity and mortality after near-drowing. Crit Care Med 14:529–534, 1986.

Chapter 17

NEUROLOGIC COMPLICATIONS OF MULTISYSTEM TRAUMA

Patients with multiple injuries are often admitted to designated surgical or trauma units, mostly because many have had early hemodynamic deterioration or have become hypoxic from direct chest or airway trauma.

In this hectic environment, cranial computed tomography (CT) scanning to detect brain injury in need of neurosurgical intervention may not seem to have priority over surgical stabilization of the patient. Decreased level of consciousness that initially appears as a direct result of hypoxemia, hypercapnia, or shock should be reassessed after resuscitation and stabilization. The threshold for additional neuroimaging should be low, particularly if the level of responsiveness does not improve within reasonable time.[1] Failure to recognize and treat head or spine injury early may have devastating consequences for neurologic outcome.

Adequate oxygenation, rapid correction of hypotension, and treatment of increased intracranial pressure are all hallmarks of emergency management, with the ultimate goal being to prevent secondary brain damage in a patient with a recently injured and vulnerable brain. These concerns are not trivial. Even transfer from the emergency room to the intensive care unit may increase the likelihood of insult from hypoxia, hypotension, or surges of increased intracranial pressure.[2] To improve the odds, appropriate triage to hospitals with neurologic or neurosurgical intensive care facilities should follow after major trauma. This determination starts at field transport with the choice between trauma center and rural hospital.[3]

The major focus of this chapter is the discussion of priorities of evaluation and management guidelines in patients with intracranial and spinal injuries. Specific neurosurgical and orthopedic interventions for spine injury are not addressed. At least in one survey, there appears to be a tendency for neurosurgeons to relegate care of patients with polytrauma to other services,[4] but for these patients with very complex disorders, trauma surgeons, neurosurgeons, and consulting neurologists should work collaboratively.

CLINICAL SPECTRUM OF HEAD INJURY

Reduced level of consciousness remains the predominant clinical feature in many patients with diffuse head injury and is best expressed in the Glasgow coma scale score (Chapter 1). The depth of coma is determined by the severity of axonal injury, which may involve bilateral hemorrhagic contusions (Plate 17–1) and even a primary brain stem lesion. Primary injury to the brain stem after trauma is considered a rare cause of coma. Many victims have additional injury at the hemispheric interface of gray matter and white matter or significant mass effect causing secondary damage to the brain stem from the effects of herniation. However, in a recent animal study, severity of coma was linked to primary axonal damage to the brain stem.[5]

In most centers, multitraumatized patients are young athletic men in coma (Glasgow coma sum score of 8 or less) with reactive pupils but with hypoxemia or shock in 10% to 20%.[7,8] In these patients with traumatic brain injury, eye opening to voice or pain and the range of motor responses and, less helpful, verbal responses (due to emergency intubation) are important initial guides to severity of the impact. An immediately present fixed and enlarged pupil from a third cranial nerve lesion invariably indicates an extracranial compressing hematoma, but a traumatic lesion in the mesencephalon or a unilateral orbital compartment syndrome (orbital blowout), often with proptosis and a "frozen globe," produce similar findings.[6–8]

Facial trauma and lacerations are common and need specific attention by a plastic surgeon. The development of "raccoon eyes" indicates basal skull fracture or fractures of the orbit or zygoma (Fig. 17–1). Retroauricular hematoma ("battle sign") is indicative of a petrosal fracture. Cerebral herniation syndromes are not expected at presentation (Chapter 1) but may emerge rapidly, almost always prompting evacuation of an enlarging hemorrhagic contusion or epidural or subdural hematoma. Dysautonomic features, such as tachycardia, tachypnea, and profuse sweating in brief periods, have been noted in very severe forms of cranial injury.[9] In less severe head injury, post-traumatic confusion (previously called "post-traumatic amnesia," or "PTA")[10] characterized by lack of attention, vigilant restlessness, and profound inability to memorize is common.

PATHOPHYSIOLOGIC MECHANISMS

Diffuse traumatic brain injury predominantly damages axons. The degree of destruction most likely depends on the force of impact.

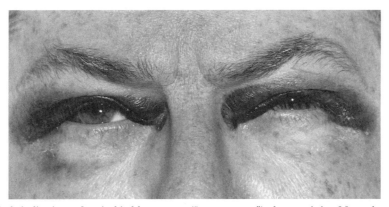

Figure 17–1. Early indications of periorbital hematoma ("raccoon eyes") characteristic of frontobasal trauma.

Separating the effects of a direct insult from secondary effects remains challenging, and primary injury was uncommon in neuropathologic studies from a trauma center in Glasgow.[11] Fragmentation of axons by mechanical shear, disconnection, and increase in axonal diameter lead to pathologically recognizable axonal bulbs. The process of axonotomy is preferentially localized in subcortical parasagittal areas, corpus callosum, and internal capsules but may also involve cerebellar folia and brain stem tracts. The process of axonotomy is time locked. Earlier changes are fixed, although recovery may occur. Protracted changes (secondary axotomy) include disorganization of the cell organization and skeleton, which progressively leads to reduced axonal transport. Loss of microtubules may be one of the main reasons for increased calcium and calcium-specific neutral proteases. Axon swelling occurs, setting the stage for apoptosis. Other pathways that lead to destruction may involve free radical and lipid peroxidation, but the clinical relevance is not known, and findings in the first clinical trials using scavengers were basically negative.[12,13] Two recent trials of the effect of drugs (tirilazad mesylate and antioxidant polyethylene glycol-conjugated superoxide dismutase) on one of these mechanisms, lipid peroxidation, were unsuccessful[12,14] (Fig. 17–2).

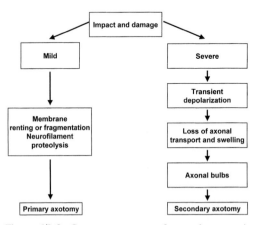

Figure 17–2. Current concepts of axonal traumatic brain injury. (Modified from Maxwell WL, Povlishock JT, Graham DL. A mechanistic analysis of nondisruptive axonal injury: a review. J Neurotrauma 14:419–440, 1997. By permission of Mary Ann Liebert Publishers.)

NEURORADIOLOGIC FINDINGS IN HEAD INJURY

After stabilization of airway, circulation, and fractures, head CT scanning is a logical next step in patients with severe trauma. Some physicians have the need for CT scanning, depending on the level of responsiveness and the type of trauma. It should be strongly argued, however, that any patient with multiple trauma or major forceful impact to the head should undergo baseline head CT scanning with additional bone-setting views. In addition, failure to obtain a CT scan of the brain in a patient with multitrauma may have medicolegal consequences.

Predictive factors for intracerebral hematomas have been identified that may guide trauma surgeons to assess the need for emergency CT scanning. These predictors are age (with a notable increase in incidence after the fourth decade), injury from fall, Glasgow coma scale sum score of less than 8 on admission, pupillary inequality, and skull fracture[15] but not unilateral or bilateral fixed pupils, trauma to multiple organs, and alcohol intoxication.[15] Computed tomography scanning may detect abnormalities that could determine management in the first hours.[1] Certain radiologic findings[16] may signal a potential for rapid neurologic deterioration[17] in, for example, patients with epidural hematomas of mixed density (suggesting continuing hemorrhage), posterior fossa epidural hematomas, subdural hematoma with mass effect, or temporal lobe or bilateral frontal lobe contusions.

Generally, the traumatic lesions that can be demonstrated on CT can be divided into diffuse axonal injury with edema, intracerebral hematoma, or a combination. Multiple lesions are common with severe head injury (Fig. 17–3), but the CT scan can be initially normal in 50% of patients admitted comatose to an emergency department. Magnetic resonance imaging (MRI), as expected, has a higher sensitivity than conventional CT, but it is not an easily available first diagnostic test in patients with acute multiple injuries.[18–24] Prospective MRI studies have demonstrated a higher incidence of intra-axial lesions and parenchymal lesions not seen on initial CT scans, but CT remains superior

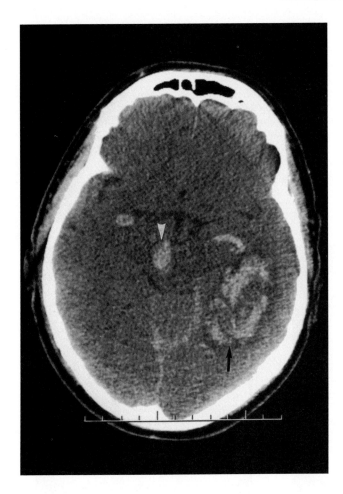

Figure 17–3. Multiple contusions, including hematoma in the left posterior temporal lobe (arrow) and a midbrain hemorrhage (arrowhead).

in demonstration of hemorrhagic lesions in the first days of trauma.[25] The most pertinent features of a proposed classification system of CT scanning in diffuse head injury are summarized in Table 17–1.[26]

Diffuse Axonal Injury

The main features of diffuse axonal injury are multiple small hemorrhagic shear lesions. Cerebral edema associated with loss of visibility of the mesencephalic and suprasellar cisterns may emerge.

Frequently found on CT scan in patients with diffuse closed head injury are small tissue-tear hemorrhages, or so-called shear lesions.[27,28] They are commonly seen at the frontal cortex and white matter interface, basal ganglia, thalamus, and internal cap-

sule. Shearing abnormalities of the corpus callosum are often associated with small lesions in the thalamus, splenium, or septum pellucidum, consistent with a fronto-occipital direction of acceleration (Fig. 17–4). Subarachnoid or intraventricular blood is noted in up to 50% of the patients.[29] Shearing injuries in multiple sites do not necessarily imply a poor outcome. Localization in both the corpus callosum and the interpeduncular midbrain, however, has been singled out as an MRI or a CT scan marker of poor outcome (Fig. 17–5) (see Chapter 19).

Isolated shearing injury in the midbrain caused by sudden displacement in the sagittal plane from a frontal or occipital impact ruptures the perforating arteries to the midbrain.[30] If shearing injury is not present in other locations, good neurologic outcome can be expected.[31] It is important to differ-

Table 17–1. Computed Tomography (CT) Classification of Diffuse Brain Injury

Category	Definition
I	No visible intracranial disease on CT scan
II	Cisterns present Midline shift of 0 to 5 mm or lesion density, or both No high- or mixed-density lesion >25 mL May include bone fragments and foreign bodies
III	Cisterns compressed or absent Midline shift of 0 to 5 mm No high- or mixed-density lesion >25 mL
IV	Midline shift >5 mm No high- or mixed-density lesion >25 mL

Modified from Marshall et al.[26] By permission of the American Association of Neurological Surgeons.

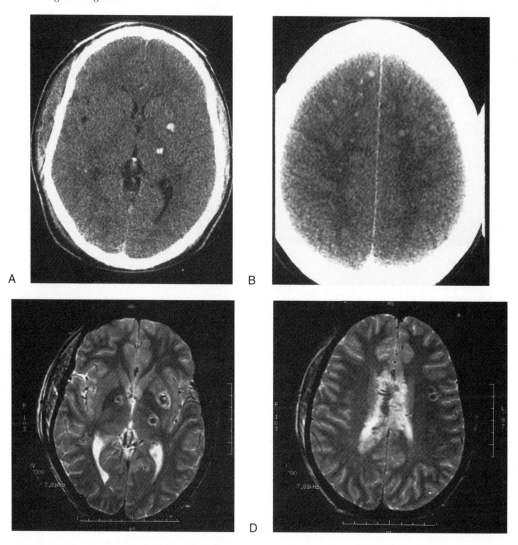

Figure 17–4. Multiple focal areas of hemorrhage corresponding to shear lesions on computed tomography scan images (*A,B*) and magnetic resonance images (*C,D*) in a comatose patient with extensor posturing after a fall from a horse. Note extensive soft tissue swelling overlying the right frontal calvaria, corresponding to the site of impact.

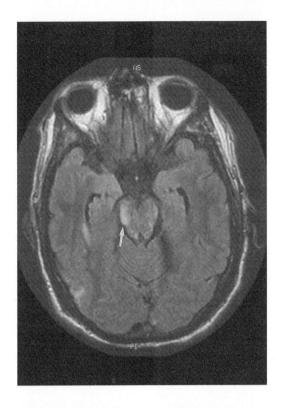

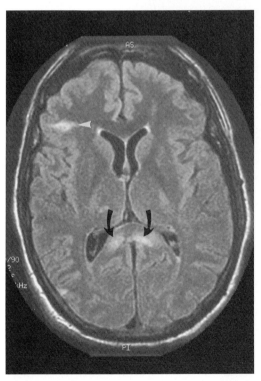

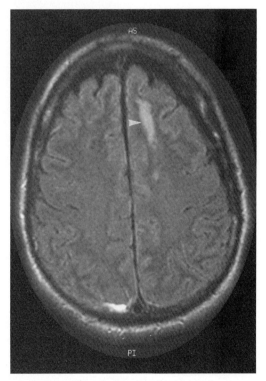

Figure 17–5. Diffuse axonal brain injury. Magnetic resonance imaging with fluid-attenuated inversion recovery shows lesions in the splenium of the corpus callosum (curved arrows), lateral midbrain (arrow), and subcortical white matter (arrowheads).

307

entiate these punctate midbrain lesions from larger acute traumatic midbrain hemorrhages, which carry a more dismal outcome. Acute traumatic midbrain hemorrhages may occur as a primary event, causing damage that occupies the ventral rim of the aqueduct to the interpeduncular fossa and extends inferiorly to the pontomesencephalic junction.[32] They often have a stellate configuration.

Traumatic Intracerebral Hematomas

Most traumatic parenchymal lesions are located in the frontal and temporal lobes. Bilateral frontal contusions are associated with a significant risk of further deterioration from massive edema and brain stem compression in the anteroposterior direction[33] (Fig. 17–6). Because of proximity to the brain stem, temporal lobe hematomas or hematomas in temporoparietal locations also increase the risk of clinical deterioration.[34] Mass effect needs to be assessed and can be a reason for early evacuation or placement of an intracranial pressure monitor. The signs are displacement of the septum pellucidum or pineal gland (>1 cm), unilateral widening of the prepontine or perimesencephalic cistern from horizontal displacement or rotation of the brain stem, and development of obstructive hydrocephalus.

Basal ganglia hemorrhages and hemorrhage in the corpus callosum[35] are traumatic hemorrhages that have been associated with shearing of midsized cerebral blood vessels. Basal ganglia hemorrhages are rare (3% in two large series) and indicate diffuse axonal and tissue shear injury.[36–39] Traumatic basal ganglia hemorrhage may be differentiated from spontaneous basal ganglia hemorrhage by its preferred location in the lenticulate

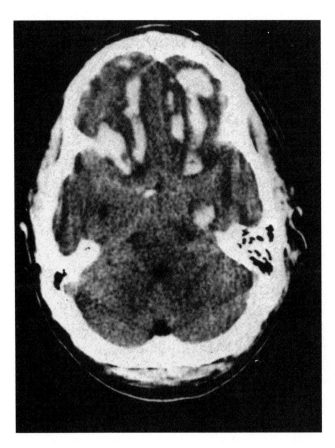

Figure 17–6. Bilateral frontal lobe contusions.

nucleus and external capsule. High-velocity trauma may rupture the lenticulostriate or anterior choroidal branches. These unusual traumatic hemorrhages are seldom isolated CT scan findings, and intraventricular, subarachnoid, or contrecoup hemorrhages are frequent. These basal ganglia hematoma are commonly documented in young patients (in Boto and associates' series,[40] the mean age was 28 years), may have a delayed presentation on CT, may enlarge, and may need evacuation if intracranial pressure is not controlled. Outcome, despite surgery, remains very poor[40] and is related to the existence of additional lesions.[36–39]

Traumatic intraventricular hematomas[41,42] are often seen in association with multiple parenchymal lesions, but rupture of subependymal veins due to pressure change from impact or a tear in the tela choroidea[43] may explain the primary location in the ventricles.

Admission CT scanning may not identify mixed-density lesions or intracerebral hematomas in patients with major head injury ("one CT in head injury is no CT"). Delayed traumatic intracerebral hematomas may occur after an initial normal CT scan, but often, an earlier hint of intracerebral hemor-

rhagic contusion is found on the initial CT scan, justifying repeat scanning within 24 hr in any such circumstance. Sudden deterioration from large intracerebral hematomas has been noted in patients with initial CT scans that showed a depressed skull fracture and small midline subdural hematoma.[44] Delayed intracerebral hematomas mostly occur in patients with initial neurologic impairment, but 20% of patients may be alert. In a series of 656 patients, 9 with delayed intracerebral hematoma were identified 8 hr to 13 days after the impact (average, within 2 days).[45,46]

Subdural or Epidural Hematoma

Subdural hematoma is easily recognized by a concave hyperdense mass on CT causing compression of sulci, white matter, and ventricles and a shift in position when size is substantial (Fig. 17–7). Computed tomography scanning may occasionally show isodense subdural hematoma in the acute phase, frequently associated with anemia (hemoglobin concentration <10 g/dL) or disseminated intravascular coagulation.[47]

Epidural hematoma is associated with a

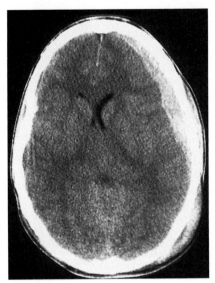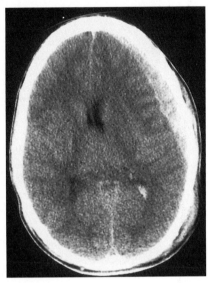

Figure 17–7. Computed tomography scan images of a left frontal and parietal subdural hematoma with associated mass effect and shift.

skull fracture and has a lentiform shape. Its mass effect is profound (Fig. 17–8). Another consistent warning radiologic sign is a radiolucent region within the denser clot, probably an indication of active bleeding.[48,49] Other, more obvious, warning signs are depressed level of consciousness, volume of hematoma, and midline shift.[48]

Another potentially dangerous location is the posterior fossa.[50,51] A traumatic hematoma in this small, contained compartment may produce rapid and at times abrupt clinical deterioration. An extradural infratentorial hematoma is most likely due to bleeding from the transverse sinus. In most cases, suboccipital craniectomy is needed because of life-threatening brain stem compression. Delayed epidural hemorrhage has been noted in patients hypotensive from multiple trauma whose condition deteriorated after correction of hypotension,[52–58] and increased blood pressure may have reopened the sealing arterial clot (Fig. 17–9).

GENERAL PRINCIPLES OF MANAGEMENT

Skull and basal skull fractures pose difficult management problems. Conservative treatment of closed skull fractures[59,60] is standard care for many neurosurgeons. Compound skull fractures generally undergo exploration, debridement, and dura mater repair. The risk of epilepsy (up to 60%) is increased when the post-traumatic confusional stage lasts more than 24 hr and a dural tear is present. Clearly, antiepileptic drugs (phenytoin, 300 mg in three divided doses) should be considered when these predictive factors are present.[61]

Cerebrospinal fluid fistulas are estimated to occur in 5% to 10% of basal skull fractures. Rhinorrhea is most likely to occur immediately after the impact and can be confirmed by glucose determination or detection of beta$_2$-transferrin and tau fractions in the cerebrospinal fluid.[62,63] The risk of

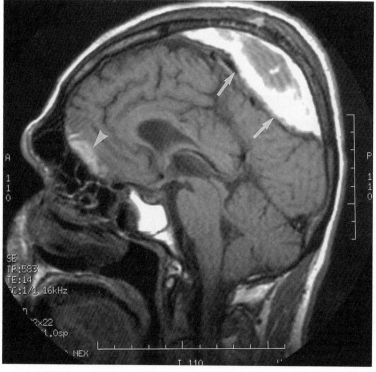

Figure 17–8. Sagittal T1-weighted magnetic resonance image showing the dramatic effects of epidural hematoma (arrows) and contrecoup frontal contusion (arrowhead).

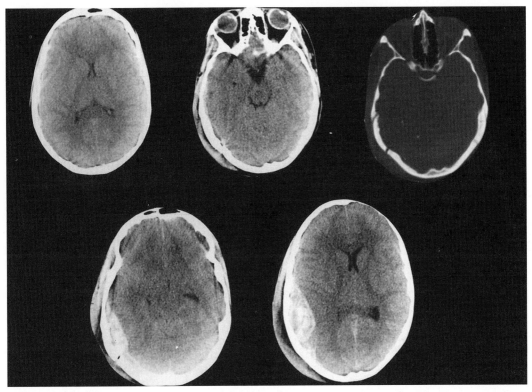

Figure 17–9. A series of computed tomography images in a patient with multiple facial injuries shows small epidural hematoma and associated skull fracture. Repeated scan confirmed a marked increase in the volume of the epidural hematoma, corresponding to sudden development of dilated fixed pupils observed during surgical repair of facial lacerations. Outcome was excellent after evacuation of the epidural hematoma.

bacterial meningitis from cerebrospinal fluid fistulas is low, and antibiotic prophylaxis is not indicated. If rhinorrhea persists, surgical repair is indicated.

Evidence-based guidelines for medical management have been published, and most trauma centers adhere to them.[7,64] Patients with multitrauma often receive large volumes of fluids. Uncontrolled fluid resuscitation may lead to massive fluid intakes and may theoretically exacerbate cerebral edema. Little is known about the ideal fluid balance in patients with severe head injuries, but there is a consensus that patients with head injury should be kept normovolemic, and free water should be restricted.

Blood pressure is very often increased as part of an adrenergic stress response with outpouring of catecholamines.[65] Guidelines for appropriate blood pressure levels are not available, because no study has addressed the effect of antihypertensive agents on cerebral perfusion pressure and outcome in severe head injury. Sedation is probably more effective than treatment with antihypertensive medication. For patients with persistent hypertension with evolving clinical signs of left ventricular failure or pulmonary edema (rales, third heart sound, or pulse deficit), a bolus of labetalol (20 mg intravenously; maximum of 300 mg) is advised. The intent is to produce a 25% decrease in mean arterial pressure below baseline, usually keeping mean arterial blood pressure below 120 mm Hg. At this juncture, intracranial pressure monitoring is needed to obtain intracranial pressure readings and to calculate cerebral perfusion pressure (cerebral perfusion pressure = mean arterial pressure − intracranial pressure). Reduction in mean arterial blood pressure should not result in a cerebral perfusion pressure of less than 70 mm Hg.

One trauma group recommends artificial increase of blood pressure to maintain cerebral perfusion pressure at 70 mm Hg or more and an emphasis on intracranial pressure.[66] A recent experimental study could not document improvement of cerebral blood flow by phenylephrine or attenuation of brain edema[67] but showed worsening neurologic deficit with phenylephrine or large volumes of saline, seriously undermining the theory that pharmacologically increased blood pressure has a favorable effect on cerebral perfusion.

Use of antiepileptic drugs is controversial, but administration of phenytoin aiming at a high therapeutic dosage range decreases the incidence of post-traumatic seizures, although its effect is noticeable only during the first week.[68] Antiepileptic therapy can be discontinued if no seizures have occurred from the time of impact until the first 2 to 3 weeks of hospital admission.

Normothermia should remain the primary goal. The effects of hypothermia are uncertain and probably minimal. Hypothermia can be induced and maintained with cooling blankets and propofol (maximum of 50 $\mu g/kg$ per minute) or atracurium (infusion of 5 $\mu g/kg$ per minute) to prevent shivering. A prospective randomized trial by Marion and co-investigators[69] suggested improved outcome at 3 and 6 months in comatose patients (Glasgow coma scale score, 5 to 7) treated with hypothermia, but none of the differences persisted at 1 year. Small single-center randomized studies confirmed these results, but the recently completed multicenter study in 392 patients (National Acute Brain Injury Study) had negative findings. Moderate hypothermia (approximately 33°C) did not have a significant effect on outcome in trauma patients but appeared beneficial in patients who were hypothermic (<35°C) at presentation. Medical complications were significantly worse in all patients older than 45 years. With current data, maintenance of normothermia (less than 37°C) and no rewarming in younger patients with hypothermia at presentation seem reasonable.[70,71] Whether hypothermia (moderate, 33°C to 35°C) could be effective in certain subpopulations in head injury remains inconclusive.

Nutrition in head-injured patients is not easily managed. The demand is high, many patients are hypercatabolic, gastric emptying is disturbed, and enteral feeding is cumbersome.[72,73] However, a recent trial comparing early versus late enteral feeding did not document differences in length of stay or infection rate.[74] In addition, full-strength, full-rate feedings are poorly tolerated in the first week. In patients with prolonged intolerance, a feeding tube should be placed in the jejunum.[75] Administration of low-residual, high-caloric, high-protein commercial enriched mixtures delivered continuously by a volumetric feeding pump should be initiated.[73] If this therapy is unsuccessful, total parenteral nutrition is indicated, because starvation decreases alertness and subsequently increases the risk of aspiration and decreases the ability to fend off nosocomial infections.

A contestable issue is management of hyperglycemia (>200 mg/dL), which is considered a result of a stress-induced increase in cortisol and catecholamines. Hyperglycemia may be beneficial to a traumatized brain with increased utilization of glucose.[76] On the other hand, fasting conditions in gerbils exposed to ischemia increased heat shock proteins (which have a neuroprotective role), which were absent under normoglycemic or hyperglycemic conditions.[77] Early hyperglycemia may also lead to excessive accumulation of lactate, facilitating tissue acidosis and secondary damage. Poor outcome is related to hyperglycemia, but the effect of manipulation of serum glucose is not known. Most trauma centers monitor blood glucose carefully and treat hyperglycemia with insulin sliding scale regimens.[78]

MANAGEMENT OF INCREASED INTRACRANIAL PRESSURE

Guidelines for placement of intracranial pressure monitoring devices are summarized in Table 17–2, but the indications may differ in various centers. Placement of a parenchymal monitoring device should be strongly considered in any patient with a motor response less than localizing or a CT scan with the absence of basal cisterns, intraventricular or subarachnoid blood, and an intracerebral hematoma. Other trauma cen-

Table 17–2. Guidelines for Intracranial Pressure (ICP) Monitoring in Patients with Multisystem Trauma and Head Injury

- Glasgow coma score ≤8
- Need for prolonged sedation and neuromuscular paralysis (such as mechanical ventilation for adult respiratory distress syndrome or lung contusion)
- Computed tomography scan abnormalities indicating increased ICP:
  Any hemorrhagic contusion with shift of the pineal gland from midline
  Bifrontal and temporal lobe contusion
  Intraventricular and subarachnoid hemorrhage
  Absence of ambient cisterns or narrowing of third ventricle due to diffuse
      brain edema

ters use Glasgow coma sum scores of 8 or less as the only cutoff point to decide whether such a device should be placed. Fiberoptic systems in which the probe is placed directly into the white matter are currently used[79,80] (Fig. 17–10). Infectious complications and intracerebral hematoma at the site of placement are rare, but contamination may occur with *Staphylococcus epidermidis,* and intracranial hematomas may develop in patients with a coagulopathy (15% of 108 insertions).[81] An important drift in intracranial pressure readings can be expected only after 5 days of placement, but intracranial pressure monitoring is often no longer indicated at that time.

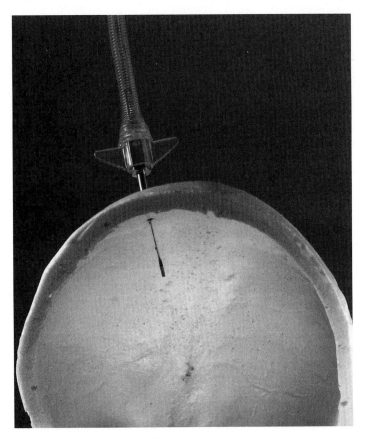

Figure 17–10. Fiberoptic device for parenchymal monitoring of intracranial pressure is shown in demonstration model (Camino Laboratories).

Increased intracranial pressure is defined as readings higher than 15 mm Hg on several occasions. Current recommendations call for immediate reduction of intracranial pressure to <20 mm Hg and maintaining cerebral perfusion pressure at >60 mm Hg. A recent post hoc analysis of 427 patients with head injury who had careful monitoring of intracranial pressure could not find any evidence that management of cerebral perfusion pressure alone influences outcome and stressed aggressive management of intracranial pressure.[82] Treatment of increased intracranial pressure should focus on the recognition of common triggers first.

Combative behavior and patient intolerance of mechanical ventilation can be counteracted by sedation, preferably with short-acting sedatives (for example, propofol, infusion of 0.3 to 0.6 mg/kg per hour) or opioids (for example, morphine, 1 to 3 mg/hr). In patients with extreme agitation and profuse sweating, neuromuscular blockade and morphine are needed occasionally to maximize oxygen delivery. Positive end-expiratory pressure mode is often necessary to ensure adequate oxygenation in patients with additional lung trauma. Positive end-expiratory pressure of <10 cm H_2O does not significantly raise intracranial pressure. Decreased lung compliance in these patients with acute lung concussion or flail chest most likely prevents transmural conductance of airway pressure to the right atrium and eventually to the cerebral venous system.[83] Endotracheal suctioning may cause important increases in intracranial pressure. These marked increases cannot be ameliorated by simple hyperoxygenation.[84] Patients with marked increases in intracranial pressure after endotracheal suctioning should receive lidocaine, 1 mg/kg, or thiopental, 0.5 to 1 mg/kg, intravenously to blunt this response. In addition, the number of suction passes should be limited to one.[84,85]

Patients with head injury should have elevation of the head to 30° in neutral position, although in some patients intracranial pressure may not change or may paradoxically increase.[86] For this reason, it is prudent to determine which position optimizes cerebral perfusion pressure in an individual patient rather than to use head elevation indiscriminately. Hydrostatic displacement of the cerebrospinal fluid from the cranial cavity to the spinal space and facilitation of venous outflow are the most likely mechanisms for decrease of intracranial pressure after head elevation.[87] After cervical spine injury is excluded with flexion and extension X-ray views, a rigid collar should be removed because it may also contribute to venous congestion.[88]

One treatment for control of increased intracranial pressure is to induce cerebral vasoconstriction and reduce cerebral blood volume by hyperventilation, with a goal of Pa_{CO_2} in the low 30s.[80,89] Experimental data suggest, however, that the effect on cerebrospinal fluid pH and ultimately vessel diameter is brief and is attenuated after 6 hr. When hyperventilation is the only mode of treatment (for example, in patients with severe renal failure), addition of tromethamine (THAM) (0.3 M at a rate of 1 mL/kg per hour)[90] can be considered. A randomized study with tromethamine found that fluctuations in intracranial pressure could be controlled, but outcome in head injury was not significantly improved.[90] There is no rationale for prophylactic hyperventilation in the first 24 hr after head injury, and there is preliminary evidence that a decreased vasoreactivity to Pa_{CO_2} changes exists on the first injury day.[91] In addition, prolonged hyperventilation (Pa_{CO_2} <25 mm Hg) in head injury in the absence of increased intracranial pressure should be avoided, and evidence suggests a higher incidence of poor outcome.[92]

Treatment with osmotic agents remains the cornerstone of intracranial pressure reduction,[80,89,93] aiming at serum osmolality of 310 to 320 mOsm/L. This can be readily achieved with mannitol in a starting dose of 0.25 to 2 g/kg. Plasma osmolality of >325 mOsm/L results in renal failure. Reduction of intracranial pressure can be expected 20 min after a bolus, and the first-pass effect may last 6 hr. A difference of <10 mOsm/kg between measured and calculated osmolality, determined as follows:

$$2[Na^+] + \frac{[glucose]}{18} + \frac{[blood\ urea\ nitrogen]}{2.8}$$

should indicate the need for an additional bolus of mannitol. A rebound effect of mannitol is seldom encountered. In one study, a rebound was demonstrated in only 12% of 65 patients and did not occur more often in patients treated with higher doses or faster infusion rates.[94]

Lack of response to treatment with the maximal dose of mannitol (2 g/kg) and no new CT scan findings other than diffuse abnormalities or cerebral edema may be followed by a more aggressive (but also potentially harmful) treatment. Hypertonic saline (23.4%) can be added and may have a more profound effect. Hypertonic saline 3% is as successful as mannitol (50 mL in 10 min).[95] Barbiturates (loading dose of pentobarbital, 10 to 20 mg/kg; maintenance dose, 1 to 3 mg/kg per hour) can be considered next, but only 50% of patients with refractory increased intracranial pressure have a response to high-dose barbiturate therapy. It reduces cerebral blood flow due to reduced cerebral metabolism, physiologic functions that are closely linked. Vasoconstriction may not be the main effect. No clinical study with barbiturates in head injury has demonstrated improved outcome. Moreover, it is not clear, but is particularly concerning, whether treatment with pentobarbital increases the number of patients with severe disability and vegetative state whose course otherwise would have been rapid deterioration to brain death.

Barbiturate treatment has significant complications. Hypotension occurred in 50% of 38 patients with severe trauma.[96] Other frequent complications were hypokalemia, hepatic and renal dysfunction, and sepsis. Barbiturates may depress lung mucociliary clearance[97] and therefore may account for an increased risk of nosocomial pulmonary infections.[98,99] Nonetheless, many neurosurgeons understandably feel compelled to use aggressive treatment with barbiturates as the last resort in young patients with head injury.

Propofol has emerged as an alternative agent for sedation and control of intracranial pressure.[100–102] A small randomized, prospective trial of propofol found an important benefit over morphine with better control of sedation.[103] Lower doses (initial infusion of 5 μg/kg per minute) may result in sedation only, and much higher doses (6 to 12 mg/kg per hour) may be needed to decrease intracranial pressure, often resulting in additional hypotension and bradycardia. Patients can be periodically assessed neurologically with propofol, an advantage that is virtually eliminated by use of barbiturates with half-lives of at least 48 hr. Interest in decompressive surgery to control brain swelling (large bifrontal craniectomy with fascial graft) as a last resort was rekindled after a report of "surprisingly good" outcomes, but evidence of properly designed trials or even cohorts is lacking.[104]

A recent report from the Cochrane database collecting evidence of therapies such as hyperventilation, mannitol, cerebrospinal fluid drainage, barbiturates, and corticosteroids concluded that the current studies were too small to support or refute any of these therapies[105,106] (Fig. 17–11). It remains a tour de force to organize such trials.

MANAGEMENT OF TRAUMATIC INTRACRANIAL HEMATOMAS

Options for trauma unit management of intracranial hematomas are presented in this section. Typically, early surgical management influences survival. A major treatment dilemma occurs when a small extracranial hematoma without appreciable shift is found.

Epidural Hematoma

It has been estimated that of the total population of patients with head injury admitted to emergency departments, 3% to 5% have epidural hematoma.[7,64] The clinical presentation is typically dramatic, with rapid onset of coma. The pupil ipsilateral to the epidural hematoma dilates and becomes fixed to light, and lack of reactivity soon follows in the opposite pupil because of direct compression, traction, or compression of the opposite oculomotor nerve against the clivus.

It has been argued whether an exploratory bur hole should be drilled before a CT scan is performed. Andrews and associates[107] reported, in a large series, that 86% of extradural hematomas could be localized by an ipsilateral bur hole. A contralateral epidural or subdural hematoma was found in 2 of

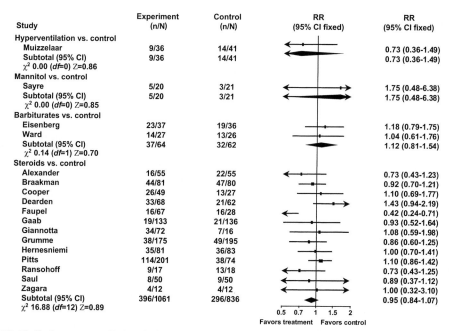

Figure 17–11. Cochrane controlled trials database. CI, confidence interval; RR, relative risk. (From Roberts I, Schierhout G, Alderson P. Absence of evidence for the effectiveness of five interventions routinely used in the intensive care management of severe head injury: a systematic review. J Neurol Neurosurg Psychiatry 65:729–733, 1998. By permission of the journal.)

56 explorations. In 33 patients, "complete" bur hole exploration (bilateral temporal, frontal, and parietal bur holes) produced negative findings. Both poor outcome and the 44% negative rate with bur hole exploration in these patients make this heroic procedure difficult to justify. In most patients, there should be enough time for a CT scan, and acquisition time is now a matter of minutes. Immediate surgical exploration at the site of pupil enlargement or skull fracture may occasionally be considered in patients with rapid loss of brain stem reflexes in the emergency department if a CT scan suite is not nearby.

Acute bilateral epidural hematomas are infrequent,[108] representing approximately 15% of all epidural hematomas. Mortality is high, usually because major trauma is needed to produce bilateral epidural hematomas. However, one report found that in patients with bilateral frontal epidural hematoma, the chance of good recovery was relatively high (60%).[109] Posterior fossa epidural hematomas are rare and seldom associated with concomitant supratentorial

contusion; outcome is excellent after immediate surgical intervention, with low mortality (12% to 18%).[110–112]

An important controversial issue is the management of small epidural hematomas that do not produce appreciable clinical signs. Knuckey and associates[49] attempted prospective medical management in 22 patients with small epidural hematomas seen within several hours after trauma. Patients with associated skull fractures that traversed the arteria meningea media or major dural vessels, such as the transverse sinus, had a 1 in 2 chance of delayed expansion requiring surgical intervention. Almost two-thirds of these patients did not have clinical deterioration in the course of conservative management. Conservative management of asymptomatic epidural hematomas may be appropriate except when CT scans show a volume of >30 mL, thickness of >15 mm, and a midline shift beyond 5 mm.[113]

Mortality in patients with epidural hematomas is extremely variable in large series, ranging from 20% to 55%. It is intuitively obvious that mortality from epidural hematoma is related to the Glasgow coma scale score before evacuation. Two-thirds of patients with an epidural hematoma and Glasgow motor score of 3 or less die or remain in a vegetative state.[114] Prognosis for good recovery is worse in patients with an associated intracerebral contusion. Good outcome can be expected in patients who have withdrawal to pain before surgical evacuation.

Subdural Hematoma

Patients with an acute subdural hematoma due to ruptured bridging veins from trauma generally present with Glasgow coma scale scores of less than 7.[115] In 7% of patients, an associated cerebral contusion is found, and outcome is presumably related to diffuse head injury rather than to the effect of brain shift alone.[116]

Interhemispheric location of subdural hematomas has been described, and conservative treatment can be considered in asymptomatic patients, particularly those with maximal Glasgow coma scale scores.[117,118] Delayed subdural hematomas are less common than epidural hematomas[119,120] and may also occur after removal of a contralateral epidural hematoma from release of its tamponade effect.[121–123]

The initial management of traumatic acute subdural hematoma may remain conservative if the thickness of the hematoma is similar to the skull bone thickness on CT scan and no midline shift is noted.[124] A discrepancy of low Glasgow coma scale scores in patients with small subdural hematomas may be attributed to additional post-traumatic lesions prone to become visible on repeat CT scans or to alcohol, drugs, or systemic factors. Therefore, it is prudent to wait and act only in case of enlargement associated with clinical deterioration. With further liquefaction over time, bur holes may be sufficient.

Acute subdural hematoma remains associated with high mortality, particularly in the elderly.[125–127] A large study of acute subdural hematomas found that old age (defined as older than 65 years) quadrupled the mortality rate.[128] None of these elderly patients with Glasgow coma scale scores of less than 13 had independent function after surgical evacuation. A later study[115] of 101 patients

with acute subdural hematomas noted a mortality of 66% and 19% functional recovery. Poor predictors for outcome were age older than 65 years, admission Glasgow coma scale score of 3 or 4, and postoperative intracranial pressure >45 mm Hg.

Intraparenchymal Hematoma

Multiple contusions are common in traumatic head injury. Large contusions on CT scan are prone to cause deterioration and thus are best handled by neurosurgical evacuation.[129] Frontal and temporal hematomas should be removed, with additional lobe resection when the location is the nondominant hemisphere. Hematomas in the deep white matter are treated medically in many large trauma centers. The management of a patient with a small intracerebral hematoma and minimal neurologic deficit is conservative, but as mentioned previously, intracranial pressure monitoring should be used in frontal and temporal lobe localizations, and sudden sustained elevation of intracranial pressure may indicate enlargement and prompt evacuation.[130]

MANAGEMENT OF TRAUMATIC CEREBRAL ANEURYSM

An arterial lesion that develops into a false aneurysm is a possibility with severe blunt or penetrating trauma to the brain.[131–134] The initial effect of trauma may seem minor, with insignificant facial lacerations or none at all. The pericallosal artery is most commonly affected because it is adjacent to the free edge of the falx cerebri. Commonly, the lesion is detected incidentally, but deterioration may occur from a newly developing frontal hematoma up to 9 weeks after the injury. Traumatic pericallosal aneurysms form because of damage to the wall, intramural hematoma, and outpouching in the ensuing weeks. The aneurysm is peripherally located (not at the branching point as in berry aneurysms) and should be surgically occluded to reduce rebleeding. In patients with a delayed hematoma, often in retrospect blood is found in the interhemispheric fissure on CT scan (Fig. 17–12).

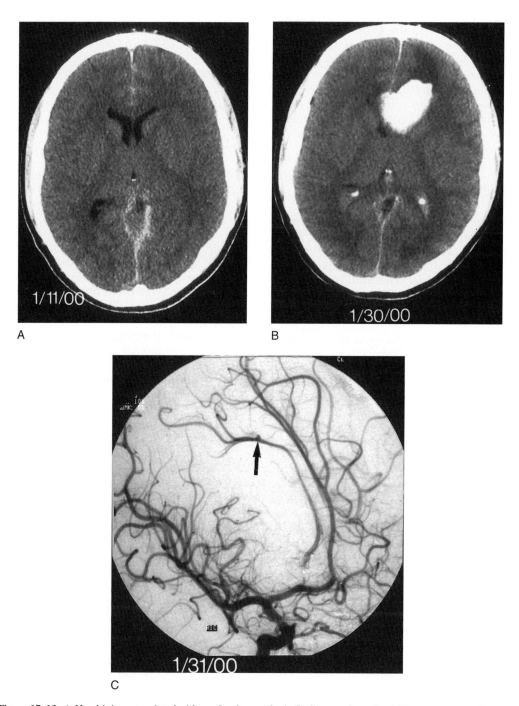

A   B

C

Figure 17–12. *A*: Head injury associated with no focal neurologic findings and maximal Glasgow coma scale score. The computed tomography scan shows blood in the interhemispheric fissure and on the tentorium. *B*: Sudden worsening in level of consciousness and confusion 19 days after initial trauma. A left frontal hematoma is adjacent to the corpus callosum. *C*: Traumatic pseudoaneurysm of the azygos pericallosal artery (arrow) demonstrated with conventional catheter angiography.

318

TRAUMA OF SPINE AND SPINAL CORD

A potential consequence of major trauma is injury to the spine and spinal cord, usually subtle and at times unaccompanied by pertinent clinical findings. Management of trauma to the spine demands proper judgment and extensive experience. This section is a practical summary of spine and spinal cord injury and initial management. Remaining interpretations and decisions can be found in several treatises[135,136] and should be left to the discretion of the consulting neurosurgeon and spine surgeon.

Most patients should be evaluated with anteroposterior, lateral, oblique, and open-mouth odontoid radiographic views. A lateral cervical spine film to "clear C-spine" is not sufficient, and 25% of cervical spine injuries can be overlooked.[137,138]

Plain cervical spine films should be scrutinized for soft tissue abnormalities, abnormalities in alignment, abnormality in disc space height, and fractures. Multiple spine fractures may occur, and three multilevel patterns have been recognized[139] (Fig. 17–13). Questionable radiologic findings should prompt further imaging with CT, but many institutions already simultaneously image head and cervical spine in patients with multisystem trauma. Important cervical spine fractures, however, may be overlooked with 4- to 10-mm slices, and occasionally a segment is not displayed on a CT scan. Computed tomography scanning has the major advantages of a lack of superimpositions and the potential for reconstruction. Because of the ability of MRI to image in multiple planes,[140] it should be considered the best method to demonstrate spinal cord damage. A recent small study predicted posterior ligamentous injury with a sensitivity of 90% and a specificity of 100%.[141]

Cervical Spine Injuries

Cervical spine injuries can be classified by mechanism of injury, which may guide choice of treatment.[135,142–145] Many trauma centers use White and Panjabi's classification for instability (Table 17–3). The most com-

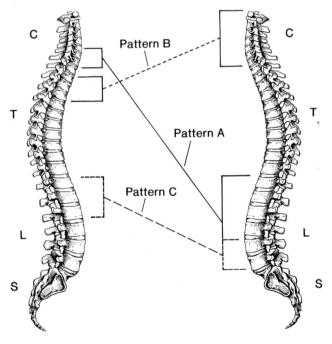

Primary Lesion   **Secondary Lesion**

Figure 17–13. Multilevel spine fractures. *Pattern A*: C5 through C7 associated with T11 through L5. *Pattern B*: T2 through T4 associated with C1 through C7. *Pattern C*: T11 through L2 associated with L4 and L5.

Table 17–3. Checklist for the Diagnosis of Clinical Instability in the Middle and Lower Cervical Spine

Element	Point Value
Anterior elements destroyed or unable to function	2
Posterior elements destroyed or unable to function	2
Positive stretch test	2
Radiographic criteria	4
A. Flexion/extension radiographs	
1. Sagittal plane translation >3.5 mm or 20% (2 points)	
2. Sagittal plane rotation >20° (2 points)	
or	
B. Resting radiographs	
1. Sagittal plane displacement >3.5 mm or 20% (2 points)	
2. Relative sagittal plane angulation >11° (2 points)	
Abnormal disc narrowing	1
Developmentally narrow spinal canal (sagittal diameter <13 mm)	1
Spinal cord damage	2
Nerve root damage	1
Dangerous loading anticipated	1
Total of 5 or more points = unstable	

Modified from White AA III, Panjabi MM. Clinical Biomechanics of the Spine, 2nd ed. Lippincott, Philadelphia, 1990, p 314. By permission of the publisher.

mon cervical spine injuries are outlined in Figure 17–14.

HYPERFLEXION INJURIES

Hyperflexion forces result in rupture of the posterior ligamentous complex, sometimes including the posterior portion of the annulus fibrosis. Rupture causes additional traumatic disc prolapse and compression fractures of the vertebral body.

Acute Anterior Subluxation (Hyperflexion Sprain) (Fig. 17–14A)

Many patients experience excruciating neck pain that limits neck flexion and extension. Neurologic findings are rarely demonstrated at the time of examination and seldom appear at later stages. Among the many posterior ligaments that can be torn with this type of injury are the supraspinous and interspinous ligaments, capsules of the interfacetal joints, and the posterior longitudinal ligament. Characteristic radiographic findings are hyperkyphotic angulation, anterior glide of vertebra with some forward subluxation of the superior facets, and, often more evident, widening of the interspinous spaces.

This type of injury is potentially unstable, because significant angulation and subluxation may occur, necessitating follow-up flexion and extension views. Most patients are initially treated with a Philadelphia collar.

Unilateral Facet Dislocation (Fig. 17–14B)

Common at C4–7 levels, this cervical spine injury is unstable. Nerve root injury may occur at the time of injury or during reduction. Radiologic features are anterior displacement of the superior vertebral body, usually within 50% of the anterior–posterior width of the vertebral body below the displaced segment. The retropharyngeal space is characteristically enlarged.

When the anterior displacement reaches 60% of the width of the underlying vertebral body, both facet joints are generally subluxed or dislocated. Impaction fractures of the interfacetal joint or articular mass may be an associated radiologic feature. Operative fixation is indicated.

Bilateral Facet Dislocation (Fig. 17–14C)

A free-floating vertebral body, seen on the lateral view, predominantly involves the C5–6 and C6–7 levels and indicates complete disruption of all soft tissue structures. This type of cervical injury is unstable, and spinal cord damage is common. Open reduction is indicated when traction results in worsening of neurologic symptoms or is unable to reduce the dislocation. Magnetic resonance imaging or CT-myelogram is indicated before open reduction to rule out an associated disc herniation. If a disc herniation is identified, the extruded fragment must be removed anteriorly before posterior reduction is done. Failure to follow this protocol may lead to spinal cord compression from the extruded fragment during reduction, with potentially devastating neurologic sequelae.[146]

Anterior Wedge Compression Fracture (Fig. 17–14D)

Wedge fractures of the C5 or C6 vertebral body are often associated with transient facet separation or other cervical injuries. This type of injury should be differentiated from a burst fracture of the vertebral body, which has a vertical fracture line and is caused by axial force rather than sudden flexion. Neurologic findings are usually absent. If there is no evidence of facet subluxation, this injury is stable and needs only radiologic follow-up to detect delayed instability.

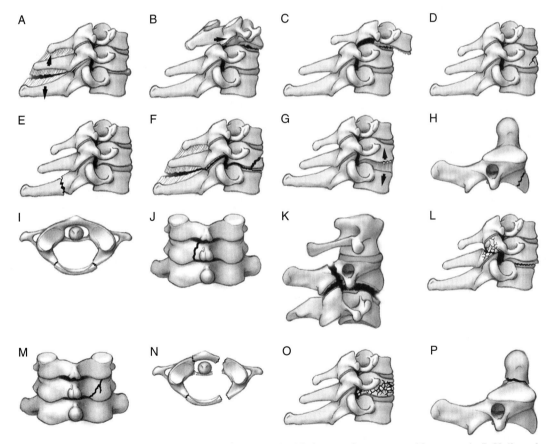

Figure 17–14. Cervical fractures. *A*: Hyperflexion sprain (stable but may become unstable; see text). *B*: Unilateral facet dislocation (unstable). *C*: Bilateral facet dislocation (unstable). *D*: Anterior wedge compression fracture (stable). *E*: Clay shoveler's fracture (stable). *F*: Teardrop fracture-dislocation (unstable). *G*: Hyperextension strain (stable). *H*: Teardrop fracture of axis (stable). *I*: Posterior arch fracture of atlas (stable). *J*: Laminar fracture (stable). *K*: Hangman's fracture (unstable). *L*: Hyperextension fracture-dislocation (unstable). *M*: Pillar fracture (stable). *N*: Jefferson C1 fracture (unstable). *O*: Burst fracture of cervical body (stable). *P*: Odontoid fracture (unstable).

Clay Shoveler's Fracture (Fig. 17–14E)

A typical hyperflexion injury occurs in approximately 15% of all patients with cervical spine injury. This spinous process avulsion fracture is frequently seen in the C7, T1, or T2 region on lateral projection films. The avulsed fragment may be small and dislocated, at times mimicking nuchal ligament calcification. Neurologic findings are absent, and this condition, if isolated, is generally stable, but radiologic follow-up with flexion and extension radiographs is necessary to detect instability.

Teardrop Fracture-Dislocation (Fig. 17–14F)

Complete disruption of all ligaments and the vertebral disc at the level of injury produces a highly unstable injury and is sometimes detected on films only by a small triangular fragment in the anteroinferior corner. Other radiologic findings are posterior kyphotic angulation, retropulsion of the posterior portion of the vertebral body, and bilateral dislocated facet joints. Displacement of the vertebral body into the spinal canal frequently causes spinal cord injury, most commonly anterior spinal cord syndrome. Operative removal of disc material or bone fragments during operative stabilization unfortunately may not improve the overall poor outcome.

HYPEREXTENSION INJURIES

Retroflexion or hyperextension injuries may produce only ligamentous or muscular injuries. In the elderly population with cervical spondylosis, these injuries produce spinal cord syndromes.

Hyperextension Strain (Fig. 17–14G)

The most important hallmark is conspicuous lack of radiologic features in a patient with otherwise severe spinal cord injury. Subtle findings are prevertebral swelling, small horizontally oriented avulsion chips from the anteroinferior margin of the vertebral body, gas phenomena or vacuum defect, and widening of a disc space. The clinical findings are striking, consisting of either a complete cord lesion or a central cord syndrome.[147] Both pincer action and vertical tearing of nervous tissue produce hemorrhage in the central cord. The typical clinical features of a central cord syndrome are arm and hand weakness more prominent than leg weakness and preservation of the sacral segments and perianal sensation.[147] Some upper arm function may return, but spasticity of the legs usually remains in some degree.

Teardrop Fracture of Axis (Fig. 17–14H)

In patients with severe osteoporosis or advanced cervical spondylosis, a large triangular fragment may chip from the body of the axis and can be recognized radiologically by larger vertical height than transverse width and by prevertebral soft tissue swelling. This fracture should be differentiated from a teardrop fracture in a flexion injury. This fracture is stable in flexion and is not associated with spinal cord damage.

Posterior Arch Fracture of Atlas (Fig. 17–14I)

Absence of bilateral displacement of lateral masses of C1 relative to C2 on the open mouth odontoid view and absence of anterior arch fracture differentiate this fracture from the Jefferson burst fracture. (The fracture line is posterior to lateral masses and the transverse atlantal ligament.) The fracture is stable and is uncommonly associated with neurologic symptoms. However, one should carefully look for associated hyperextension fractures and type II odontoid fractures.

Laminar Fractures (Fig. 17–14J)

Hyperextension injuries are most common in elderly persons with spondylosis. Neurologic abnormalities can be expected only when laminar fragments are displaced into the spinal canal. A CT scan may be more sensitive than plain films for diagnosis. This injury is stable because the anterior column and facet joints are intact.

Traumatic Spondylolisthesis of C2 (Hangman's Fracture) (Fig. 17–14K)

This uncommon cervical spine injury (7% of all cervical injuries) is caused by abrupt deceleration and is frequently accompanied by severe closed head injury, facial trauma, and lung contusion. Traumatic spondylolisthesis seldom produces neurologic signs. In a series of 181 patients, 8 (4%) had some neurologic findings, but 6 of the 8 completely recovered.[148]

The degree and type of displacement of the anterior fragment are important. Type I fractures are isolated hairline fractures of the axis ring with minimal displacement. The disc space between C2 and C3 is normal, and the injury at this stage is stable. In type II fractures, the disc space C2–3 is abnormal and the body of C2 is displaced. The body of C2 usually shows some anterior angulation. Type III fractures are characterized by definite displacement and flexion of the body of C2 and bilateral interfacetal dislocation of C2 and C3.

Both types II and III fractures are considered unstable and are frequently treated with closed reduction with traction before halo vest placement. Type III fractures often require operative intervention. This flexion-distraction injury pattern is unstable in traction, and stretch of the spinal cord may occur. Direct application of a halo vest without traction is the appropriate form of management of this injury.[149]

Hyperextension Fracture-Dislocation (Fig. 17–14L)

Anterior displacement of the vertebral body (usually at the C4–7 level), horizontal rotation of the fractured articular pillar, and anterior displacement of the pillar into the intervertebral foramen are typical radiologic findings. Either the facet is severely comminuted or the inferior facet of the superior vertebra is driven upward. The condition is unstable, largely because the facet joints are disrupted.

Pillar Fracture (Fig. 17–14M)

Simultaneous hyperextension and bending to one side may cause vertical fractures of the articular mass that may extend into the transverse process of the pedicle or posteriorly into the lamina. Pillar views or CT scanning is necessary to demonstrate this fracture, which occasionally produces an acute radiculopathy.

VERTICAL COMPRESSION

Typically, heavy weights dropped on top of the skull or, more commonly, hitting of the skull on the bottom of a swimming pool causes vertical compression fractures.

Jefferson C1 Fracture (Fig. 17–14N)

This uncommon fracture complex consists of two fractures on each side involving the anterior and posterior sides of the arch of C1. Prevertebral soft tissue swelling may be prominent, and with disruption of the transverse ligament, one of the lateral masses may spread more than 7 mm.

Widening of the lateral atlantodental interval is another feature of disruption of the transverse ligament (>3 mm). The involvement of the transverse ligament determines instability of the injury.

In a review of 15 patients from the Northwestern University Acute Spine Center, 4 had spinal cord injury.[136] Management is generally conservative, but posterior C1–2 fusion (after healing of the C1 fracture) is an option in unstable injuries with disruption of the transverse ligament.

Burst Fracture of the Cervical Body (Fig. 17–14O)

All ligamentous structures are intact; therefore, the bony lesion is stable, but spinal cord injury is common because disc material and fragments are forced into the spinal canal. Surgical removal and bone grafting are frequently done when canal intrusion is significant.

MISCELLANEOUS CERVICAL SPINE INJURIES

The mechanisms underlying these injuries are not understood. Most likely, multiple vector forces contribute.

Odontoid Fractures (Fig. 17–14P)

Odontoid fractures can be classified into three types.[150–152] Type I is an avulsion of the tip, type II (the most common) is a fracture through the neck of the odontoid, and type III is a fracture extending into the body of C2.

Most patients have only neck stiffness, pain, or torticollis, which may occur weeks after injury. Surgical fixation is often required in type II fractures. Other types heal successfully with conservative treatment.

A common pitfall is os odontoideum—presumed congenital or due to past trauma—in type II fractures. Radiologic differences are difficult to interpret, but in os odontoideum, the ossicle is rounded and widely separated from the base of the odontoid.

Thoracolumbar Spine Injuries

Many algorithms have been proposed for management of thoracolumbar fractures.[153] In many of them, CT, myelographic, or MRI demonstration of cord compression with more than 50% narrowing of the bone canal is an indication for decompression and fusion.

COMPRESSION FLEXION FRACTURE (FIG. 17–15A)

Neurologic findings can be expected in patients with fractures that cause narrowing of the spinal canal. The neurologic signs and symptoms may also progressively worsen over time, usually within 2 days after the onset of trauma. The chance of cord damage, however, remains relatively small, approximately 10%. (This type of fracture should be differentiated from a burst fracture, which is invariably caused by axial damage and has an up to 60% chance of cord injury; in general, if the canal is narrowed, it is most likely a burst fracture.) Operative treatment is indicated only in the most severe compression fractures.

DISTRACTIVE FLEXION FRACTION (FIG. 17–15B)

This fracture is well known because of its association with lap seatbelt injury. The impact often causes rupture of a hollow viscus, such as the duodenum. Radiologically, a wide disruption through the body, spinous process, and disc is seen, at times associated with fracture of the spinous process—so-called chance fracture. Most injuries are ligamentous and do not involve the bone. Bony injuries often heal with bracing, whereas ligamentous injuries generally require surgery.

LATERAL FLEXION FRACTURE (FIG. 17–15C)

An acute lateral bending of the spine causes shortening of the vertebral body. Neurologic involvement is rare.

FRACTURE-DISLOCATIONS (FIG. 17–15D)

A high incidence of spinal cord injury can be expected if fractures are located in the thoracic area. Transection is less common in the lumbar area because the spinal canal is wider.

ROTATION DISLOCATION (FIG. 17–15E)

Tension and compression may cause a very unstable fracture of the thoracolumbar spine severe enough to produce complete transection of the spinal cord. Operative stabilization is mandatory.

BURST FRACTURE (FIG. 17–15F)

Many of these types of fractures are located between T10 and L2,[154] and the vertical impact frequently causes lower extremity fractures, particularly of the knee and calcaneus. Whether the approach should be conservative or operative is controversial. The proponents of surgical stabilization[155,156] have reasoned that post-traumatic kyphosis and progressive neurologic deterioration may occur with the conservative approach. Nevertheless, even with compression of the spinal canal, neurologic deterioration does not necessarily occur.

MISCELLANEOUS THORACOLUMBAR INJURIES

Rare fractures of the thoracic and lumbar spine are distractive extension and lumbosacral dislocation, both with infrequent neurologic damage.

Isolated chip fractures of the transverse

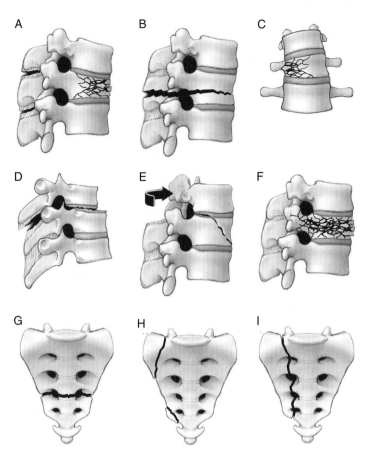

Figure 17–15. Thoracolumbar and sacral fractures. *A*: Compression flexion fracture. *B*: Distractive flexion fracture. *C*: Lateral flexion fracture. *D*: Fracture-dislocation. *E*: Rotation dislocation. *F*: Burst fracture. *G*: Transverse sacral fracture. *H,I*: Vertical sacral fractures.

processes or spinous processes may be found but do not produce any nerve damage, except that T1–2 transverse fractures may damage the brachial plexus.

Sacral Fractures

Sacral fractures are almost invariably associated with pelvic fractures.[157,158] The mechanism of neurologic injury may involve direct bony compression of nerve roots at the level of the foramina entry, stretching and avulsion of plexus lumbosacral roots, or a cauda equina lesion. The incidence of neurologic involvement depends on the type of sacral fracture.[159–163]

TRANSVERSE SACRAL FRACTURES (FIG. 17–15G)

Most transverse sacral fractures are at the level of the os coccyx, so that neurologic function remains intact. Higher level fractures are unstable, and their proximity to the foramina produces nerve root damage in most patients.

VERTICAL SACRAL FRACTURES (FIG. 17–15H,I)

Denis and associates[163] divided sacral fractures into three zones. Zone I fractures are avulsion fractures of the sacrotuberous ligament or alar fractures, both with a low incidence of nerve root or bladder function damage. Zone II involves a fracture line through the foramina. In one series, L5 involvement was most frequent, resulting in footdrop. Bladder involvement occurred in 4 of 23 patients.[163] Fractures into the central canal (zone III) may spare nerve roots in 50% of the patients, but bowel, bladder, and sexual dysfunction are common. Operative decompression may result in significant improvement in ambulation and bladder function.

ACUTE SPINAL CORD INJURY

Fractures and dislocations of the spine may contuse the spinal cord,[164–167] but direct forces may injure the cord over several segments as well. Complete transection of the cord is rare. Patients who enter the trauma ICU may have maximal deficits from spinal shock rather than permanent immediate complete damage. Likewise, pharmacologic treatment of acute spinal cord injury assumes that additional biochemical damage is causing secondary injury that can potentially be arrested or ameliorated. The pathophysiology of secondary spinal cord injury is not elucidated, but many investigators in this field have postulated that lipid peroxidation leads to neuronal damage through release of free radicals and excitatory amino acids and that the post-traumatic microvascular injury results from vasoconstriction, platelet aggregation, and edema. Animal experiments have supported the existence of complex cascades of tissue injuries, and the reader is referred to scholarly reviews on this subject.[168–170] Early randomized trials have already resulted in promising agents for treatment, such as methylprednisolone and ganglioside GM_1.[171–173]

Spinal cord injury is very dramatic in presentation and should not have to remain unrecognized in emergency trauma units. Neurologic assessment of the level of cord damage should be done immediately. Several key points in motor and sensory examination may assist in localization (Fig. 17–16). High-level cervical spinal cord injury (above the C3 level) instantaneously paralyzes the respiratory muscles. The generation of sufficient tidal volumes is impossible because diaphragmatic expansion and abdominal muscle function are lost.[174,175] In patients with cervical cord injury above C3, paradoxical inward movement of the rib cage and excessive use of neck muscles can be observed, but most patients are already intubated and mechanically ventilated. (Guidelines for intubation, with use of fiberoptic bronchoscopy, in presumed cervical spine injury have been described.[176,177]) More commonly, however, respiratory function in patients with multisystem trauma is compromised because pneumothorax is present. Neurogenic pulmonary edema may occur in acute spinal cord injury,[178–182] but cardiac or lung contusion may be a more common mechanism. In lower cervical spinal cord injury, respiration is characterized by postural dependence of breathing, and vital capacity increases in the supine position secondary to the pressure effect of the abdominal contents. Abdominal binders are needed for mobilization. Neurologic involvement between the C1 and T6 segments results in sympathetic loss, hypotension, hypothermia, and bradycardia from unopposed vagal function. Hypotension may theoretically increase secondary spinal cord injury[183] and should be aggressively treated with anti-Trendelenburg positioning, fluid administration, dopamine, or phenylephrine.[184,185] Differentiation from hypovolemic shock remains difficult in the acute stage. In spinal shock, peritoneal signs and symptoms may be absent. However, in many trauma centers, when hypotension is present an abdominal tap, echocardiogram, or abdominal CT scan is done in patients with multitrauma.

Bradyarrhythmias refractory to atropine or β-adrenergic agonists may require cardiac pacing, but this situation seldom occurs.[186]

In the flaccid paralysis of spinal shock, fecal and urinary retention occurs, but it may disappear in some patients after months. In an atonic bladder, an indwelling catheter should be immediately placed.[187] A nasogastric tube should also be placed, because gastric atony may result in a considerable risk of aspiration.

Medical treatment of spinal cord injury has been advanced by the results of the National Acute Spinal Cord Injury Study (NASCIS), which showed that recovery was significantly greater in patients treated with methylprednisolone within 8 hr after cord damage (intravenous bolus of 30 mg/kg followed by infusion with 5.4 mg/kg per hour for 23 hr).[171,172] Ganglioside GM_1 is effective as well but not yet routinely used.[173]

POST-TRAUMATIC NEUROPATHIES ASSOCIATED WITH FRACTURES

Isolated nerve injuries and plexopathies are uncommon in patients with multitrauma and require the expertise of neurosurgeons and

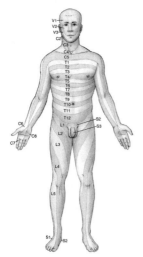

Figure 17–16. Distribution of sensory segments. Landmarks are nipple (T4) and navel (T10).

orthopedic surgeons. Clinical decision making often focuses on whether to explore the injured area or wait for spontaneous recovery.

Brachial Plexopathies

Traumatic brachial plexus palsy is frequently seen in young patients after motorcycle accidents.[188] In the initial assessment of brachial plexus injuries, careful evaluation of the magnitude of nerve damage is important, because secondary deterioration may be associated with the development of a false aneurysm or an arteriovenous fistula in an axillary artery that needs immediate surgical intervention. Closed brachial plexus injuries may be approached by differentiating patients who have a proximal injury from those who have a postganglionic injury.

Proximal brachial plexus injury is manifested by Horner's syndrome (C8 to T1), winging of the scapula, and paralysis of the rhomboids. Diaphragmatic paralysis is occasionally present. Electromyographic and sensory nerve studies are usually performed 6 to 8 weeks after the initial insult and may differentiate a preganglionic from a postganglionic lesion. Normal sensory conduction from the anesthetic median or radial nerve area of the hand strongly suggests a preganglionic injury at the C6–7 level. Somatosensory studies may also be helpful. Subsequently, myelography, CT myelography, or MRI[189] is done to exclude rootlet avulsion in case plexus repair is considered. (In most patients, 3 months must have elapsed without spontaneous improvement.)

Similarly, in postganglionic injuries of the brachial plexus, operative repair is considered if no clinical or electromyographic improvement is found after 3 months. Detailed discussion of nerve repair techniques can be found in textbook and review articles.[190–192] Nerve root avulsion of the brachial plexus is the most devastating injury, and only palliative therapy and control of pain, which may be excrutiating in some patients, are possible. Complete paralysis or some remaining flicker of movement in the deltoid, supraspinus, or biceps muscle may be found, and all sensation is lost. A recent provocative study in 10 patients examined the effects of reimplantation of avulsed ventral roots through slits in the pia mater and spinal cord surface. Three of the 10 patients had a small degree of recovery, with resistance in some muscles and biceps strength to overcome gravity. Joint position improved in some, and pain was reduced.[193]

Lumbosacral Plexus Injury

Far less common than traumatic brachial plexus lesions, lumbosacral plexus injury can result from compression or stretching of the plexus in sacral and pelvic fractures.[194] External iliac artery injury occasionally accompanies the nerve damage.[195] A MRI may be useful in establishing lumbosacral nerve root avulsion,[196] which precludes operative correction. Outcome of traumatic lumbosacral plexus injury is unpredictable but often poor.

Miscellaneous Isolated Neuropathies Associated with Fractures

Fractures of the ulna have been associated with complete paralysis of the anterior interosseous nerve, a motor branch of the me-

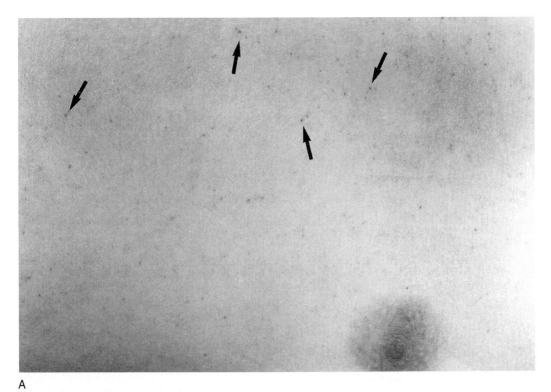

A

B

Figure 17–17. Fat embolism syndrome. *A*: Petechiae (arrows) on the chest. *B*: Photomicrograph showing fat droplets (arrows) within capillary vessels.

dian nerve. A characteristic feature is weakness of the flexor pollicis longus or flexor digitorum profundus and pronator quadratus without any sensory deficit. Patients may notice abnormal pinching, which can easily be demonstrated when they are asked to make a circle with thumb and index finger. Complete recovery may take months.[197]

Acute median nerve damage may also occur in wrist fractures[198] (for example, Colles' fractures) or may be exacerbated after immobilization of wrist fractures in marked flexion.[199] Entrapment of the ulnar nerve at the elbow region may occur in supracondylar humeral fractures.[200] Neurolysis with anterior transposition has resulted in satisfactory outcomes, but a comparison with conservative management is not available.[201]

Radial nerve paralysis associated with fractures of the humerus has been frequently reported, usually with fractures of the distal part of the humerus. Excellent recovery was reported in a series of 62 patients, 95% of whom regained normal radial nerve function.[202] Clinical recovery occurred within 1 month in one-third of the patients, and the remainder improved within 6 months. Other peripheral nerve injuries are axillary nerve damage (anterior dislocation of the shoulder) and damage to the sciatic nerve (dislocation of the acetabulum of the pelvis), both with potential for complete recovery.

Treatment of all the above-mentioned fractures in patients with head injury should be timely.

FAT EMBOLISM SYNDROME

Embolization of fat and fatty acids from bone marrow of long bones that have been fractured probably occurs in most patients with multitrauma, but a typical clinical fat embolism syndrome develops in only a minority (3% to 4%).[203] In general, 12 to 75 hr after the initial traumatic impact, the patient's condition deteriorates in parallel with laboratory changes.

Sudden tachypnea and tachycardia, fever, and development of a large A–a gradient are the first clinical indicators of the lodging of fat globules in the pulmonary vasculature. A pleural friction rub may be heard, but this sign is almost always absent. A pathognomonic sign, present in 50% of patients, is a petechial rash appearing suddenly on the chest (Fig. 17–17A), axillary folds, and, occasionally, conjunctiva. Cotton-wool spots, petechial hemorrhages, and intravascular fat globules may be seen in the fundi but only in patients with widespread skin petechiae and thrombocytopenia. Neuropathologic studies in patients with central nervous system involvement have repeatedly demonstrated fat droplets in arteries supplying both white and gray matter and multiple microinfarcts (Fig. 17–17B). Petechiae are often found in the centrum semiovale, brain stem, and cerebellum.[204]

Central nervous system involvement is most often manifested by an acute confusional state,[203,205–209] but focal signs and generalized tonic–clonic seizures may be

Table 17–4. **Clinical Criteria for Fat Embolism Syndrome**

Major	Minor
Axillary or subconjunctival petechiae	Tachycardia >110/min
$Pa_{O_2} < 60$ mm Hg, $F_{IO_2} \leq 0.4$	Temperature >38.5°C
Central nervous system symptoms	Retinal emboli
Pulmonary edema, acute respiratory distress syndrome	Fat in urine
	Fat in sputum
	Decreased hematocrit and platelets, increased erythrocyte sedimentation rate

Modified from Gurd AR. Fat embolism: an aid to diagnosis. J Bone Joint Surg Br 52:732–737, 1970. By permission of the British Editorial Society of Bone and Joint Surgery.

temporarily seen. Laboratory findings that support the diagnosis are urinary fat droplets identified by Sudan red staining. The diagnostic criteria for fat embolism syndrome are summarized in Table 17–4. The clinical diagnosis becomes fairly certain when at least one major and four minor criteria are present. Bronchoalveolar lavage has been shown to rapidly confirm the diagnosis, and this may become the preferred diagnostic test in patients with unexplained neurologic deterioration after multitrauma and fractures.[210]

In patients without pulmonary symptoms, cerebral fat embolization can at times be explained by a patent foramen ovale. In other patients, however, the pathway of fat globules small enough to pass through the lungs is presumably similar to that of air emboli.

Imaging studies of the brain are often nondiagnostic, but multiple hypodensities in the frontal white matter[211] have been noted on a CT scan. A massive pontine hemorrhagic infarct was reported in a patient with nontraumatic fat embolism.[212] Multiple scattered spotty white matter lesions resembling demyelination have been documented on T2-weighted MRI, with potential for complete resolution.[213–215]

Fat embolism syndrome can be rapidly fatal, but in most patients clinical signs resolve within 24 hr. Treatment should be focused on immediate stabilization of the fracture. Early repair of the fracture decreases the risk of fat embolization.

CONCLUSIONS

Management of patients with multitrauma begins in the field. The most challenging patient is the one who "talks and deteriorates" after normal findings on the initial CT scan. Important causes are subdural or epidural hematoma, fat embolization, and delayed hemorrhagic frontal or temporal lobe contusion. In patients with limited subdural or epidural hematoma, placement of a fiberoptic monitor may detect increasing intracranial pressure if emergency surgery for reasons other than head injury is contemplated (for example, abdominal exploration, orthopedic surgery). Ideally, patients with multitrauma and head and spine injuries should also be cared for by neurosurgeons and neurointensive care specialists, who can appreciate delicate changes in neurologic condition and interpret imaging studies of the brain and spine.

REFERENCES

1. Rockswold GL, Leonard PR, Nagib MG. Analysis of management in thirty-three closed head injury patients who "talked and deteriorated." Neurosurgery 21:51–55, 1987.
2. Andrews PJ, Piper IR, Dearden NM, Miller JD. Secondary insults during intrahospital transport of head-injured patients. Lancet 335:327–330, 1990.
3. Nicholl J, Turner J. Effectiveness of a regional trauma system in reducing mortality from major trauma: before and after study. BMJ 315:1349–1354, 1997.
4. Valadka AB, Andrews BT, Bullock MR. How well do neurosurgeons care for trauma patients? A survey of the membership of the American Association for the Surgery of Trauma. Neurosurgery 48:17–24, 2001.
5. Smith DH, Nonaka M, Miller R, et al. Immediate coma following inertial brain injury dependent on axonal damage in the brainstem. J Neurosurg 93:315–322, 2000.
6. Holt GR, Holt JE. Management of orbital trauma and foreign bodies. Otolaryngol Clin North Am 21:35–52, 1988.
7. Ghajar J. Traumatic brain injury. Lancet 356:923–929, 2000.
8. Bailes JE, Cantu RC. Head injury in athletes. Neurosurgery 48:26–45, 2001.
9. Boeve BF, Wijdicks EFM, Benarroch EE, Schmidt KD. Paroxysmal sympathetic storms ("diencephalic seizures") after severe diffuse axonal head injury. Mayo Clin Proc 73:148–152, 1998.
10. Stuss DT, Binns MA, Carruth FG, et al. The acute period of recovery from traumatic brain injury: posttraumatic amnesia or posttraumatic confusional state? J Neurosurg 90:635–643, 1999.
11. Teasdale GM, Graham DI. Craniocerebral trauma: protection and retrieval of the neuronal population after injury. Neurosurgery 43:723–737, 1998.
12. Young B, Runge JW, Waxman KS, et al. Effects of pegorgotein on neurologic outcome of patients with severe head injury. A multicenter, randomized controlled trial. JAMA 276:538–543, 1996.
13. Muizelaar JP, Marmarou A, Young HF, et al. Improving the outcome of severe head injury with the oxygen radical scavenger polyethylene glycol-conjugated superoxide dismutase: a phase II trial. J Neurosurg 78:375–382, 1993.
14. Marshall LF, Maas AI, Marshall SB, et al. A multicenter trial on the efficacy of using tirilazad mesylate in cases of head injury. J Neurosurg 89:519–525, 1998.
15. Teasdale GM, Murray G, Anderson E, et al. Risks

of acute traumatic intracranial haematoma in children and adults: implications for managing head injuries. BMJ 300:363–367, 1990.

16. Thornbury JR, Masters SJ, Campbell JA. Imaging recommendations for head trauma: a new comprehensive strategy. AJR Am J Roentgenol 149: 781–783, 1987.

17. Lobato RD, Rivas JJ, Gomez PA, et al. Head-injured patients who talk and deteriorate into coma. Analysis of 211 cases studied with computerized tomography. J Neurosurg 75:256–261, 1991.

18. Gentry LR, Godersky JC, Thompson B. MR imaging of head trauma: review of the distribution and radiopathologic features of traumatic lesions. AJR Am J Roentgenol 150:663–672, 1988.

19. Gentry LR, Godersky JC, Thompson B, Dunn VD. Prospective comparative study of intermediate-field MR and CT in the evaluation of closed head trauma. AJR Am J Roentgenol 150:673–682, 1988.

20. Hadley DM, Teasdale GM, Jenkins A, et al. Magnetic resonance imaging in acute head injury. Clin Radiol 39:131–139, 1988.

21. Hesselink JR, Dowd CF, Healy ME, Hajek P, Baker LL, Luerssen TG. MR imaging of brain contusions: a comparative study with CT. AJR Am J Roentgenol 150:1133–1142, 1988.

22. Tanaka T, Sakai T, Uemura K, Teramura A, Fujishima I, Yamamoto T. MR imaging as predictor of delayed posttraumatic cerebral hemorrhage. J Neurosurg 69:203–209, 1988.

23. Wilberger JE Jr, Deeb Z, Rothfus W. Magnetic resonance imaging in cases of severe head injury. Neurosurgery 20:571–576, 1987.

24. Jaicks RR, Cohn SM, Moller BA. Early fracture fixation may be deleterious after head injury. J Trauma 42:1–5, 1997.

25. Snow RB, Zimmerman RD, Gandy SE, Deck MD. Comparison of magnetic resonance imaging and computed tomography in the evaluation of head injury. Neurosurgery 18:45–52, 1986.

26. Marshall LF, Marshall SB, Klauber MR, et al. A new classification of head injury based on computerized tomography. J Neurosurg 75 Suppl:S14–S20, 1991.

27. Besenski N, Jadro-Santel D, Grcevic N. Patterns of lesions of corpus callosum in inner cerebral trauma visualized by computed tomography. Neuroradiology 34:126–130, 1992.

28. Levi L, Guilburd JN, Lemberger A, Soustiel JF, Feinsod M. Diffuse axonal injury: analysis of 100 patients with radiological signs. Neurosurgery 27: 429–432, 1990.

29. Wilberger JE Jr, Rothfus WE, Tabas J, Goldberg AL, Deeb ZL. Acute tissue tear hemorrhages of the brain: computed tomography and clinicopathological correlations. Neurosurgery 27:208–213, 1990.

30. Takenaka N, Mine T, Suga S, et al. Interpeduncular high-density spot in severe shearing injury. Surg Neurol 34:30–38, 1990.

31. Meyer CA, Mirvis SE, Wolf AL, Thompson RK, Gutierrez MA. Acute traumatic midbrain hemorrhage: experimental and clinical observations with CT. Radiology 179:813–818, 1991.

32. Ropper AH, Miller DC. Acute traumatic midbrain hemorrhage. Ann Neurol 18:80–86, 1985.

33. Statham PF, Johnston RA, Macpherson P. Delayed deterioration in patients with traumatic frontal contusions. J Neurol Neurosurg Psychiatry 52:351–354, 1989.

34. Andrews BT, Chiles BW III, Olsen WL, Pitts LH. The effect of intracerebral hematoma location on the risk of brain-stem compression and on clinical outcome. J Neurosurg 69:518–522, 1988.

35. Shigemori M, Kojyo N, Yuge T, Tokutomi T, Nakashima H, Kuramoto S. Massive traumatic haematoma of the corpus callosum. Acta Neurochir (Wien) 81:36–39, 1986.

36. Colquhoun IR, Rawlinson J. The significance of haematomas of the basal ganglia in closed head injury. Clin Radiol 40:619–621, 1989.

37. Katz DI, Alexander MP, Seliger GM, Bellas DN. Traumatic basal ganglia hemorrhage: clinicopathologic features and outcome. Neurology 39: 897–904, 1989.

38. Lee JP, Wang AD. Post-traumatic basal ganglia hemorrhage: analysis of 52 patients with emphasis on the final outcome. J Trauma 31:376–380, 1991.

39. Macpherson P, Teasdale E, Dhaker S, Allerdyce G, Galbraith S. The significance of traumatic haematoma in the region of the basal ganglia. J Neurol Neurosurg Psychiatry 49:29–34, 1986.

40. Boto GR, Lobato RD, Rivas JJ, Gomez PA, de la Lama A, Lagares A. Basal ganglia hematomas in severely head injured patients: clinicoradiological analysis of 37 cases. J Neurosurg 94:224–232, 2001.

41. Fujitsu K, Kuwabara T, Muramoto M, Hirata K, Mochimatsu Y. Traumatic intraventricular hemorrhage: report of twenty-six cases and consideration of the pathogenic mechanism. Neurosurgery 23: 423–430, 1988.

42. Jayakumar PN, Kolluri VR, Basavakumar DG, Arya BY, Das BS. Prognosis in traumatic intraventricular haemorrhage. Acta Neurochir (Wien) 106:48–51, 1990.

43. Berry K, Rice J. Traumatic tear of tela choroidea resulting in fatal intraventricular hemorrhage. Am J Forensic Med Pathol 15:132–137, 1994.

44. Elsner H, Rigamonti D, Corradino G, Schlegel R Jr, Joslyn J. Delayed traumatic intracerebral hematomas: "Spat-Apoplexie." Report of two cases. J Neurosurg 72:813–815, 1990.

45. Diaz FG, Yock DH Jr, Larson D, Rockswold GL. Early diagnosis of delayed posttraumatic intracerebral hematomas. J Neurosurg 50:217–223, 1979.

46. Gudeman SK, Kishore PR, Miller JD, Girevendulis AK, Lipper MH, Becker DP. The genesis and significance of delayed traumatic intracerebral hematoma. Neurosurgery 5:309–313, 1979.

47. Boyko OB, Cooper DF, Grossman CB. Contrast-enhanced CT of acute isodense subdural hematoma. AJNR Am J Neuroradiol 12:341–343, 1991.

48. Hamilton M, Wallace C. Nonoperative management of acute epidural hematoma diagnosed by CT: the neuroradiologist's role. AJNR Am J Neuroradiol 13:853–859, 1992.

49. Knuckey NW, Gelbard S, Epstein MH. The management of "asymptomatic" epidural hematomas. A prospective study. J Neurosurg 70:392–396, 1989.

50. Firsching R, Frowein RA, Thun F. Intracerebellar haematoma: eleven traumatic and non-traumatic

cases and a review of the literature. Neurochirurgia (Stuttg) 30:182–185, 1987.

51. St John JN, French BN. Traumatic hematomas of the posterior fossa. A clinicopathological spectrum. Surg Neurol 25:457–466, 1986.

52. Ashkenazi E, Constantini S, Pomeranz S, Rivkind AI, Rappaport ZH. Delayed epidural hematoma without neurologic deficit. J Trauma 30:613–615, 1990.

53. Bucci MN, Phillips TW, McGillicuddy JE. Delayed epidural hemorrhage in hypotensive multiple trauma patients. Neurosurgery 19:65–68, 1986.

54. Di Rocco A, Ellis SJ, Landes C. Delayed epidural hematoma. Neuroradiology 33:253–254, 1991.

55. Domenicucci M, Signorini P, Strzelecki J, Delfini R. Delayed post-traumatic epidural hematoma. A review. Neurosurg Rev 18:109–122, 1995.

56. Lee ST, and Lui TN: Delayed intracranial haemorrhage in patients with multiple trauma and shock-related hypotension. Acta Neurochir (Wien) 113:121–124, 1991.

57. Nelson AT, Kishore PR, Lee SH. Development of delayed epidural hematoma. AJNR Am J Neuroradiol 3:583–585, 1982.

58. Smith HK, Miller JD. The danger of an ultra-early computed tomographic scan in a patient with an evolving acute epidural hematoma. Neurosurgery 29:258–260, 1991.

59. Braakman R. Depressed skull fracture: data, treatment, and follow-up in 225 consecutive cases. J Neurol Neurosurg Psychiatry 35:395–402, 1972.

60. van den Heever CM, van der Merwe DJ. Management of depressed skull fractures. Selective conservative management of nonmissile injuries. J Neurosurg 71:186–190, 1989.

61. Jennett B, Miller JD, Braakman R. Epilepsy after nonmissile depressed skull fracture. J Neurosurg 41:208–216, 1974.

62. Oberascher G. Cerebrospinal fluid otorrhea—new trends in diagnosis. Am J Otol 9:102–108, 1988.

63. Fransen P, Sindic CJ, Thauvoy C, Laterre C, Stroobandt G. Highly sensitive detection of beta-2 transferrin in rhinorrhea and otorrhea as a marker for cerebrospinal fluid (C.S.F.) leakage. Acta Neurochir (Wien) 109:98–101, 1991.

64. Brain Trauma Foundation, American Association of Neurological Surgeons, Joint Section on Neurotrauma and Critical Care. Guidelines for the management of severe head injury. J Neurotrauma 13:639–734, 1996.

65. Shiozaki T, Taneda M, Kishikawa M, et al. Transient and repetitive rises in blood pressure synchronized with plasma catecholamine increases after head injury. Report of two cases. J Neurosurg 78:501–504, 1993.

66. Rosner MJ, Rosner SD, Johnson AH. Cerebral perfusion pressure: management protocol and clinical results. J Neurosurg 83:949–962, 1995.

67. Talmor D, Merkind V, Artru AA, et al. Treatments to support blood pressure increases bleeding and/or decreases survival in a rat model of closed head trauma combined with uncontrolled hemorrhage. Anesth Analg 89:950–956, 1999.

68. Temkin NR, Dikmen SS, Wilensky AJ, Keihm J, Chabal S, Winn HR. A randomized, double-blind study of phenytoin for the prevention of post-traumatic seizures. N Engl J Med 323:497–502, 1990.

69. Marion DW, Penrod LE, Kelsey SF, et al. Treatment of traumatic brain injury with moderate hypothermia. N Engl J Med 336:540–546, 1997.

70. Jiang J-Y, Yu M-K, Zhu C. Effect of long-term mild hypothermia therapy in patients with severe traumatic brain injury: 1-year follow-up review of 87 cases. J Neurosurg 93:546–549, 2000.

71. Clifton GL, Miller ER, Choi SC, et al. Lack of effect of induction of hypothermia after acute brain injury. N Engl J Med 344:556–563, 2001.

72. Clifton GL, Robertson CS, Grossman RG, Hodge S, Foltz R, Garza C. The metabolic response to severe head injury. J Neurosurg 60:687–696, 1984.

73. Hadley MN, Grahm TW, Harrington T, Schiller WR, McDermott MK, Posillico DB. Nutritional support and neurotrauma: a critical review of early nutrition in forty-five acute head injury patients. Neurosurgery 19:367–373, 1986.

74. Minard G, Kudsk KA, Melton S, Patton JH, Tolley EA. Early versus delayed feeding with an immune-enhancing diet in patients with severe head injuries. JPEN J Parenter Enteral Nutr 24:145–149, 2000.

75. Ott L, Young B, Phillips R, et al. Altered gastric emptying in the head-injured patient: relationship to feeding intolerance. J Neurosurg 74:738–742, 1991.

76. Bergsneider M, Hovda DA, Shalmon E, et al. Cerebral hyperglycolysis following severe traumatic brain injury in humans: a positron emission tomography study. J Neurosurg 86:241–251, 1997.

77. Garnier P, Bertrand N, Flamand B, Beley A. Preischemic blood glucose supply to the brain modulates HSP(72) synthesis and neuronal damage in gerbils. Brain Res 836:245–255, 1999.

78. Lam AM, Winn HR, Cullen BF, Sundling N. Hyperglycemia and neurological outcome in patients with head injury. J Neurosurg 75:545–551, 1991.

79. Crutchfield JS, Narayan RK, Robertson CS, Michael LH. Evaluation of a fiberoptic intracranial pressure monitor. J Neurosurg 72:482–487, 1990.

80. Lyons MK, Meyer FB: Cerebrospinal fluid physiology and the management of increased intracranial pressure. Mayo Clin Proc 65:684–707, 1990.

81. Martinez-Manas RM, Santamarta D, de Campos JM, Ferrer E. Camino intracranial pressure monitor: prospective study of accuracy and complications. J Neurol Neurosurg Psychiatry 69:82–86, 2000.

82. Juul N, Morris GF, Marshall SB, Marshall LF. Intracranial hypertension and cerebral perfusion pressure: influence on neurological deterioration and outcome in severe head injury. The Executive Committee of the International Selfotel Trial. J Neurosurg 92:1–6, 2000.

83. Cooper KR, Boswell PA, Choi SC. Safe use of PEEP in patients with severe head injury. J Neurosurg 63:552–555, 1985.

84. Rudy EB, Turner BS, Baun M, Stone KS, Brucia J. Endotracheal suctioning in adults with head injury. Heart Lung 20:667–674, 1991.

85. Rudy EB, Baun M, Stone K, Turner B. The rela-

tionship between endotracheal suctioning and changes in intracranial pressure: a review of the literature. Heart Lung 15:488–494, 1986.

86. Ropper AH, O'Rourke D, Kennedy SK. Head position, intracranial pressure, and compliance. Neurology 32:1288–1291, 1982.

87. Feldman Z, Kanter MJ, Robertson CS, et al. Effect of head elevation on intracranial pressure, cerebral perfusion pressure, and cerebral blood flow in head-injured patients. J Neurosurg 76:207–211, 1992.

88. Hunt K, Hallworth S, Smith M. The effects of rigid collar placement on intracranial and cerebral perfusion pressures. Anaesthesia 56:511–513, 2001.

89. Borel C, Hanley D, Diringer MN, Rogers MC. Intensive management of severe head injury. Chest 98:180–189, 1990.

90. Wolf AL, Levi L, Marmarou A, et al. Effect of THAM upon outcome in severe head injury: a randomized prospective clinical trial. J Neurosurg 78:54–59, 1993.

91. Carmona Suazo JA, Maas AI, van den Brink WA, van Santbrink H, Steyerberg EW, Avezaat CJ. CO_2 reactivity and brain oxygen pressure monitoring in severe head injury. Crit Care Med 28:3268–3274, 2000.

92. Muizelaar JP, Marmarou A, Ward JD, et al. Adverse effects of prolonged hyperventilation in patients with severe head injury: a randomized clinical trial. J Neurosurg 75:731–739, 1991.

93. Smith HP, Kelly DL Jr, McWhorter JM, et al. Comparison of mannitol regimens in patients with severe head injury undergoing intracranial monitoring. J Neurosurg 65:820–824, 1986.

94. Node Y, Nakazawa S. Clinical study of mannitol and glycerol on raised intracranial pressure and on their rebound phenomenon. Adv Neurol 52:359–363, 1990.

95. Qureshi AI, Suarez JI. Use of hypertonic saline solutions in treatment of cerebral edema and intracranial hypertension. Crit Care Med 28:3301–3313, 2000.

96. Sato M, Tanaka S, Suzuki K, Kohama A, Fujii C. Complications associated with barbiturate therapy. Resuscitation 17:233–241, 1989.

97. Forbes AR, Gamsu G. Depression of lung mucociliary clearance by thiopental and halothane. Anesth Analg 58:387–389, 1979.

98. Rockoff MA, Marshall LF, Shapiro HM. High-dose barbiturate therapy in humans: a clinical review of 60 patients. Ann Neurol 6:194–199, 1979.

99. Schalen W, Messeter K, Nordstrom CH. Complications and side effects during thiopentone therapy in patients with severe head injuries. Acta Anaesthesiol Scand 36:369–377, 1992.

100. Farling PA, Johnston JR, Coppel DL. Propofol infusion for sedation of patients with head injury in intensive care. A preliminary report. Anaesthesia 44:222–226, 1989.

101. Herregods L, Verbeke J, Rolly G, Colardyn F. Effect of propofol on elevated intracranial pressure. Preliminary results. Anaesthesia 43 Suppl:107–109, 1988.

102. Pinaud M, Lelausque JN, Chetanneau A, Fauchoux N, Menegalli D, Souron R. Effects of propofol on cerebral hemodynamics and metabolism in patients with brain trauma. Anesthesiology 73:404–409, 1990.

103. Kelly DF, Goodale DB, Williams J, et al. Propofol in the treatment of moderate and severe head injury: a randomized, prospective double-blind pilot trial. J Neurosurg 90:1042–1052, 1999.

104. Guerra WK, Gaab MR, Dietz H, Mueller JU, Piek J, Fritsch MJ. Surgical decompression for traumatic brain swelling: indications and results. J Neurosurg 90:187–196, 1999.

105. Dearden NM, Gibson JS, McDowall DG, Gibson RM, Cameron MM. Effect of high-dose dexamethasone on outcome from severe head injury. J Neurosurg 64:81–88, 1986.

106. Roberts I, Schierhout G, Alderson P. Absence of evidence for the effectiveness of five interventions routinely used in the intensive care management of severe head injury: a systematic review. J Neurol Neurosurg Psychiatry 65:729–733, 1998.

107. Andrews BT, Pitts LH, Lovely MP, Bartkowski H. Is computed tomographic scanning necessary in patients with tentorial herniation? Results of immediate surgical exploration without computed tomography in 100 patients. Neurosurgery 19:408–414, 1986.

108. Arienta C, Baiguini M, Granata G, Villani R. Acute bilateral epidural hematomas. Report of two cases and review of the literature. J Neurosurg Sci 30:139–142, 1986.

109. Dharker SR, Bhargava N. Bilateral epidural haematoma. Acta Neurochir (Wien) 110:29–32, 1991.

110. Lui TN, Lee ST, Chang CN, Cheng WC. Epidural hematomas in the posterior cranial fossa. J Trauma 34:211–215, 1993.

111. Pozzati E, Tognetti F, Cavallo M, Acciarri N. Extradural hematomas of the posterior cranial fossa. Observations on a series of 32 consecutive cases treated after the introduction of computed tomography scanning. Surg Neurol 32:300–303, 1989.

112. Rivano, Borzone CM, Altomonte M, Capuzzo T. Traumatic posterior fossa extradural hematomas. Neurochirurgia (Stuttg) 35:43–47, 1992.

113. Chen TY, Wong CW, Chang CN, et al. The expectant treatment of "asymptomatic" supratentorial epidural hematomas. Neurosurgery 32:176–179, 1993.

114. Seelig JM, Marshall LF, Toutant SM, et al. Traumatic acute epidural hematoma: unrecognized high lethality in comatose patients. Neurosurgery 15:617–620, 1984.

115. Wilberger JE Jr, Harris M, Diamond DL. Acute subdural hematoma: morbidity, mortality, and operative timing. J Neurosurg 74:212–218, 1991.

116. Cervantes LA. Concurrent delayed temporal and posterior fossa epidural hematomas. Case report. J Neurosurg 59:351–353, 1983.

117. Delfini R, Santoro A, Innocenzi G, Ciappetta P, Salvati M, Zamponi C. Interhemispheric subdural hematoma (ISH). Case report. J Neurosurg Sci 35:217–220, 1991.

118. Vaz R, Duarte F, Oliveira J, Cerejo A, Cruz C. Traumatic interhemispheric subdural haematomas. Acta Neurochir (Wien) 111:128–131, 1991.

119. Borovich B, Braun J, Guilburd JN, et al. Delayed onset of traumatic extradural hematoma. J Neurosurg 63:30–34, 1985.

120. Piepmeier JM, Wagner FC Jr. Delayed posttraumatic extracerebral hematoma. J Trauma 22:455–460, 1982.

121. Feuerman T, Wackym PA, Gade GF, Lanman T, Becker D. Intraoperative development of contralateral epidural hematoma during evacuation of traumatic extraaxial hematoma. Neurosurgery 23:480–484, 1988.

122. Meguro K, Kobayashi E, Maki Y. Acute brain swelling during evacuation of subdural hematoma caused by delayed contralateral extradural hematoma: report of two cases. Neurosurgery 20:326–328, 1987.

123. Starr AJ, Hunt JL, Chason DP, Reinert CM, Walker J. Treatment of femur fracture with associated head injury. J Orthop Trauma 12:38–45, 1998.

124. Pozzati E, Tognetti F. Spontaneous healing of acute extradural hematomas: study of twenty-two cases. Neurosurgery 18:696–700, 1986.

125. Jones NR, Blumbergs PC, North JB. Acute subdural haematomas: aetiology, pathology and outcome. Aust N Z J Surg 56:907–913, 1986.

126. Phonprasert C, Suwanwela C, Hongsaprabhas C, Prichayudh P, O'Charoen S. Extradural hematoma: analysis of 138 cases. J Trauma 20:679–683, 1980.

127. Rivas JJ, Lobato RD, Sarabia R, Cordobes F, Cabrera A, Gomez P. Extradural hematoma: analysis of factors influencing the courses of 161 patients. Neurosurgery 23:44–51, 1988.

128. Howard MA III, Gross AS, Dacey RG Jr, Winn HR. Acute subdural hematomas: an age-dependent clinical entity. J Neurosurg 71:858–863, 1989.

129. Gutman MB, Moulton RJ, Sullivan I, Hotz G, Tucker WS, Muller PJ. Risk factors predicting operable intracranial hematomas in head injury. J Neurosurg 77:9–14, 1992.

130. Bullock R, Golek J, Blake G. Traumatic intracerebral hematoma—which patients should undergo surgical evacuation? CT scan features and ICP monitoring as a basis for decision making. Surg Neurol 32;181–187, 1989.

131. Nakstad P, Nornes H, Hauge HN. Traumatic aneurysms of the pericallosal arteries. Neuroradiology 28:335–338, 1986.

132. Soria ED, Paroski MW, Schamann ME. Traumatic aneurysms of cerebral vessels: a case study and review of the literature. Angiology 39:609–615, 1988.

133. Parkinson D, West M. Traumatic intracranial aneurysms. J Neurosurg 52:11–20, 1980.

134. Senegor M. Traumatic pericallosal aneurysm in a patient with no major trauma. Case report. J Neurosurg 75:475–477, 1991.

135. Errico TJ, Bauer RD, Waugh T (eds). Spinal Trauma. JB Lippincott, Philadelphia, 1991.

136. Meyer PR Jr (ed). Surgery of Spine Trauma. Churchill Livingstone, New York, 1989.

137. Ross SE, Schwab CW, David ET, Delong WG, Born CT. Clearing the cervical spine: initial radiologic evaluation. J Trauma 27:1055–1060, 1987.

138. Harris MB, Waguespack AM, Kronlage S. 'Clearing' cervical spine injuries in polytrauma patients:

is it really safe to remove the collar? Orthopedics 20:903–907, 1997.

139. Powell JN, Waddell JP, Tucker WS, Transfeldt EE. Multiple-level noncontiguous spinal fractures. J Trauma 29:1146–1150, 1989.

140. Perovitch M, Perl S, Wang H. Current advances in magnetic resonance imaging (MRI) in spinal cord trauma: review article. Paraplegia 30:305–316, 1992.

141. Emery SE, Pathria MN, Wilber RG, Masaryk T, Bohlman HH. Magnetic resonance imaging of posttraumatic spinal ligament injury. J Spinal Disord 2:229–233, 1989.

142. Allen BL Jr, Ferguson RL, Lehmann TR, O'Brien RP. A mechanistic classification of closed, indirect fractures and dislocations of the lower cervical spine. Spine 7:1–27, 1982.

143. Cloward RB. Acute cervical spine injuries. Clin Symp 32:1–32, 1980.

144. Fielding JW. Injuries to the upper cervical spine. Instr Course Lect 36:483–494, 1987.

145. Harris HJ Jr, Edeiken-Monroe B. Radiology of Acute Cervical Spine Trauma, 2nd ed. Williams & Wilkins, Baltimore, 1987.

146. Eismont FJ, Arena MJ, Green BA. Extrusion of an intervertebral disc associated with traumatic subluxation or dislocation of cervical facets. Case report. J Bone Joint Surg Am 73:1555–1560, 1991.

147. Morse SD. Acute central cervical spinal cord syndrome. Ann Emerg Med 11:436–439, 1982.

148. Francis WR, Fielding JW, Hawkins RJ, Pepin J, Hensinger R. Traumatic spondylolisthesis of the axis. J Bone Joint Surg Br 63B:313–318, 1981.

149. Levine AM, Edwards CC. The management of traumatic spondylolisthesis of the axis. J Bone Joint Surg Am 67:217–226, 1985.

150. Anderson LD, D'Alonzo RT. Fractures of the odontoid process of the axis. J Bone Joint Surg Am 56:1663–1674, 1974.

151. Fujii E, Kobayashi K, Hirabayashi K. Treatment in fractures of the odontoid process. Spine 13:604–609, 1988.

152. Hanssen AD, Cabanela ME. Fractures of the dens in adult patients. J Trauma 27:928–934, 1987.

153. Aebi M, Mohler J, Zach G, Morscher E. Analysis of 75 operated thoracolumbar fractures and fracture dislocations with and without neurological deficit. Arch Orthop Trauma Surg 105:100–112, 1986.

154. Atlas SW, Regenbogen V, Rogers LF, Kim KS. The radiographic characterization of burst fractures of the spine. AJR Am J Roentgenol 147:575–582, 1986.

155. Krompinger WJ, Fredrickson BE, Mino DE, Yuan HA. Conservative treatment of fractures of the thoracic and lumbar spine. Orthop Clin North Am 17:161–170, 1986.

156. Weinstein JN, Collalto P, Lehmann TR. Thoracolumbar "burst" fractures treated conservatively: a long-term follow-up. Spine 13:33–38, 1988.

157. Byrnes DP, Russo GL, Ducker TB, Cowley RA. Sacrum fractures and neurological damage. Report of two cases. J Neurosurg 47:459–462, 1977.

158. Carl A, Delman A, Engler G. Displaced transverse sacral fractures. A case report, review of the liter-

ature, and the CT scan as an aid in management. Clin Orthop 194:195–198, 1985.

159. Chiaruttini M. Transverse sacral fracture with transient neurologic complication. Ann Emerg Med 16:111–113, 1987.

160. Dowling T, Epstein JA, Epstein NE. S1–S2 sacral fracture involving neural elements of the cauda equina. A case report and review of the literature. Spine 10:851–853, 1985.

161. Patterson FP, Morton KS. Neurologic complications of fractures and dislocations of the pelvis. Surg Gynecol Obstet 112:702–706, 1961.

162. Sabiston CP, Wing PC. Sacral fractures: classification and neurologic implications. J Trauma 26: 1113–1115, 1986.

163. Denis F, Davis S, Comfort T. Sacral fractures: an important problem. Retrospective analysis of 236 cases. Clin Orthop 227:67–81, 1988.

164. Bedbrook GM. Treatment of thoracolumbar dislocation and fractures with paraplegia. Clin Orthop 112:27–43, 1975.

165. Bedbrook GM. Spinal injuries with tetraplegia and paraplegia. J Bone Joint Surg Br 61B:267–284, 1979.

166. Bedbrook G, Clark WB. Thoracic spine injuries with spinal cord damage. J R Coll Surg Edinb 26: 264–271, 1981.

167. Waters RL, Adkins RH, Yakura JS. Definition of complete spinal cord injury. Paraplegia 29:573–581, 1991.

168. Hall ED. The neuroprotective pharmacology of methylprednisolone. J Neurosurg 76:13–22, 1992.

169. Tator CH, Fehlings MG. Review of the secondary injury theory of acute spinal cord trauma with emphasis on vascular mechanisms. J Neurosurg 75: 15–26, 1991.

170. Amar AP, Levy ML. Pathogenesis and pharmacological strategies for mitigating secondary damage in acute spinal cord injury. Neurosurgery 44:1027–1039, 1999.

171. Bracken MB, Shepard MJ, Collins WF, et al. A randomized, controlled trial of methylprednisolone or naloxone in the treatment of acute spinal-cord injury. Results of the Second National Acute Spinal Cord Injury Study. N Engl J Med 322: 1405–1411, 1990.

172. Bracken MB, Shepard MJ, Collins WF Jr, et al. Methylprednisolone or naloxone treatment after acute spinal cord injury: 1-year follow-up data. Results of the second National Acute Spinal Cord Injury Study. J Neurosurg 76:23–31, 1992.

173. Geisler FH, Dorsey FC, Coleman WP. Recovery of motor function after spinal-cord injury—a randomized, placebo-controlled trial with GM-1 ganglioside. N Engl J Med 324:1829–1838, 1991.

174. Ledsome JR, Sharp JM. Pulmonary function in acute cervical cord injury. Am Rev Respir Dis 124: 41–44, 1981.

175. Mansel JK, Norman JR. Respiratory complications and management of spinal cord injuries. Chest 97:1446–1452, 1990.

176. Doolan LA, O'Brien JF. Safe intubation in cervical spine injury. Anaesth Intensive Care 13:319–324, 1985.

177. King HK, Wang LF, Khan AK, Wooten DJ. Transla-

178. Brisman R, Kovach RM, Johnson DO, Roberts CR, Ward GS. Pulmonary edema in acute transection of the cervical spinal cord. Surg Gynecol Obstet 139:363–366, 1974.

179. Carter RE. Respiratory aspects of spinal cord injury management. Paraplegia 25:262–266, 1987.

180. Kiker JD, Woodside JR, Jelinek GE. Neurogenic pulmonary edema associated with autonomic dysreflexia. J Urol 128:1038–1039, 1982.

181. Reines HD, Harris RC. Pulmonary complications of acute spinal cord injuries. Neurosurgery 21: 193–196, 1987.

182. Winslow EB, Lesch M, Talano JV, Meyer PR Jr. Spinal cord injuries associated with cardiopulmonary complications. Spine 11:809–812, 1986.

183. Marshall LF, Knowlton S, Garfin SR, et al. Deterioration following spinal cord injury. A multicenter study. J Neurosurg 66:400–404, 1987.

184. Alexander S, Kerr FW. Blood pressure responses in acute compression of the spinal cord. J Neurosurg 21:485–491, 1964.

185. Lambert DH, Deane RS, Mazuzan JE Jr. Anesthesia and the control of blood pressure in patients with spinal cord injury. Anesth Analg 61:344–348, 1982.

186. Evans DE, Kobrine AI, Rizzoli HV. Cardiac arrhythmias accompanying acute compression of the spinal cord. J Neurosurg 52:52–59, 1980.

187. Comarr AE. Neurourology of spinal cord-injured patients. Semin Urol 10:74–82, 1992.

188. Gebarski KS, Glazer GM, Gebarski SS. Brachial plexus: anatomic, radiologic, and pathologic correlation using computed tomography. J Comput Assist Tomogr 6:1058–1063, 1982.

189. Gupta RK, Mehta VS, Banerji AK, Jain RK. MR evaluation of brachial plexus injuries. Neuroradiology 31:377–381, 1989.

190. Alnot JY. Traumatic brachial plexus palsy in the adult. Retro- and infraclavicular lesions. Clin Orthop 237:9–16, 1988.

191. Kline DG, Judice DJ. Operative management of selected brachial plexus lesions. J Neurosurg 58: 631–649, 1983.

192. Leffert RD. Brachial-plexus injuries. N Engl J Med 291:1059–1067, 1974.

193. Carlstedt T, Anand P, Hallin R, Misra PV, Norén G, Seferlis T. Spinal nerve root repair and reimplantation of avulsed ventral roots into the spinal cord after brachial plexus injury. J Neurosurg 93: 237–247, 2000.

194. Sidhu JS, Dhillon MK. Lumbosacral plexus avulsion with pelvic fractures. Injury 22:156–158, 1991.

195. Birchard JD, Pichora DR, Brown PM. External iliac artery and lumbosacral plexus injury secondary to an open book fracture of the pelvis: report of a case. J Trauma 30:906–908, 1990.

196. Freedy RM, Miller KD Jr, Eick JJ, Granke DS. Traumatic lumbosacral nerve root avulsion: evaluation by MR imaging. J Comput Assist Tomogr 13:1052–1057, 1989.

197. Mirovsky Y, Hendel D, Halperin N. Anterior interosseous nerve palsy following closed fracture of the proximal ulna. A case report and review of the

literature. Arch Orthop Trauma Surg 107:61–64, 1988.

198. Aro H, Koivunen T, Katevuo K, Nieminen S, Aho AJ. Late compression neuropathies after Colles' fractures. Clin Orthop 233:217–225, 1988.

199. Gelberman RH, Szabo RM, Mortensen WW. Carpal tunnel pressures and wrist position in patients with Colles' fractures. J Trauma 24:747–749, 1984.

200. Maye U, Hacke W. Anterior interosseous nerve syndrome following supracondylar lesions of the median nerve: clinical findings and electrophysiological investigations. J Neurol 229:91–96, 1983.

201. Barrios C, Ganoza C, de Pablos J, Canadell J. Post-traumatic ulnar neuropathy versus non-traumatic cubital tunnel syndrome: clinical features and response to surgery. Acta Neurochir (Wien) 110: 44–48, 1991.

202. Shah JJ, Bhatti NA. Radial nerve paralysis associated with fractures of the humerus. A review of 62 cases. Clin Orthop 172:171–176, 1983.

203. Levy D. The fat embolism syndrome. A review. Clin Orthop 261:281–286, 1990.

204. Kamenar E, Burger PC. Cerebral fat embolism: a neuropathological study of a microembolic state. Stroke 11:477–484, 1980.

205. Fabian TC, Hoots AV, Stanford DS, Patterson CR, Mangiante EC. Fat embolism syndrome: prospective evaluation in 92 fracture patients. Crit Care Med 18:42–46, 1990.

206. Findlay JM, DeMajo W. Cerebral fat embolism. Can Med Assoc J 131:755–757, 1984.

207. Gossling HR, Pellegrini VD Jr. Fat embolism syndrome: a review of the pathophysiology and physiological basis of treatment. Clin Orthop 165:68–82, 1982.

208. Hagley SR, Lee FC, Blumbergs PC. Fat embolism syndrome with total hip replacement. Med J Aust 145:541–543, 1986.

209. Jacobson DM, Terrence CF, Reinmuth OM. The neurologic manifestations of fat embolism. Neurology 36:847–851, 1986.

210. Chastre J, Fagon JY, Soler P, et al. Bronchoalveolar lavage for rapid diagnosis of the fat embolism syndrome in trauma patients. Ann Intern Med 113:583–588, 1990.

211. Sakamoto T, Sawada Y, Yukioka T, Yoshioka T, Sugimoto T, Taneda M. Computed tomography for diagnosis and assessment of cerebral fat embolism. Neuroradiology 24:283–285, 1983.

212. McCarthy M, Norenberg MD. Pontine hemorrhagic infarction in nontraumatic fat embolism. Neurology 38:1645–1647, 1988.

213. Saito A, Meguro K, Matsumura A, Komatsu Y, Oohashi N. Magnetic resonance imaging of a fat embolism of the brain: case report. Neurosurgery 26:882–884, 1990.

214. Takahashi M, Suzuki R, Osakabe Y, et al. Magnetic resonance imaging findings in cerebral fat embolism: Correlation with clinical manifestations. J Trauma 46:324–327, 1999.

215. Yoshida A, Okada Y, Nagata Y, Hanaguri K, Morio M. Assessment of cerebral fat embolism by magnetic resonance imaging in the acute stage. J Trauma 40:437–440, 1996.

Chapter 18

NEUROLOGIC COMPLICATIONS OF ORGAN TRANSPLANTATION

Despite the worrisome scarcity of organs and the substantial cost to society, transplantation has become firmly established as a viable cure for vital organ failure and not only for the fortunate few. The lives of many people are affected by transplantation, and most patients rate their quality of life as good or excellent.[1] Most academic institutions have meticulously organized transplantation programs, yet several teams share the responsibility for care of the transplant patient. Currently, patients are admitted to surgical units specially equipped for transplant recipients.

Transplantation has profoundly changed the spectrum of neurologic consultations in the intensive care unit (ICU), and a bewildering new array of neurologic complications has appeared. Neurologists should expect to be frequently consulted in the perioperative period. When they appear, neurologic complications are confined largely to use of immunosuppressive drugs or to infectious complications in immunocompromised patients. Other neurologic complications, particularly peripheral nerve damage, are related to the surgical procedure and are less specific in most instances.

Currently, the kidney, pancreas, liver, heart, and lung, alone or in combination, are successfully transplanted. Although in a sense not strictly an organ, hematopoietic stem cell is included here. Neurologic complication from transplantation occurs in approximately 10% of patients, but the frequency may depend on motivation of transplant teams to consult a neurologist. Prospective incidence studies may not capture all the postoperative events, and to be accurate, they would require a neurologist on daily rounds. Neurologic complications may be major when they involve recurrent seizures, postoperative failure to awaken, immunosuppression neurotoxicity, or acute disabling neuromuscular disease, all of which are addressed in this chapter. A monograph richer in detail on the neurologic complications in organ transplant recipients can be consulted for more in-depth coverage.[2]

GENERAL CONSIDERATIONS IN TRANSPLANTATION

Transplantation programs may have subtle differences in procedures, postoperative care, and immunosuppression regimens, but most critical care aspects are uniform. A brief overview of the first postoperative weeks in each of these transplantations may help in understanding the circumstances in which neurologic complications occur.

Kidney and Pancreas Transplantation

The recipient of a renal graft is least likely to have a prolonged intensive care stay. Most patients do well, are already extubated a few hours after surgery, and have graft function without major clinical intervention. Occasionally, cadaver kidneys take hours to resume production of urine. Deterioration of the renal graft results in oliguria, increasing creatinine, fever, and hypertension. Uremia may occur suddenly, most frequently from acute tubular necrosis, acute accelerated rejection, or renal vein thrombosis, but these conditions are rare. Wound infection and renal artery thrombosis may also result in loss of the graft. The most life-threatening complication—hemorrhage in the transplant bed when the suture line of the vascular anastomosis is insufficient—may result in hypovolemic shock and a need for urgent exploration.

Chronic rejection occurs in up to 50% of renal transplant recipients by histologic criteria and remains a major cause for graft loss 1 year after transplantation. Graft rejection is countered with high doses of corticosteroids, and if this treatment is unsuccessful, muromonab-CD3, tacrolimus, or mycophenolate mofetil (CellCept) is given. Mycophenolate mofetil prevents the glycosylation of adhesion molecules needed for lymphocytes to attach to endothelium and in combination with corticosteroids is a powerful agent against rejection, with more than 80% graft preservation.[3]

Pancreas transplantation is typically combined with renal transplantation, invariably in patients with secondary effects of diabetes mellitus. A significant halt in organ damage from vascular complications and even improvement in nerve conduction have been established in patients with insulin-dependent diabetes mellitus. Uncommon complications of pancreas transplantation are pancreatitis due to procurement or reperfusion injury, fistula and abscesses from anastomosis, leak of pancreatic fluids and urologic complications in patients with bladder-draining grafts. However, the incidence of surgical complications is declining, probably because of improved antimicrobial therapy and intensive care. The largest single center experience, from the University of Minnesota, reported a significant improvement in overall outcome except for increased bleeding complications due to prophylaxis with heparin and aspirin. No neurologic complications were reported.[4]

Heart and Lung Transplantation

The hemodynamic function of the cardiac graft in the first postoperative days determines care in the ICU. One may theoretically expect a large increase in cardiac output and relative hypertension when a poorly functioning heart has been replaced by an adequate muscle pump. In clinical practice, however, a tendency to become hypotensive is the rule. The transplanted heart may have been subjected to insults during procurement. Massive sympathetic outpouring before the diagnosis of brain death in the donor became established may have resulted in myocardial injury from contraction band necrosis. However, ventricular dysfunction is more likely to be due to prolonged ischemic time. Additionally, the denervated heart cannot adjust easily to marked changes in filling pressure, and cardiac output is frequently maintained with inotropic agents. Nonetheless, use of cyclosporine and increasing doses of inotropic agents may cause overcompensation to hypertension. Cardiac arrhythmias are a major postoperative concern, and a temporary pacemaker has been indicated in instances of complete heart block. Rejection of the transplanted heart may be manifested by fever and hypotension. In other patients, the clinical manifestations include extreme fatigue and dyspnea. Less severe rejection is asymptomatic and is demonstrated only by endomyocardial biopsy.

The number of lung transplantations is increasing, but the critical care experience is still limited. Early complications include cytomegalovirus pneumonitis and obstructive bronchiolitis, which may lead to loss of the graft. Many of the neurologic manifestations in lung transplantations in the early postoperative course may be related to severe hypoxemia caused by airway obstruction. Postoperative hypotension may occur because of strict fluid management to prevent pulmonary edema. However, two recent studies on neurologic complications in lung transplantation did not record any specific complications and emphasized seizures, neurotoxicity of cyclosporine, and infection.[5,6] Occasionally, transient brachial plexopathy occurs from forceful splitting of the rib cage during thoracotomy. Phrenic nerve damage and diaphragmatic failure may be associated with hilar dissection, but damage to the nerve is generally avoided by the transplant surgeon.[7]

Liver Transplantation

Chronic liver failure (for example, primary biliary cirrhosis, primary sclerosing angiitis, alcoholic cirrhosis, and hepatitis C infection), primary liver cancer, and fulminant hepatic failure are accepted indications for liver transplantation. Recently, liver transplantation in selected patients with amyloidosis, Wilson's disease, and Crigler-Najjar syndrome[8] has led to significant improvement in the neurologic manifestations.

The fundamentals of postoperative care in liver recipients include management of coagulopathy, pulmonary care, and management of blood pressure and fluids.[9,10] The production of clotting factors (for example, factor V) is one of the indicators of graft function, but severe coagulopathy may persist in the first postoperative days. Infusion of fresh-frozen plasma and platelets is often needed. In the first postoperative days, fluid loss from third space sequestration and protein loss from drains are common, but fluid status may rapidly switch into hypervolemia associated with hypertension.

The perioperative phase of liver transplantation is full of challenges to the integrity of the brain. Severe bleeding may occur during hepatectomy. Venovenous bypass during the anhepatic phase may increase damage to the portal vein or injure the axillary vein, resulting in profound rapid blood loss and shock.

The postoperative period in liver transplantation is frequently dominated by nosocomial infections that may cause death from sepsis. Selective gut decontamination and antifungal prophylaxis may limit the risk of infection, but the multiplicity of lines, catheters, and drains also predisposes to infection and emphasizes the need for strict sterile techniques.

Hematopoietic Stem Cell Transplantation

Use of hematopoietic transplantation, effective in hematologic malignant disorders, is increasing. In the pretransplantation period, neurologic side effects, including seizures, transverse myelitis, leukoencephalopathy, meningitis, and isolated cranial nerve palsies, can occur from high doses of multiple chemotherapeutic agents.[11,12] The specific toxicities of chemotherapy and radiotherapy regimens are outside the scope of this chapter. Details can be found in reviews.[13,14]

Three types of bone marrow transplants are in vogue: allogeneic bone marrow transplant (bone marrow from HLA-identical sibling of the patient obtained under general anesthesia), allogeneic peripheral blood stem cell transplant (mobilizing stem cells in donor using granulocyte colony-stimulating factor), and autologous peripheral blood stem cell transplant (patient's own bone marrow, same procedure as allogeneic but no graft-versus-host disease prophylaxis). After hematopoietic stem cell infusion, pancytopenia is expected for 2 to 5 weeks before a significant response is mounted. As expected, infectious complications of the central nervous system are particularly common at the stage of pancytopenia. During this critical period, gram-negative sepsis, bleeding from thrombocytopenia, and disseminated intravascular coagulation are the most feared complications.[11]

A potentially devastating complication (although mild in some cases) is graft-versus-host disease (GVHD),[15] which is diagnosed by skin biopsy, but many other organs can be involved in various degrees. A poorly characterized encephalopathy and seizures were common in a prospective study of bone marrow transplantation, mostly in patients with GVHD.[16]

NEUROLOGIC COMPLICATIONS IN TRANSPLANTATION

Within the range of transplantation-related complications, neurologic manifestations should be considered infrequent. Among the patients with neurologic complications, neurologists must confront difficult issues, the most pressing of which is whether the usually excellent outcome of organ transplantation has been compromised. The effects of neurotoxicity of immunosuppressive agents and seizures are reversible if recognized in time, and to a limited extent, this

may also apply to intracranial infections. Pattern recognition has become a major part of the initial assessment in this well-defined population of patients in the ICU[2] (Table 18–1).

Neurotoxicity of Immunosuppressive Agents

Most transplantation programs have adopted triple drug therapy, but with the introduction of new and possibly less toxic immunosuppressive agents, protocols are continuously adjusted. In liver transplant recipients, cyclosporine typically is administered intravenously, because initially insufficient bile production results in erratic absorption. A recently engineered microemulsion of cyclosporine (Neoral) allows absorption without bile in patients with liver transplantation. Tacrolimus has now been used as a primary

Table 18–1. Neurologic Complications after Transplantation: Classification by Neurologic Signs and Symptoms and Common Diagnostic Considerations

Sign or Symptom	Consideration
Failure to awaken	Hypoxic–ischemic encephalopathy, central pontine myelinolysis, anesthetic agents, air embolism, acute uremia, acute graft failure, multiple intracranial abscesses
Loss of consciousness	Intracranial hemorrhage, fulminant meningitis, seizures, drug toxicity
Confusional state	Immunosuppressive toxicity, acute hypoglycemia, hyperglycemia, corticosteroids, fungal meningitis
Seizures	Cyclosporine or tacrolimus toxicity, intracranial hemorrhage, lymphoma, meningitis, chemotherapeutic agents
Mute or stuttering	Cyclosporine or tacrolimus toxicity, cerebral infarct
Cortical blindness	Cardiac arrest, cyclosporine toxicity, cardiac catheterization, hypertensive encephalopathy
Hemiparesis	Brachial plexopathy, ischemic or hemorrhagic stroke, neoplasm, brain abscess
Tremors	Immunosuppressive drugs
Myoclonus	Hypoxic–ischemic encephalopathy, ketamine or cephalosporin intoxication
Asterixis	Acute liver, renal, or pulmonary disease
Rigidity	Haloperidol overdose, malignant hyperthermia
Muscle weakness	Acute critical illness polyneuropathy, polymyositis, corticosteroids, associated myopathy, neuromuscular blocking agents
Headaches	Fungal meningitis, muromonab-CD3 toxicity, cyclosporine or tacrolimus use, lymphoma, astrocytoma

From Wijdicks EFM. Neurologic complications in transplant recipients: a bird's-eye view. In: Wijdicks EFM (ed). Neurologic Complications in Organ Transplant Recipients. Butterworth-Heinemann, Boston, 1999, pp 57–62. By permission of Mayo Foundation.

immunosuppressive agent, and structural variants of the agent (for example, sirolimus[17]) with a possibly better safety profile are currently under study in clinical trials. Azathioprine and corticosteroids are part of the commonly used immunosuppressive initiation program, but mycophenolate mofetil may replace azathioprine. Its effect is based on inhibition of T and B lymphocytes by the blocking of purine synthesis.

The neurologic manifestations of immunosuppressive agents can be nonspecific, such as acute confusional state, seizures, and diminished alertness, but more typical adverse effects have been reported with all of these agents. The incidence may have changed artificially, because yesterday's side effects may be today's accepted nuisances. Neurologic manifestations have not been reported with use of antithymocyte globulin and azathioprine.

CYCLOSPORINE

Cyclosporine, a cyclic oligopeptide extracted from fungi, mainly inhibits T-lymphocyte maturation, but reduction of interleukin-2 production in helper T cells is equally important.[18] The discovery of immunosuppressive metabolites of *Trichoderma polysporum refai* in a Norwegian soil sample led to cyclosporine. (Sandoz employees on vacation were typically asked to collect soil samples that could harbor microorganisms with antifungal or antibacterial activity.[19]) Cyclosporine has greatly advanced the success rate of organ transplantation.

The systemic side effects of cyclosporine are reversible. These are nephrotoxicity from its vasoconstrictive effect and severe hypertension, either alone or in combination with nephrotoxicity. Neurotoxicity associated with cyclosporine most often develops within the first 2 weeks after transplantation,[20–28] a time when the patient is loaded with the drug to target levels.

Cyclosporine neurotoxicity has been linked to several clinical syndromes with striking abnormalities on neuroimaging.[29] It has been a major cause of the posterior reversible encephalopathy syndrome. Initially, white matter changes were deemed responsible, but cortical involvement is common.[30]

Table 18–2. **Drugs That Increase Cyclosporine Bioavailability and the Risk of Toxicity***

Erythromycin	Ciprofloxacin
Itraconazole	Norfloxacin
Ketoconazole	Oral contraceptives
Diltiazem	Danazol
Nicardipine	Colchicine
Verapamil	Sulindac
Metoclopramide	Fluconazole
Cimetidine	Trimethoprim
Ranitidine	Sulfamethoxazole

*High-fat diet and grapefruit juice increase the risk of neurotoxicity.[31,32]

Hypertensive encephalopathy, which undoubtedly has many features of cyclosporine toxicity in its presentation (see Chapter 9), should be dismissed as a potential mechanism because malignant hypertension (mean arterial pressure >130 mm Hg) and papilledema rarely occur and hypertension occurs months after grafting and is seldom severe in the preoperative period. Predisposing factors that have received considerable attention are aluminum overload, hypomagnesemia, and high doses of corticosteroids, but they may be covariants, and the possibility of important interactions with commonly used drugs should be carefully investigated (Table 18–2).

PATHOPHYSIOLOGIC MECHANISMS

Major theories of cyclosporine toxicity have been proposed, but they are largely speculative.[33–38] Cyclosporine may have a direct damaging effect on the vascular endothelium, causing vasoconstriction from increased plasma endothelium levels or from an altered balance of prostacyclin and thromboxane. Recent evidence suggests that the injury to the brain capillary endothelial cells may inhibit the expression of P-glycoprotein, which has been recognized as a drug efflux pump.[33] Another attractive, but unproven, hypothesis[39] suggests that cyclosporine is transported into the neurons by the low-density lipoprotein receptor, but it applies only to patients with liver transplants. Cholesterol levels are low in recent recipients of liver transplantation, and they may not be restored quickly after grafting. This delay favors binding of cyclosporine to low-density lipoprotein fractions. The low-density lipoprotein receptors in the brain may be sensitized and up-regulated, particularly in patients with low cholesterol levels, and thus bind low-density lipoprotein particles containing cyclosporine. This theory assumes a disturbed blood–brain barrier and low cholesterol levels; both have been inconsistently demonstrated in series of patients with liver transplantation and cyclosporine neurotoxicity. Moreover, cyclosporine neurotoxicity has been described after intralipid infusion, which lowers the low-density lipoprotein fraction and increases the free fraction of cyclosporine, casting more doubt on this mechanism.[40]

Breakdown of the blood–brain barrier is needed for cyclosporine to enter, because no lipoprotein transport system exists. Cyclosporine is very lipophilic from aliphatic groups but cannot cross the blood–brain barrier because of tight junctions.[41] How crossing occurs remains a major mystification. Perhaps impairment of the blood–brain barrier is facilitated by surgery-associated ischemic insults due to hypotension. The predilection of the posterior areas of the brain may also be related to a less developed blood–brain barrier that quickly opens when challenged. Oligodendroglia are more susceptible than astrocytes.[34] This characteristic fits nicely with the largely white matter lesions on magnetic resonance imaging (MRI).[29,38]

The pathway of neurotoxicity associated with cyclosporine or tacrolimus has not been resolved at a molecular level. Both immunosuppressive drugs bind to an immunophilin, a protein with an affinity for both drugs, and consequently trigger a cascade of actions that include blockade of calcineurin. Calcineurin is involved in cell signaling and maintenance of cytoskeletal protein function, particularly in oligodendrocytes. Inhibition of calcineurin activity, therefore, may lead to neuronal death or apoptosis.[34] It remains very likely, however, that extremely high doses in the earlier

days of transplantation due to unfamiliarity with the drugs have had a major role. This possibility is also supported by the very low incidence of cyclosporine neurotoxicity in the oral preparation, resulting in stable blood levels and avoidance of extreme blood levels during intravenous loading.[42] The earliest abnormality seems to be neurotoxicity from fluid extravasation (vasogenic edema) and not cell destruction (cytotoxic edema).[38] Very limited data on pathology suggest demyelination.[25,43] A possible mechanism is shown in Figure 18–1.

Mild side effects of cyclosporine almost always are manifested by fine positional tremor in the fingers,[35] sometimes associated with paresthesias, and resolve after the dose of cyclosporine is reduced. Cyclosporine-associated headaches have been regularly reported and are often refractory to common analgesics. Other typically dose-related side effects are confusional states with delusions and hallucinations. Bizarre behavior with echolalia, a panic state, and paranoia may color its presentation, but increasing lack of interest and lethargy are often the first indicators of cyclosporine toxicity and should not be explained simply by a trivial metabolic derangement. Insomnia may also point to cyclosporine toxicity, but this side effect has not been studied in sleep laboratories.

As early as the first postoperative day, patients may become inactive, and expressive aphasia with paraphasic errors and naming difficulties may appear and progressively worsen within hours.[44,45] Some patients have nonsensical rambling speech or stuttering or become completely mute.[46,47] Visual hallucinations,[45] often with bright colors, may occur intermittently. Some patients may have cortical blindness,[48–51] almost always with corresponding bilateral parieto-occipital increased T2 signal on MRI.[32] In patients with cortical blindness, months may be required for visual acuity to return to normal.[52,53] In autopsy studies, blindness was linked to demyelination and petechial hemorrhage, but edema is more likely in other instances.

When neurotoxicity is unrecognized, patients may lapse into coma or cerebellar or spinal cord symptoms develop. Severe spas-

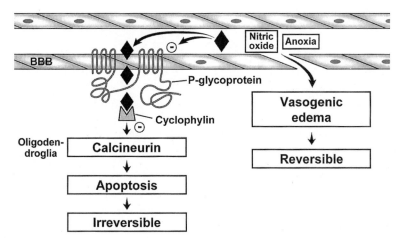

Figure 18–1. Proposed mechanism of cyclosporine neurotoxicity. Damage to the blood–brain barrier (BBB) may lead to vasogenic edema, but prolonged exposure may trigger apoptosis (see text). Black diamonds indicate cyclosporine. (From Wijdicks.[35] By permission of the American Association for the Study of Liver Diseases.)

ticity with brisk reflexes and Babinski's sign is invariably found and resolves after withdrawal of cyclosporine. Oculogyric crises, grimacing, and tongue protrusion as part of severe orofacial dyskinesia were reported in three patients, two of whom recovered completely.[54] In one of these three patients, central pontine myelinolysis was subsequently found on MRI, and incomplete recovery was related to extrapontine locations in the basal ganglia.[54] These manifestations probably are incidental and have been a consequence of early trials with the drug. In our experience, such dramatic presentations are now exceptional.

Many reports have demonstrated virtually complete resolution of neurologic symptoms after administration of cyclosporine was discontinued or the dose significantly reduced. Surprisingly, neurologic symptoms did not recur after rechallenge with lower doses of cyclosporine.[22]

Magnetic resonance imaging is most sensitive in demonstrating cyclosporine neurotoxicity. Mere use of cyclosporine does not produce lesions. In 10 asymptomatic patients treated with cyclosporine, no abnormalities were found by MRI and single-photon emission computed tomography (CT).[55] Typically, abnormalities are predominantly to white matter areas in the occipital lobes[29] but may involve other locations and deeper

structures (Fig. 18–2). Other MRI changes are cerebellar edema and interhemispheric subdural hematomas, which may be related to trauma of the hemispheres against the falx in a patient with coexisting coagulopathy after seizures. Subcortical white matter involvement is typical, but in one fluid-attenuated inversion recovery study, many patients, particularly those with milder toxicity, had cortical lesions.[30] However, cyclosporine neurotoxicity may occur without these MRI abnormalities and must remain a strong contender when changes in level of consciousness or behavior emerge in a patient who recently began receiving immunosuppressive agents.

A well-recognized phenomenon is the poor correlation of neurotoxicity with cyclosporine plasma trough levels. Even more complicated is the situation in which symptoms occur during loading of cyclosporine in an attempt to reach a satisfactory blood level (usually 300 to 400 ng/mL for cyclosporine) in a patient in whom an acute confusional state could have a different origin.

Discontinuation of cyclosporine administration is often entertained first. If the patient has renal failure, recovery from cyclosporine toxicity may require days. Treatment of agitation due to cyclosporine neurotoxicity may include haloperidol (2 to 4 mg intravenously). Switching to another immuno-

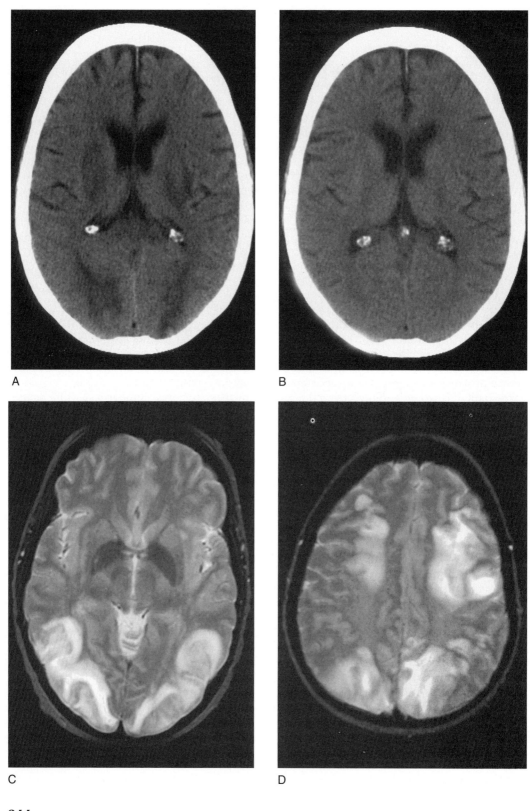

A

B

C

D

Figure 18–2. *A* and *B*: Serial computed tomography scans in a liver transplant patient with cyclosporine toxicity. *A*: Marked hypodensity in the occipital lobes and bilateral lentiform nuclei with some hemorrhagic component due to marked platelet reduction. *B*: Complete resolution after discontinuation of cyclosporine. *C* and *D*: Magnetic resonance image (fluid-attenuated inversion recovery) in a recent patient with severe cyclosporine neurotoxicity following bone marrow transplantation. The presentation was visual hallucinations and a generalized tonic–clonic seizure. Marked hyperintensities are evident in the posterior occipital regions and in areas in the frontal lobes of the brain.

←――――――――――――

suppressive agent is recommended. There is no evidence that rejection is more common with change to another agent. Switching to cyclosporine in patients with tacrolimus neurotoxicity, and vice versa, has been studied in two large series, with resolution in virtually all cases but with a rejection rate of approximately 30% to 40%.[56,57]

Headaches are challenging to treat, but propranolol (20 mg every 6 to 8 hr) has been very effective in most patients, who otherwise may need narcotics for pain control.[58] Headache may be aborted with standard antimigraine therapy because the nature of the throbbing may suggest a vascular type of headache; sumatriptan or a high dose of aspirin (1500 mg) can be considered.[59] Administration of verapamil should be discouraged because of its enhancement of cyclosporine levels. Switching to tacrolimus was successful in one striking case.[59,60]

TACROLIMUS

A promising and possibly less toxic immunosuppressive agent, introduced as FK 506, is now known as tacrolimus.[43,61,62] Tacrolimus suppresses T-lymphocyte activation and inhibits the synthesis of cytokines. Experience is already substantial, and results of the first trials are very favorable in liver transplantation. Hypertension is 50% less than that with cyclosporine, but nephrotoxicity and glucose intolerance remain undesirable effects.[61,62]

Again, certain drugs increase the serum levels of tacrolimus, and they have to be replaced by alternative agents (Table 18–3). Although the chemical structure of tacrolimus is totally different, many clinical features of tacrolimus neurotoxicity, including abnormalities on MRI, are similar to those of cyclosporine.[52,63,64] Many patients have hand tremors. Some severe tremor results in difficulty writing and inability to sign checks and contracts[65] (Fig. 18–3). Tremor is not associated with plasma trough levels and appears to be an all-or-nothing phenomenon. Tremor may become less troublesome with reduction of the dosage but never completely disappears. Painful dysesthesias in the hands and feet sometimes occur without objective neurologic or electrophysiologic findings of small fiber neuropathy. This "tingling hands and restless feet" syndrome has emerged as a common patient complaint with tacrolimus, but response to temazepam (30 mg at night) is good. Speech apraxia or mutism[66] occasionally occurs. Initial studies suggest that vowel distortion is characteristic ("foreign accent syndrome"). Characteristically, some patients have intact auditory comprehension of language, but simple oral nonspeech motor acts (for example, whistling) cannot be performed. A recent positron emission tomography scan image suggested that the abnormality can be traced to the cingulate gyrus.[66] The defect may resolve completely, but stuttering speech may

Table 18–3. **Drugs That Increase Tacrolimus Bioavailability and Chances of Toxicity**

Erythromycin
Clotrimazole
Danazol
Fluconazole

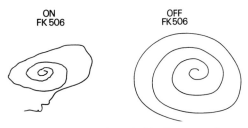

Figure 18–3. Archimedes spiral in liver transplant recipient with "therapeutic" levels of tacrolimus (FK 506) (*left*) and after administration of the drug was discontinued (*right*). Note marked improvement in skilled movement.

Table 18–4. Neurotoxicity of Tacrolimus in 44 Consecutive Patients with Orthotopic Liver Transplantation

Clinical Characteristics	No. of Patients
Tremors	10
Tingling hands and feet	3
Mood swings and psychosis	3
Apraxia of speech	3
Seizures	2

Data from Wijdicks et al.[65]

remain for months.[65] Other significant reported signs are seizures, florid nightmares, bizarre behavior, severe mood swings, inappropriate crying, and acoustic hallucinations (Table 18–4).

A MRI may show increased T2 signals in white matter, representing edema, or remain normal.[65] Diffusion mapping MR may show increased diffusion on the ADC map highly suggestive of vasogenic edema. Abnormalities on MRI have been uncommon in our experience, but we have noted well-documented cases of posterior reversible encephalopathy syndrome. In one report, bilateral thalamic hypodensities not known in cyclosporine neurotoxicity were found, and we had a similar case[64,67] (Fig. 18–4).

Although blood and plasma levels of tacrolimus are usually similar in patients with and without neurotoxicity, peak plasma levels may have a better correlation. Deciding whether neurotoxicity of tacrolimus can explain the clinical symptoms should not depend on tacrolimus plasma trough levels. In all patients, dose reduction results in striking clinical improvement.[65] In one study, tacrolimus neurotoxicity was dramatically reduced in maintenance doses of 0.075 mg/kg twice a day. Reducing the dosage, switching to cyclosporine, and treating symptomatically until clinical resolution are advised.

MUROMONAB-CD3

Muromonab-CD3 (OKT3) is a rescue agent for failing grafts in patients unresponsive to high doses of corticosteroids or antilymphocyte globulin but may also serve as a primary agent, particularly in heart and lung transplantation programs.[68–70] This agent consists of a monoclonal IgG antibody against the T3 receptor of T lymphocytes and blocks recognition of classes I and II major histocompatibility complex antigens.

Its adverse effects are considerable but, as with many other immunosuppressive agents, are self-limiting. Usually, within 1 hr after the first or any subsequent dose, nonspecific signs, such as fever, chills, vomiting, diarrhea, wheezing, and dyspnea, may develop in some patients, but others predominantly have myalgias, rigors, and headache.[71]

The neurotoxicity of muromonab-CD3 involves an aseptic meningitis and, now much less commonly, a severe toxic encephalopathy. Muromonab-CD3 aseptic meningitis may resemble any of the bacterial or fungal meningitides in immunosuppressed patients with nonspecific clinical signs such as fever, meningism, and headache. The spinal fluid formula with polymorphic or mononuclear cells appears to coincide with the degree of fever.[72,73] The true incidence of this meningitis is not known, and if the cerebrospinal fluid (CSF) is not examined for lymphocytic pleocytosis in suspicious cases, the disorder may remain undetected.[74,75] Aseptic meningitis has been found immediately after the first dose, but Adair and associates[72] noted onset of meningitis 5 to 16 days after completion of daily administration of muromonab-CD3. At the Mayo Clinic, muromonab-CD3 is used for induction therapy in heart and lung transplantation. In approximately 200 cases, only three instances of aseptic meningitis were observed (Dr. C. G. A. McGregor, personal communication).

A more dramatic toxic leukoencephalopathy may emerge in muromonab-CD3 administration. Several patients with wild psychotic episodes, hallucinations, multifocal myoclonus, asterixis, and seizures have been reported.[71,76] Out-of-body experience, preoccupation with death, aggressive response to hallucinated objects, and auditory hallucinations occurred before the patients' level of consciousness became impaired 24 to 75 hr after initiation of muromonab-CD3 therapy.[77]

Two reports of muromonab-CD3 encephalopathy highlighted cerebral edema diag-

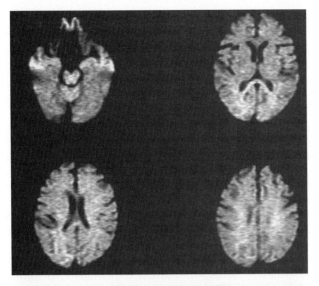

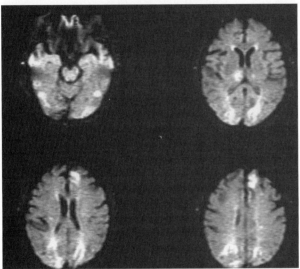

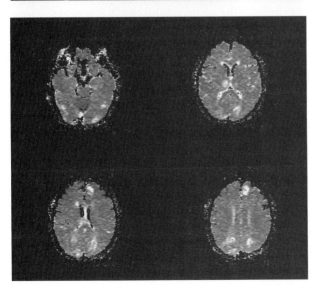

Figure 18–4. Magnetic resonance imaging in a patient with tacrolimus neurotoxicity. Note scattered white matter lesions, with the most severe abnormalities in the occipital parietal areas but abnormalities also in the thalamus and frontal lobe. The upper image includes the isotropic diffusion-weighted images, with b = 1000. The middle image is the corresponding b = 0, FLAIR prepared echoplanar images. The lower image has the apparent diffusion coefficients (ADC) maps. Note that the involved areas are relatively isointense to adjacent brain parenchyma on the isotropic images but have increased signal on the b = 0 images and increased ADC. Findings are consistent with vasogenic edema. A follow-up magnetic resonance image was normal.

347

nosed on computed tomography (CT) and increased CSF opening pressures.[78,79] Patchy gadolinium enhancement and diffuse confluent lesions were observed. Complete resolution was noted after 3 days.[80] Chan and associates[81] found that patients receiving renal transplants who had muromonab-CD3 encephalopathy had been premedicated with indomethacin, which is known to cause an aseptic meningoencephalitis. Drugs that predispose to aseptic meningitis should not be combined with muromonab-CD3 (see Table 6–1 for a complete list). That muromonab-CD3 encephalopathy did not develop in any patient treated at the heart transplant center at the Mayo Clinic could be a consequence of careful blood T-cell monitoring during initiation.

Central Nervous System Infections

Immunocompromised patients have an enhanced susceptibility to systemic infection but less commonly within the 1-month duration of immunosuppression.[82] Nosocomial infections, such as those caused by gram-negative organisms, *Staphylococcus*, and *Candida albicans*, are as frequent in transplant recipients as in any other critically ill patients and are related to contamination of central intravenous catheters and surgical wound sepsis. Many transplantation centers preempt early immunosuppression-associated infection by using trimethoprim-sulfamethoxazole prophylaxis.

This section is divided into brief discussions of the most relevant central nervous system (CNS) infections in the post-transplantation period (Table 18–5). Anecdotal reports of rare parasital or fungal CNS infections, which may occur only in highly endemic areas, are not relevant to most patients and are not discussed in this text.

PARASITIC INFECTIONS

Many parasite species can gain access to the CNS. Some are endemic, and others have a widespread geographic prevalence. *Toxoplasma gondii* remains the most common agent in the immunosuppressed population, but strongyloidiasis, cysticercosis, and *Trypanosoma cruzi* (Chagas' disease) have been reported in renal transplantation.[83,84]

Toxoplasma gondii

One of the most serious parasitic infections in compromised hosts is caused by *Toxoplasma gondii*.[85–88] The CNS involvement may occur in up to 25% of the patients, typically with systemic features at presentation. Several instances of acute toxoplasma encephalitis have been reported, mostly in patients with heart, renal,[85] or bone marrow[87] transplantation. A primary infection in which the graft contains the infection is common in heart transplantation. The dormant organisms in cysts relapse several months after transplantation.

Diagnosis of CNS toxoplasma remains complicated. Clinical symptoms can be minimal with a mild hemiparesis or absent despite multiple abscesses on a CT scan. Headache, low-grade fever, and confusion may be the only findings. Cerebellar signs from a proclivity to lodge in the cerebellum may be found when abscesses reach a critical size. Toxoplasmic abscesses are also often located in the basal ganglia but surprisingly rarely produce movement disorders. Chorioretinitis is infrequently seen, and ophthalmoscopy cannot assist in the diagnosis. In others, acute, fatal toxoplasma encephalitis occurs, and patients may also die from infestation in the myocardium that leads to refractory cardiac arrhythmias.

Before the CT scan era, the diagnosis of CNS toxoplasma was very rarely confirmed, because toxoplasma tachyzoites almost never appear in the CSF. The CSF typically shows a profound mononuclear pleocytosis with a marked increase in protein concentration but a normal glucose value. Toxoplasmosis occurs more often in seropositive patients, but serologic tests in immunocompromised patients are not always helpful. In one study, 23 of 25 bone marrow transplant recipients with disseminated toxoplasmosis had unchanged IgG titers, and specific IgM antibody response was detected in only 2 patients.[89] The sensitivity of polymerase chain reaction is high (around 90%) in untreated patients but its diagnostic value is

Table 18–5. Opportunistic Central Nervous System Infections in Transplant Recipients

Organism	Time from Tx (months)	Presentation	CT or MRI	CSF	Diagnosis	Therapy
Listeria monocytogenes	1–6	Headache, stupor (prior abdominal cramps and diarrhea)	Meningeal enhancement only; commonly brain stem involvement	May be normal	CSF culture	Ampicillin, 10–12 g/day IV; gentamicin, 1.0–1.5 mg/kg IV every 8 hr
Nocardia asteroides	1–6	Localizing findings: headache, stupor	Abscesses (may be solitary)	Pleocytosis	Biopsy, CSF blood culture	Trimethoprim-sulfamethoxazole, 2.5–10.0 mg/kg twice a day
Aspergillus	1–6	Rapidly developing coma, seizures (prior lung infection)	Ring lesion, scattered hemorrhages	Pleocytosis	Biopsy, blood culture	Amphotericin B, 1.0–1.5 mg/kg per day
Cryptococcus neoformans	>6	Unexplained headache, fever, cognitive changes, rarely focal signs	Thalamus, basal ganglia; widespread miliary; no edema	Pleocytosis; may be normal	CSF antigen	Amphotericin B, 1.0–1.5 mg/kg per day
Toxoplasma gondii	>6	Seizures, stupor, rarely focal signs	Multiple lesions, subcortical meninges spared	Pleocytosis; may be normal	Brain biopsy, SPECT	Trimethoprim-sulfamethoxazole, 2.5–10.0 mg/kg twice a day

CSF, cerebrospinal fluid; CT, computed tomography; IV, intravenously; MRI, magnetic resonance imaging; SPECT, single-photon emission computed tomography; Tx, transplantation.

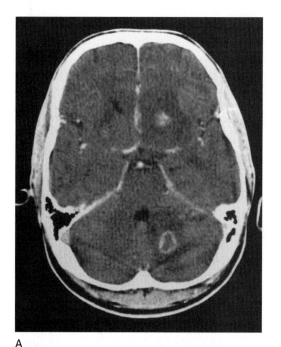
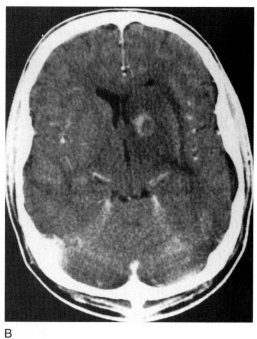

A

B

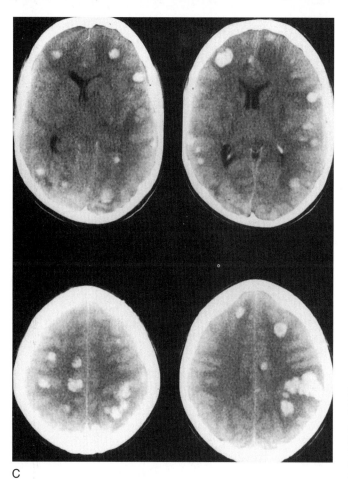

C

Figure 18–5. Computed tomography scans in two patients with toxoplasmosis. Typical predilection sites with ringlike abscesses in cerebellum (*A*) and basal ganglia (*B*). *C*: Multiple hemorrhages. (Panel *C* from Wijdicks et al.[88] By permission of the American Neurological Association.)

markedly reduced when specific treatment has begun.[90]

The CT scan findings are fairly typical. Ring-enhancing necrotic abscesses (Fig. 18–5A) are multiple but can be single on CT scan. In acute fulminant toxoplasmosis, the CT scan is negative or may demonstrate multiple abscesses, brain edema, or multiple rounded hemorrhages[88] (Fig. 18–5B). MRI usually additionally demonstrates abscesses that are not visualized by CT scan and should reveal sparing of the leptomeninges, ependyma, and corpus callosum. MRI may document a small nodule within the wall of the abscess.

Treatment (trimethoprim-sulfamethoxazole) is very effective, and apart from clinical improvement, the abscesses may markedly decrease in size within 10 to 14 days.

VIRAL INFECTIONS

Systemic viral infections may emerge after transplantation but most often are expected 1 month to 6 months after grafting. A systemic viremia is often present in patients with CNS involvement. Some viral infections in immunocompromised patients can cause fulminant and lethal disseminated infections. The most plausible mechanism is reactivation or infection introduced by the graft itself. These viral infections are seen months after transplantation. The virus that causes progressive multifocal leukoencephalopathy, JC virus, is not further considered.[91,92] The presentation is visual loss or frontal lobe dementia, often more than 6 months after transplantation. White matter changes on MRI may involve the parieto-occipital lobe symmetrically but are more often in one location at presentation. This site of predilection is similar to that in immunosuppression neurotoxicity, and differentiation may require brain biopsy when patients are seen several months after transplantation.[93] A polymerase chain reaction is available for diagnosis.[94] Cidofovir may be considered, but mortality remains high.[95]

Cytomegalovirus

Cytomegalovirus is perhaps the most common viral infection after organ transplanta-

tion, but a cytomegalovirus encephalitis is seldom diagnosed during life. Ganciclovir may be effective not only in eradication of the virus but also in prevention. Its use is advocated in many transplantation protocols, particularly among recipients of bone marrow. Unfortunately, strains of cytomegalovirus resistant to conventional treatment with ganciclovir have been reported.

The incidence of cytomegalovirus infection of the brain may have been underestimated. Microglial nodules in cerebral and cerebellar cortex have been reported in recipients of renal, liver, and hematopoietic stem cell transplants and confirmed with in situ hybridization and polymerase chain reaction.

The clinical presentation of cytomegalovirus encephalitis is nonspecific and may include severe refractory headache with profound vomiting, behavior changes, slowly developing memory deficits, and seizures. In a large series of neurologic complications of hematopoietic stem cell transplantation, six patients had neuropathologic evidence of cytomegalovirus infection and, in retrospect, signs of encephalopathy.[96] Convincing cases of cytomegalovirus encephalitis after organ transplantation diagnosed during life are seldom reported.

Cytomegalovirus may also cause Guillain-Barré syndrome or acute transverse myelitis. In these patients, the diagnosis of disseminated cytomegalovirus infection was confirmed by positive cultures of buffy coat and bronchoalveolar lavage fluid and a marked (16-fold) rise in IgG antibody titer. Paraparesis and urinary retention completely resolved with therapy.[97]

Varicella Zoster Virus

Prophylactic administration of antiviral agents after grafting has reduced the occurrence of varicella zoster virus infections. Reactivation of latent infection of sensory ganglion neurons with varicella zoster virus may occur in transplant recipients. Many patients have a dermatomal zoster (shingles), which may disseminate over extensive cutaneous areas. Oral therapy with famciclovir is advocated, but it may not eliminate postherpetic pain.

Less common neurologic manifestations include meningoencephalitis, acute transverse myelitis, and, in some patients, involvement of only a single cranial nerve. Varicella zoster virus infection becomes rapidly more generalized and life threatening due to multiple organ involvement and intravascular coagulation. The standard dose of acyclovir is 10 mg/kg every 8 hr. Detailed neuropathologic studies in transplant recipients have not been reported.

Epstein-Barr Virus

Epstein-Barr virus is involved not only in the development of lymphoma from B-cell proliferation but also in causing a lymphoproliferative disorder.[98] Post-transplantation lymphoproliferative disorder is an unbridled lymphoproliferation induced by Epstein-Barr virus. Constitutional symptoms are similar to those in mononucleosis, with cervical lymphadenopathy, fever, malaise, and pharyngitis, but occasionally jaundice, headache, and nuchal rigidity are found. Lymphoproliferative disease associated with Epstein-Barr virus can be very extensive, involving the entire neuraxis. Overwhelming lymphomatous invasion of the CNS is always part of a systemic dissemination that causes multiple granulomas in many other organs. It occurs in 2% to 3% of solid organ transplants (Fig. 18–6).

An abdominal CT scan confirms the diagnosis. Post-transplantation lymphoproliferative disorder may result in solitary lesions and localized periventricular regions on a brain CT scan. Necrosis and hemorrhage are common, as is ring enhancement. The prognosis is much worse with CNS lesions. Prognosis depends on the morphology, with high mortality in the monomorphic monoclonic types.[99,100]

Human Herpesvirus 6

Human herpesvirus 6 infection can be transmitted through the graft and cause a life-

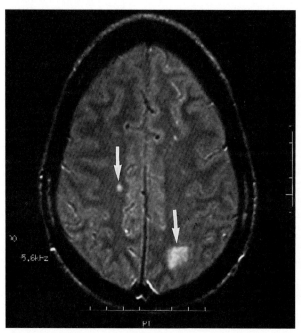
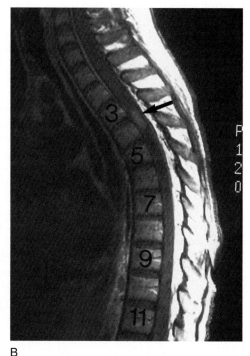

A   B

Figure 18–6. Multiple lesions (arrows) on magnetic resonance images of the brain (*A*) and spine (*B*) in post-transplantation lymphoproliferative disorder.

threatening disseminated infection.[101] Encephalitis occurring within a month after transplantation may be due to human herpesvirus 6.[102] There are clinical similarities with immunosuppression neurotoxicity, but MRI shows multiple nonenhancing, low-attenuation lesions in gray matter without any predilection for a certain localization. Fever may occur in 25% of patients, but most patients are confused, hallucinate, and have progression to coma. The diagnosis can be established by a recently developed polymerase chain reaction. Foscarnet has been successful in some cases, but mortality is high.[101,102]

Adenovirus

Adenovirus infection is frequent after hematopoietic stem cell transplantation,[103] and invasive infection has been reported in 20% of patients. Many patients have severe liver failure, gross hematuria, and pneumonia. Adenovirus can be cultured from a variety of specimens.

An acute meningoencephalitis initially characterized by headache and drowsiness and progressing with seizures, status epilepticus, and coma occurs, and ultrastructurally intranuclear viral aggregates have been reported. There is no effective treatment when this fulminant, uniformly fatal complication occurs.[103]

FUNGAL INFECTIONS

Cryptococcus neoformans and *Aspergillus fumigatus* are most frequently involved in transplant recipients who have fungal meningitis or brain abscesses.[104] Many anecdotal reports are on record of other fungal infections in patients who were immunosuppressed and visited or lived in endemic areas. Coccidioidomycosis is endemic in the southwestern United States, Mexico, and parts of South America, and an increased incidence of infections has been reported in Native Americans, African-Americans, and Filipinos.[105]

Coccidioidal meningitis has been reported in heart transplant recipients and is rapidly fatal. Central nervous system histoplasmosis has a worldwide distribution but is rare in transplant recipients; it may result in subacute or chronic meningitis.[82] Granulomatous meningitis from coccidioidomycosis, histoplasmosis, and blastomycosis can be very difficult to diagnose, often proved only by cultures of a brain biopsy specimen. Only the most common fungal infections in transplant recipients are discussed herein.

Cryptococcus neoformans

Cryptococcosis first appears as a primary pulmonary infection followed by hematogenous dissemination.[106,107] The most typical manifestation of *Cryptococcus* infestation is a meningitis. Clinical symptoms are very often absent, subtle, or fluctuating in severity. Persistent headache may be the only symptom that points to cryptococcal meningitis. Focal neurologic signs, neck stiffness, and papilledema may be absent unless mass lesions emerge. A CSF examination can yield high opening pressures, normal cell count, and findings expected in a fungal meningitis, such as lymphocytic pleocytosis and reduced glucose. In 95% of patients, the diagnosis can be confirmed by CSF culture, positive India ink preparation outlining the capsule, and serologic detection of cryptococcal antigen titers of 1:32 or more.

Parenchymal cryptococcoma and hydrocephalus may be spotted on a CT scan. Cryptococcomas produce hypodense lesions with a predilection for the basal ganglia, thalamus, and periventricular white matter, commonly in a miliary pattern but without appreciable perilesional edema. However, a study of patients with intracranial cryptococcal infection showed normal CT scan findings in 43%, diffuse atrophy in 34%, mass lesions in 11%, and hydrocephalus in 9%, with diffuse cerebral edema in one patient.[108] A MRI may help in recognition by demonstration of multiple enhancing nodules not seen by conventional CT scanning.[109]

Standard treatment for *Cryptococcus neoformans* meningitis or abscesses is amphotericin B intravenously in high doses (1 to 1.5 mg/kg daily) for 4 to 6 weeks while clearance of the CSF cryptococcal antigen is awaited. Fluconazole (400 to 800 mg/day) or itraconazole (200 to 600 mg/day) is given after the first signs of improvement.[110,111] Evidence that recurrence of cryptococcal meningitis results from persistence of the initial strain should influence the decision to use more aggressive combination therapies.[112]

Aspergillus fumigatus

Evolving *Aspergillus* infection in transplant recipients may go unnoticed, and, unfortunately, CNS inoculation is seldom diagnosed before death. Boon and associates[113] emphasized a relatively high incidence (9 of 44 autopsied brains) in liver transplant recipients. In only two patients with CNS aspergillosis, the diagnosis was made shortly before death.

Aspergillus tends to cause meningoencephalitis, but brain abscesses may develop.[114–117] Hemorrhagic necrosis resulting in often fatal intracerebral hematoma is frequently a feature of *Aspergillus* infestation.[115] Therefore, intracerebral hematomas appearing suddenly after transplantation may have resulted from aspergillosis, and this association has been described in heart–lung and bone marrow transplantation.

A large pathology series of 22 patients from Pittsburgh documented seizures in 41%.[115] Rapid onset of coma was associated with generalized tonic–clonic seizures in approximately half the patients. Meningeal signs were uncommon. Of particular interest in the Pittsburgh series was the frequent combination of *Aspergillus* infection in patients with antirejection therapy and retransplantation.[114] At the Mayo Clinic, CNS aspergillosis occurred in 4 of 430 liver transplantations. All instances were fatal. One patient had a solitary abscess at presentation with evidence of hemorrhage on MRI. Systemic aspergillosis became more evident later with pulmonary involvement. Recurrent seizures and, finally, multiorgan failure preceded death. Another patient presented with multiple abscesses and a large ganglionic hemorrhage (Fig. 18–7).

Finally, *Aspergillus* infection can be manifested as a spinal cord syndrome from an epidural abscess.[118] Similarly, progression is rapidly fatal.

Possibly, increased awareness of this devastating fungal infection may increase sur-

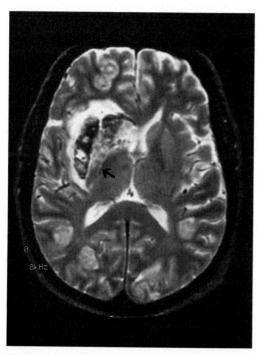 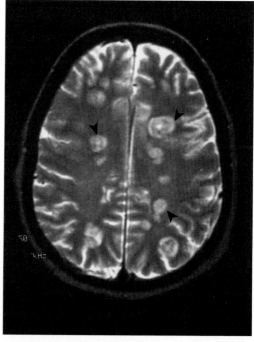

Figure 18–7. Magnetic resonance imaging scans of *Aspergillus* abscess (arrowheads) in a patient with liver transplantation. Multiple abscesses with large basal ganglia hemorrhage are shown (arrow).

vival if treatment with high doses of amphotericin B (up to 1.5 mg/kg per day) is initiated early. Tolkhoff-Rubin and associates[119] suggested the addition of rifampin, 600 to 900 mg/day, in patients with CNS involvement, with success in several cases.

BACTERIAL INFECTIONS

Mundane bacterial infection in the ICU can be expected in the days after transplantation, but immunocompromised transplant recipients are particularly susceptible to *Listeria monocytogenes* and *Nocardia asteroides*.

Listeria monocytogenes

Systemic listeriosis is a well-recognized clinical entity in transplant recipients. In one report, most renal transplant recipients were infected within 1 month after transplantation,[120] but *Listeria* abscess with a delay of 6 months to years after renal transplantation is more likely.[121] Patients with *Listeria* infection were possibly predisposed because of treatment with additional monoclonal antibodies and high doses of steroids to counteract acute rejection.

Listeria may infect transplant recipients through contaminated dairy products and is commonly manifested by cramps and diarrhea. When the CNS becomes involved after bacteremia, the most frequent clinical presentation of listeriosis is acute meningitis with fever and headache. Hydrocephalus may occur, causing stupor. Bulbar signs with dysarthria and dysphagia may be due to a predilection of *Listeria* for the brain stem. Nuchal rigidity is usually difficult to appreciate in immunosuppressed patients and is absent in almost 75% of the cases.[120] Bacteremia is often present, and blood cultures may already identify *Listeria* before CSF results are available. Stereotactic neurosurgical intervention may be necessary to isolate the organism, and some patients need a ventriculostomy to drain hydrocephalus. Magnetic resonance imaging may show meningeal enhancement, hydrocephalus, and scattered lesions in the brain stem. *Listeria* may cause brain abscesses, frequently accompanied by focal signs, and when this happens, mortality doubles. Multiple abscesses like those in toxoplasmosis are infrequent, although the preferred location in basal ganglia is similar.[121,122] *Listeria* meningitis may also lead to arterial occlusion.[123,124] The outcome can be good after adequate treatment with ampicillin (10 to 12 g/day) or gentamicin (1.0 to 1.5 mg/kg intravenously three times a day) for 3 weeks.

Patients with *Listeria* meningitis may experience recurrence, and any patient who had one episode during rejection should have prophylactic antibiotic treatment when increasing doses of immunosuppressive agents are needed.[125]

Nocardia

Patients with ring-like and hemorrhagic parenchymal lesions may have nocardial abscess, especially if they have bilateral pleural effusions, pulmonary nodules, or pulmonary abscesses. It has also been suggested that skin lesions predict disseminated disease and cerebral lesions.[126,127]

Medical treatment of brain abscesses can be successful with a combination of amikacin, ciprofloxacin, and amoxicillin with clavulanic acid.[127] However, one should perform a brain parenchymal and meningeal biopsy on an intracranial mass lesion in a transplant recipient. A differential diagnosis of mass lesions in immunosuppressed transplant recipients is presented in Table 18–6.

Cerebrovascular Complications

Successful grafting can be offset by a devastating stroke[131,132] (Table 18–7). Causes of stroke vary, but the perioperative circumstances may play a crucial role.[134,135]

Table 18–6. **Differential Diagnosis of Mass Lesions in Patients with Transplants**[82,93,128–130]

Nocardia asteroides
Toxoplasma gondii
Cryptococcus neoformans
Listeria monocytogenes
Mycobacteria
Lymphoma
Progressive multifocal leukoencephalopathy

If an ischemic stroke occurs in heart transplants, it is frequently related to effects of cardiac bypass, retained thrombi within the graft, or catheterization of the right side of the heart for endomyocardial biopsy (see Chapter 5). However, Adair and colleagues[131] noted that a history of stroke and preoperative carotid stenosis of more than 50% significantly increase the risk for ischemic stroke after heart transplantation. Ischemic strokes after surgery therefore may not have a specific cause but may represent the overall risk in major surgical procedures. Stroke remains an important cause of morbidity after heart transplantation despite an overall decrease in neurologic complications.[136]

Intracerebral hemorrhages, often in multiple intracranial compartments, are more common in liver transplantation and hematopoietic stem cell transplantation. Many cases in the literature, however, have been linked to *Aspergillus* inoculation,[132,133,135,137–140] coagulopathy, or hypertension.[139]

In the Mayo liver transplantation program, 10 patients had intracerebral hemorrhages (4%) (Fig. 18–8). Two of the 10 had subdural hematomas. In one patient, a *Candida*-associated mycotic aneurysm was found. In another patient, hemorrhage was associated with systemic aspergillosis. When these patients were compared with a control series of patients without intracerebral hemorrhage and liver transplantation, no statistically significant differences were found in the incidence of extracranial bleeding sites or cyclosporine toxicity, but bacteremia or fungemia and coagulopathy were more common, suggesting that intracerebral hematoma may have an origin in overwhelming infection.[141] In a study of 1573 patients who received renal transplants at the Mayo Clinic, CT documented that 10 patients had lobar, cerebellar, or putaminal hemorrhage. Autosomal dominant polycystic kidney disease and diabetes increased the risk tenfold and fourfold, respectively.[139]

In the cytopenic stage of hematopoietic stem cell transplantation, intracranial hemorrhages may occur and are often fatal.[142] In a series of 105 hematopoietic stem cell transplantations, subarachnoid hemorrhage occurred in 13% of the patients, subdural hematoma in 10%, and intraparenchymal hematoma in 5%.[143] Subarachnoid hemorrhage is often localized in the sulci and, as alluded to earlier, is typical of a coagulopathy (Fig. 18–9). None of our patients with subarachnoid hemorrhage associated with hematopoietic stem cell transplantation harbored an aneurysm. Thrombocytopenia is common, and platelet infusions are needed. Bleeding from other sites is present as well (for example, pulmonary epistaxis, alveolar hemorrhages). Mortality remains high if bleeding cannot be controlled. Ischemic strokes have been poorly characterized in bone marrow recipients but may occur with

Table 18–7. Cerebrovascular Complications after Transplantation

Series	Year	Total Patients (No.)	TX	PATIENTS (NO.)			
				ICH	SDH	SAH	IS
Andrews et al.[132]	1990	90	Heart	2	0	0	3
Estol et al.[133]	1991	1357	Liver	3*	2	3	5
Adair et al.[131]	1992	275	Heart	1	0	0	3
Adams et al.[134]	1986	467	Kidney	3	1	1†	2
Mayo series, unpublished	1994	505	Liver	9	2	0	3
Coplin et al.[135]	2001	1245	HSCT	21	0	0	15

ICH, intracerebral hematoma; HSCT, hematopoietic stem cell transplantation; IS, ischemic stroke; SAH, subarachnoid hemorrhage; SDH, subdural hematoma; TX, transplanted organ.

*Five patients had ICH-SDH and ICH-SAH combinations.

†No evidence of polycystic kidney disease.

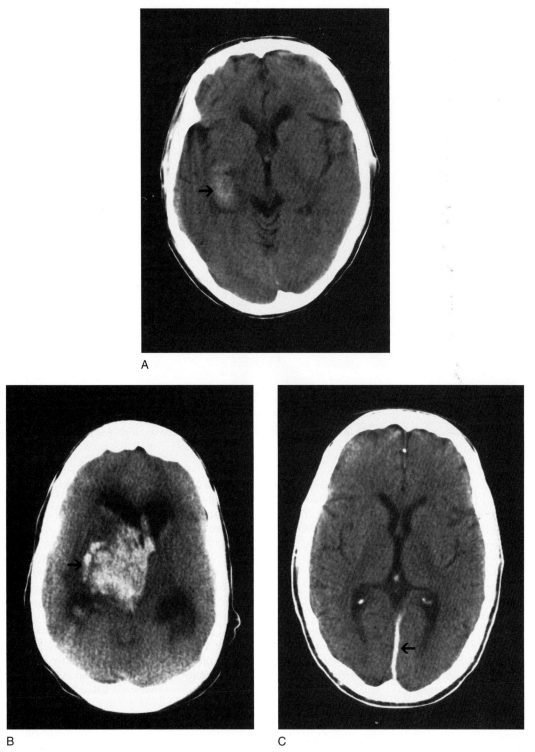

A

B   C

Figure 18–8. Types of intracranial hemorrhages in liver transplantation.[141] *A*: Small intracerebral hematoma (arrow) associated with mycotic aneurysm demonstrated at autopsy. *B*: Massive putaminal hemorrhage (arrow) with acute hydrocephalus. No cause was found. *C*: Small subdural rim of blood (arrow). No cause was found except a flurry of seizures from cyclosporine toxicity.

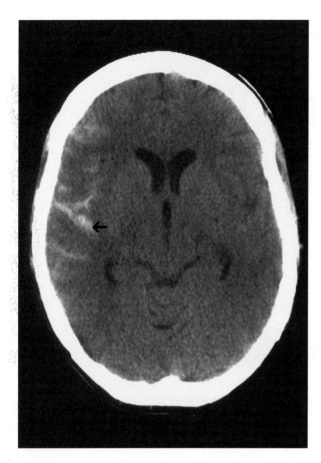

Figure 18–9. Subarachnoid hemorrhage after hematopoietic stem cell transplantation. Note sulci (arrow) filled with blood. Results of magnetic resonance angiography were normal.

nonbacterial thrombotic endocarditis as a consequence of a hypercoagulable state. Chemotherapy may additionally contribute to nonbacterial thrombotic endocarditis[144] when it is used in the conditioning pre-transplantation regimen. Echocardiography is needed to detect vegetations.

Seizures

The highly selected population of transplant recipients is at risk for seizures (see Chapter 3). The most commonly reported circumstances are outlined in Table 18–8.[146–151] New-onset seizures may have multiple causes, but in transplant recipients, seizures could be the first indication that the immunosuppressive agent has reached toxic levels or the beginning of a virulent CNS infection.[150]

The incidence of seizures frequently is high in liver transplant recipients. Our study sug-

gested a high correlation with neurotoxicity from immunosuppressive agents.[150] It is difficult to be certain that cyclosporine is truly responsible for seizures. However, most seizures in liver transplantation occur in the perioperative phase during adjustment of immunosuppressive drugs,[150] a clear suggestion of a link with neurotoxicity, and late seizures when cyclosporine levels are stable are very uncommon. Focal complex partial or generalized tonic–clonic seizures with epileptiform activity on electroencephalograms (interictal spike and sharp waves) in these patients could also indicate severe ischemic–anoxic damage, subdural hemorrhage, or subarachnoid hemorrhage.[151]

Management of seizures in transplant recipients could be guided by four criteria: no structural CNS lesion (for example, abscess, lymphoma, or meningitis), corrected metabolic cause, low probability of drug toxicity, and no epileptiform abnormalities on elec-

Table 18–8. **Potential Causes of Early New-Onset Seizures in Transplant Recipients**

Type of Transplant	Incidence (%)	Toxicity or Acute Metabolic Derangement	Structural
Liver	10–20	Hypocalcemia, hyponatremia, hypomagnesemia, hyperglycemia Cyclosporine, tacrolimus toxicity	Ischemic–anoxic encephalopathy, subdural hematoma, intracerebral hemorrhage, subarachnoid hemorrhage, extrapontine myelinolysis, fungal or bacterial abscess
Kidney	1–5	Acute uremia, hyponatremia	Intracranial hemorrhage, fungal or bacterial abscess
Heart	10–15	Cyclosporine toxicity	Ischemic stroke, air emboli, *Toxoplasma* or *Aspergillus* abscess
HSCT	5–10	Drug-related*	Cortical venous thrombosis, intracerebral hemorrhage, GVHD

*Drugs used before bone marrow transplantation, such as busulfan in high doses.[145]
GVHD, graft-versus-host disease; HSCT, hematopoietic stem cell transplantation.

troencephalograms. If none of these factors is present, long-term management with antiepileptic agents is not needed. If any of these four is present in the short term (1 to 2 months), phenytoin should be considered. Recurrence of seizures is very uncommon.[150]

De Novo Central Nervous System Malignant Lesions

The incidence of post-transplantation malignant lesions involving the CNS is low. Most CNS tumors are B-cell lymphomas, but glioblastoma multiforme with a rapidly fatal course may develop, usually years after transplantation. Astrocytomas have been reported in bone marrow transplantation and heart transplantation[152] (Fig. 18–10), and in some reports another predisposing factor, such as prophylactic cranial irradiation.[153]

Penn[154,155] noticed in his transplant tumor registry that the incidence of lymphomas has increased and that lymphomas have occurred earlier. The interval to the onset of lymphoma was an average of 32 months (3 weeks to 248.5 months) (Fig. 18–11) in the Cincinnati Transplant Tumor Registry.[156] Lymphoma of the brain occurs in 7% of transplant recipients. Most post-transplantation lymphomas are monoclonal B-cell lymphomas, but multiclonal B-cell lymphomas

(from different progenitor cells) or T-cell lymphomas have been reported.[157,158] The addition of both muromonab-CD3 and cyclosporine or the use of any intensive immunosuppressive therapy to counteract rejection of the graft has been tentatively linked to higher incidences of lymphoma and lymphoproliferative disease.[159] On the other hand, risk of post-transplantation lymphoma is not higher in patients who require a second transplantation.

Epstein-Barr virus infection has been linked to B-cell lymphoma because the genome DNA of the virus could be demonstrated in tumor tissue in some patients.[160,161] Serologic evidence of active Epstein-Barr virus infection is present in 80% to 90% of patients with B-cell lymphoma after transplantation. In T-cell lymphoma, human T-cell lymphotrophic virus 1 may have a role, but data are contradictory.

The clinical manifestations of CNS lymphoma may include brain and spinal cord involvement. Localization in other organs is absent in most patients.

The symptoms at presentation are often behavioral changes with visual hallucinations and hemiparesis. Headache is noted by one-third of the patients and points to meningeal involvement. The lack of localizing neurologic signs and preponderance of personality changes in patients with intracranial lym-

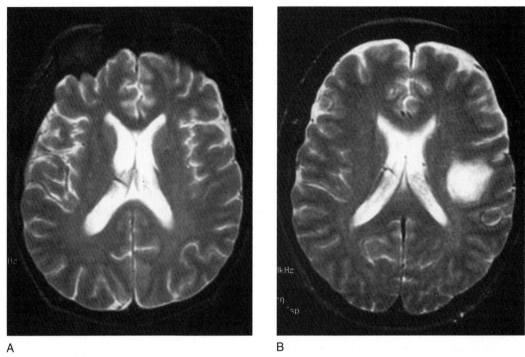

A   B

Figure 18–10. Heart transplant recipient. *A*: Pretransplantation magnetic resonance image is normal. *B*: Magnetic resonance image 2 years later shows mass lesion due to astrocytoma.

phoma may delay detection. Although brain biopsy should be performed to confirm suspected lymphoma, the risk of biopsy-related intracranial hematoma may be comparatively high, possibly because of increased vascular-

ity of the tumor. A CT scan or MRI shows a solitary mass lesion in the periventricular region[162] (Fig. 18–12). Multiple localizations, sometimes with diffuse subependymal nodules, can occur, and MRI increases their yield.

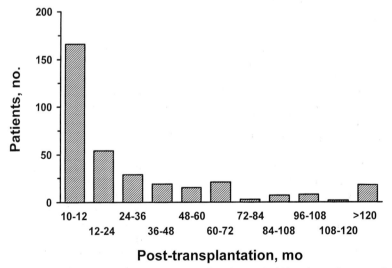

Figure 18–11. Time of appearance of central nervous system lymphomas in 342 patients after transplantation. (From Penn.[156] By permission of Mayo Foundation.)

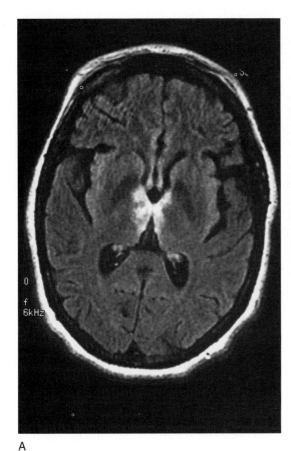

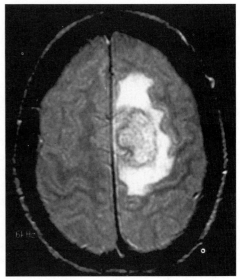

B

A

Figure 18–12. Examples of lymphoma in transplant recipients. *A*: Periventricular enhancement. *B*: Mass lesion.

Aggressive treatment with radiation may result in complete resolution of the lesion on CT scanning and of the neurologic findings in both types of lymphomas, but the prospect of long-term survival is low.

Neuropathies

Peripheral nerves are ideally situated to become damaged after grafting, but the limited studies available have suggested a very low risk. The overall incidence of peripheral nerve injuries in the general surgical population is around 0.1%.[163,164] The perioperative incidence may be higher in more complex surgical procedures, such as transplantation, particularly when additional instruments and devices are used. Mononeuropathies may be due to direct damage from cannulation (Chapter 5), to coagulopathy-induced compressive hematoma (Chapter 11), or as a consequence of immunosuppression, predominantly a flare-up of herpes zoster. Polyneuropathies are less understood and have been only sporadically reported.

Perioperative compression may result in ulnar, radial, and peroneal nerve injury and have reached 4% in transplantation cohorts.[165,166] Postoperative ulnar neuropathy is noted often days after surgery, a finding questioning the link with poor operative positioning. Compression may have occurred at the upper humerus site or at the elbow (condylar groove or cubital tunnel), and protection of the ulnar nerve by padding does not eliminate this complication.[164,167] Heterotopic ossification or formation of bone within muscle or soft connective tissue has been reported as a cause of ulnar neuropathy in liver and lung transplant recipients.

Clinical recognition of ulnar neuropathy is determined by the demonstration of diminished pinprick and light touch over the fifth and half of the fourth fingers and weakness of the abductor digiti minimi (abduction of the little finger), flexor carpi ulnaris (flexion; ulnar deviation of hand at wrist), flexor digitorum profundus of the fourth and fifth fingers (flexion of distal phalanx with other phalanges extended), interossei (spreading and closing of extended fingers), and adductor pollicis (adduction of the thumb in the plane of the palm, holding paper firm between thumb and edge of index finger, or so-called Froment's sign). Severe involvement does not bode well for recovery, but sensory involvement alone after surgery seems to have a good prospect for recovery.[164]

Radial nerve injury detected by a wrist drop is usually from direct compression at the spiral groove and may occur from poor positioning against a pole supporting thoracic cage retractors. With liver transplantation, a lesion in the axilla may occur from placement of the venovenous bypass in the axillary vein, causing direct damage, but it is very uncommon because this practice has been largely abandoned. Weakness of the triceps muscle differentiates a lesion in the axilla from one on the upper arm. In some cases of compression at the upper arm, decreased sensation is joined at the dorsal part of the hand and limited to the thumb, index finger, and half of the middle finger.

Femoral neuropathy may occur due to coagulopathy-associated psoas hematoma (Chapter 11), compression from medial and inferior retractor blades during kidney transplantation,[168] and direct cannulation of the saphenous vein. Femoral neuropathy is diagnosed by a sensory deficit in the cutaneous branch of the femoral nerve (anterior thigh) or saphenous nerve (medial tibia); weakness of the iliopsoas (flexion of hips), quadriceps (extension of leg), and hip adductors (separation of knees); and absent patellar reflex. Peroneal neuropathy is diagnosed when weakness is found in the foot everter, toe extensors, and dorsiflexion. Sensory loss is expected in the anterolateral skin of the lower leg and dorsum of the foot and toes.

The peroneal nerves are at risk in malnourished end-stage renal or kidney transplants, and damage may be bilateral. Operative positioning may contribute when anesthetized patients lie on the operating table with legs turned outward, a position favoring compression of the common peroneal nerve against the tibular head. Obviously, walking may be very difficult after surgery, but most reported patients recover fully after 1 to 2 months and can remove their splints.[169]

Brachial plexopathies after transplantation are typically neuropraxis injuries from malpositioning of the arm or compression between clavicle and first rib during heart transplantation (Chapter 16). Improvement is expected within 3 months. Lumbosacral plexopathies are very uncommon clinically, but fresh hemorrhages in a patient with a transplanted liver have been reported at autopsy.[169]

Polyneuropathies in transplant recipients may have an origin in sepsis (Chapter 6). They have also been associated with tacrolimus use,[170,171] but the relation with cyclosporine and tacrolimus has not been established. This relation seems very unlikely because of increasing use of tacrolimus in transplant recipients and lack of a simultaneous increase in reports of polyneuropathy. Careful pathologic studies are scarce. Inflammatory demyelinating polyneuropathy with profound weakness but good response to intravenous immunoglobulin has been associated with hepatitis B relapse and a decrease in the dose of cyclosporine.[172]

NEUROLOGIC COMPLICATIONS OF GRAFT-VERSUS-HOST DISEASE

In GVHD, viable immunocompetent donor bone marrow cells react to certain target organs, resulting in dermatitis, enteritis, and hepatitis. Acute GVHD is usually apparent 20 to 100 days after infusion of bone marrow–derived stem cells. Survival is determined by infectious complications. The incidence of GVHD may reach 50% to 70% in bone marrow transplants. A chronic form of GVHD may occur as early as 3 months after hematopoietic stem cell transplantation. Chronic GVHD strongly resembles any of the vasculitis syndromes, such as systemic lupus erythematosus, scleroderma, and sicca syndrome. Both forms are still incompletely understood but require complex interactions of immunocompetent donor cells (T lymphocytes, monocytes, and dendritic cells) and cytokines (such as tumor necrosis factor-α, interleukin 1 and 6, and interferon-γ) released by both donor and recipient tissue, the latter induced by conditioning of the transplant recipient by means of chemotherapy or total body irradiation. The principal neurologic complications of GVHD are polymyositis and myasthenia gravis.[96,173,174] Peripheral nerve abnormalities have been sporadically described, including herpes zoster neuralgia, Guillain-Barré syndrome,[175] and mononeuritis multiplex involving the peroneal and cutaneous femoral lateral nerves.[96,173] A chronic demyelinating polyneuropathy 3 years after autologous bone marrow transplantation was successfully treated with plasma exchange.[176]

Polymyositis

Polymyositis may appear 2 to 54 months after allogeneic bone marrow transplantation.[177-183] It is not common in autologous bone marrow transplantation, and only one patient with polymyositis treated for recurrent Hodgkin's disease is known.[179]

Clinical presentation is similar to that in any other patient with polymyositis, although the initial experience suggests that early contractures are frequent and most likely associated with marked skin involvement. Many patients complain of stiffness with movement and pain in proximal shoulder muscles. These symptoms are often followed by marked weakness and wasting of neck flexors and shoulder girdle muscles. Many patients have a low-grade fever. Serum creatine phosphokinase levels are increased but could be within normal range in patients with minimal weakness and nontender muscles. Muscle biopsies invariably demonstrate necrotic fibers with endomysial lymphocytes and phagocytosis but without immunoglobulin deposits or blood vessel abnormalities.

Outcome is good if the patient survives the devastating consequences of chronic GVHD. Excellent return of muscle function has been reported after treatment with prednisone (1 to 3 mg/kg of body weight), prednisone with antithymocyte globulin (7 mg of IgG/kg), or azathioprine (100 mg daily).[182,183]

Myasthenia Gravis

Nine isolated cases of myasthenia gravis have been published.[184–189] It has been speculated that patients with HLA-B7 and HLA-DR2 antigens are at risk.[190] Six of the nine patients had bone marrow transplantation for aplastic anemia. All features known in typical myasthenia gravis have been described. Weakness in the jaw, face, and proximal arm and leg muscles can be demonstrated, with rapid fatigability after repeated testing. Ptosis may begin unilaterally but becomes bilateral in all patients. Oropharyngeal involvement may occur, and diaphragmatic failure requiring support by mechanical ventilation develops in some patients. Patients with myasthenia gravis as part of GVHD were comparatively young (range, 9 to 26 years; mean, 18 years). The clinical impression of myasthenia gravis is usually confirmed by edrophonium chloride test (positive result in all reported patients with myasthenia gravis associated with bone marrow transplantation) and conventional or single-fiber electromyography.

Acetylcholine receptor antibody concentrations are increased[186,191,192] but can be negative. An association with thymoma has not been reported. One study found that levels of IgG acetylcholine receptor antibody were increased 2 to 13 months after bone marrow transplantation in 20% of patients who otherwise did not have clinical myasthenia gravis.[191] In another study,[192] even 41% of the patients had anti-acetylcholine receptor antibodies. Prednisone and azathioprine are successful in treatment, but tapering of the dosage may lead to exacerbation, and long-term maintenance therapy is crucial.

CONCLUSIONS

The transplantation literature is rife with neurologic manifestations of the major immunosuppressive agents: cyclosporine, tacrolimus, and, less often, muromonab-CD3. The likelihood of toxicity from cyclosporine or tacrolimus is substantial in patients with agitation, nonsensical speech, seizures, and tremor ("rage, ramble, shake, and shiver").

Opportunistic CNS infections and lymphoma may occur in the postoperative months. There is a low probability of cerebrovascular complications at any time after organ transplantation. Intracranial hemorrhages may be associated with fungal infections, particularly those caused by *Aspergillus.*

An intracranial mass may be manifested by new-onset seizures or focal signs. Malignant lymphoma, astrocytoma, nocardia, toxoplasma, and progressive multifocal leukoencephalopathy are possible causes. Brain biopsy may yield a final diagnosis.

REFERENCES

1. Riether AM, Smith SL, Lewison BJ, Cotsonis GA, Epstein CM. Quality-of-life changes and psychiatric and neurocognitive outcome after heart and liver transplantation. Transplantation 54:444–450, 1992.
2. Wijdicks EFM (editor). Neurologic Complications in Organ Transplant Recipients. Butterworth-Heinemann, Boston, 1999.
3. The Mycophenolate Mofetil Acute Renal Rejection Study Group. Mycophenolate mofetil for the treatment of a first acute renal allograft rejection: Three-year follow-up. Transplantation 71:1091–1097, 2001.
4. Humar A, Kandaswamy R, Granger D, Gruessner RW, Gruessner AC, Sutherland DE. Decreased surgical risks of pancreas transplantation in the modern era. Ann Surg 231:269–275, 2000.
5. Wong M, Mallory GB Jr, Goldstein J, Goyal M, Yamada KA. Neurologic complications of pediatric lung transplantation. Neurology 53:1542–1549, 1999.
6. Goldstein LS, Haug MT III, Perl J II, et al. Central nervous system complications after lung transplantation. J Heart Lung Transplant 17:185–191, 1998.
7. Sheridan PH Jr, Cheriyan A, Doud J, et al. Incidence of phrenic neuropathy after isolated lung transplantation. The Loyola University Lung Transplant Group. J Heart Lung Transplant 14:684–691, 1995.
8. Whitington PF, Emond JC, Heffron T, Thistlethwaite JR. Orthotopic auxiliary liver transplantation for Crigler-Najjar syndrome type 1. Lancet 342:779–780, 1993.
9. Carton EG, Rettke SR, Plevak DJ, Geiger HJ, Kranner PW, Coursin DB. Perioperative care of the liver transplant patient: part 1. Anesth Analg 78:120–133, 1994.
10. Carton EG, Plevak DJ, Kranner PW, Rettke SR, Geiger HJ, Coursin DB. Perioperative care of the liver transplant patient: part 2. Anesth Analog 78:382–399, 1994.
11. Champlin RE, Gale RP. The early complications of bone marrow transplantation. Semin Hematol 21:101–108, 1984.
12. Gallardo D, Ferra C, Berlanga JJ, et al. Neurologic complications after allogeneic bone marrow transplantation. Bone Marrow Transplant 18:1135–1139, 1996.
13. Delattre J-Y, Posner JB. Neurological complications of chemotherapy and radiation therapy. In: Aminoff MJ (ed). Neurology and General Medicine. Churchill Livingstone, New York, 1989, pp 365–387.
14. Kaplan RS, Wiernik PH. Neurotoxicity of antineoplastic drugs. Semin Oncol 9:103–130, 1982.
15. Sullivan KM, Shulman HM, Storb R, et al. Chronic graft-versus-host disease in 52 patients: adverse natural course and successful treatment with combination immunosuppression. Blood 57:267–276, 1981.
16. Antonini G, Ceschin V, Morino S, et al. Early neurologic complications following allogeneic bone marrow transplant for leukemia: a prospective study. Neurology 50:1441–1445, 1998.
17. Ingle GR, Sievers TM, Holt CD. Sirolimus: continuing the evolution of transplant immunosuppression. Ann Pharmacother 34:1044–1055, 2000.
18. de Groen PC. Cyclosporine: a review and its specific use in liver transplantation. Mayo Clin Proc 64:680–689, 1989.
19. Borel JF, Kis ZL. The discovery and development of cyclosporine (Sandimmune). Transplant Proc 23:1867–1874, 1991.
20. Bohlin AB, Berg U, Englund M, et al. Central nervous system complications in children treated with ciclosporin after renal transplantation. Child Nephrol Urol 10:225–230, 1990.
21. de Groen PC, Aksamit AJ, Rakela J, Forbes GS, Krom RA. Central nervous system toxicity after liver transplantation. The role of cyclosporine and cholesterol. N Engl J Med 317:861–866, 1987.
22. Vazquez de Prada JA, Martin-Duran R, Garcia-Monco C, et al. Cyclosporine neurotoxicity in heart transplantation. J Heart Transplant 9:581–583, 1990.
23. Lind MJ, McWilliam L, Jip J, Scarffe JH, Morgenstern GR, Chang J. Cyclosporine associated demyelination following allogeneic bone marrow transplantation. Hematol Oncol 7:49–52, 1989.
24. McManus RP, O'Hair DP, Schweiger J, Beitzinger J, Siegel R. Cyclosporine-associated central neurotoxicity after heart transplantation. Ann Thorac Surg 53:326–327, 1992.
25. Reece DE, Frei-Lahr DA, Shepherd JD, et al. Neurologic complications in allogeneic bone marrow transplant patients receiving cyclosporin. Bone Marrow Transplant 8:393–401, 1991.
26. Scheinman SJ, Reinitz ER, Petro G, Schwartz RA, Szmalc FS. Cyclosporine central neurotoxicity following renal transplantation. Report of a case using magnetic resonance images. Transplantation 49:215–216, 1990.
27. Pujol A, Graus F, Rimola A, et al. Predictive factors of in-hospital CNS complications following liver transplantation. Neurology 44:1226–1230, 1994.
28. Hauben M. Cyclosporine neurotoxicity. Pharmacotherapy 16:576–583, 1996.
29. Truwit CL, Denaro CP, Lake JR, DeMarco T. MR imaging of reversible cyclosporin A-induced neu-

rotoxicity. AJNR Am J Neuroradiol 12:651–659, 1991.

30. Casey SO, Sampaio RC, Michel E, Truwit CL. Posterior reversible encephalopathy syndrome: utility of fluid-attenuated inversion recovery MR imaging in the detection of cortical and subcortical lesions. AJNR Am J Neuroradiol 21:1199–1206, 2000.

31. Zylber-Katz E. Multiple drug interactions with cyclosporine in a heart transplant patient. Ann Pharmacother 29:127–131, 1995.

32. Kane GC, Lipsky JJ. Drug-grapefruit juice interactions. Mayo Clin Proc 75:933–942, 2000.

33. Takeguchi N, Ichimura K, Koike M, Matsui W, Kashiwagura T, Kawahara K. Inhibition of the multidrug efflux pump in isolated hepatocyte couplets by immunosuppressants FK506 and cyclosporine. Transplantation 55:646–650, 1993.

34. McDonald JW, Goldberg MP, Gwag BJ, Chi SI, Choi DW. Cyclosporine induces neuronal apoptosis and selective oligodendrocyte death in cortical cultures. Ann Neurol 40:750–758, 1996.

35. Wijdicks EFM. Neurotoxicity of immunosuppressive drugs. Liver Transplant 7:937–942, 2001.

36. Bechstein WO. Neurotoxicity of calcineurin inhibitors: impact and clinical management. Transpl Int 13:313–326, 2000.

37. Kochi S, Takanaga H, Matsuo H, et al. Induction of apoptosis in mouse brain capillary endothelial cells by cyclosporin A and tacrolimus. Life Sci 66:2255–2260, 2000.

38. Coley SC, Porter DA, Calamante F, Chong WK, Connelly A. Quantitative MR diffusion mapping and cyclosporine-induced neurotoxicity. AJNR Am J Neuroradiol 20:1507–1510, 1999.

39. de Groen PC. Cyclosporine, low-density lipoprotein, and cholesterol. Mayo Clin Proc 63:1012–1021, 1988.

40. De Klippel N, Sennesael J, Lamote J, Ebinger G, de Keyser J. Cyclosporin leukoencephalopathy induced by intravenous lipid solution [letter]. Lancet 339:1114, 1992.

41. Begley DJ, Squires LK, Zlokovic BV, et al. Permeability of the blood–brain barrier to the immunosuppressive cyclic peptide cyclosporin A. J Neurochem 55:1222–1230, 1990.

42. Wijdicks EFM, Dahlke LJ, Wiesner RH. Oral cyclosporine decreases severity of neurotoxicity in liver transplant recipients. Neurology 52:1708–1710, 1999.

43. Small SL, Fukui MB, Bramblett GT, Eidelman BH. Immunosuppression-induced leukoencephalopathy from tacrolimus (FK506). Ann Neurol 40:575–580, 1996.

44. Palmer BF, Toto RD. Severe neurologic toxicity induced by cyclosporine A in three renal transplant patients. Am J Kidney Dis 18:116–121, 1991.

45. Steg RE, Garcia EG. Complex visual hallucinations and cyclosporine neurotoxicity. Neurology 41:1156, 1991.

46. Laureno R, Karp BP. Cyclosporine mutism [letter]. Neurology 48:296–297, 1997.

47. Valldeoriola F, Graus F, Rimola A, et al. Cyclosporine-associated mutism in liver transplant patients. Neurology 46:252–254, 1996.

48. Ghalie R, Fitzsimmons WE, Bennett D, Kaizer H.

49. Rubin AM. Transient cortical blindness and occipital seizures with cyclosporine toxicity. Transplantation 47:572–573, 1989.

50. Wijdicks EFM, Wiesner RH, Krom RA. Neurotoxicity in liver transplant recipients with cyclosporine immunosuppression. Neurology 45:1962–1964, 1995.

51. Drachman BM, DeNofrio D, Acker MA, Galetta S, Loh E. Cortical blindness secondary to cyclosporine after orthotopic heart transplantation: a case report and review of the literature. J Heart Lung Transplant 15:1158–1164, 1996.

52. Lopez OL, Martinez AJ, Torre-Cisneros J. Neuropathologic findings in liver transplantation: a comparative study of cyclosporine and FK 506. Transplant Proc 23:3181–3182, 1991.

53. Rubin AM, Kang H. Cerebral blindness and encephalopathy with cyclosporin A toxicity. Neurology 37:1072–1076, 1987.

54. Bird GL, Meadows J, Goka J, Polson R, Williams R. Cyclosporin-associated akinetic mutism and extrapyramidal syndrome after liver transplantation. J Neurol Neurosurg Psychiatry 53:1068–1071, 1990.

55. Sheth TN, Ichise M, Kucharczyk W. Brain perfusion imaging in asymptomatic patients receiving cyclosporin. AJNR Am J Neuroradiol 20:853–856, 1999.

56. Jain A, Brody D, Hamad I, Rishi N, Kanal E, Fung J. Conversion to neoral for neurotoxicity after primary adult liver transplantation under tacrolimus. Transplantation 69:172–176, 2000.

57. Emre S, Genyk Y, Schluger LK, et al. Treatment of tacrolimus-related adverse effects by conversion to cyclosporine in liver transplant recipients. Transpl Int 13:73–78, 2000.

58. Gryn J, Goldberg J, Viner E. Propranolol for the treatment of cyclosporine-induced headaches. Bone Marrow Transplant 9:211–212, 1992.

59. Rozen TD, Wijdicks EFM. Headache in organ transplant recipients. Headache Q 8:214–218, 1997.

60. Rozen TD, Wijdicks EFM, Hay JE. Treatment-refractory cyclosporine-associated headache: relief with conversion to FK-506. Neurology 47:1347–1348, 1996.

61. Hooks MA. Tacrolimus, a new immunosuppressant—a review of the literature. Ann Pharmacother 28:501–511, 1994.

62. Todo S, Fung JJ, Starzl TE, et al. Liver, kidney, and thoracic organ transplantation under FK 506. Ann Surg 212:295–305, 1990.

63. Eidelman BH, Abu-Elmagd K, Wilson J, et al. Neurologic complications of FK 506. Transplant Proc 23:3175–3178, 1991.

64. Freise CE, Rowley H, Lake J, Hebert M, Ascher NL, Roberts JP. Similar clinical presentation of neurotoxicity following FK 506 and cyclosporine in a liver transplant recipient. Transplant Proc 23:3173–3174, 1991.

65. Wijdicks EFM, Wiesner RH, Dahlke LJ, Krom RA. FK506-induced neurotoxicity in liver transplantation. Ann Neurol 35:498–501, 1994.

Cortical blindness: a rare complication of cyclosporine therapy. Bone Marrow Transplant 6:147–149, 1990.

66. Bronster DJ, Gurkan A, Buchsbaum MS, Emre S. Tacrolimus-associated mutism after orthotopic liver transplantation. Transplantation 70:979–982, 2000.

67. Reyes J, Gayowski T, Fung J, Todo S, Alessiani M, Starzl TE. Expressive dysphasia possibly related to FK506 in two liver transplant recipients. Transplantation 50:1043–1045, 1990.

68. Wain JC, Wright CD, Ryan DP, Zorb SL, Mathisen DJ, Ginns LC. Induction immunosuppression for lung transplantation with OKT3. Ann Thorac Surg 67:187–193, 1999.

69. Stapleton DD, Ventura HO, Grundtner SE, et al. Induction immunosuppression with the monoclonal antibody OKT3 after cardiac transplantation. Am J Med Sci 306:16–19, 1993.

70. Flechner SM, Goldfarb DA, Fairchild R, et al. A randomized prospective trial of low-dose OKT3 induction therapy to prevent rejection and minimize side effects in recipients of kidney transplants. Transplantation 69:2374–2381, 2000.

71. Thistlethwaite JR Jr, Stuart JK, Mayes JT, et al. Complications and monitoring of OKT3 therapy. Am J Kidney Dis 11:112–119, 1988.

72. Adair JC, Woodley SL, O'Connell JB, Call GK, Baringer JR. Aseptic meningitis following cardiac transplantation: clinical characteristics and relationship to immunosuppressive regimen. Neurology 41:249–252, 1991.

73. Martin MA, Massanari RM, Nghiem DD, Smith JL, Corry RJ. Nosocomial aseptic meningitis associated with administration of OKT3. JAMA 259: 2002–2005, 1988.

74. Emmons C, Smith J, Flanigan M. Cerebrospinal fluid inflammation during OKT3 therapy [letter]. Lancet 2:510–511, 1986.

75. Roden J, Klintmalm GB, Husberg BS, Nery J, Olson LM. Cerebrospinal fluid inflammation during OKT3 therapy [letter]. Lancet 2:272, 1987.

76. Capone PM, Cohen ME. Seizures and cerebritis associated with administration of OKT3. Pediatr Neurol 7:299–301, 1991.

77. Marks WH, Perkal M, Bia M, Lorber MI. Aseptic encephalitis and blindness complicating OKT3 therapy. Clin Transplant 5:435–438, 1991.

78. Thomas DM, Nicholls AJ, Feest TG, Riad H. OKT3 and cerebral oedema [letter]. Br Med J 295:1486, 1987.

79. Parizel PM, Snoeck H-W, van den Hauwe L, et al. Cerebral complications of murine monoclonal CD3 antibody (OKT3): CT and MR findings. AJNR Am J Neuroradiol 18:1935–1938, 1997.

80. Coleman AE, Norman DJ. OKT3 encephalopathy. Ann Neurol 28:837–838, 1990.

81. Chan GL, Weinstein SS, Wright CE, et al. Encephalopathy associated with OKT3 administration. Possible interaction with indomethacin. Transplantation 52:148–150, 1991.

82. Fishman JA, Rubin RH. Infection in organ-transplant recipients. N Engl J Med 338:1741–1751, 1998.

83. DeVault GA Jr, King JW, Rohr MS, Landreneau MD, Brown ST III, McDonald JC. Opportunistic infections with *Strongyloides stercoralis* in renal transplantation. Rev Infect Dis 12:653–671, 1990.

84. Riarte A, Luna C, Sabatiello R, et al. Chagas' disease in patients with kidney transplants: 7 years of experience 1989–1996. Clin Infect Dis 29:561–567, 1999.

85. Tsanaclis AM, de Morais CF. Cerebral toxoplasmosis after renal transplantation. Case report. Pathol Res Pract 181:339–343, 1986.

86. Fisher MA, Levy J, Helfrich M, August CS, Starr SE, Luft BJ. Detection of *Toxoplasma gondii* in the spinal fluid of a bone marrow transplant recipient. Pediatr Infect Dis J 6:81–83, 1987.

87. Löwenberg B, van Gijn J, Prins E, Polderman AM. Fatal cerebral toxoplasmosis in a bone marrow transplant recipient with leukemia. Transplantation 35:30–34, 1983.

88. Wijdicks EFM, Borleffs JC, Hoepelman AI, Jansen GH. Fatal disseminated hemorrhagic toxoplasmic encephalitis as the initial manifestation of AIDS. Ann Neurol 29:683–686, 1991.

89. Derouin F, Devergie A, Auber P, et al. Toxoplasmosis in bone marrow-transplant recipients: report of seven cases and review. Clin Infect Dis 15: 267–270, 1992.

90. Rodriguez JC, Martinez MM, Martinez AR, Royo G. Evaluation of different techniques in the diagnosis of *Toxoplasma* encephalitis. J Med Microbiol 46:597–601, 1997.

91. Flomenbaum MA, Jarcho JA, Schoen FJ. Progressive multifocal leukoencephalopathy fifty-seven months after heart transplantation. J Heart Lung Transplant 10:888–893, 1991.

92. Hall WA, Martinez AJ, Dummer JS. Progressive multifocal leukoencephalopathy after cardiac transplantation. Neurology 38:995–996, 1988.

93. Aksamit AJ Jr, de Groen PC. Cyclosporine-related leukoencephalopathy and PML in a liver transplant recipient. Transplantation 60:874–876, 1995.

94. Dorries K, Arendt G, Eggers C, Roggendorf W, Dorries R. Nucleic acid detection as a diagnostic tool in polyomavirus JC induced progressive multifocal leukoencephalopathy. J Med Virol 54:196–203, 1998.

95. Segarra-Newnham M, Vodolo KM. Use of cidofovir in progressive multifocal leukoencepahlopathy. Ann Pharmacother 35:741–744, 2001.

96. Patchell RA, White CL III, Clark AW, Beschorner WE, Santos GW. Neurologic complications of bone marrow transplantation. Neurology 35:300–306, 1985.

97. Spitzer PG, Tarsy D, Eliopoulos GM. Acute transverse myelitis during disseminated cytomegalovirus infection in a renal transplant recipient. Transplantation 44:151–153, 1987.

98. Randhawa PS, Markin RS, Starzl TE, Demetris AJ. Epstein-Barr virus–associated syndrome in immunosuppressed liver transplant recipients. Clinical profile and recognition on routine allograft biopsy. Am J Surg Pathol 14:538–547, 1990.

99. Pickhardt PJ, Siegel MJ, Hayashi RJ, Kelly M. Post-transplantation lymphoproliferative disorder in children: clinical, histopathologic, and imaging features. Radiology 217:16–25, 2000.

100. Patel PR. Post-transplant lymphoproliferative disorders. Clin Oncol (R Coll Radiol) 11:118–122, 1999.

101. Rossi C, Delforge M-L, Jacobs F, et al. Fatal primary infection due to human herpesvirus 6 vari-

ant A in a renal transplant recipient. Transplantation 71:288–292, 2001.

102. Singh N, Paterson DL. Encephalitis caused by human herpesvirus-6 in transplant recipients: relevance of a novel neurotropic virus. Transplantation 69:2474–2479, 2000.

103. Davis D, Henslee PJ, Markesbery WR. Fatal adenovirus meningoencephalitis in a bone marrow transplant patient. Ann Neurol 23:385–389, 1988.

104. Treseler CB, Sugar AM. Fungal meningitis. Infect Dis Clin North Am 4:789–808, 1990.

105. Drutz DJ, Catanzaro A. Coccidioidomycosis. Part II. Am Rev Respir Dis 117:727–771, 1978.

106. Kong NC, Shaariah W, Morad Z, Suleiman AB, Wong YH. Cryptococcosis in a renal unit. Aust N Z J Med 20:645–649, 1990.

107. White M, Cirrincione C, Blevins A, Armstrong D. Cryptococcal meningitis: outcome in patients with AIDS and patients with neoplastic disease. J Infect Dis 165:960–963, 1992.

108. Popovich MJ, Arthur RH, Helmer E. CT of intracranial cryptococcosis. AJNR Am J Neuroradiol 11:139–142, 1990.

109. Tien RD, Chu PK, Hesselink JR, Duberg A, Wiley C. Intracranial cryptococcosis in immunocompromised patients: CT and MR findings in 29 cases. AJNR Am J Neuroradiol 12:283–289, 1991.

110. Byrne WR, Wajszczuk CP. Cryptococcal meningitis in the acquired immunodeficiency syndrome (AIDS): successful treatment with fluconazole after failure of amphotericin B. Ann Intern Med 108:384–385, 1988.

111. Denning DW, Tucker RM, Hanson LH, Hamilton JR, Stevens DA. Itraconazole therapy for cryptococcal meningitis and cryptococcosis. Arch Intern Med 149:2301–2308, 1989.

112. Spitzer ED, Spitzer SG, Freundlich LF, Casadevall A. Persistence of initial infection in recurrent *Cryptococcus neoformans* meningitis. Lancet 341:595–596, 1993.

113. Boon AP, Adams DH, Buckels J, McMaster P. Cerebral aspergillosis in liver transplantation. J Clin Pathol 43:114–118, 1990.

114. Polo JM, Fabrega E, Casafont F, et al. Treatment of cerebral aspergillosis after liver transplantation. Neurology 42:1817–1819, 1992.

115. Torre-Cisneros J, Lopez OL, Kusne S, et al. CNS aspergillosis in organ transplantation: a clinicopathological study. J Neurol Neurosurg Psychiatry 56:188–193, 1993.

116. Cox J, Murtagh FR, Wilfong A, Brenner J. Cerebral aspergillosis: MR imaging and histopathologic correlation. AJNR Am J Neuroradiol 13:1489–1492, 1992.

117. Davenport C, Dillon WP, Sze G. Neuroradiology of the immunosuppressed state. Radiol Clin North Am 30:611–637, 1992.

118. Parker SL, Laszewski MJ, Trigg ME, Smith WL. Spinal cord aspergillosis in immunosuppressed patients. Pediatr Radiol 20:351–352, 1990.

119. Tolkoff-Rubin NE, Hovingh GK, Rubin RH. Central nervous system infections. In: Wijdicks EFM (ed). Neurologic Complications of Organ Transplant Recipients. Butterworth-Heinemann, Boston, 1999, pp 141–168.

120. Skogberg K, Syrjänen J, Jahkola M, et al. Clinical presentation and outcome of listeriosis in patients with and without immunosuppressive therapy. Clin Infect Dis 14:815–821, 1992.

121. Dee RR, Lorber B. Brain abscess due to *Listeria monocytogenes*: case report and literature review. Rev Infect Dis 8:968–977, 1986.

122. Viscoli C, Garaventa A, Ferrea G, Manno G, Taccone A, Terragna A. *Listeria monocytogenes* brain abscesses in a girl with acute lymphoblastic leukaemia after late central nervous system relapse. Eur J Cancer 27:435–437, 1991.

123. Békássy NA, Cronqvist S, Garwicz S, Wiebe T. Arterial occlusion due to *Listeria* meningoencephalitis in an immunocompromised boy. Scand J Infect Dis 19:485–489, 1987.

124. Nau R, Brück W, Bollensen E, Prange HW. Meningoencephalitis with septic intracerebral infarction: a new feature of CNS listeriosis. Scand J Infect Dis 22:101–103, 1990.

125. Larner AJ, Conway MA, Mitchell RG, Forfar JC. Recurrent *Listeria monocytogenes* meningitis in a heart transplant recipient. J Infect 19:263–266, 1989.

126. Miksits K, Stoltenburg G, Neumayer HH, et al. Disseminated infection of the central nervous system caused by *Nocardia farcinica*. Nephrol Dial Transplant 6:209–214, 1991.

127. Raby N, Forbes G, Williams R. *Nocardia* infection in patients with liver transplants or chronic liver disease: radiologic findings. Radiology 174:713–716, 1990.

128. Selby R, Ramirez CB, Singh R, et al. Brain abscess in solid organ transplant recipients receiving cyclosporine-based immunosuppression. Arch Surg 132:304–310, 1997.

129. Penn I, Porat G. Central nervous system lymphomas in organ allograft recipients. Transplantation 59:240–244, 1995.

130. Johnson BA, Fram EK, Johnson PC, Jacobowitz R. The variable MR appearance of primary lymphoma of the central nervous system: comparison with histopathologic features. AJNR Am J Neuroradiol 18:563–572, 1997.

131. Adair JC, Call GK, O'Connell JB, Baringer JR. Cerebrovascular syndromes following cardiac transplantation. Neurology 42:819–823, 1992.

132. Andrews BT, Hershon JJ, Calanchini P, Avery GJ II, Hill JD. Neurologic complications of cardiac transplantation. West J Med 153:146–148, 1990.

133. Estol CJ, Pessin MS, Martinez AJ. Cerebrovascular complications after orthotopic liver transplantation: a clinicopathologic study. Neurology 41:815–819, 1991.

134. Adams HP Jr, Dawson G, Coffman TJ, Corry RJ. Stroke in renal transplant recipients. Arch Neurol 43:113–115, 1986.

135. Coplin WM, Cochran MS, Levine SR, Crawford SW. Stroke after bone marrow transplantation. Frequency, aetiology and outcome. Brain 124:1043–1051, 2001.

136. Jarquin-Valdivia AA, Wijdicks EFM, McGregor C. Neurologic complications following heart transplantation in the modern era: Decreased incidence, but postoperative stroke remains prevalent. Transplant Proc 31:2161–2162, 1999.

137. Adams DH, Ponsford S, Gunson B, et al. Neuro-

logical complications following liver transplantation. Lancet 1:949–951, 1987.

138. Ang LC, Gillett JM, Kaufmann JC. Neuropathology of heart transplantation. Can J Neurol Sci 16: 291–298, 1989.

139. Wijdicks EFM, Torres VE, Schievink WI, Sterioff S. Cerebral hemorrhage in recipients of renal transplantation. Mayo Clin Proc 74:1111–1112, 1999.

140. Vogt DP, Lederman RJ, Carey WD, Broughan TA. Neurologic complications of liver transplantation. Transplantation 45:1057–1061, 1988.

141. Wijdicks EFM, de Groen PC, Wiesner RH, Krom RA. Intracerebral hemorrhage in liver transplant recipients. Mayo Clin Proc 70:443–446, 1995.

142. Pomeranz S, Naparstek E, Ashkenazi E, et al. Intracranial haematomas following bone marrow transplantation. J Neurol 241:252–256, 1994.

143. Mohrmann RL, Mah V, Vinters HV. Neuropathologic findings after bone marrow transplantation: an autopsy study. Hum Pathol 21:630–639, 1990.

144. Jerman MR, Fick RB Jr. Nonbacterial thrombotic endocarditis associated with bone marrow transplantation. Chest 90:919–922, 1986.

145. Ghany AM, Tutschka PJ, McGhee RB Jr, et al. Cyclosporine-associated seizures in bone marrow transplant recipients given busulfan and cyclophosphamide preparative therapy. Transplantation 52:310–315, 1991.

146. Grigg MM, Costanzo-Nordin MR, Celesia GG, et al. The etiology of seizures after cardiac transplantation. Transplant Proc 20 (Suppl 3):937–944, 1988.

147. Azuno Y, Yaga K, Kaneko T, Kaku K, Oka Y. Chronic graft-versus-host disease and seizure [letter]. Blood 91:2626–2628, 1998.

148. Baliga R, Etheredge EE. Cyclosporine-associated convulsions in a child after renal transplantation. Transplantation 51:1126–1128, 1991.

149. Kunzendorf U, Brockmöller J, Jochimsen F, Keller F, Walz G, Offermann G. Cyclosporin metabolites and central-nervous-system toxicity [letter]. Lancet 1:1223, 1988.

150. Wijdicks EFM, Plevak DJ, Wiesner RH, Steers JL. Causes and outcome of seizures in liver transplant recipients. Neurology 47:1523–1525, 1996.

151. Appleton RE, Farrell K, Teal P, Hashimoto SA, Wong PK. Complex partial status epilepticus associated with cyclosporin A therapy. J Neurol Neurosurg Psychiatry 52:1068–1071, 1989.

152. Schiff D, O'Neill B, Wijdicks EFM, Antin JH, Wen PY. Glioma arising in organ transplant recipients: an unrecognized complication of transplantation? Neurology 57:1486–1488, 2001.

153. Sanders J, Sale GE, Ramberg R, Clift R, Buckner CD, Thomas ED. Glioblastoma multiforme in a patient with acute lymphoblastic leukemia who received a marrow transplant. Transplant Proc 14: 770–774, 1982.

154. Penn I. Cancers complicating organ transplantation [editorial]. N Engl J Med 323:1767–1769, 1990.

155. Penn I. The changing pattern of posttransplant malignancies. Transplant Proc 23:1101–1103, 1991.

156. Penn I. De novo malignant lesions of the central nervous system. In: Wijdicks EFM (ed). Neuro-logic Complications in Organ Transplant Recipients. Butterworth-Heinemann, Boston, 1999, pp 217–227.

157. Grant JW, von Deimling A. Primary T-cell lymphoma of the central nervous system. Arch Pathol Lab Med 114:24–27, 1990.

158. Hacker SM, Knight BP, Lunde NM, Gratiot-Deans J, Sandler H, Leichtman AB. A primary central nervous system T cell lymphoma in a renal transplant patient. Transplantation 53:691–692, 1992.

159. Swinnen LJ, Costanzo-Nordin MR, Fisher SG, et al. Increased incidence of lymphoproliferative disorder after immunosuppression with the monoclonal antibody OKT3 in cardiac-transplant recipients. N Engl J Med 323:1723–1728, 1990.

160. Hochberg FH, Miller DC. Primary central nervous system lymphoma. J Neurosurg 68:835–853, 1988.

161. Hochberg FH, Miller G, Schooley RT, Hirsch MS, Feorino P, Henle W. Central-nervous-system lymphoma related to Epstein-Barr virus. N Engl J Med 309:745–748, 1983.

162. Jack CR Jr, O'Neill BP, Banks PM, Reese DF. Central nervous system lymphoma: histologic types and CT appearance. Radiology 167:211–215, 1988.

163. Dylewsky W, McAlpine FS. Peripheral nervous system. In: Martin JT, Warner MA (eds). Positioning in Anesthesia and Surgery, 3rd ed. WB Saunders, Philadelphia, 1997, pp 299–318.

164. Warner MA, Warner DO, Matsumoto JY, Harper CM, Schroeder DR, Maxson PM. Ulnar neuropathy in surgical patients. Anesthesiology 90:54–59, 1999.

165. Campellone JV, Lacomis D, Giuliani MJ, Kramer DJ. Mononeuropathies associated with liver transplantation. Muscle Nerve 21:896–901, 1998.

166. Campellone JV, Lacomis D. Neuromuscular complications. In: Wijdicks EFM (ed). Neurologic Complications in Organ Transplant Recipients. Butterworth-Heinemann, Boston, 1999, pp 169–192.

167. Stoelting RK. Postoperative ulnar nerve palsy—is it a preventable complication? Anesth Analg 76: 7–9, 1993.

168. Vaziri ND, Barton CH, Ravikumar GR, Martin DC, Ness R, Saiki J. Femoral neuropathy: a complication of renal transplantation. Nephron 28:30–31, 1981.

169. Wijdicks EFM, Litchy WJ, Wiesner RH, Krom RA. Neuromuscular complications associated with liver transplantation. Muscle Nerve 19:696–700, 1996.

170. Wilson JR, Conwit RA, Eidelman BH, Starzl T, Abu-Elmagd K. Sensorimotor neuropathy resembling CIDP in patients receiving FK506. Muscle Nerve 17:528–532, 1994.

171. Bronster DJ, Yonover P, Stein J, Scelsa SN, Miller CM, Sheiner PA. Demyelinating sensorimotor polyneuropathy after administration of FK506. Transplantation 59:1066–1068, 1995.

172. Taylor BV, Wijdicks EFM, Poterucha JJ, Weisner RH. Chronic inflammatory demyelinating polyneuropathy complicating liver transplantation. Ann Neurol 38:828–831, 1995.

173. Nelson KR, McQuillen MP. Neurologic complications of graft-versus-host disease. Neurol Clin 6: 389–403, 1988.

174. Adams C, August CS, Maguire H, Sladky JT. Neuromuscular complications of bone marrow transplantation. Pediatr Neurol 12:58–61, 1995.

175. Bulsara KR, Baron PW, Tuttle-Newhall JE, Clavien PA, and Morgenlander J. Guillain-Barré syndrome in organ and bone marrow transplant patients. Transplantation 71:1169–1172, 2001.

176. Griggs JJ, Commichau CS, Rapoport AP, Griggs RC. Chronic inflammatory demyelinating polyneuropathy in non-Hodgkin's lymphoma. Am J Hematol 54:332–334, 1997.

177. Anderson BA, Young PV, Kean WF, Ludwin SK, Galbraith PR, Anastassiades TP. Polymyositis in chronic graft vs host disease. A case report. Arch Neurol 39:188–190, 1982.

178. Reyes MG, Noronha P, Thomas W Jr, Heredia R. Myositis of chronic graft versus host disease. Neurology 33:1222–1224, 1983.

179. Schmidley JW, Galloway P. Polymyositis following autologous bone marrow transplantation in Hodgkin's disease. Neurology 40:1003–1004, 1990.

180. Slatkin NE, Sheibani K, Forman SJ, et al. Myositis as the major manifestation of chronic graft versus host disease (GVHD) [abstract]. Neurology 37 (Suppl 1):205, 1987.

181. Urbano-Márquez A, Estruch R, Grau JM, et al. Inflammatory myopathy associated with chronic graft-versus-host disease. Neurology 36:1091–1093, 1986.

182. Parker P, Chao NJ, Ben-Ezra J, et al. Polymyositis as a manifestation of chronic graft-versus-host disease. Medicine (Baltimore) 75:279–285, 1996.

183. Graus F, Saiz A, Sierra J, et al. Neurologic complications of autologous and allogeneic bone marrow transplantation in patients with leukemia: a comparative study. Neurology 46:1004–1009, 1996.

184. Bolger GB, Sullivan KM, Spence AM, et al. Myasthenia gravis after allogeneic bone marrow transplantation: relationship to chronic graft-versus-host disease. Neurology 36:1087–1091, 1986.

185. Grau JM, Casademont J, Monforte R, et al. Myasthenia gravis after allogeneic bone marrow transplantation: report of a new case and pathogenetic considerations. Bone Marrow Transplant 5:435–437, 1990.

186. Seely E, Drachman D, Smith BR, Antin JH, Ginsburg D, Rappeport JM. Post bone marrow transplantation (BMT) myasthenia gravis: evidence for acetylcholine receptor (ACh R) abnormality [abstract]. Blood 64 (Suppl 1):221a, 1984.

187. Smith CI, Aarli JA, Biberfeld P, et al. Myasthenia gravis after bone-marrow transplantation. Evidence for a donor origin. N Engl J Med 309:1565–1568, 1983.

188. Dowell JE, Moots PL, Stein RS. Myasthenia gravis after allogeneic bone marrow transplantation for lymphoblastic lymphoma. Bone Marrow Transplant 24:1359–1361, 1999.

189. Mackey JR, Desai S, Larratt L, Cwik V, Nabholtz JM. Myasthenia gravis in association with allogeneic bone marrow transplantation: clinical observations, therapeutic implications and review of literature. Bone Marrow Transplant 19:939–942, 1997.

190. Melms A, Faul C, Sommer N, Wietholter H, Muller CA, Ehninger G. Myasthenia gravis after BMT: identification of patients at risk? [letter]. Bone Marrow Transplant 9:78–79, 1992.

191. Baron F, Sadzot B, Wang F, Beguin Y. Myasthenia gravis without chronic GVHD after allogeneic bone marrow transplantation. Bone Marrow Transplant 22:197–200, 1998.

192. Lefvert AK, Björkholm M. Antibodies against the acetylcholine receptor in hematologic disorders: implications for the development of myasthenia gravis after bone marrow grafting [letter]. N Engl J Med 317:170, 1987.

Part III

Outcome in Central Nervous System Catastrophes

Chapter 19

OUTCOME OF ACUTE INJURY TO THE CENTRAL NERVOUS SYSTEM

The delivery of care for critically ill patients has profoundly changed, and there is an incentive to control costs. A sudden major neurologic complication, often producing coma, typically prompts a reassessment of the level of care. In some, dropping all elements of support may be justified; in others, the original plan of critical care should remain unchanged because a functional outcome can be anticipated. Precision in determining outcome is necessary because finite intensive care unit (ICU) resources should not be sacrificed to patients with disorders that are inevitably disastrous.

In many ICUs, outcome determination in critically ill patients has been modeled by the acute physiology and chronic health evaluation (APACHE)[1] score, but this system is not problem-free, and interobserver variability is substantial.[2] The score is largely determined by age, temperature, blood pressure, electrolytes, acid–base balance, creatinine, white blood cell count, and Glasgow coma scale score. Increasing scores are positively correlated with hospital mortality. The APACHE scores are considered objective means of predicting outcome, but a comparative study illustrated that clinical assessment of hospital mortality risk was just as accurate as use of several laboratory variables.[3]

The APACHE III version, introduced in 1991, is an expanded modification of the Glasgow coma scale score and thus offers a better assessment of the consequence of neurologic catastrophes on hospital mortality.[1,2] Significant differences between prediction and observation remain in patients admitted to ICUs with acute myocardial infarction, multiple trauma, or traumatic brain injury without surgical intervention.[4,5]

This chapter focuses on outcome of major neurologic complications, mostly those involving coma, and may serve as a reference and guide for management decisions. Each of the conclusions is supported by the best available evidence. Only major categories are discussed, and outcome in more specific complications can be found in other chapters.

DESCRIPTION OF OUTCOME CATEGORIES AFTER COMA

At its simplest, outcome can be defined as death, persistent vegetative state, moderate or severe disability, or good recovery. Detailed cognitive evaluation is not available in most neurologic conditions, and only broad categories can be used (Fig. 19–1). These components are frequently used in widely accepted rating systems, including the Glasgow outcome scale. In the category of severely disabled patients, persistent vegetative state is least common, largely because mortality after 3 years is more than 80%.

Persistent vegetative state is defined as no awareness of person or surroundings but eyes are open ("awake but not aware"); lack of sustained, reproducible, purposeful, or voluntary behavioral responses to any stimuli; mutism but with occasional sounds or expressions, such as yawning, lip smacking, and grimacing; and withdrawal from painful stimuli (see also Chapter 1). Automatic and stereotypical behavior may occur. Primitive auditory or visual orienting reflexes with head turning may perplex family members and can incorrectly suggest awareness, but they are not reproducible. Visual tracking to large moving objects or response, such as blinking, to visual threat is characteristically absent. Startle myoclonus, teeth-grinding, tear-shedding, and autonomic functions remain preserved. Respiratory function may be normal. Persistent vegetative state becomes evident 1 month after the insult, but it may take 1 year to confidently reclassify it as permanent. Recovery to a minimal condition of communication has been documented in a few cases. Persistent vegetative state may occur in critically ill patients after major traumatic head injury, cardiac resuscitation, or fat emboli.

Akinetic mutism should be considered a variant of the vegetative state, but suffering is experienced. Patients remain mute and motionless but may notice the speech of visitors and nursing staff. In contrast to persistent vegetative state, visual fixation and tracking may occur to movement of objects shown to the patient and confrontation with sound may startle the patient. Akinetic mutism is rare but has been reported with toxic doses of cyclosporine, amphotericin B, and baclofen and after irradiation and chemotherapy in bone marrow transplantation.[6–8] The differences between these states are shown in Table 19–1.[9]

Severe disability is usually applied to patients with residual cognitive or motor deficits that prevent them from functioning independently. Active rehabilitation training programs may produce significant gains in physical independence, but generally if no spontaneous improvement has emerged within 1 year, return to gainful employment should be considered an unrealistic expectation. However, continued improvement has been reported in patients with severe disability after head injury.

In the category *moderate disability*, the patient may have significant neurologic impairment, but these patients are able to return to their previous employers, often with

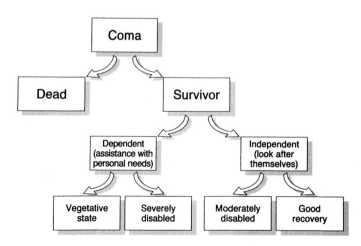

Figure 19–1. Major categories of outcome after coma.

Table 19–1. **Neurologic Conditions That Produce or Mimic Unresponsiveness**

Condition	Prognosis for Neurologic Recovery
Persistent vegetative state*	Traumatic PVS (1-year outcome): PVS, 15% of patients; dead, 33%; GR, 7%; MD, 17%; SD, 28%
	Nontraumatic PVS (1-year outcome): PVS, 32% of patients; dead, 53%; GR, 1%; MD, 3%; SD, 11%
Brain death[†]	Equals death
Locked-in syndrome	Recovery unlikely; patients remain quadriplegic; prolonged survival possible
Akinetic mutism	Recovery very unlikely and depends on cause

GR, good recovery; MD, moderately disabled; PVS, persistent vegetative state; SD, severely disabled.
*Adults only.
[†]Profound hypothermia or drug intoxication may produce similar presentations (Chapter 1).
Modified from the Multi-Society Task Force on PVS.[9] By permission of the Massachusetts Medical Society.

adjustments to much lower job levels. *Good recovery* refers to complete return to baseline function without forced retirement, major impediments due to depression, lack of productivity, or loss of originality. Minor fixed, nondisabling neurologic deficits may be present.

OUTCOME IN METABOLIC ENCEPHALOPATHIES

Clinical observation alone most likely remains the mainstay of prognostication in metabolic encephalopathies. Careful neurologic examination with daily follow-up should include some elements of cognitive testing, assessment of brain stem reflexes, and motor response to noxious stimuli. Without confounding sedative agents, lack of improvement of the motor component of the Glasgow coma scale alone over a certain observation period is often indicative of poor outcome. In a large series of patients with nontraumatic coma caused by acute metabolic derangements or hypoxia, longitudinal evaluation for 1 week proved to be already very sensitive in the prediction of outcome.[10] Overall, only 16% of the 500 patients in coma recovered to an independent living. Viewed in the context of critical illness, the underlying disorder may determine mortality.

Postresuscitation (Anoxic–Ischemic) Encephalopathy

In many patients, a confident decision on withdrawal of support cannot be made within 72 hr after cardiopulmonary resuscitation. Generally, at least 6 hr must have passed before clinical neurologic signs can be used for prognostication. Not infrequently, neurologists are asked to assess the patient during resuscitation to determine whether a continuous effort of cardiac compression is necessary. Obviously, at the time of resuscitation, nonreactive pupils and absent motor responses associated with a global decrease in cerebral blood flow do not necessarily indicate permanent neuronal damage in the cortical layers.

Awakening within the first day after cardiac resuscitation and interactive conversational speech (incidence of 15% to 20% in large series) predict good outcome. In these fortunate patients, permanent cognitive deficits are unusual,[11–14] but underlying cardiac disease limits performance, and a significant proportion of these survivors of previous cardiopulmonary resuscitation may still die suddenly in the first year (Fig. 19–2). Patients who remain comatose after resuscitation have a very high chance of dying in the hospital because of recurrent arrhythmias or withdrawal of support initiated by family members honoring the patient's previously voiced wishes.

Generally, patients who remain comatose after 24 hr have a very small chance (approximately 6%) of recovery to independent living. After 3 days from the time of cardiopulmonary resuscitation, independent functioning is achieved only by those who improve the motor response to at least withdrawal to pain. The rules of prognostication may be different in patients who were resuscitated as a result of submersion and hypothermia, but they can be used as a guideline (see Chapter 16).

Prognosticators of poor outcome have been identified; if they are present, severe disability, persistent vegetative state, or death is very likely (approximately 95% probability, or 1 in 20 instances wrong) (Table 19–2). However, the percentage of patients with absent scalp somatosensory evoked potentials, myoclonus status epilepticus, and certainly fixed pupils in the first day is relatively small, and definitive prognostication often must be postponed until the third day after return of circulation. The guidelines from a prospective study by Levy and associates[10] are useful and have remained unchallenged[15,16] (Fig. 19–3).

The chance of awakening decreases remarkably in the first week (50% in the first day, 25% in the third day, and 10% at the end of the first week). Awakening after more than 3 days of coma due to postresuscitation encephalopathy is very frequently associated with severe disability. The neuropsychologic sequelae have been studied in detail, and of 54 survivors of cardiac arrest, 26 (48%) had severe cognitive deficits and 22 (41%) had additional evidence of depression.[17] Patients with severe disability after postresuscitation encephalopathy often remain in a tragic state. Dramatic recovery from a severely disabled state after 1 month is rarely seen, and 6-month outcome is not much different from that in the first month.

Cognitive function can be relatively spared, but action myoclonus may determine disability in patients with a major insult. Sudden shock-like involuntary movements in all limbs, caused by active muscular contractions, are precipitated by movement or action. Action myoclonus emerges after awakening and often coincides with severe ataxia.

Action myoclonus, also called Lance and Adams syndrome, is perhaps more often seen in asphyxia and must be differentiated from myoclonus status epilepticus.[18] During coma, an electroencephalogram (EEG) shows slowing of background rhythm, which is different from the characteristic burst–suppression abnormality in myoclonus status epilepticus. In patients with action myoclonus evoked potentials, computed tomography (CT) and magnetic resonance imaging (MRI) scans are frequently normal.

Administration of clonazepam or 5-hydroxytryptophan with carbidopa is the first line of treatment.[19–22] Additional treatment with valproate sodium, primidone, or fluoxetine may be considered, but with polytherapy sedation often becomes a limiting factor. A

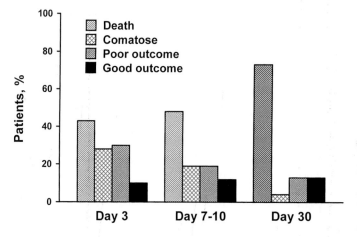

Figure 19–2. Estimate of neurologic outcome in postresuscitation coma (data were collected from several large series of patients studied after cardiac arrest).

Table 19–2. **Prognosticators of Poor Outcome in Coma after Cardiac Arrest**

Clinical	Laboratory
• Pupils fixed to light • Myoclonus status epilepticus • Sustained upward gaze • Withdrawal to pain or worse at 3 days	• Absence of bilateral cortical response on somatosensory evoked potentials • Burst-suppression pattern on electroencephalogram • Magnetic resonance imaging documentation of multiple areas of cortical laminar necrosis

placebo-controlled, randomized study that included many causes of cortical myoclonus found that piracetam (4 grams daily, 10-day increment to maximal dose of 24 grams daily) significantly improved disability, in some patients with dramatic results, when used in combination with other drugs.[19]

Isolated cognitive deficits, including an

amnesic syndrome, may occur in the first weeks after resuscitation but are very uncommon. Patients with normal intellectual function but impaired recall, intact long-term memory, and intact recognition have been recognized.[23] Amnesic syndromes may be permanent.[24] Very frequently in amnesic syndrome, a combination of apraxia and

Initial Examination

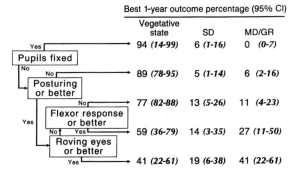

3 Days After CPR

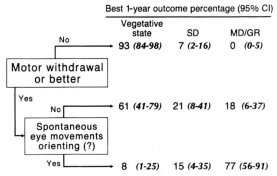

Figure 19–3. Algorithms for prognostication after cardiopulmonary resuscitation (CPR). Data are based on 210 prospectively studied patients. The percentage of patients is given in each subcategory. (Note the wide confidence intervals [CI] caused by the small number of studied patients in each outcome category; these limit the robustness of the data.) SD, severely disabled; MD, moderately disabled; GR, good recovery. (Data from Levy et al.[10])

motor aphasia is found, and this condition does not notably improve over the years. Although extrapyramidal syndromes have been largely reported with cyanide or carbon monoxide poisoning associated with hypoxia,[25–27] they are also noted after cardiac arrest.[28,29] An akinetic rigid syndrome develops as early as 1 week and as late as 1 year[29] after cardiopulmonary resuscitation and may evolve into progressive generalized dystonia with severe oromandibular dystonia and blepharospasms.

The predilection for basal ganglia involvement after hypoxic–ischemic insult may possibly stem from increased vulnerability due to its vast glutaminergic input. Glutamine may have been released in excess after this insult and become excitotoxic. Calcification in the lentiform nuclei can be documented on neuroimaging in these patients as early as several weeks (Fig. 19–4). Disablement in these patients necessitates a wheelchair or confinement in bed, but some may improve.[29] This extranigral, drug-resistant clin-

ical disorder may be successfully treated with bilateral posteroventral pallidotomy.[30]

Uremic Encephalopathy

Associated systemic conditions determine outcome in patients with uremic encephalopathy. Thus, mortality from acute renal failure is low (approximately 10%) when serious complications such as sepsis, massive gastrointestinal bleeding, acute myocardial infarction, and acute respiratory failure are absent. Under these circumstances, outcome in uremic encephalopathy can be excellent.

The clinical signs of uremic encephalopathy may completely disappear after dialysis. In a few patients, improvement in uremic encephalopathy after dialysis is offset by generalized muscle weakness and muscle cramps. The transient muscle cramps that often occur immediately after dialysis are not related to electrolyte abnormalities, and the mechanism has not been elucidated.

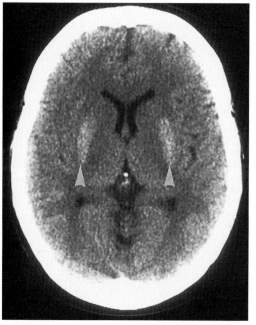

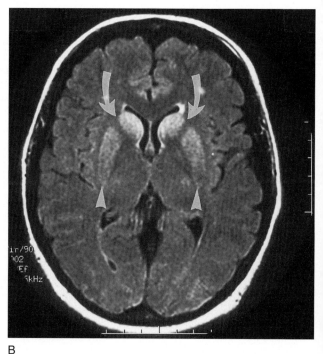

A   B

Figure 19–4. In a patient with a delayed parkinsonian syndrome after cardiac resuscitation, computed tomography (*A*) shows calcification in the lentiform nuclei (arrowheads) and magnetic resonance imaging (*B*) shows further involvement of the caudate nucleus (curved arrows).

Profound persistent weakness may be caused by hypophosphatemia related to antacid administration and hemodialysis.

Systematic clinical neurologic studies of recovery in patients with acute renal failure and uremic encephalopathy have not been published, but anecdotal experience suggests that most patients, if not all, recover without sequelae. Patients may vividly remember a psychotic experience at the time of severe renal failure. Resolution of the clinical signs and symptoms of uremic encephalopathy, often in reverse order of appearance, has also been noted during the diuretic phase of acute renal failure but only when the concentrating ability of the kidney decreases serum urea and creatinine values. In fact, in the early polyuric phase of recovery, the excretion of urea and creatinine is not yet established and an increase in serum levels is more common.

Failure to improve could point to additional ischemic damage from conditions that are secondary to acute renal failure. During dialysis, hypotension may occur in 30% of the patients and may, despite immediate intervention, be an additional challenge to cerebral perfusion pressure. Failure to recover from uremic encephalopathy also occurs when acute renal failure is associated with shock damaging the brain and kidney simultaneously and other types of systemic disease, such as the systemic vasculitides (see Chapter 12) and thrombotic thrombocytopenic purpura (see Chapter 11). These patients with associated conditions and renal failure do poorly if they do not awaken within 1 week after resolution of uremia by dialysis. Bilateral subdural hematoma is a very unusual cause but may halt recovery and must be considered when severe coagulopathy is present or when heparin is used during hemodialysis. It may be provoked by severe thrombocytopenia, which is common during dialysis and is induced either by heparin treatment or from contact with the dialysis membrane. Long-term outcome in patients with chronic renal failure is determined by the potential development of dialysis encephalopathy.

In general, intellectual deterioration is uncommon in patients undergoing long-term dialysis, and many patients do not have significant changes in neuropsychologic performance when tested over the years. Dialysis dementia is rare, occurring only after 2 years of dialysis treatment. It is characterized by severe dysarthria, apraxia of speech, and rapid decline in cognitive function until death 6 months after diagnosis. Although serum levels of aluminum correlate poorly with its occurrence, aluminum exposure probably causes this devastating complication. Renal transplantation had a significant positive effect on cognitive function and even resulted in reversal when patients with long-term dialysis were tested.[31] A comprehensive review of dialysis dementia is found in Bolton and Young's monograph on renal disease.[32]

Hepatic Encephalopathy

Outcome in patients with hepatic encephalopathy depends on the nature of the liver disease.[33] Many patients with hepatic encephalopathy admitted to ICUs have either fulminant hepatic failure or sudden worsening of long-standing cirrhosis. The fatality rate is considerable in fulminant hepatic failure, but outcome can be better in patients with liver cirrhosis punctuated by an acute episode of gastrointestinal bleeding that evolves into acute portosystemic encephalopathy.[34]

Fulminant hepatic failure is frequently fatal without emergency liver transplantation. In a recent retrospective survey in the U.S. involving 295 patients in 12 transplant centers, 25% of the patients survived spontaneously, 41% underwent transplantation, and 34% died before transplantation.[35] Outcome may be more favorable in patients with drug-induced hepatitis (for example, acetaminophen overdose) and non-A, non-B associated hepatic necrosis, but outcome in patients with rapid progression to stage III or IV encephalopathy without transplantation is poor. This is largely due to brain edema in higher stages of encephalopathy in fulminant hepatic failure. Brain edema may be resistant to any traditional management of intracranial pressure and result in brain herniation and brain death (see Chapter 10). In others, despite successful treatment of intracranial pressure and resolution of clinical and radiologic signs, outcome may still be guarded from complications of liver transplantation and immunosuppression. But patients who survive do well and are expected to have normal intellectual performance. In our experience, patients in whom encephalopathy reaches stage IV tend to have a greater chance of severe cognitive deficits, but data on long-term outcome in patients within this category are only anecdotal.

Hepatic encephalopathy in patients admitted to medical ICUs can be precipitated by bleeding from varices, spontaneous bacterial peritonitis, or use of diuretic agents. Therefore, blood transfusion, correction of associated metabolic abnormalities, and administration of lactulose and neomycin may result in a striking improvement in level of consciousness. As discussed in Chapter 10, a weak linear relationship exists between stages of encephalopathy and arterial level of ammonia,[36] but increased arterial ammonia level may precede coma by several days, and a decrease in ammonia concentration may precede improvement in the stage of hepatic encephalopathy.

Of patients who become comatose or stuporous from hepatic encephalopathy, only one-third regain independent function; the remaining 60% of patients die without regaining consciousness.[10,37] Prognosticators of poor outcome in hepatic coma in patients with cirrhosis are ascites, low prothrombin index, and development of hepatorenal syndrome. In one study, outcome in patients comatose from hepatic encephalopathy was worse when it was caused by gastrointestinal bleeding than when it was associated with other triggers.[34]

Many patients who recover from hepatic encephalopathy remain impaired in alertness and performance. Much of the day may be spent sleeping, yawning, and remaining inactive.

Sepsis-Associated Encephalopathy

When acute respiratory distress syndrome, disseminated intravascular coagulation, or multiorgan failure emerges in patients with sepsis, mortality is high. It is not clear whether sepsis-associated encephalopathy is an independent predictor of mortality. Brain function most likely fails with multiple organ failure, but even so, it is likely that severe hypotension is an important contributor to sepsis-associated encephalopathy, in contrast to the assumption that the brain is a separate organ system that fails in sepsis.

In a series of 14 patients with severe sepsis-associated encephalopathy, only 3 recovered,[38] and patients who lacked motor responses died. In the assessment of outcome in these patients, however, one should be aware of the long-standing effects of the neuromuscular blocking agents frequently used in this situation and other evidence of a critical illness polyneuropathy or myopathy.

In a series of 50 patients, the degree of coma measured by Glasgow coma score, increased APACHE II scores, and renal failure affected mortality. Mortality was 20% with a Glasgow coma score of 13 or 14 and 63% with a score of less than 8.[39] In these patients, EEG recordings, although nonspecific, may be helpful to assess brain damage. Mortality in sepsis-associated encephalopathy has been shown to correlate with EEG abnormalities. Young[40] reported no deaths in patients with normal EEG findings, 19% mortality with theta activity, 36% with delta activity, 50% with triphasic waves, and 67% with burst–suppression activity. Periodic lateralized epileptiform discharges did not have a predictive value. Systematic studies of outcome in septic encephalopathy are needed, but in all likelihood, the rules in postresuscitation encephalopathy probably also apply to septic encephalopathy.

An EEG or somatosensory evoked potentials could be used for further confirmation in patients who fail to awaken after sepsis syndrome. Clearly, there are two categories of patients: first, patients with acute confusional states and abnormal consciousness during the progression of sepsis syndrome, and second, patients who rapidly become comatose while experiencing barely controllable shock and downward spiraling coagulation abnormalities, all multiplying to permanent damage.

Diabetic Comas

Mortality in patients with hyperosmolar nonketotic derangement varies from 20% to

60%, and death occurs in half the patients in the first 3 days.[41–44] Prognosticators of poor outcome have not been consistently identified, but severity of hyperglycemia, hyperosmolarity, or uremia at presentation does not have predictive value.[43] Beyond that, hypovolemia and cardiogenic shock may be more relevant.

In contrast to nonketotic hyperosmolar states, diabetic ketoacidosis seldom produces prolonged coma.[45] Many patients, often young, completely recover after treatment. In certain instances, hypoglycemia-induced coma can be devastating and may result in a persistent vegetative state or severe disability.[46–48] Selective damage in the hippocampus may occur in hypoglycemia, but in many patients hypoxia plays an additional role[49,50] (see Chapter 8). Why so many patients recover, even after long episodes of hypoglycemia, has not been adequately explained. In addition, a cohort study found that cognitive decline based on scores on the Mini-Mental State Examination did not occur in patients with frequent hypoglycemic episodes.[51] A more recent study from Edinburgh, however, documented increased frequency of depression and poor performance in the digit symbol and Stroop tests in patients with recurrent hypoglycemia.[52] This topic needs further clinical evaluation and longitudinal study.

OUTCOME IN STROKE

Prognostic factors have been identified in various types of stroke but remain largely unexplored in patients in whom critical illness has been complicated by a stroke. Weaning from a ventilator may be complicated because of reduced alertness and ventilatory drive. In other patients, issues of concern pertain to risk of deep venous thrombosis in a paralyzed limb, risk of aspiration, oropharyngeal dysfunction and nutrition, and seizures or confusion causing repeated dislodgment of central or arterial catheters.

Intracerebral Hematoma

Factors that influence outcome in the entire population of patients with intracerebral hemorrhage are summarized in Table 19–3.[53–56] Mortality is high in patients with hematoma of large volume, intraventricular extension, and midline shift. Coma caused by intracerebral hemorrhage with volumes of >50 mL is likely to result in death.[58] It is not known how many patients deteriorate from continued bleeding, but increase in volume up to 400% has been noted.[59] The total volume of intraventricular clot, however, is equally important.[56]

Drowsiness, limb weakness, and advanced age are all factors that determine low probability of good recovery. Patients who are comatose when transferred out of the ICU have virtually no chance of full recovery unless other systemic factors are depressing the level of consciousness. The mechanism of hemorrhage probably does not influence survival, although hemorrhages associated with tissue plasminogen activator and anticoagulation are more often associated with severe disability. Bleeding into multiple intracranial compartments and continued bleeding may account for this outcome. Of the surviving patients with supratentorial intracerebral hematomas due to thrombolysis, half will have major deficits.[60]

The site of intracerebral hematoma may be more important in prognostication. Ganglionic hemorrhages (thalamus, putamen) often extend into the ventricular system, and the development of hydrocephalus together with coma (Glasgow coma scale score <8) significantly increases the chance of early (30-day) mortality. Outcome is not improved with ventriculostomy.[57,61] Lobar hemorrhages (frontal, temporal, or parietal) are devastating if size approaches 40 mL and the patient is stuporous, and outcome seems hopeless in comatose patients with a septum pellucidum shift of >6 mm on CT scan.[62] Emergency evacuation should be considered, but morbidity is not known in this subset of patients. In our experience, many of the critically ill patients in whom an intracerebral hematoma developed were past cure from multiple organ failure.

Cerebellar hemorrhages are considered neurologic emergencies. Prompt neurosurgical evacuation in a patient with a cerebellar hematoma of >3 cm, brain stem distortion, and extension to the vermis is warranted, because the risk of rapid deteri-

Table 19–3. Prognosticators of Poor Outcome in Intracerebral Hemorrhage

Older than 70 years
Decreased level of consciousness after ictus (each grade)
Limb paresis (each grade)
Hyperglycemia after ictus
Intracranial hemorrhage volume >60 mL
Intraventricular blood volume ≥20 mL
Midline shift of the septum pellucidum or pineal gland (6-10 mm) on CT scan
Acute hydrocephalus (putaminal hemorrhage)

Data from Daverat et al.,[53] Fieschi et al.,[54] and Phan et al.[57]

oration is substantial. Lack of corneal reflexes in a comatose patient with a cerebellar hematoma portends a very poor outcome.[63] Pontine hemorrhages are rarely seen in the ICU, and they are typically immediately fatal. Pontine hemorrhages in surviving patients are managed conservatively, but the destruction they cause can result in substantial morbidity from diplopia and gait ataxia. Survival is very uncommon if they are associated with hyperthermia, acute hydrocephalus, or extension of the hemorrhage into the midbrain and thalamus.[64]

Ischemic Stroke

Outcome in patients with infarcts in the distribution of the anterior cerebral circulation is different from that in patients with infarcts in the posterior cerebral circulation. Hemispheric infarcts cause a high rate of death, certainly in patients with stem (M1) occlusions of the middle cerebral artery. Prog-

nosticators of poor outcome have been identified, and these factors may also predict brain swelling (Table 19–4). Hemorrhagic transformation on CT scan does not necessarily imply a risk of clinical worsening or higher probability of permanent disability. Many patients with middle cerebral artery territory stroke improve, but major functional improvement is not expected after the first 3 to 6 months. Intensive rehabilitation programs, however, may produce improvement of functional ability beyond this time limit.[66] In nondominant hemispheric strokes, neglect disappears within 1 year. Recovery of motor function may begin 2 weeks after onset. Hand and arm movement within 1 to 2 weeks in a previously plegic extremity predicts a high likelihood of recovery to a functional state. In dominant hemisphere strokes, aphasia may be supplanted by increasing fluency, but deficits are likely to persist in patients who presented with global aphasia.[67]

Early seizure (within 2 weeks) in acute

Table 19–4. Prognosticators of Poor Outcome in Ischemic Stroke Involving the Anterior Cerebral Circulation

Decreased level of consciousness after ictus
Gaze palsy, gaze preference, pupillary asymmetry
Hypodensity >50% of arterial territory, brain swelling or early midline shift on CT scan
Need for reintubation and mechanical ventilation[65]

stroke is associated with a significant chance of recurrence.[68,69] A seizure disorder develops in one-third of the patients with an ischemic stroke and a seizure at the beginning.[70] Thus, antiepileptic drugs are recommended in this subset of patients. In one study, however, most of the patients who had recurrent seizures had phenytoin coverage, a finding that suggests that treatment and monitoring after a single seizure should be more aggressive.[69]

Many infarcts in the posterior cerebral circulation are from penetrating artery disease, and thus the area of the infarcted tissue is smaller. Brain stem syndromes that involve small perforating arteries are associated with a good chance of survival and recovery to independent function.[71] Outcome correlates with the number of infarcts, particularly those involving the pons and thalamus.[72] In patients with ischemic stroke in the posterior cerebral circulation, outcome is also determined by localization[73] (Table 19–5). Cerebellar stroke has a good potential for recovery but less so in patients with a superior cerebellar artery occlusion, whose outcome may be related to more common brain stem compression.[74]

Embolus to the basilar artery that causes coma or locked-in syndrome is associated with high mortality and no recovery to independent function unless an early attempt at intra-arterial thrombolysis is possible.[75] Outcome in locked-in syndrome from any cause is very poor, and significant improvement has been reported only very occasionally. A review of 117 patients from the literature noted a mortality of 67%.[76] Home placement, permanent gastrostomy, tracheostomy, indwelling urine catheters, and bowel programs, all requiring 24-hr skilled nursing care, are possible, with survival up to 12 years.[77] Communication is achieved only through very sophisticated electronic devices that signal vertical eye movements. However, locked-in syndrome may be incomplete and patients with some retained bulbar function and limb function may still have substantial improvement.

OUTCOME IN HEAD INJURY

Although numerous clinical variables determine the outcome in head injuries, trauma data banks have consistently identified factors with high predictive power. The Glasgow coma scale, since its introduction in the early 1970s, remains a strong clinical predictor, and many of the laboratory tests do not add any value.[78] In addition, attempts to modify the Glasgow coma scale have not increased the predictive value.[79] Poor outcome can be expected in patients who have the clinical features and CT scan abnormalities outlined in Table 19–6.

Patients with minimal Glasgow coma sum scores of 3 or 4 after stabilization of airway and hemodynamic resuscitation in the emergency department have a poor outcome irrespective of mass lesions or shift on CT scan. In many data banks, prediction of good or poor outcome was more powerful than prediction of moderate to severe disability. Moreover, continued improvement over the first 6 months can be expected. Three courses of recovery in surviving patients with initial Glasgow coma scale sum scores of 8 or less (equivalent to coma) have been identified. One-third of these patients have significant improvement in 6 months that is followed by some deterioration in performance that may be linked to depressive symptoms. Half the patients improved in the

Table 19–5. Prognosticators of Poor Outcome in Ischemic Stroke Involving the Posterior Cerebral Circulation

Basilar artery occlusion causing locked-in syndrome or coma
Cerebellar infarction with brain stem compression and hydrocephalus
Bilateral thalamic infarcts

Data from Nadeau et al.[73]

Table 19–6. **Prognosticators of Poor Outcome in Traumatic Brain Injury**

Postresuscitation Glasgow coma score of 3

Older than 65 years

Abnormal pupil or pupils for at least one observation

Shock on admission (blood pressure <80 mm Hg) and during hospital stay

Persistent increased intracranial pressure (>20 mm Hg)

Hypoxia on admission (Po_2 <60 mm Hg)

Computed tomography scan abnormalities (absent cisterns, intraventricular hemorrhage, midline shift, shearing in corpus callosum)

Data from Jennett et al.,[78] Pal et al.,[79] Ross et al.,[80] Alberico et al.,[81] and Choi et al.[82]

first 6 months and had only minimal gains in the following 6 to 12 months. No improvement was seen in the remaining patients, but many had additional documented hypoxia, again suggesting that the initial traumatic impact may have been worsened by other factors, such as hypoxia and hypothermia.[79]

Advanced age has been consistently identified as an independent predictor of poor outcome in patients with severe injury. Elderly patients do very poorly. In a retrospective analysis of a series of 195 patients older than 65, comatose patients had only a 10% chance of survival and a 4% chance of independent functional outcome.[80] Elderly patients more often have extradural hematomas, associated cerebrovascular disease, or multitrauma that jeopardizes recovery.

Computed tomographic scan abnormalities have also been described as potential indicators of poor outcome, and the findings of compressed basal cisterns and midline shift from hemorrhagic contusion are predictors of poor outcome.[81] Intraventricular hemorrhage also predicts poor outcome but is not an independent prognostic factor.[83] The MRI findings have not been systematically studied, but one study claimed a very poor outcome when corpus callosum lesions appeared in conjunction with brain stem lesions.[84] Moderate disability seemed to be related more to frontotemporal lesions by MRI.[85]

Patients who become severely disabled after severe head injury may be able to return to work in sheltered workplaces, usually with responsibilities far inferior to those before

the injury; only a relative minority are cared for in nursing homes.[86]

Many prediction trees in diffuse brain injury have been developed to determine outcome. Complementary examples are shown in Figures 19–5 and 19–6 for patients with polytrauma.

OUTCOME IN TRAUMATIC SPINE INJURY

Prognostication in spine injury is extraordinarily difficult. Reliable predictive factors are not available, and only general estimates apply. High C1 to C3 level lesions abolish respiration, and mechanical ventilation is permanently needed. It has been observed that in a patient with complete cord lesion, some motor or sensory function must return within 2 days or there is no chance of clinically significant recovery.[88] Complete thoracic spine lesions also have less potential for recovery than complete cervical or lumbar lesions. It may take 3 months to decide whether a complete lesion remains complete. In incomplete lesions, recovery can still be expected up to 18 months.

Bladder function is permanently lost in complete quadriplegia. Suprapubic catheters must be placed. Hyperreflexic bladder appears later, and voiding can be accomplished with manual external pressure. Anticholinergic agents may improve bladder capacity if reflex bladder is too easily triggered. Bowel function can be accomplished by use of suppositories and digital stimulation. Sexual function is lost, but many mod-

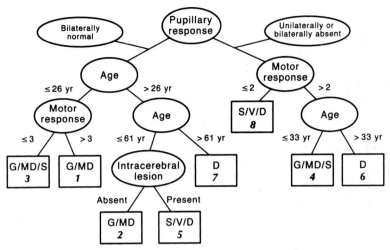

Figure 19–5. Outcome in severe head injury. Prediction tree is based on 555 patients with head injury. The predicted 12-month outcome is defined by the Glasgow coma scale. G, good recovery; MD, moderately disabled; S, severely disabled; V, persistent vegetative state; D, death. The number in each terminal prognostic subgroup (square) represents the prognostic rank of that subgroup according to the proportion of good (G or MD) outcomes. Subgroup 1 is the group with the best prognostic pattern, and subgroup 8 is the group with the worst prognostic pattern. (From Choi et al.[82] By permission of the American Association of Neurological Surgeons.)

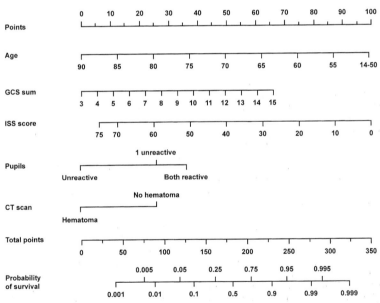

Figure 19–6. Nomogram for predicted probability of survival at 1 year in patients with traumatic brain injury. For each of the five variables, points are calculated by reading from the top scale. The total point score is then translated into a probability of survival by using the bottom two scales. For example, a patient of age 70 (50 points) with a Glasgow coma scale score (GCS) of 12 (50 points), an injury severity score (ISS) of 20 (75 points), reactive pupils (35 points), and no hematoma on computed tomography (CT) (25 points) has a total score of 235 points and a corresponding probability of survival at 1 year of about 0.93. The ISS is an anatomical scoring system for multiple injuries[87] and is calculated by adding together the squares of the three highest abbreviated injury scale scores in the most severely injured body areas. These body areas are head or neck, face, chest, abdomen and pelvic contents, bony pelvis and limbs, and body surface. The severity is graded as 1, minor; 2, moderate; 3, severe, not life-threatening; 4, severe, life-threatening, survival probable; and 5, critical, survival uncertain. (From Signorini DF, Andrews PJ, Jones PA, Wardlaw JM, and Miller JD. Predicting survival using simple clinical variables: A case study in traumatic brain injury. J Neurol Neurosurg Psychiatry 66:20–25, 1999. By permission of the journal.)

ifications can result in acceptable alternatives. A comprehensive discussion can be found in Trieschman's text.[89]

CONCLUSIONS

A practical approach is early identification of signs of poor or favorable prognosis. High probability of poor outcome (persistent vegetative state, severe disability) should influence decisions on management and must reduce prolongation of futile treatments. Neurologists should identify what kind of outcome can be expected in any neurologic catastrophe, although in some situations, outcome studies are either conflicting or simply not available and categorical statements about outcome may thus be unfounded. Neuroimaging studies (particularly MRI) and somatosensory evoked potentials may be helpful additional tests to confirm the clinical impression of a poor prospect for recovery in a functional state of health.

REFERENCES

1. Knaus WA, Wagner DP, Draper EA, et al. The APACHE III prognostic system. Risk prediction of hospital mortality for critically ill hospitalized adults. Chest 100:1619–1636, 1991.
2. Polderman KH, Thijs LG, Girbes AR. Interobserver variability in the use of APACHE II scores. Lancet 353:380, 1999.
3. Kruse JA, Thill-Baharozian MC, Carlson RW. Comparison of clinical assessment with APACHE II for predicting mortality risk in patients admitted to a medical intensive care unit. JAMA 260:1739–1742, 1988.
4. Cho DY, Wang YC. Comparison of the APACHE III, APACHE II and Glasgow Coma Scale in acute head injury for prediction of mortality and functional outcome. Intensive Care Med 23:77–84, 1997.
5. Zimmerman JE, Wagner DP, Draper EA, Wright L, Alzola C, Knaus WA. Evaluation of acute physiology and chronic health evaluation III predictions of hospital mortality in an independent database. Crit Care Med 26:1317–1326, 1998.
6. Rubin DT, So EL. Reversible akinetic mutism possibly induced by baclofen. Pharmacotherapy 19:468–470, 1999.
7. Walker RW, Rosenblum MK. Amphotericin B–associated leukoencephalopathy. Neurology 42:2005–2010, 1992.
8. Devinsky O, Lemann W, Evans AC, Moeller JR, Rottenberg DA. Akinetic mutism in a bone marrow transplant recipient following total-body irradiation and amphotericin B chemoprophylaxis. A positron

emission tomographic and neuropathologic study. Arch Neurol 44:414–417, 1987.
9. The Multi-Society Task Force on PVS. Medical aspects of the persistent vegetative state (part 1). N Engl J Med 330:1499–1508, 1994.
10. Levy DE, Bates D, Caronna JJ, et al. Prognosis in nontraumatic coma. Ann Intern Med 94:293–301, 1981.
11. Bertini G, Margheri M, Giglioli C, et al. Prognostic significance of early clinical manifestations in postanoxic coma: a retrospective study of 58 patients resuscitated after prehospital cardiac arrest. Crit Care Med 17:627–633, 1989.
12. Edgren E, Hedstrand U, Nordin M, Rydin E, Ronquist G. Prediction of outcome after cardiac arrest. Crit Care Med 15:820–825, 1987.
13. Mullie A, Verstringe P, Buylaert W, et al. Predictive value of Glasgow coma score for awakening after out-of-hospital cardiac arrest. Cerebral Resuscitation Study Group of the Belgian Society for Intensive Care. Lancet 1:137–140, 1988.
14. Niskanen M, Kari A, Nikki P, et al. Acute physiology and chronic health evaluation (APACHE II) and Glasgow coma scores as predictors of outcome from intensive care after cardiac arrest. Crit Care Med 19:1465–1473, 1991.
15. Zandbergen EG, de Haan RJ, Stoutenbeek CP, Koelman JH, Hijdra A. Systematic review of early prediction of poor outcome in anoxic-ischaemic coma. Lancet 352:1808–1812, 1998.
16. Krieger DW. Evoked potentials not just to confirm hopelessness in anoxic brain injury. Lancet 352:1796–1797, 1998.
17. Roine RO, Kajaste S, Kaste M. Neuropsychological sequelae of cardiac arrest. JAMA 269:237–242, 1993.
18. Lance JW, Adams RD. The syndrome of intention or action myoclonus as a sequel to hypoxic encephalopathy. Brain 86:111–136, 1963.
19. Brown P, Steiger MJ, Thompson PD, et al. Effectiveness of piracetam in cortical myoclonus. Mov Disord 8:63–68, 1993.
20. Fahn S. Newer drugs for posthypoxic action myoclonus: observations from a well-studied case. Adv Neurol 43:197–199, 1986.
21. Kanoti GA, Gombeski WR Jr, Gulledge AD, Konrad D, Collins R, Medendorp SV. The effect of do-not-resuscitate orders on length of stay. Cleve Clin J Med 59:591–594, 1992.
22. Obeso JA, Artieda J, Rothwell JC, Day B, Thompson P, Marsden CD. The treatment of severe action myoclonus. Brain 112:765–777, 1989.
23. Volpe BT, Hirst W. The characterization of an amnesic syndrome following hypoxic ischemic injury. Arch Neurol 40:436–440, 1983.
24. Finklestein S, Caronna JJ. Amnestic syndrome following cardiac arrest [abstract]. Neurology 28:389, 1978.
25. Hawker K, Lang AE. Hypoxic–ischemic damage of the basal ganglia. Case reports and a review of the literature. Mov Disord 5:219–224, 1990.
26. Schwartz A, Hennerici M, Wegener OH. Delayed choreoathetosis following acute carbon monoxide poisoning. Neurology 35:98–99, 1985.
27. Uitti RJ, Rajput AH, Ashenhurst EM, Rozdilsky B. Cyanide-induced parkinsonism: a clinicopathologic report. Neurology 35:921–925, 1985.

28. Bhatt MH, Obeso JA, Marsden CD. Time course of postanoxic akinetic-rigid and dystonic syndromes. Neurology 43:314–317, 1993.

29. Boylan KB, Chin JH, DeArmond SJ. Progressive dystonia following resuscitation from cardiac arrest. Neurology 40:1458–1461, 1990.

30. Goto S, Kunitoku N, Soyama N, et al. Posteroventral pallidotomy in a patient with parkinsonism caused by hypoxic encephalopathy. Neurology 49: 707–710, 1997.

31. Kramer L, Madl C, Stockenhuber F, et al. Beneficial effect of renal transplantation on cognitive brain function. Kidney Int 49:833–838, 1996.

32. Bolton CF, Young GB. Neurological Complications of Renal Disease. Butterworths, Boston, 1990.

33. Komori H, Hirasa M, Takakuwa H, et al. Concept of the clinical stages of acute hepatic failure. Am J Gastroenterol 81:544–549, 1986.

34. Christensen E, Krintel JJ, Hansen SM, Johansen JK, Juhl E. Prognosis after the first episode of gastrointestinal bleeding or coma in cirrhosis. Survival and prognostic factors. Scand J Gastroenterol 24: 999–1006, 1989.

35. Schiodt FV, Atillasoy E, Shakil AO, et al. Etiology and outcome for 295 patients with acute liver failure in the United States. Liver Transpl Surg 5:29–34, 1999.

36. Stahl J. Studies of the blood ammonia in liver disease: its diagnostic, prognosis, and therapeutic significance. Ann Intern Med 58:1–24, 1963.

37. Bates D, Caronna JJ, Cartlidge NEF, et al. A prospective study of nontraumatic coma: methods and results in 310 patients. Ann Neurol 2:211–220, 1977.

38. Wijdicks EFM, Stevens M. The role of hypotension in septic encephalopathy following surgical procedures. Arch Neurol 49:653–656, 1992.

39. Eidelman LA, Putterman D, Putterman C, Sprung CL. The spectrum of septic encephalopathy. Definitions, etiologies, and mortalities. JAMA 275:470–473, 1996.

40. Young GB. The EEG in coma. J Clin Neurophysiol 17:473–485, 2000.

41. Greene DA. Acute and chronic complications of diabetes mellitus in older patients. Am J Med 80: 39–53, 1986.

42. Small M, Alzaid A, MacCuish AC. Diabetic hyperosmolar non-ketotic decompensation. Q J Med 66:251–257, 1988.

43. Wachtel TJ, Silliman RA, Lamberton P. Prognostic factors in the diabetic hyperosmolar state. J Am Geriatr Soc 35:737–741, 1987.

44. Wachtel TJ, Tetu-Mouradjian LM, Goldman DL, Ellis SE, O'Sullivan PS. Hyperosmolarity and acidosis in diabetes mellitus: a three-year experience in Rhode Island. J Gen Intern Med 6:495–502, 1991.

45. Faich GA, Fishbein HA, Ellis SE. The epidemiology of diabetic acidosis: a population-based study. Am J Epidemiol 117:551–558, 1983.

46. Agardh CD, Rosen I, Ryding E. Persistent vegetative state with high cerebral blood flow following profound hypoglycemia. Ann Neurol 14:482–486, 1983.

47. Malouf R, Brust JC. Hypoglycemia: causes, neurological manifestations, and outcome. Ann Neurol 17:421–430, 1985.

48. Miller SI, Wallace RJ Jr, Muscher DM, Septimus EJ, Kohl S, Baughn RE. Hypoglycemia as a manifestation of sepsis. Am J Med 68:649–654, 1980.

49. Kalimo H, Olsson Y. Effects of severe hypoglycemia on the human brain. Neuropathological case reports. Acta Neurol Scand 62:345–356, 1980.

50. Simon RP, Meldrum BS, Schmidley JW, Swan JH, Chapman AG. Mechanisms of selective vulnerability: hypoglycemia. Cerebrovasc Dis 15:13–24, 1987.

51. Kramer L, Fasching P, Madl C, et al. Previous episodes of hypoglycemic coma are not associated with permanent cognitive brain dysfunction in IDDM patients on intensive insulin treatment. Diabetes 47:1909–1914, 1998.

52. Strachan MW, Deary IJ, Ewing FM, Frier BM. Recovery of cognitive function and mood after severe hypoglycemia in adults with insulin-treated diabetes. Diabetes Care 23:305–312, 2000.

53. Daverat P, Castel JP, Dartigues JF, Orgogozo JM. Death and functional outcome after spontaneous intracerebral hemorrhage. A prospective study of 166 cases using multivariate analysis. Stroke 22:1–6, 1991.

54. Fieschi C, Carolei A, Fiorelli M, et al. Changing prognosis of primary intracerebral hemorrhage: results of a clinical and computed tomographic follow-up study of 104 patients. Stroke 19:192–195, 1988.

55. Hemphill JC III, Bonovich DC, Besmertis L, Manley GT, Johnston SC: The ICH score: a simple, reliable grading scale for intractable hemorrhage. Stroke 32:891–897, 2001.

56. Young WB, Lee KP, Pessin MS, Kwan ES, Rand WM, Caplan LR. Prognostic significance of ventricular blood in supratentorial hemorrhage: a volumetric study. Neurology 40:616–619, 1990.

57. Phan TG, Koh M, Vierkant RA, Wijdicks EFM. Hydrocephalus is a determinant of early mortality in putaminal hemorrhage. Stroke 31:2157–2162, 2000.

58. Broderick JP, Brott TG, Duldner JE, Tomsick T, Huster G. Volume of intracerebral hemorrhage. A powerful and easy-to-use predictor of 30-day mortality. Stroke 24:987–993, 1993.

59. Wijdicks EFM, Fulgham JR. Acute fatal deterioration in putaminal hemorrhage. Stroke 26;1953–1955, 1995.

60. Gore JM, Granger CB, Simoons ML, et al. Stroke after thrombolysis. Mortality and functional outcomes in the GUSTO-I trial. Global Use of Strategies to Open Occluded Coronary Arteries. Circulation 15:2811–2818, 1995.

61. Diringer MN, Edwards DF, Zazulia AR. Hydrocephalus: a previously unrecognized predictor of poor outcome from supratentorial intracerebral hemorrhage. Stroke 29:1352–1357, 1998.

62. Flemming KD, Wijdicks EFM, Li H. Can we predict poor outcome at presentation in patients with lobar hemorrhage? Cerebrovasc Dis 11:183–189, 2001.

63. St Louis EK, Wijdicks EFM, Li H, Atkinson JD. Predictors of poor outcome in patients with a spontaneous cerebellar hematoma. Can J Neurol Sci 27: 32–36, 2000.

64. Wijdicks EFM, St Louis E. Clinical profiles predictive of outcome in pontine hemorrhage. Neurology 49:1342–1346, 1997.

65. Wijdicks EFM, Scott JP. Causes and outcome of mechanical ventilation in patients with hemispheric ischemic stroke. Mayo Clin Proc 72:210–213, 1997.

66. Ferrucci L, Bandinelli S, Guralnik JM, et al. Recovery of functional status after stroke. A postrehabilitation follow-up study. Stroke 24:200–205, 1993.

67. Turney TM, Garraway WM, Whisnant JP. The natural history of hemispheric and brainstem infarction in Rochester, Minnesota. Stroke 15:790–794, 1984.

68. Gupta SR, Naheedy MH, Elias D, Rubino FA. Postinfarction seizures. A clinical study. Stroke 19:1477–1481, 1988.

69. Kilpatrick CJ, Davis SM, Hopper JL, Rossiter SC. Early seizures after acute stroke. Risk of late seizures. Arch Neurol 49:509–511, 1992.

70. So EL, Annegers JF, Hauser WA, O'Brien PC, Whisnant JP. Population-based study of seizure disorders after cerebral infarction. Neurology 46:350–355, 1996.

71. Norrving B, Cronqvist S. Lateral medullary infarction: prognosis in an unselected series. Neurology 41:244–248, 1991.

72. Schwarz S, Egelhof T, Schwab S, Hacke W. Basilar artery embolism. Clinical syndrome and neuroradiologic patterns in patients without permanent occlusion of the basilar artery. Neurology 49:1346–1352, 1997.

73. Nadeau S, Jordan J, Mishra S. Clinical presentation as a guide to early prognosis in vertebrobasilar stroke. Stroke 23:165–170, 1992.

74. Kelly PJ, Stein J, Shafqat S, et al. Functional recovery after rehabilitation for cerebellar stroke. Stroke 32:530–534, 2001.

75. Phan TG, Wijdicks EFM. Intra-arterial thrombolysis for vertebrobasilar circulation ischemia. Crit Care Clin 15:719–742, 1999.

76. Haig AJ, Katz RT, Sahgal V. Locked-in syndrome: review. Curr Concepts Rehabil Med 2:12–16, 1986.

77. Haig AJ, Katz RT, Sahgal V. Mortality and complications of the locked-in syndrome. Arch Phys Med Rehabil 68:24–27, 1987.

78. Jennett B, Teasdale G, Braakman R, Minderhoud J, Heiden J, Kurze T. Prognosis of patients with severe head injury. Neurosurgery 4:283–289, 1979.

79. Pal J, Brown R, Fleiszer D. The value of the Glasgow Coma Scale and Injury Severity Score: predicting outcome in multiple trauma patients with head injury. J Trauma 29:746–748, 1989.

80. Ross AM, Pitts LH, Kobayashi S. Prognosticators of outcome after major head injury in the elderly. J Neurosci Nurs 24:88–93, 1992.

81. Alberico AM, Ward JD, Choi SC, Marmarou A, Young HF. Outcome after severe head injury. Relationship to mass lesions, diffuse injury, and ICP course in pediatric and adult patients. J Neurosurg 67:648–656, 1987.

82. Choi SC, Muizelaar JP, Barnes TY, Marmarou A, Brooks DM, Young HF. Prediction tree for severely head-injured patients. J Neurosurg 75:251–255, 1991.

83. Lee JP, Lui TN, Chang CN. Acute post-traumatic intraventricular hemorrhage analysis of 25 patients with emphasis on final outcome. Acta Neurol Scand 84:85–90, 1991.

84. Kampfl A, Schmutzhard E, Franz G, et al. Prediction of recovery from post-traumatic vegetative state with cerebral magnetic-resonance imaging. Lancet 351:1763–1767, 1998.

85. van der Naalt J, Hew JM, van Zomeren AH, Sluiter WJ, Minderhoud JM. Computed tomography and magnetic resonance imaging in mild to moderate head injury: early and late imaging related to outcome. Ann Neurol 46:70–78, 1999.

86. Groswasser Z, Sazbon L. Outcome in 134 patients with prolonged posttraumatic unawareness. Part 2. Functional outcome of 72 patients recovering consciousness. J Neurosurg 72:81–84, 1990.

87. Baker SP, O'Neill B, Haddon W, Long WB. The injury severity score: A method for describing patients with multiple injuries and evaluating emergency care. J Trauma 14:187–196, 1974.

88. Donovan WH. Spinal cord injury. In: Evans RW, Baskin DS, Yatsu FM (eds). Prognosis of Neurological Disorders. Oxford University Press, New York, 1992, pp 109–118.

89. Trieschman RB. Spinal Cord Injuries: Psychological, Social, and Vocational Rehabilitation, 2nd ed. Demos Publications, New York, 1988, pp 158–185.

Chapter 20

WITHDRAWING LIFE SUPPORT IN THE INTENSIVE CARE UNIT: A NEUROLOGIST'S PERSPECTIVE

Major cultural, religious, and societal differences determine the level of care. Van den Noort[1] writes, and few would argue, "There is a philosophy that is particularly American of 'do something' with little regard to the probability of success, the cost of the achievement or the consequences of such focused efforts on society as a whole." In the U.S. health care system, there is a tendency to provide all available technical care and later determine its justification. Often riven by emotion, attending physicians and advising consultants sometimes may cringe at absurd demands of family members who have lost all sense of proportion. In other countries, conditions with a likelihood of irreversibility would not even warrant care in an intensive care unit (ICU). The time may come when physicians cannot be realistically hopeful, and remedies are replaced by comfort and palliation.

Families of these unfortunate patients should not be left in the dark by overcautious physicians, and decisions should not become too protracted. In such instances, the decision to stop treatment in a hopeless situation may be postponed because family members have only a vague idea of the expected disability. Families may have received discordant information—one bit of information that bodes well and another that bodes poorly—which may have reflected conflicting goals of care between consultants.[2] Most family members understand that sustained medical care in a patient with a major neurologic insult may create a situation that may be more penetrating emotionally than an acute tragic death. Many family members clearly understand the demoralizing effect for caregivers, waste of resources, and unnecessary high technologic care. They may carry the burden of care of a severely disabled person and should know what to expect when aggressive treatment is continued. No one can know with perfect certainty what the outcome will be, but in some central nervous system catastrophes, prognostic factors have been explicitly identified.

Recent in-depth studies from several countries showed that withdrawal of treatment is common in the ICU, with relevant differences between community and teaching hospitals. Initiation of withdrawal by physicians was more common in teaching hospitals.[3] A recent prospective survey in 167 ICUs associated with all U.S. training programs in critical care medicine or pulmonary and critical care medicine revealed that 13% of patients had some form of life support withheld before death and that 33% of deaths followed complete withdrawal.[4] The most common reason to withdraw support, however, is imminent death.[5]

Neurologists are commonly involved in decisions to limit life support, which could be partly a reflection of the high prevalence of neurologic catastrophies in patients with a critical illness. A survey on withholding or withdrawal of support in critically ill patients that involved 1719 patients admitted to ICUs in San Francisco found that 66 of 115 patients (57%) had intracranial lesions, although in this series, 15 patients were brain dead.[6]

After the review of outcome for most pertinent neurologic complications in critical illness in Chapter 19, this chapter deals with the inevitable consequences of a poor outcome and the assessment of level of support.

GENERAL CONSIDERATIONS

There are unique features to withdrawal of support in patients with neurologic complications. First, prediction of poor outcome remains very difficult except in a few well-defined disorders with an established poor outcome. With these conditions (Table 20–1), most neurologists, given adequate time for observation, would feel comfortable in withdrawing support, a decision not likely to con-

flict with the professional judgment of the attending intensive care specialist.

Second, patient autonomy may not exist, because the structural lesion of the brain affects any expression of the patient's wishes. A neurologic condition often renders the patient unable to think clearly and participate in treatment decisions.

Third, clinical judgment may be very difficult in acute situations that require adaptation by the patient. For example, the decision to withdraw the mechanical ventilator in a patient with acute traumatic high cervical quadriplegia is unsettling, and studies suggest a major shift in the patient's judgment over time.[8,9]

However, any decision about cessation of therapy is based largely on family preferences. This was clearly outlined by M. Angell[10] in an editorial on vegetative state: " . . . the judgment about whether to keep such patients alive, once the medical facts are established, requires no medical expertise."

LEGAL ASPECTS OF WITHDRAWAL OF CARE

Many states in the U.S. carry the possibility of obtaining a living will. The quality of the text varies, and so does ambiguity. In these documents, the definition of care beyond cardiopulmonary resuscitation is often inadequate to guide therapy, and clear discus-

---

Table 20–1. **Coma and No Hope for Good Recovery**

- Myoclonus status epilepticus and brain swelling after cardiac arrest
- Multiple territorial infarcts and brain swelling after cardiac surgery
- Basilar artery occlusion
- Multiple intracranial hemorrhages associated with tissue plasminogen activator
- Pontine hemorrhage with hyperthermia and extension to midbrain and thalamus
- Multiple hemorrhagic contusions and associated extradural hematoma and brain swelling
- Gunshot wounds to the head with intraventricular and intracerebral hemorrhage and disseminated intravascular coagulation
- Complete cervical cord transection with apnea

Data from Wijdicks EFM, 2000.[7]

sions with the family and occasionally with patients are needed for clarification. Advance directives may include clear statements on cardiopulmonary resuscitation; mechanical ventilation; defibrillation; nutritional assistance, whether intravenous, parenteral, or enteral; and blood transfusion or plasma expanders.[11] A do-not-resuscitate order specifies no resuscitation in the event of cardiac or respiratory arrest and may also include no intravenous drugs for acute cardiac arrhythmias, invasive monitoring devices, hemodialysis, cardiac pacemakers, endotracheal tubes, cardioversion, chest tubes, or bronchoscopy. Although many U.S. states recognize advance directives from other states, some do not. Three types of directives are known.[12,13]

A *living will* gives specific directions on health care or appoints an agent or proxy to make decisions on the patient's behalf in the event of terminal illness. A living will should instruct in broad terms to surrogate decision makers any wishes to withhold or withdraw treatment in situations at the end of life, and it may include religious preferences.

Durable power of attorney for health care authorizes another person (agent or proxy) to make decisions on the patient's behalf even though the patient may not be terminally ill.

A *mental health declaration* provides specific direction or designates a proxy to make decisions about intrusive mental health treatment (for example, electroshock therapy and neuroleptic medications).

Doctors cannot decline to accept advance directives or claim to be acting in good faith and in accordance with good professional practice. Generally, there is a low rate of completion of advance directives. Pollack's review of the literature[14] claimed that 90% of patients do not have an advance directive and suggested that the information be included on the Medicare card.

The situation of withdrawal of support is more problematic when the physician concludes that life-sustaining treatment is futile and the family demands continued treatment. The major issues and legality of futile treatment were elegantly summarized by Helft et al. in an article entitled "The Rise and Fall of the Futility Movement." The authors noted " . . . the reason the courts have not upheld the right of physicians to make unilateral judgments about the futility of medical care is that the medical community could not agree on underlying principles."[15] It should be noted that in a recent survey, 38% of U.S. neurologists were concerned about the legality of withdrawal of support despite established jurisdiction.[16] The American Academy of Neurology has summarized end-of-life care in a position paper.[17] The statement emphasized the patient's right to refuse life-sustaining treatment. Neurologists are obligated to honor these requests for withdrawal or withholding of care and to provide palliative care. But it is *not* the neurologists' duty to provide assisted suicide or active euthanasia at the request of their patients.[18] As emphasized before, continuous communication with family, full disclosure, and documentation of these interactions remain a noble strategy. Impartial review by a hospital ethics committee may be helpful.

DECISIONS IN WITHDRAWAL OF CARE

If the outcome is established and communication with the family (and, if possible, the patient) results in a consensus, a plan to withdraw life support can be made.

Studies into the attitudes and biases of general physicians found that certain medical treatments were more easily withdrawn.[19] From most likely to least likely to be withdrawn, they are as follows: blood products, hemodialysis, intravenous vasopressors, total parenteral nutrition, antibiotics, mechanical ventilation, tube feedings, and intravenous fluids.[19] Other important biases are reluctance to withdraw support in an iatrogenic situation, to withdraw recently instituted therapies, and to withdraw forms of support that would cause delayed death rather than imminent death. Gender, religion, rank, specialty, time spent in clinical practice, and total number of patients from whom life support had been withdrawn did not influence decision making by physicians. Age of the patient was a criterion, however, in a survey from Sweden that claimed age per se strongly influenced care,[20] a finding that may be in contrast with those from other countries.

One should consider, for example, the inconclusive relationship between time spent in the ICU and quality of life. Prolonged length of stay in the ICU, defined as more than 2 weeks, results in functional survival in a considerable proportion of patients,[21-23] including the elderly (more than 70 years old).[24] Other studies have found that major functional impairment can be expected.[25]

Neurologists must be part of an ad hoc decision-making team. Otherwise, the practice of consultation may result in cursory encounters or notes in the chart that may not be communicated. These teams (for example, physicians, clergy, nursing staff) have to deal specifically with the certainty of the patient's disability after they have made valiant but ineffective attempts to save the patient.

It would be naive to capture the complexity of the encounter with the family in a few paragraphs. Neurologists need to be experienced to understand the family's grief and to guide a sensitive dialogue toward an understanding of what they believe are the patient's best interests.[26]

When futility of care seems highly likely, the family should be approached directly with the question of why we have to persist in the pursuit of mechanical ventilation, nutrition, and fluids to maintain a person in a permanently unconscious state or with a major handicap. It is true that the physician's ability to convey the prognosis influences decisions by the family, but often families and physician agree early on the course to be taken.[27]

The neurologist should have families articulate what they believe the patient wants or what they think is in the patient's interest. If the patient can communicate, preferences at the moment have priority over wishes expressed earlier or in an advance directive. In addition, the family should be told explicitly that when comfort care is given, the perceived hastening of death by sedation or pain relief is an unintended consequence of the primary purpose of comfort and becomes irrelevant ("double effect"). In certain circumstances, the family should be prepared for imminent death.[26,27] In others, timing cannot be controlled and the course may be slower, and when comfort is maximal, physicians should not be pressed to increase narcotics or sedation to hasten the time of death. If death is expected within 1 day, comfort care should be provided in the ICU rather than in the ward. The sudden change in sophistication of care by transfer to the ward may be perceived by some family members as lack of compassion.

WITHDRAWAL OF CARE

Several issues need to be articulated. Management of some specific situations is summarized in Table 20–2.

After withdrawal of supportive intravenous drugs, mechanical ventilation and endotracheal intubation are commonly considered for withdrawal of support in a neurologic catastrophe. Extubation, however, seldom leads to rapid respiratory arrest. The degree of brain herniation and thus brain stem dysfunction predicts respiratory drive. Pontine stages of herniation result in a rapid tachypnea interrupted by apneas or, more typically, Cheyne-Stokes breathing. Breathing may be noisy and rattling and a source of great distress for families. When a change in head and body position is unsuccessful, glycopyrrolate or subcutaneous scopolamine (hyoscine) or a patch can be used. Scopolamine relaxes the smooth muscles, and both drugs dry up the secretions of the exocrine glands.[28-31]

Terminal dry mouth is managed with oral hygiene every 2 to 4 hr, smoothing the lips with vaseline, and moist air. Terminal vomiting from increased intracranial pressure can be treated with 25 to 50 mg of promethazine rectally, metoclopramide, haloperidol, or ondansetron, 32 mg intravenously. Hiccups can be relieved with baclofen (10 mg oral dose) before withdrawal of the gastrointestinal tube. Extreme agitation may be treated with 0.4 to 2 mg of lorazepam intravenously, midazolam, or propofol infusion.

Seizures may reoccur in patients when antiepileptic drugs are discontinued, but this possibility can be anticipated by administering fosphenytoin (300 mg) intramuscularly before extubation. The family should be told that this drug is now used for careful palliation. Transient myoclonus status epilepticus may be very distressful and suggest suffering and pain to family members. Because we have not been successful with any of the antiepileptic drugs, piracetam, or midazolam, we proceed with propofol infusion for 1 day, discontinue it, and then withdraw support.

Table 20–2. **Palliative Pharmacologic End-of-Life Care of the Neurologic Patient**

Signs	Therapy
Coughing	Humidification with steam inhalation Morphine, 2.5–5 mg Atropine, 1–2 mg IM Midazolam, 2.5–5 mg IM
Hiccups	Metoclopramide, 10 mg push IV; repeat q4h Baclofen, 5 mg p.o. t.i.d. Chlorpromazine, 25–50 mg t.i.d. IM
Rattling	Scopolamine patch, 1.5 mg Atropine, 1 mg IM
Nausea and vomiting	Metoclopramide, 1–2 mg IV Haloperidol infusion, 1.5 mg IV/24 hr Ondansetron, 8 mg IV
Seizures	Lorazepam, 4 mg IV Fosphenytoin, 300 mg IM
Panic and anxiety	Midazolam, 2–10 mg/day IM Propofol infusion, 10–20 mg/hr Haloperidol, 0.5–1.5 mg IM
Pain (severe)	Morphine, 5–10 mg IV every 10 min

IM, intramuscularly; IV, intravenously.

Terminal sedation ought to be permissible and part of palliation, and the administration of opiates for palliation is ethical and legal in all U.S. states. In one study, the average amounts of benzodiazepines and opiates in the 24 hr before withdrawal were 2.2 mg/hr for diazepam and 3.3 mg/hr for morphine sulfate and in the 24 hr thereafter were 9.8 mg/hr and 11.2 mg/hr, respectively. No evidence exists that these drugs hasten death.[32]

Carefully constructed compassionate guidelines have been published by the American College of Physicians–American Society of Internal Medicine End-of-Life Care Consensus Panel. Additional guiding principles for care in the final hours are summarized in Table 20–3.[33]

WITHDRAWAL OF CARE IN SPECIAL NEUROLOGIC CIRCUMSTANCES

Several comparatively common dilemmas pose major management problems. Amyotrophic lateral sclerosis (ALS) is diagnosed in medical ICUs when patients are admitted with respiratory distress and often, in retrospect, have had generalized weakness. The preferences toward withdrawal of care are not known.[34] One study in Oregon and Washington state, biased toward white, college-educated male patients, only 2% of whom were receiving mechanical ventilation, suggested that 56% would consider assisted suicide if it were legal.[35] Other patients want to live as long as possible; in 22% of patients with long-term ventilation, life was prolonged for 8 to 17 years. Many claimed a high quality of life, and locked-in syndrome occurred in only 10%.[36,37]

A recent study of patients with ALS receiving long-term mechanical ventilation provides further insight.[38] Only three-fourths of the 75 patients with advanced ALS were aware that respiratory failure was likely to develop, and fewer than half had discussed their decision with their physician. Only 42% had made their decision before the emergency of respiratory failure despite an average of 3 years with the disease, and approximately one-third of the patients consented in an emergency. The family burden was rated as very stressful and fully depen-

Table 20–3. **Ways in Which Intensive Care Units Can Simulate a Home Environment for Dying Patients**

Transportable Aspect of a Patient's Home	Ways to Provide this Aspect in the Intensive Care Unit
Privacy	Provide a private room
	Close doors and curtains
Ready access to family	Suspend restrictive visiting hours
	Provide comfortable chairs, recliners, and cots for family members in the patient's room
Access to patient's own possessions and amenities	Allow family to bring in favorite music, clothes, religious icons, food, and pets
Family serving as personal caregivers	When appropriate, allow family to assist with patient care
Access to religious rituals and spiritual support	Provide religious and spiritual resources
	Encourage religious and other family rituals at the bedside before and after death

From Faber-Langendoen et al.[33] By permission of the American College of Physicians–American Society of Internal Medicine.

dent on adequate insurance. It is often not clear who should begin the discussion of long-term mechanical ventilation or withdrawal of ventilatory support, and thus it may not occur at all. When mechanical ventilation is required, the patient should be informed about progression of the disorder. The functional status of 50 ventilated patients with ALS was quadriplegic in 46%, feeding tube placed in 72%, some use of arms in 36%, communication with talking or mouthing of words in 42%, and assisted communication (computers or boards) and eye blinks in 58%.[38]

In deciding whether to withdraw support, it is important to exclude intermittent pulmonary infections or other disorders that may contribute to the patient's state. When a patient decides to discontinue ventilation, removal of the ventilator may be very uncomfortable to the patient and cause air hunger. Slow weaning with supplemental oxygen produces further retention of carbon dioxide and eventually coma, and this method seems preferable in addition to several doses of morphine to counter possible signaled discomfort.

The ethical questions in patients with traumatic quadriplegia and ventilator dependency are more difficult, and the morality of withdrawal is debatable.[39,40] Complete cervical transection with apnea usually precludes

recovery, but 28% to 57% of patients with injuries at the C3 level or lower may recover.[41]

It is unusual for a patient with full knowledge of the consequences to ask emphatically to have the ventilator removed. In follow-up interviews at rehabilitation centers, remarks were predominantly positive, with up to 93% of the patients "glad to be alive." Although many patients express some degree of hopelessness and despondency about the remaining years of life, many also change their mind with the passage of time.

Whether to honor the request when requests to turn off the ventilator continue requires ethical analysis by an ethics committee. Often the effects of an antidepressant have to be evaluated.

It is difficult to judge whether the patient's request is a rational choice and whether the patient is capable of autonomous choice. The patient should be presented with all relevant facts and rehabilitation options. Postponing the decision is wise, but patients may continue to forcefully reject any such suggestion. The family should be told that it is the patient's decision alone. The ventilator can be withdrawn if the patient refuses to reconsider, because the patient may exercise the right to refuse life-sustaining treatment.

Withdrawal in patients who are brain dead is done when organ donation is not possible or is refused by family members. Some family members may accept only cardiac arrest, not brain death, as the universality of death, possibly because of religious or cultural preferences. Cardiac arrest and treatment-refractory hypotension occur in most patients because critical functions of the brain are lost.

CONCLUSIONS

Studies describing neurologic circumstances in which specific forms of life support have been withdrawn are scarce. Neurologic conditions with a bleak outlook in patients with critical illness have been identified and in fact are often a consequence of a terminal critical medical condition. When the critical illness can be stabilized, discussions about quality of life and the need for long-term care soon emerge, and withdrawal of support is commonly considered in severely brain-damaged patients. In the United States, all states permit refusal by capable patients, and many states allow surrogates to make decisions when patients are not competent.[42] The neurologist has an important if not pivotal role and may provide additional compassion to reach out to devastated families.

Medical opinion may be divided in specific disorders. Problems of diagnosis, the unmeasurable and unpredictable powers of recovery, erratic judgment, and, perhaps most difficult, the inherent arbitrariness of value judgments on the quality of life are examples of the complexity.

REFERENCES

1. van den Noort S. Ethical aspects of unproved therapies in multiple sclerosis, amyotrophic lateral sclerosis, and other neurologic diseases. Semin Neurol 4:83–86, 1984.
2. Asch DA, Hansen-Flaschen J, Lanken PN. Decisions to limit or continue life-sustaining treatment by critical care physicians in the United States: conflicts between physicians' practices and patients' wishes. Am J Respir Crit Care Med 151:288–292, 1995.
3. Keenan SP, Busche KD, Chen LM, Esmail R, Inman KJ, Sibbald WJ. Withdrawal and withholding of life support in the intensive care unit: a comparison of teaching and community hospitals. The Southwestern Ontario Critical Care Research Network. Crit Care Med 26:245–251, 1998.
4. Prendergast TJ, Claessens MT, Luce JM. A national survey of end-of-life care for critically ill patients. Am J Respir Crit Care Med 158:1163–1167, 1998.
5. Manara AR, Pittman JA, Braddon FE. Reasons for withdrawing treatment in patients receiving intensive care. Anaesthesia 53:523–528, 1998.
6. Smedira NG, Evans BH, Grais LS, et al. Withholding and withdrawal of life support from the critically ill. N Engl J Med 322:309–315, 1990.
7. Wijdicks EFM. Neurologic catastrophes in the Emergency Department. Butterworth-Heinemann, Boston, 2000.
8. Maynard FM, Muth AS. The choice to end life as a ventilator-dependent quadriplegic. Arch Phys Med Rehabil 68:862–864, 1987.
9. Maynard FM. Responding to requests for ventilator removal from patients with quadriplegia. West J Med 154:617–619, 1991.
10. Angell M. After Quinlan: the dilemma of the persistent vegetative state (editorial). N Engl J Med 330:1524–1525, 1994.
11. Emanuel LL. Advance directives: do they work? J Am Coll Cardiol 25:35–38, 1995.
12. Samuels A. The advance directive (or living will). Med Sci Law 36:2–8, 1996.
13. Silverman HJ, Vinicky JK, Gasner MR. Advance directives: implications for critical care. Crit Care Med 20:1027–1031, 1992.
14. Pollack S. A new approach to Advance Directives. Crit Care Med 28:3146–3148, 2000.
15. Helft PR, Siegler M, Lantos J. The Rise and Fall of the Futility Movement. N Engl J Med 2000:343:293–296.
16. Carver AC, Vickrey BG, Bernat JL, Keran C, Ringel SP, Foley KM. End-of-life care: a survey of US neurologists' attitudes, behavior, and knowledge. Neurology 53:284–293, 1999.
17. The American Academy of Neurology Ethics and Humanities Subcommittee. Palliative care in neurology. Neurology 46:870–872, 1996.
18. Bernat JL, Cranford RE, Kittredge FI Jr, Rosenberg RN. Competent patients with advanced states of permanent paralysis have the right to forgo life-sustaining therapy. Neurology 43:224–225, 1993.
19. Christakis NA, Asch DA. Biases in how physicians choose to withdraw life support. Lancet 342:642–646, 1993.
20. Melltorp G, Nilstun T. Age and life-sustaining treatment. Attitudes of intensive care unit professionals. Acta Anaesthesiol Scand 40:904–908, 1996.
21. Heyland DK, Konopad E, Noseworthy TW, Johnston R, Gafni A. It is 'worthwhile' to continue treating patients with a prolonged stay (>14 days) in the ICU? An economic evaluation. Chest 114:192–198, 1998.
22. Konopad E, Noseworthy TW, Johnston R, Shustack A, Grace M. Quality of life measures before and one year after admission to an intensive care unit. Crit Care Med 23:1653–1659, 1995.
23. Niskanen M, Ruokonen E, Takala J, Rissanen P, Kari A. Quality of life after prolonged intensive care. Crit Care Med 27:1132–1139, 1999.
24. Montuclard L, Garrouste-Orgeas M, Timsit JF, Misset B, De Jonghe B, Carlet J. Outcome, functional autonomy, and quality of life of elderly patients with a long-term intensive care unit stay. Crit Care Med 28:3389–3395, 2000.
25. Jacobs CJ, van der Vliet JA, van Roozendaal MT, van

der Linden CJ. Mortality and quality of life after intensive care for critical illness. Intensive Care Med 14:217–220, 1988.

26. Curtis JR, Patrick DL, Shannon SE, Treece PD, Engelberg RA, Rubenfeld GD. The family conference as a focus to improve communication about end-of-life care in the intensive care unit: opportunities for improvement. Crit Care Med 29(Suppl):N26–N33, 2001.

27. O'Callahan JG, Fink C, Pitts LH, Luce JM. Withholding and withdrawing of life support from patients with severe head injury. Crit Care Med 23:1567–1575, 1995.

28. Bennett MI. Death rattle: An audit of hyoscine (scopolamine) use and review of management. J Pain Symptom Manage 12:229–233, 1996.

29. Voltz R, Borasio GD. Palliative therapy in the terminal stage of neurological disease. J Neurol 244 (Suppl 4):S2–S10, 1997.

30. Watts T, Jenkins K, Back I. Problem and management of noisy rattling breathing in dying patients. Int J Palliat Nursing 3:245–252, 1997.

31. Hughes AC, Wilcock A, Corcoran R. Management of 'death rattle.' J Pain Symptom Manage 12:271–272, 1996.

32. Wilson WC, Smedira NG, Fink C, McDowell JA, Luce JM. Ordering and administration of sedatives and analgesics during the withholding and withdrawal of life support from critically ill patients. JAMA 267:949–953, 1992.

33. Faber-Langendoen K, Lanken PN, for the ACP-ASIM End-of-Life Care Consensus Panel. Dying patients in the intensive care unit: forgoing treatment, maintaining care. Ann Intern Med 133:886–893, 2000.

34. Goldblatt D, Greenlaw J. Starting and stopping the ventilator for patients with amyotrophic lateral sclerosis. Neurol Clin 7:789–806, 1989.

35. Ganzini L, Johnston WS, McFarland BH, Tolle SW, Lee MA. Attitudes of patients with amyotrophic lateral sclerosis and their care givers toward assisted suicide. N Engl J Med 339:967–973, 1998.

36. Mcdonald ER, Hillel A, Wiedenfeld SA. Evaluation of the psychological status of ventilatory-supported patients with ALS/MND. Palliat Med 10:35–41, 1996.

37. Rowland LP. Assisted suicide and alternatives in amyotrophic lateral sclerosis [editorial]. N Engl J Med 339:987–989, 1998.

38. Moss AH, Oppenheimer EA, Casey P, et al. Patients with amyotrophic lateral sclerosis receiving long-term mechanical ventilation. Advance care planning and outcomes. Chest 110:249–255, 1996.

39. Ohry A. Ethical questions in the treatment of spinal cord injured patients. Paraplegia 25:293–295, 1987.

40. Whiteneck GG, Carter RE, Charlifue SW, et al. A Collaborative Study of High Quadriplegia. Englewood, Colorado, Craig Hospital, 1985.

41. Wicks AB, Menter RR. Long-term outlook in quadriplegic patients with initial ventilator dependency. Chest 90:406–410, 1986.

42. Luce JM, Alpers A. End-of-life care: What do the American courts say? Crit Care Med 29(Suppl):N40–N45, 2001.

INDEX